Sourcebook of Rehabilitation
and
Mental Health Practice

Plenum Series in Rehabilitation and Health

SERIES EDITORS
Michael Feuerstein
Uniformed Services University of the Health Sciences (USUHS)
Bethesda, Maryland
and
Anthony J. Goreczny
Chatham College
Pittsburgh, Pennsylvania

ENABLING ENVIRONMENTS: Measuring the Impact of Environment on
Disability and Rehabilitation
Edited by Edward Steinfeld and Gary Scott Danford

HANDBOOK OF HEALTH AND REHABILITATION PSYCHOLOGY
Edited by Anthony J. Goreczny

INTERACTIVE STAFF TRAINING: Rehabilitation Teams that Work
Patrick W. Corrigan and Stanley G. McCracken

SOCIAL RELATIONS AND CHRONIC PAIN
Ranjan Roy

SOURCEBOOK OF OCCUPATIONAL REHABILITATION
Edited by Phyllis M. King

SOURCEBOOK OF REHABILITATION AND
MENTAL HEALTH PRACTICE
Edited by David P. Moxley and John R. Finch

A Continuation Order Plan is available for this series. A continuation order will bring delivery of each new volume
immediately upon publication. Volumes are billed only upon actual shipment. For further information please contact
the publisher.

Sourcebook of Rehabilitation and Mental Health Practice

Edited by

David P. Moxley

Wayne State University
Detroit, Michigan

and

John R. Finch

Rehabilitation Consultant
Columbus, Ohio

Kluwer Academic/Plenum Publishers

New York • Boston • Dordrecht • London • Moscow

MT

Library of Congress Cataloging-in-Publication Data

ISBN: 0-306-47745-9
© 2003 Kluwer Academic Publishers
233 Spring Street, New York, New York 10013

http://www.wkap.nl

10 9 8 7 6 5 4 3 2 1

A C.I.P. Catalogue record for this book is available from the Library of Congress

Permissions for books published in Europe: *permissions@wkap.nl*
Permissions for books published in the United States of America:
permissions@wkap.com

Printed in the United States of America

List of Contributors

JOHN B. ALLEN JR., Director, Bureau of Recipient Affairs Office of Mental Health, Albany, NY.

LARRY ABRAMSON, Director of the Back to Work Program, St Luke's House, Bethesda, Maryland.

ANN ROSEGRANT ALVAREZ, Wayne State University School of Social Work, Detroit, Michigan.

ROBERT BAER, Outreach Center for Innovation in Transition and Employment, Kent State University, Kent, Ohio.

CREIGS BEVERLY, Wayne State University School of Social Work, Detroit, Michigan.

BEVERLY M. BLACK, Wayne State University School of Social Work, Detroit, Michigan.

MARGARET BRUNHOFER, Wayne State University School of Social Work, Detroit, Michigan.

MATTHEW BURNS, Vinfen Corporation, Boston, Massachusetts.

JOHN CORRIGAN, Department of Rehabilitation and Physical Medicine, College of Medicine and Public Health, Ohio State University, Columbus, Ohio

WILLIAM CRIMANDO, Rehabilitation Administration and Services Program, Rehabilitation Institute, Southern Illinois University, Carbondale, Illinois.

GARY M. CUSICK, Administrator of Planning and Research, Louisville & Jefferson County Health Department, Louisville, Kentucky.

ELIZABETH DANTO, Hunter College School of Social Work, City University of New York, New York, New York.

ROBERT ERLANDSON, Wayne State University College of Engineering, Detroit, Michigan.

ELLEN FABIAN, CAPS Department, University of Maryland, College Park, Maryland.

MARIANNE FARKAS, World Health Organization Collaborating Center, Boston University Center for Psychiatric Rehabilitation, Boston, Massachusetts.

ALISON FAVORINI, Huntington Woods, Michigan.

JOHN R. FINCH, Rehabilitation Consultant, Columbus, Ohio.

STUART FORMAN, Wayne State University, Detroit, Michigan.

CHERYL GAGNE, Boston University Center for Psychiatric Rehabilitation, Boston, Massachusetts.

GREGORY G. GARSKE, Division of Intervention Services, Bowling Green State University, Bowling Green, Ohio.

CHARLES GARVIN, University of Michigan School of Social Work, Ann Arbor, Michigan.

BARBARA GRANGER, The Matrix Center at Horizon House, Inc., Philadelphia, Pennsylvania.

LAURIE R. GWILLIAM, Department of Rehabilitation and Physical Medicine, College of Medicine and Public Health, Ohio State University, Columbus, Ohio.

JAMES J. HENNESSY, Fordham University Graduate School of Education, New York, New York.

LOREN HOFFMAN, Wayne State University School of Social Work, Detroit, Michigan.

PAMELA S. HYDE, Secretary, New Mexico, Department of Human Services, Santa Fe, New Mexico.

CHRISTINE HYDUK, Marygrove College Department of Social Work, Detroit, Michigan.

EVETTE JACKSON, The Technical Assistance Collaborative, Inc., Boston, Massachusetts.

GERALYN L. JANECZKO, Director of Support Services, Southfield Public Schools, Southfield, Michigan.

MARTHA B. KNISLEY, Director of the District of Columbia Department of Mental Health, Washington, D.C.

MARTIN KOEHLER, Boston University Center for Psychiatric Rehabilitation, Boston, Massachusetts.

KATHY KUSTOWSKI, Visiting Nurses Association of Southeast Michigan, Detroit, Michigan.

KRISTA MAGAW, Tecumseh Land Trust, Yellow Springs, Ohio.

PAMELA K. MANELA, Southfield Public Schools, Southfield, Michigan.

ROGER W. MANELA, Detroit Public Schools, Detroit, Michigan.

ERNESTINE MOORE, Wayne State University School of Social Work, Detroit, Michigan.

DAVID P. MOXLEY, Wayne State University School of Social Work, Detroit, Michigan.

DEBBIE NICOLELLIS, World Health Organization Collaborating Center, Boston University Center for Psychiatric Rehabilitation, Boston, Massachusetts.

JERRY OLSHESKI, Department of Counseling and Higher Education, Ohio University, Athens, Ohio.

NATHANIEL J. PALLONE, Rutgers, The State University of New Jersey, New Brunswick, New Jersey.

JANET L. PRAY, Gallaudet University Department of Social Work, Washington, D.C.

DENISE RABOLD, NeuroRehab, Inc., Columbus, Ohio.

MELVYN RAIDER, Wayne State University School of Social Work, Detroit, Michigan.

RICHARD SCHELAT, Ohio Bureau of Vocational Rehabilitation, Athens, Ohio.

SANDRA SCHIFF, Wayne State University School of Social Work, Detroit, Michigan.

LEROY SPANIOL, Senior Director of the Boston University Center for Psychiatric Rehabilitation, Boston, Massachusetts.

PATRICK SULLIVAN, Indiana University School of Social Work, Indianapolis, Indiana.

JAMES TRIPP, Wayne State University School of Social Work, Detroit, Michigan.

WAYNE TYRELL, Boston University Department of Rehabilitation Sciences, Boston, Massachusetts.

NOELLE VAN DER TUIN, Migrant Health Promotion, Progresso, Texas.

JOSEPH WALSH, Virginia Commonwealth University School of Social Work, Richmond, Virginia.

MARGARET S. WALSH, State Human Rights Director, Commonwealth of Virginia Department of Mental Health, Mental Retardation, and Substance Abuse Services, Richmond, Virginia.

ARLENE N. WEISZ, Wayne State University School of Social Work, Detroit, Michigan.

SHARI WILLIS, CAPS Department, University of Maryland, College Park, Maryland.

ANTHONY ZIPPLE, Vinfen Corporation, Boston, Massachusetts.

Preface

We live in a day and age in which many fields come together to define new ones, and out of these newly defined areas come innovative practices, and emergent ways of thinking. The *Sourcebook on Rehabilitation and Mental Health Practice* documents one of these new fields, one formed by the coalescence of rehabilitative and mental health services and employment. Only recently have human service practitioners, policy makers, and administrators recognized that there is a growing synergy among these areas once separated by great gulfs of differences in culture, perspectives and values, and technologies.

It is not happenstance that rehabilitation, mental health, and employment are becoming increasingly integrated in contemporary human services. There is considerable interest in work in contemporary society although different values and perspectives mediate this interest. For people with disabilities, an interest in work often comes from deep frustration—from not having ready access to work, and from not having enough of it to facilitate an acceptable quality of life or independent living. Some people find work to be a source of problems that negatively affects their functioning. They find the workplace stressful and unsupportive, or they feel that work exacts too much from them, reducing their quality of life and setting into motion numerous negative personal effects (Beck, 2000).

Over the past several decades, American society has accelerated its expectations of work and of those who engage in it. The decade of the 1970s saw economic upheaval in American society, an acceleration of inflation and the emergence of stagflation. Other countries, most notably Japan, overtook the United States in productivity and quality. In the 1980s, expectations of worker performance heightened and the workplace was restructured through new management and work engineering practices, quality management approaches, and new workplace expectations of employees for autonomy, self-sufficiency, and technical mastery (Appelbaum & Batt, 1994). These changes to the workplace continued into the decade of the 1990s, but the American economy took off, some say because of the macro-economic policies of the 1980s, while others underscore the ingenuity of American enterprise, and still others point to the great investment workers have made. But all was not right in the 1980s and 1990s. Despite societal assertions that people ought to work and work a lot, workers themselves felt more insecure about the permanence of work. The fall out of restructuring and the re-engineering of the workplace took its toll not only at the lower echelons of corporate enterprises, but also at mid-level echelons, and within the ranks of professionals, once areas of employment thought secure and permanent (Meyer, 1995). The restructuring of performance expectations, pensions, and salaries meant that work was increasingly more performance-based and subject to competitive forces.

Perhaps the net effect of these changes in the workplace were the feelings that work was as much a potential problem to people as it was a positive area of human development that could foster personal identity and meaning. Workplace violence, harassment of workers, and job stress were stark reminders that employment could create negative mental health consequences and that people may need to seek human services to cope with the consequences of work and to sustain their performance on the job (Ryan & Oestreich, 1998). The emergence of work-related services for employees, such as employee assistance programs, critical incident intervention, and substance abuse treatment and counseling, have become standard practices in many areas of business and industry.

During the decades of the 1970s, 1980s, and 1990s, human services were not insulated from the necessity to prepare people for work, to help people sustain work, and to facilitate their performance on the job. Of course, there had always been models of rehabilitation and employment that emulated work, such as sheltered workshops, industrial enclaves, and work adjustment that focused on the preparation of people for work and on the facilitation of work readiness. Yet, over these three decades there was a critique emerging within human services that these models only simulated the real thing and only served to create deviance and stigma by amplifying people's disabilities and preventing them from enjoying involvement in real-life work settings.

Many people with disabilities, particularly those with developmental disabilities or serious mental illness, had difficulty getting work and sustaining it. This was not because they were unfit for involvement in employment, but employer and organizational attitudes; the structure and engineering of work; and disability benefits literally coalesced into major barriers to employment. To this day, people with disabilities, particularly serious ones, are underrepresented in the workforce and this lack of representation may reinforce prevailing societal stereotypes that people with disabilities do not make good employees or do not want to work.

Movements developed within fields such as serious mental illness, developmental disabilities, and physical disabilities that emphasized normalization, inclusion, and community support. The availability of work in real work settings in which people with disabilities could work alongside people without disabilities were seen as the policy and practice aims of many innovations in human services including supported employment, self-employment, and competitive employment. The achievement of social integration, from this perspective, required people to be involved in real work and in nothing less. To be deprived of employment was seen as a violation of human rights. From this perspective the competence of human services was situated in the ability of systems of services to facilitate the participation of people with disabilities in mainstream community employment. Major policy products in the 1980s and 1990s and into the first decade after 2000 underscored the importance of the availability of work and the transition and movement of people with disabilities into employment.

So, the field we speak of in this book, rehabilitation and mental health practice, is linked to employment from at least two vantage points. First, there is work as a source of problems that can create negative consequences for functioning and mental health. Second, there is the facilitation of the involvement in work of people who often can experience deprivation in this area of human development or exclusion because of their physical, cognitive, emotional, or social qualities.

Within this first segment of the field one may find rehabilitation and mental health services that address the negative consequences of work by:

1. facilitating a better fit between individuals and their work settings or between individuals and their specific work responsibilities;
2. bolstering the skills and competencies of individuals so they perform more effectively; and
3. helping individuals reduce the scope and severity of negative consequences.

Within this second segment of the field one may find rehabilitation and mental health supports that facilitate access to employment and that, in the words of psychiatric rehabilitation professionals, help people to "choose, get, and keep employment." Strategies that compose this segment of the field may be accommodative in their focus and aims. That is, they help people to make the requisite changes to their environments that support their vocational development or their achievement of employment outcomes and vocational success. Other strategies may facilitate changes in the person so that he/she gains the skills, competencies, and capacities to work successfully in the work settings of a competitive and market-oriented society that values self-sufficiency and autonomy.

It is the purpose of the *Sourcebook* to illuminate the practices that form the field of rehabilitation and mental health. We, as editors, understand that this field is complex, emergent, and growing and so it is difficult to cover it exhaustively. However, we feel that we capture in the *Sourcebook* a large portion of the contemporary domain through the diverse array of authors—practitioners, administrators, and academics who are active in the field of rehabilitation and mental health practice—who write from different substantive areas of practice and from different perspectives.

Through five sections the contributing authors illuminate many of the thematic areas of rehabilitation and mental health practice that are significant to today's practice as well as to the practice of the near future. This coverage is of great enough scope to justify the idea that this book truly is a sourcebook, a volume that is deep and broad enough to serve as a textbook and reference for students preparing for practice, and yet relevant to experienced practitioners looking for insight and new understanding. We will save the overview of chapters for those introductions we incorporate within major sections. But let us underscore that each section and the chapters that compose them offer frameworks, practices, and perspectives that will enable the reader to obtain a good understanding of the field of rehabilitation and mental health practice.

Section I, "The Promise and Challenges of Employment," is composed of six chapters that give the reader a sense of why employment is important to human development and the conditions that influence employment, for better or worse. The four chapters of Section II, "Service Roles and Contexts in Rehabilitation and Mental Health Practice," offer a broad review of professional roles and systems devoted to the integration of rehabilitation and mental health service for the purpose of achieving employment outcomes. In Section III, we devote six chapters to the development of readiness for employment in which rehabilitation and mental health services are brought together for individuals to facilitate their involvement in work. Section IV offers seven chapters that focus on the themes of sustaining employment and developing self-employment options, two areas that have considerable contemporary relevance. The nine chapters of Section V, "Responding to Rehabilitation, Mental Health and Employment Needs," address service strategies for specific populations with a special focus on the arrangements and resources that influence the facilitation of employment for these groups and the issues that practitioners and recipients must address to achieve successful outcomes. The authors of these chapters seek to assemble promising or best mental health and rehabilitation practices that are relevant to the achievement of employment outcomes within the context of specific service situations.

Contributing authors represent the spectrum of professionals and disciplines that compose the field of rehabilitation and mental health practice. The reader will find represented among the contributing authors the disciplines of social work, engineering, psychology, rehabilitation counseling, nursing, law, sociology, and business. No one discipline can claim rehabilitation and mental health practice as an exclusive domain. It is truly an interdisciplinary field benefiting from the ideas and practice of professionals from a diversity of backgrounds and educational preparation. The combination of this diversity makes this a vibrant and evolving field of human service inquiry and practice.

We welcome you to the *Sourcebook* and hope you find it to be a resource that is relevant to the advancement of your own practice. This is our aim and this is our hope.

DAVID P. MOXLEY
Detroit, Michigan

JOHN R. FINCH
Columbus, Ohio

REFERENCES

Appelbaum, E., & Batt, R. (1994). *The new American workplace: Transforming work systems in the United States.* Ithaca, NY: Cornell University Press.

Beck, U. (2000). *The brave new world of work.* Cambridge, UK: Polity Press.

Meyer, G. J. (1995). *Executive blues: Down and out in corporate America.* New York: Dell.

Ryan, K. D., & Oestreich, D. K. (1998). *Driving fear out of the workplace.* San Francisco: Jossey-Bass.

Contents

1. Introduction: The Coalescence of Rehabilitation and
Mental Health Practice 1
David P. Moxley and John R. Finch

I. THE PROMISE AND CHALLENGES OF EMPLOYMENT 9

2. Americans at Work: A Developmental Approach 11
Elizabeth Danto

3. Employment and Empowerment of People with Disabilities:
A Social Development Perspective 27
Creigs Beverly and Ann Rosegrant Alvarez

4. The Recovery Framework in Rehabilitation and Mental Health 37
LeRoy Spaniol, Cheryl Gagne, and Martin Koehler

5. Business and Legal Conditions Supporting the Employment of
Individuals with Disabilities 51
Robert Erlandson

6. Reasonable Job Accommodations for People with
Psychiatric Disabilities 61
Jerry Olsheski and Richard Schelat

7. Strategic Career Development for People with Disabilities 77
David P. Moxley, John R. Finch, James Tripp, and Stuart Forman

II. SERVICE ROLES AND CONTEXTS IN REHABILITATION
AND MENTAL HEALTH PRACTICE 93

8. The Role of Vocational Rehabilitation Counselors in
Mental Health Services 95
Gregory G. Garske

9.   The Role of Mental Health Professionals in Responding to
        Employment Needs 105
        Joseph Walsh and Margaret S. Walsh

10. State Rehabilitation Authorities and Their Role in Responding to
        the Employment Needs of People with Serious Mental Illness 117
        Ellen Fabian, Larry Abramson, and Shari Willis

11. Involvement of State and Local Mental Health Authorities in
        Addressing the Employment Needs of People with Serious
        Mental Illness 127
        Martha B. Knisley, Pamela S. Hyde, and Evette Jackson

        III.   DEVELOPING READINESS FOR EMPLOYMENT   143

12. Fostering Readiness for Rehabilitation and Employment 145
        Marianne Farkas and Debbie Nicolellis

13. Cognitive Remediation for Increasing Functional Independence 161
        Laurie R. Gwilliam, Denise Rabold, and John Corrigan

14. Utilization of Group Approaches to Address Employment Issues 171
        Charles Garvin

15. The Vocational Development Functions of the Clubhouse 185
        Krista Magaw

16. Benefit Advisement for Mental Health Consumers
        Seeking Employment 199
        Gary M. Cusick

17. Workplace Socialization of People with Disabilities: Implications for Job
        Development and Placement 207
        David P. Moxley, John R. Finch, and Stuart Forman

        **IV.   SUSTAINING EMPLOYMENT AND DEVELOPING
                SELF-EMPLOYMENT OPTIONS   219**

18. Organizing Supports in the Workplace to Sustain Employment 221
        Wayne Tyrell, Matthew Burns, and Anthony Zipple

19. Accessible Design and Employment of People with Disabilities 235
        Robert Erlandson

20. Clinical Interventions into Employment-Related Mental
        Health Concerns 253
        Melvyn Raider, Alison Favorini, and Margaret Brunhofer

21. | Mental Health Case Management and Employment Outcomes 269
Patrick Sullivan

22. | Addressing Substance Abuse Problems in the Workplace 283
Alison Favorini

23. | Sustaining Employment during Acute Mental Health Episodes 303
Loren Hoffman, Roger W. Manela, and Sandra Schiff

24. | Helping People with Psychiatric Disabilities Start and
Develop Consumer-Run Businesses 319
John B. Allen Jr. and Barbara Granger

**V. RESPONDING TO REHABILITATION, MENTAL HEALTH, AND
EMPLOYMENT NEEDS   333**

25. | Planning and Supporting the Transition of Secondary School Students
from School to Adult Life 335
Roger W. Manela, Pamela K. Manela, and Geralyn L. Janeczko

26. | Mental Health and Community Support Strategies for Fostering
Employment of People Who Are Deaf and Hard of Hearing 351
Janet L. Pray

27. | Supporting the Employment of People with Serious Mental Illness 363
Robert Baer

28. | Addressing the Employment Needs of Persons with Physical Disabilities:
Implications for Rehabilitation and Mental Health Service Workers ... 379
William Crimando

29. | Meeting the Employment and Mental Health Needs of Immigrants 401
Noelle Van der Tuin

30. | Helping People Coping with HIV and AIDS Manage Employment 417
Christine Hyduk and Kathy Kustowski

31. | Responding to Mental Health Concerns of People Transitioning from
Welfare to Work 433
Ernestine Moore

32. | Mental Health and Rehabilitation Issues in the
Employment of Women 445
Arlene N. Weisz and Beverly M. Black

33. | Rehabilitation Services for Criminal Offenders 459
Nathaniel J. Pallone and James J. Hennessy

Index 481

CHAPTER 1

Introduction

The Coalescence of Rehabilitation and Mental Health Practice

DAVID P. MOXLEY AND JOHN R. FINCH

INTRODUCTION

Coalescence requires the creation of a unity out of disparate parts and, as we underscore in the Preface, there is a coalescence occurring between the fields of rehabilitation and mental health as it pertains to helping people address the role of work and employment in their lives. Looking forward to the coming decade, no American or no member of the world community can discount the importance of work and its precarious nature (Aronowitz & DiFazio, 1994; Meyer, 1995). Work, its availability, content, amount, and quality, has emerged as one of the most controversial areas of society (Ciulla, 2000). Whole groups of humanity are on the move within nation states and across national and international boundaries in search of employment (Kaplan, 2000) and many countries, most notably the United States, are dealing with the consequences in the changes to the nature of work.

The United States is one of the largest hosts in the world to newcomers who are in search of employment—particularly work that they can sustain—and that offers the benefits that make work so desirable, namely health care, insurance, and retirement, to name just a few of the more tangible benefits. European communities face considerable challenges in hosting newcomers and in integrating such newcomers into their work forces. On both continents one need only to read the daily news or watch cable news stations to see the latest upheavals that bring newcomers into host countries in search of employment (French, 2000; Kaplan, 2000). Work often is seen as a "right" and fully enfranchised citizens may even engage in violent actions to demonstrate their disapproval of immigrants and migrants taking jobs away from those who consider themselves legitimate citizens.

DAVID P. MOXLEY • Wayne State University School of Social Work, Detroit, Michigan.
JOHN R. FINCH • Rehabilitation Consultant, Columbus, Ohio.

MODELS IN ACTION

The history of human services has been sensitive to the facilitation of employment among newcomers and whole employment models have been developed to help them to get and keep employment. Two models in particular, Jewish Vocational Service and the settlement house, were created in the fields of rehabilitation and social work to facilitate employment among immigrants as a means to foster their integration into American society. The vision of both of these models was to offer not only employment services but also an array of other human and educational services that would support the immigrants' quest for social inclusion since involvement in work requires a cultural awareness of social norms and mores.

The area of immigration has been a model for the coalescence of rehabilitation and mental health services. During the 1980s and 1990s Jewish Vocational Services facilitated the settlement of Russian Jews in the United States and helped many immigrating Russian professionals to take their skill sets and use them to secure productive work or to enhance their credentials to stay in the professions in which they were originally educated, such as engineering. Although the settlement house model has faded in salience, there remain many settlement houses located in urban areas that now focus on issues of poverty rather than immigration. Such a model remains robust, since people seeking to escape poverty face many of the same kinds of issues as people who are seeking to accommodate to a new culture. In many cases they must acquire a new language, new dress, and new attitudes and skills among other assets in order to move into the workforce which, to them, may seem like a foreign country.

In southeastern Michigan, the home of one of the *Sourcebook* authors, there are three "models in action" that stand out as exemplars of serving people on the move: ACCESS, Freedom House, and Migrant Health Promotion. We are sure they have counterparts in many of the geographical areas in which our readers reside. ACCESS (the Arab Community Center for Economic and Social Services) facilitates the immigration of people of Arab and Chaldean descent to the United States and facilitates their inclusion in the new culture. This innovative agency understands that people are coming from many different cultures since being of Arab descent does not involve a monolithic cultural block. Indeed, there are well over 20 countries in what the United States labels as the Middle East. The agency recognizes that the transition from the home of origin to the United States requires people to accommodate their identities to a new culture. The agency does not facilitate assimilation but rather accommodation in which people become Arab Americans who blend their cultures of origin with a new culture adding to the diverse mix of what it means to be American.

Freedom House, located adjacent to the bridge linking Detroit, Michigan, to Windsor, Ontario, a concrete and steel structure that brings two countries together, facilitates the journeys of people who are fleeing economic and political oppression in their home countries and who are making their way to the United States or Canada. Freedom House offers a mix of legal and immigration, residential, mental health, health, and social services that people who are displaced require for survival and resettlement. A seasoned human service professional can easily imagine the kinds of community supports people who are displaced require. It is difficult for the agency to pull its services apart because they must be bundled and integrated to produce the kinds of resettlement outcomes people require.

A third exemplar is the Migrant Health Promotion, located in Saline, Michigan and Progreso, Texas. The agency works directly with seasonal migrants who travel between Michigan and Texas for work. Families make major seasonal moves in order to follow the cycle of nature and the harvesting of crops. The agency works with individuals and families to facilitate their well-being, to foster their health, and to address the many economic, mental health, social service, and educational needs such form of employment creates. Like ACCESS and Freedom House, this agency must bundle its services, work closely with people who are in transition, and facilitate their accommodation to circumstances that are ever changing.

THE EMERGENCE OF A NEW PARADIGM

These models in action reflect a paradigm of the coalescence of rehabilitation and mental health services. They have a synergistic quality to them. The people who offer services and the people who receive services are members of an effort to produce quality of life outcomes and employment is one of these vital outcomes. The services are bundled and not easily divisible and the program offers them to participants in a friendly and informal manner. The success of the program may require the understanding of a professional staff member who has a first-hand understanding of the situation of recipients that can be gained only through direct experience. Thus, the staffing of these programs is not only a mix of health, social service, rehabilitation, and mental health personnel, but also people who have direct personal experience with the so-called problem area who may find careers for themselves in these kinds of organizations.

The paradigm is a robust one. One can see these model programs in a variety of different fields of rehabilitation and mental health service. To name a few: Fairweather Lodges, microenterprises, clubhouses for people coping with serious mental illness, social clubs for people who are deaf, centers of independent living for people with physical disabilities, and job clubs for people seeking to escape poverty. These models are group-based and many of them operate as clubs hosting their members, who work together and with professionals to explore, choose, search for, and sustain employment. These various programmatic models serve as support systems with their own cultures. These support systems may be jumping-off points for people who feel that they must recover from life-transforming or horrific experiences and prepare themselves for entry or re-entry into the greater culture. Or, these support systems may be sustaining cultures in that they insulate people from what they see as negative forces emanating from the greater culture. These cultures themselves may offer the social networks to sustain the economic, housing, educational, and socialization requirements of participants.

Such model programs can teach practitioners a great deal about how work and career unfold within a person's life space. The fashion of the day within many rehabilitation and mental health programs is to view employment as a discrete outcome that is easily separated from the life space of individuals. Even recipients fall into this fallacy: "Just get me a job and everything will be ok." Professionals may assert that it all comes down to employment—just get people working. We, the editors, understand the importance of employment but we also understand that employment is part of a larger life matrix.

THE CENTRALITY OF VOCATIONAL
DEVELOPMENT AND RECOVERY

This paradigm suggests that employment is part of a process of recovery, particularly for people who experience oppression within the greater society. The vocational development of homeless individuals, for example, requires that affordable housing and supportive social services are in place and that there is some semblance of permanent income for individuals as they move forward in employment and career. Of course, immediate employment is important for individuals who are homeless, but if housing does not come first, then it is likely that participation in employment will be transient or itinerant at best.

People recovering from serious mental illness may want and need a period of confidence-building that enables them to contemplate how work and career fit into their life styles that must take into consideration the realities of long-term illness or disabilities. The effectiveness of the service setting lies in its ability to support the self-exploration, inquiry, and episodes of experimentation the person undertakes with work and career and in its ability to support the person once he or she makes a decision about an employment direction. In this kind of setting, rehabilitation and mental health service are not discrete products or programmatic elements. They combine synergistically and transform themselves as people move forward in their vocational development and in their involvement in the world of work.

Programmatic models must offer a variety of supports to help people coping with mental illness to move from the contemplation of employment into transitional employment. It is the purpose of these innovations to support people; that is, to help them make sense of their experiences, to troubleshoot and resolve barriers to employment, and to gain support to sustain their employment. The matrix of services and supports is complex, but requires integration if people are to get the supports they either want or need to become successful in the world of work.

The paradigm we identify incorporates the view that rehabilitation and mental health practice in relation to employment coalesces around the process of vocational development and the process of the engagement of the individual in employment. There is ample criticism of contemporary rehabilitation models suggesting that they are too outcome-focused, short term in nature, and fail to incorporate a holistic range of supports. Criticisms of vocational rehabilitation identify the absence of career development perspectives and the short-circuiting of the rehabilitation process. Some commentators emphasize that the vocational rehabilitation process needs to be retooled to allow for the introduction of a post-employment period to facilitate a focus on continuous career development. Currently, most state vocational rehabilitation processes end when a person is placed in employment and sustains a job for several months.

EMPLOYMENT AS PART OF A LIFE PROCESS

It is indeed a challenge for rehabilitation and mental health professionals to view the preparation for employment and the achievement of employment as a process and not just an outcome. The importance of this process orientation comes up in a number of different chapters in the *Sourcebook*. The chapter on recovery, for example, suggests that as people emerge from being ill, disabled, or dispossessed the desire to become involved in employment becomes a natural expression of moving forward in one's life. Thus, it is likely that as people move forward in their own process of recovery they will begin to contemplate and reflect on themes pertaining to their involvement in work, the development of a career, and/or the acquisition of training and education that enables them to become productively employed. A sound rehabilitation and mental health service process anticipates recovery from the beginning and facilitates contemplation about and reflection on the role of work in one's life. Recovery reminds practitioners that work is a developmental process that is an expression of a person's identity and conception of self (Gamst, 1995).

Within this process the sequencing of rehabilitation and mental health activities may deviate from more traditional models. The paradigm of rehabilitation and mental health practice suggests that service activities can be sequenced in diverse ways. The achievement of employment is not a linear process but very well may be a circuitous one, much influenced by the nature of the social issue people are addressing in their lived experience.

Some people may acquire immediate employment and then receive the training they require to perform effectively in their current and future jobs. People coping with substance use challenges may get a job and then address their treatment needs post-employment, making use of employee assistance programs and industrial social services to resolve issues that pertain to their recovery. Other candidates for employment may go through several transitional work experiences so that they come to learn about the world of work first hand or rekindle their knowledge of work requirements, knowledge that may be lost after a protracted period of illness. The idea of transition, from being ill to being healthy, from being without a job to having a job, and from not possessing a career to having a career, is an important element of the contemporary paradigm of rehabilitation and mental health practice.

Thinking about employment as a process requires rehabilitation and mental health professionals to understand how environments can be modified to accommodate the unique abilities and skill sets of individuals. The coalescence of rehabilitation and mental health practice suggests a sophisticated perspective on the engineering of "micro-work environments," including the introduction of creative on-the-job and off-the-job support systems, the introduction of new technologies to facilitate work productivity, reasonable job accommodations, and the modification of benefits to facilitate participation in employment. These environmental changes are introduced strategically by practitioners who are able to position supports that strengthen the resilience of people who want to participate in work. The old models—those that seek to change the person to fit the job—are fading quickly and what is emerging are those models of rehabilitation and mental health practice that follow a theory of person–environment fit. Through the use of affirmative and accessible technologies work environments can be engineered to facilitate the inclusion of people with a diversity of skills, abilities, and qualities.

Mental health and rehabilitation practitioners focusing on employment can become quite sophisticated about business conditions at a policy level. Thus, environmental support of employment can incorporate advocacy work that fosters supportive business and legal conditions, offers new kinds of income support and job accommodations, and creates new types of career ladders and opportunities. In the post-Affirmative Action environment of the United States, advocacy that seeks to change the structure of work so that it is more supportive and developmental may be the most important actions rehabilitation and mental health practitioners can take to facilitate employment, yet practitioners may not operate in flexible ways on behalf of the people they serve (Miller, 1991).

There is no one pathway for the rehabilitation and mental health practitioners who seek to help people to become employed. There are multiple pathways leading to a diversity of employment outcomes suggesting that effective systems of rehabilitation and mental health practice incorporate a diverse set of strategies to facilitate employment. The readers, therefore, will find considerable content in the *Sourcebook* on environmental supports and work-related accommodations.

The process of rehabilitation and mental health practice focusing on employment will recognize that work does not stand alone from other areas of people's lives. Rehabilitation and mental health services are vital aspects of any effort to help people assimilate into employment settings or to introduce the identity of worker into their conceptions of themselves. Preparation for employment, involvement in employment, career development, and ongoing skill development and education cannot be easily separated. The models in action we describe earlier in this chapter illuminate the importance of bringing many discrete elements together into one programmatic focus or into one organizational form. The orchestration of these discrete elements enables people to participate in the full spectrum of services or supports and enables them to increase the probability that they will be successful on the job.

The models comprising the new paradigm help people to address the consequences of their employment, such as the agency that brings together those resources that facilitate the well-being of migrant workers. Other models may facilitate the development of jobs and the placement of jobs in people's communities. It is these models that take advantage of employment within their host communities and work closely with employers of established businesses. Still other models may underscore the importance of helping people to create their own employment or to collaborate with other people in similar circumstances to create their own enterprises. The agency that reaches out to people coping with serious mental illness or homelessness may incubate a consumer business and help people choose roles in such a business that fit their preferences and their career directions.

Rehabilitation and/or mental health systems increasingly form alliances with those agencies or organizations whose mission is to facilitate employment. Rehabilitation systems may be interested in how these programs can help recipients to achieve employment outcomes while mental health systems may be interested in how they prepare people for work as part of the recipients' recovery process. Rehabilitation professionals may find that they must become increasingly conversant in ancillary services, such as health, mental health, and social services, while mental health professionals must take their recipients' yearnings for employment seriously and help people to overcome personal and situational barriers to work. Psychiatrists who are adept at using medication strategies to facilitate the stabilization of people with psychiatric disabilities may find that they need to adopt new strategies to facilitate the participation of the people they serve in work and employment. If these professionals do not address their clients' or patients' aspirations for employment and for careers, or dismiss these yearnings as unrealistic, they may find themselves irrelevant to people who want to work.

Many mental health professionals will increasingly work with their recipients around issues or needs that directly involve employment, particularly as societies demand higher levels of performance and as work changes in its availability, amount, and quality. It is a bold assertion to suggest that many mental health concerns are rooted in work—its dominance in a person's life or its unavailability. However, work has always figured into positive mental health and the achievement of well being cannot be often separated from the role of work in people's lives.

INTEGRATION OF REHABILITATION AND MENTAL HEALTH

The chapters of the *Sourcebook* taken collectively suggest ways of practicing and ways of thinking about the integration of rehabilitation and mental health service delivery the purpose of which is ultimately to facilitate employment or to promote readiness and preparation for employment. We devote one whole section to specific populations and the rehabilitation, mental health, and employment challenges members of these populations face and must resolve to improve the quality of their lives. It is one thing to talk about a new paradigm of rehabilitation and mental health service. It is another thing to discuss this paradigm in the context of a specific group of people.

People coping with HIV and AIDS, for example, are a group whose employment needs is becoming salient in the field of rehabilitation and mental health practice. New medical technologies, medications, and health management programs are making it possible to extend lives and the quality of lives in an area that was once pervaded by pessimism. Innovations in the provision of social services are as important as advances in medical care. Like other groups people coping with HIV and AIDS have benefited from case management, community support, affordable housing, mutual support, and self-help. As people deal with the crisis of diagnosis, and learn to cope with the acute phases of their illnesses, they likely become interested in work, career, and education.

Some individuals find new conceptions of themselves in the provision of self-help, mutual support, and advocacy that help them acquire the identity, skills, and competencies relevant to careers in human services. As in other areas of human services, people with HIV and AIDS pioneered many of the mental health and social services that have become the best practices of contemporary service systems. And, people with HIV and AIDS may find new work roles within this matrix of human service delivery.

There are chapters on employment and deafness, people who are immigrants, people who are coping with serious mental illness, people transitioning from welfare to work, and people who struggle with substance abuse. These chapters, taken as a whole, suggest cross-cutting themes of a meta-model of rehabilitation and mental health practice. People experience stigma and discrimination, lose confidence, and perhaps decline in their functioning; they begin the process of recovery, and begin to emerge out of "it" through involvement in a matrix of services, mutual support, and advocacy.

Ultimately true integration of rehabilitation and mental health occurs at the individual level in which professionals and recipients collaborate to make a service process work for an individual who is seeking employment or who is addressing the negative consequences of employment in their personal lives. Integration of services around work outcomes may be one of the most powerful strategies to develop readiness for work and to facilitate entry into and retention of employment.

CONCLUSION

The desire for gainful work and engagement with the greater society through employment, training, and/or education takes on personal importance and may make individuals more willing to risk involvement in vocational development and employment. Recovery then may take on a different meaning in which social participation often is mediated through a person's involvement in work.

A good rehabilitation and mental health process facilitates the development of readiness, fosters the development of vocational maturity and vocational self-concept, and enables people to gain the support to follow through in the search for employment. Throughout this process, astute practitioners listen closely to people in recovery, help them to frame their needs and desires, and help them to identify the vocational direction they wish to take. Astute practitioners will listen closely to the fears and anxieties people in recovery have about work since the positive resolution of these concerns can help people to move forward to getting and keeping employment.

In the new paradigm, the service process, as many of these chapters suggest, is person-centered and not system-centered. This simply means that individuals direct the process of rehabilitation and mental health service delivery as well as determine its ends in a collaborative process with rehabilitation and mental health professionals. Astute practitioners are facilitators of a change process that involves substantial change in personal conceptions of self, in the manner in which services are organized and arranged, in the employment environment, and in the settings in which vocational development and the preparation for employment take place. Traditional rehabilitation and mental health service processes may fail if the system tries to push its conception of process on people. The new paradigm suggests that individuals who are seeking employment influence the service process as much as possible and, perhaps, even control it.

Some mental health and rehabilitation professionals may take umbrage with this portrayal of a new paradigm. Many service systems today, such as state rehabilitation programs and mental health providers, control much of the process. However, other systems of service do not exercise this kind of control. They seek to help people to develop in a manner that is consistent with their own sense of personal development, growth, and change. The new paradigm recognizes that contemporary society wants its adult members to work and to be productive. Service systems and service processes cannot ignore such a strong cultural norm (Miller, 1991). But practitioners of the new paradigm recognize what years of rehabilitation and mental health practice has revealed: identity as a worker develops over the human life span and people move through numerous stages and transitions in their vocational and career development (Brown, Brooks, & Associates, 1996). The recognition of this developmental process is fundamental to the coalescence of rehabilitation and mental health services.

REFERENCES

Aronowitz, S., & DiFazio, W. (1994). *The jobless future*. Minneapolis, MN: University of Minneapolis Press.

Brown, D., Brooks, L., & Associates (1996). *Career choice and development* (3rd ed.). San Francisco, CA: Jossey–Bass.

Ciulla, J. B. (2000). *The working life: The promise and betrayal of modern work*. New York, NY: Times Business.

French, H. (2000). *Vanishing borders: Protecting the planet in the age of globalization*. New York, NY: Norton.

Gamst, F. C. (1995). Considerations of work. In F. C. Gamst (Ed.), *Meanings of work: Considerations for the 21st century* (pp. 1–45). Albany, NY: SUNY Press.

Kaplan, R. D. (2000). *The coming anarchy: Shattering the dreams of the post cold war*. New York, NY: Vintage.

Meyer, G. J. (1995). *Executive blues: Down and out in corporate America*. New York, NY: Dell.

Miller, G. (1991). *Enforcing the work ethic*. Albany, NY: SUNY Press.

THE PROMISE AND CHALLENGES OF EMPLOYMENT

The six chapters of Section I address many of the social dimensions of work that foster the integration of rehabilitation and mental health service delivery. In Chapter 2, "Americans at Work: A Developmental Approach," Danto examines the role of work in human development and illustrates the importance of work over the human life span. She emphasizes that work is a fundamental aspect of a person's mental health and the absence of work jeopardizes a person's functioning, particularly in a society that emphasizes the work ethic. The author shows how work is grounded in early development and then unfolds as the human being matures and explores vocation during the life stages of latency, early adolescence, adolescence, and adulthood. This is an appropriate lead chapter for the entire book since what joins rehabilitation and mental health services is the idea that employment itself is central to self-definition and self-regard.

Beverly and Alvarez expand the framework of employment within the context of social development theory in Chapter 3: "Employment and Empowerment of People with Disabilities: A Social Development Perspective." Development in this context does not only mean the development of individuals but rather the development of community and societal institutions to support the involvement of people in work. These authors underscore the reality that the disability rights movement is global and that the promotion of people's access to gainful employment is a fundamental focus of this movement. Beverly and Alvarez identify a number of different work alternatives within the context of group and community life that can result in the empowerment of people with disabilities.

Spaniol and his colleagues outline in Chapter 4 the importance of recovery from disability by focusing on the issues people coping with serious mental illness must navigate to move forward in their lives. They point to the importance of people making sense of their situations and they highlight the importance of work to the process of recovery. Ultimately, according to these authors, recovery involves the achievement of a new identity that enables people coping with mental illness to lead lives they find satisfying. Employment is one of these important outcomes that can add greatly to a person's achievement of personal satisfaction.

Although as an engineer experienced in the development of technologies to facilitate accessible work environments for people with severe disabilities, Erlandson does not overlook the critical role of the business and legal conditions that are in place to facilitate the use of such technologies. In Chapter 5, "Business and Legal Conditions Supporting the Employment of Individuals with Disabilities," he offers an overview of the policy matrix within which the accessibility of work for people with disabilities unfolds. Perhaps one of the most provocative observations he makes is that contemporary business and disability policy needs to catch up with the availability of technologies that can expand the inclusiveness of employment.

In Chapter 6, Olsheski and Schelat offer an in-depth analysis of how work environments can offer specific and reasonable job accommodations to people with disabilities. While Erlandson's chapter illustrates the business and legal conditions that facilitate employment of people with disabilities, Olsheski and Schelat show how these mandates can be addressed in the workplace through the implementation of technologies that enable people to work. The authors underscore an important observation: practical changes to the work environment can go a long way in facilitating employment. Making environmental modifications, modifying the job, and fitting jobs to people offer rehabilitation and mental health professionals powerful tools to make employment not only possible but also a reality.

The authors of Chapter 7 focus on career development and discuss the necessity to focus not only on helping people to get and keep work but also helping people to develop careers within the context of a changing society. Moxley, Finch, and Forman point to the reality that a career is possibly a person's most important life asset. And they note that to neglect the development of this asset may result in someone failing to find personal meaning and reward in an immediate job. The authors suggest that it is increasingly difficult to define what constitutes a career but, nevertheless, the growing ambiguity in this area offers rehabilitation and mental health professionals new opportunities to work with recipients in creative and innovative ways.

So these chapters taken together reflect a principal theme of the volume. Employment offers much promise to people and is fundamental to their development as fully realized human beings. However, getting and keeping employment is a challenge and requires rehabilitation and mental health professionals to work strategically to expand resources, benefits, and institutional supports that help people to find a form of employment in which they will thrive. Employment is so important to human development that people should not labor in unfulfilling jobs. Rather, they should find their fullest potential in work. Work should and can be fulfilling. It should empower people as active contributors to the quality of community life. And, work experience can coalesce into a career that offers people a strong sense of self as vital and empowered citizens. These are the promises and challenges of employment.

CHAPTER 2

Americans at Work

A Developmental Approach

Elizabeth Danto

"So you are off to London, David, to begin the world on your own account," said Mr. Murstone. Though I quite understood that the purpose of this announcement was to get rid of me, I have no distinct remembrance whether it pleased me or frightened me. My impression is, that in a state of confusion about it, and oscillating between the two points, touched neither.

Charles Dickens, *David Copperfield*

Here is David, an adolescent boy, about to enter the world of work. One foot in the family and the other in the factory, David is struggling with one of the most significant developmental tasks of human life: the transition from school to work. Perhaps though this is only the best known signpost of the place of work in the life cycle. We have childhood memories of parents and grandparents at work or changing jobs, retiring, or losing work. "Someday," we are told, "you will become a doctor, a painter, a politician" and each occupational name is loaded with moral charge and the weight of gender and class. We move from one stage to the next in paradigmatic fashion, our progress in life defined by attainment and our happiness generally contingent on the fulfillment of work responsibilities.

What follows is an overview of this paradigm and an attempt to explore both the sociological and the psychological sides of the meaning of work in human life. Some fundamental issues underlie this exploration of "work" as a psychological entity and work as a sociocultural construct. These points are: the nature of a specifically American culture of work and its intersection with concepts of social class, stigma, and personal responsibility; the constitution of work including employment, underemployment, and unemployment; the role of work and its developmental impact from infancy through old age; and the function of work in mental health with a focus on individual identity and social values.

Elizabeth Danto • Hunter College School of Social Work, City University of New York, New York, New York.

THE CULTURE OF WORK

The United States is a country of workers for whom the idea of "work" is far more important and complex than mere economic well-being. As individuals our psychological sense of self is bound up with who we are as workers. In groups, our social identity is defined by our affiliated work institutions. Our family life is regulated by work life: who goes to work and when is intertwined with childcare plans, care of the elderly, even location and type of housing. Work also determines the boundaries of our communities: educators define college towns, government employees settle state capitols, and ranchers establish farmland. While the idea of work is clearly central to our identity as people and as a society, our relationship to work—employed, unemployed, well employed, volunteer, underemployed—is even more important because it defines for us and for others our position in the social structure. This relationship is so important throughout the life span, and work is experienced at such a meaningful level in our psychology, that it now can serve as an "essential other." The term "essential other" was coined by modern social scientists to convey "our experience of other people and entities in the environment that support the sense of a coherent and vigorous self and its development" (Galatzer-Levy & Cohler, 1993).

Work takes many forms but workplaces are the physical spaces where these forms take shape. The workplace provides workers with direct benefits (wages) and, often equally impor-tant, indirect benefits. These include social support, professional status, relationships, and collegiality. The workplace can be a family support system providing flexible scheduling of work hours, part-time work on a full-time basis, maternity and paternity leave, and sponsored childcare and other measures that support family cohesion (Swick & Rotter, 1981). But the workplace can also be a source of stress and dissatisfaction that intrudes on family life, reinforces racial and gender discrimination, and fails to meet human needs for respect and autonomy. Work tends to reflect educational status and to define economic status, so people need jobs that are both interesting and that pay adequately. But one sphere often supercedes the other, resulting in either personal or social conflict. Yet we value the idea of work above all else, and it is not long before we question whether "problems at work" result more from personal psychological dysfunction than from organizational problems.

THE WORK ETHIC: HISTORY AND THE CULTURE OF INDIVIDUALISM

How did we develop such a passion for work? Work has become the defining value of our culture. Known virtually worldwide as the "American model," this culture dominated by individual ambition and competitiveness is both admired and mocked. To convey the mean-ing of work in our culture, I am using concepts developed by the pioneering anthropologist, Clyde Kluckhohn. Culture is a "product; is historical; includes ideas, patterns and values; is selective; is learned; is based upon symbols; and is an abstraction from behavior and the products of behavior" (Kroeber & Kluckhohn, 1955). While on one level we may believe that work and society are separate, in truth no individual lives outside of their environmental context. The two aspects of our lives, the social and the personal, co-exist in a dialectical paradigm called "person-in-environment." Table 2-1 employs the "person-in-environment" paradigm to show how each of Kluckhohn's variables of culture has both an environmental

TABLE 2-1. Variables of Work in American Society

Variable of culture	Idea of work: social	Idea of work: personal
Product	Job description	Tasks and skills
Historical	Colonialism	Winning
Ideas	Responsibility of society	Personal responsibility
Patterns	Stratification	Personal motivation
Values	Human nature is moral	Human nature is selfish
Selectivity	Individual need	Individual achievement
Social learning	Dependence	Independence
Symbolic content	Preserve the status quo	Change brings progress
Behavioral basis	Interdependence	Free will

or social side, and a personal or individual side. The table helps us deconstruct the idea, or theme, of work in American society.

To illustrate two components of the table, I will examine the meaning of the terms "ideas" and "patterns" in relation to the central concept of "work." In American (meaning U.S.) culture, work lives are highly influenced by the *pattern* of social stratification and by the *idea* of responsibility. Considered by sociologists perhaps the most profoundly significant aspect of the entire discipline, stratification influences every dimension of our lives from education and housing to health care and vacation plans. Work is no exception. One's choice of occupation, ability to pursue meaningful goals, confidence to strive for self-actualization, motivation to enhance one's individual and family life, and social skills to succeed in complex organizations, all depend largely on the culture of the social group (or class) into which one is born. For many, education represents the vehicle for social mobility, and thus a better paying or more prestigious occupation. Yet even among internally driven individuals with a high degree of personal motivation, access to a chosen occupation is easily blocked by race and gender discrimination, oppression, and social stigma. In his examination of social identity and stigma, Goffman (1963) observed that "some jobs in America cause holders without the expected college education to conceal this fact; other jobs, however, can lead the few of their holders who have a higher education to keep this a secret, lest they be marked as failures and outsiders." For example, a middle-class person feels comfortable in a library (a middle-class institution) but a criminal (socially defined as lower class) feels ostracized. Thus, library use, initially, is far less influenced by personal motivation and responsibility than by social class and the attribution of stigma. So here we encounter the *idea* of responsibility. Culturally, a working person is considered responsible and a non-working person is viewed as irresponsible unless they have "earned" the right not to work through physical disability or retirement from service or employment. Poverty tends to be viewed more as a defect in individual, personal responsibility than in the structure of the economy and the society. The spectacle of poor people as failed human beings too lazy to work was concretized in Federal legislation with the 1996 passage of the Personal Responsibility and Work Opportunity Reconciliation Act euphemistically known as "welfare reform." Ruth Sidel (1998), whose pioneering sociological studies of women and children reveal the spurious nature of the correlation between poverty and personal responsibility, concluded that underlying this legislation is a basic assumption: "only through work outside the home can the poor become responsible, upright citizens worthy of respect."

THE CONTINUUM OF WORK

Employment

At its simplest, employment means the exchange of labor for wages. In fact, employment encompasses far more because work forms, as we have seen, the core of our psychological and social existence. Employment means participating systematically in the economy and, from this participation, deriving personal identity and social status. Structurally, people who are employed are counted as members of the labor force. Employment of the civilian labor force, at 145.8 million is considered "standard" today and the employment–population ratio is stable at 62.3% (BLS, 2002). Though more people are employed today than four years ago the labor force participation rate has decreased from its high of 67% in 1999 to 66.2% in 2002. Just being employed, however, is not enough. Because work means so much to us, the idea of "job quality" has become as essential to today's workers as the wages we earn. Following decades of economic restructuring of the workplace, job quality has emerged as the most important labor phenomenon of the 1980s and 1990s (Champlin, 1995). The most important features of job quality are defined as meaningful participation in decision-making, humane and responsive management, and the primacy of team leadership and responsibility. Interestingly, job quality continues to preserve the hierarchical nature and structured environment of the traditional Western workplace.

Unemployment

Generally relegated to the realms of statistics, unemployment refers quite specifically to the condition of being jobless and actively looking for a job for the four weeks previous to the one counted. The extent of actual unemployment is probably underestimated by the Bureau of Labor Statistics because migrant workers, day workers, long-term unemployed people, and homeless people are not counted. Unemployment has risen to 6.8% (8.4 million workers) from its historical low of 4.2%, just four years ago, among civilians 16 years and older (BLS, 2002). High unemployment, relatively low inflation, and low interest rates have made way for today's stagnant economy. Volunteer workers and unpaid interns (people who presumably elect to work without pay) as well as retirees are technically unemployed—but morally salaried.

Underemployment

There is a difference between work and meaningful work. Meaningful work matches an individual's talents and skills with an appropriate job. Many people, however, have income-producing jobs that are unfulfilling or lack meaning, for which they are over-qualified or which they find morally suspect. The PhD-trained art historian driving a taxi is a classic example of underemployment. But what of the same art historian who teaches six courses a term as adjunct (pay-per-course) faculty? One of the most significant developments in the American labor market since the 1950s has been the dramatic increase in part-time and temporary workers at all levels of the workforce. Temporary workers, whether bricklayers or college teachers, do much the same work as their full-time colleagues but share in few of the rewards such as sick and vacation time, pension plans, or even the sense of support and collegiality that stems from the daily interaction with peers. Perhaps even more than unemployed people, underemployed people suffer from feeling powerless, meaningless, and isolated.

EMPLOYMENT AND WORK
THROUGHOUT THE LIFE SPAN

Individual human development cannot be separated from the impact of culture, and most cultures differ in the degree to which they emphasize "person" and "work." Because American culture is essentially fused with the idea of work and maximum human productivity, we have developed a classification that links stages of human physiological development with stages of work life pretty much from birth to death. Accordingly, we have typical presentations of childhood, adolescence, adulthood, and old age, each of which carries a rather specific "natural" equivalency between the developmental stage, the person as worker, and the worker as productivity. Such generalizations may serve society as an economic whole, but often undervalue large groups such as the elderly both as human beings and as organizational resources (Noor Al-Deen, 1997). Nevertheless, psychological development does occur and it behooves us to examine it in sequence.

Infancy and Early Childhood

Work may not begin at birth literally. Yet from infancy through early childhood, many of the interactions between children and their caretakers lay the foundation for patterns later found in the workplace. Culturally, work is closely associated with the characteristics of human autonomy, that is, psychological birth. Placing a tremendously high value on self-sufficiency reinforces social norms of individualism whereby the person depends on him/herself for survival, not on the family or the social group. The developmental psychologist Margaret Mahler (Mahler, Pine, & Bergman, 1975) posited that the course of the normal human life cycle begins with a gradual, multi-stage process by which the infant separates from the adult (the mother) and thus individuates. By inference, Mahler is pointing to the infant's task of achieving a special cultural norm: in order to become an individual person, one must separate psychologically from the mother, the family, the group. The identity of the self is, again, individual, and the healthier self is that which is separate from the family. In contrast, the infant psychiatrist Daniel Stern (1985) argues that infants are differentiated from birth. The sense of self develops progressively throughout the life cycle, as a result of increasingly complex relationships between caregiver and infant. Issues of attachment, trust, and dependency (and their opposites, separation and independence) are not confined to infancy. In Stern's theory, the work-related task is social: the healthy individual is one who can relate to others and whose sense of self thrives on interdependence.

While only one decade apart, these two theory sets mirror many of the changes that have transformed the American workplace in the last decade. The 1980s saw the demise of classic bureaucracy where workers' status in an organization was denoted by the size and location of their workspace, and by the degree of privacy they held. Office space was earned according to a hierarchy, but also a merit system whereby individuals who achieved the most on their own were considered the most successful, and therefore the most deserving of a separate, let's say individuated, office. This replicated social stratification as well, since the lowest level of employees occupied the most public spaces—claims workers in rows of desks, factory workers on the assembly line. But these structures have changed considerably. "Not only have the factories, smokestack industries and manufacturing plants of the 1980s been transformed, but the nature of work itself barely resembles what Americans have known and taken for granted" (Kurzman & Akabas, 1993, p. 386). Physically, today's workplace is far more open, informal, and personalized. The team is prized above the individual. Office walls have given way to work stations and networks. The relationship between employees, and between workers and managers, is evolving into a far more participatory, mutually responsive system. The physical construction of the workplace and its consequent psychological transformations seems to duplicate many of the changes in our understanding of infant psychology, as seen in the theoretical differences between Mahler and Stern.

Childhood

Also known as middle childhood, the dramatic shift that occurs between the ages of five and seven has a profound psychological, neuro-biological, and social impact on human development. Here, most children move from a family of origin into the larger world and experience new cognitive capacities and new ways of managing anxiety (Galatzer-Levy & Cohler, 1993). Language skills are refined. Behavior can be controlled internally (the self) as well as externally (the caretakers). Self-concept and social cognition become more focused as children are increasingly able to understand other people's thoughts, feelings, and intentions. This, in turn, facilitates interpersonal awareness and interpersonal relationships (Ashford, Lecroy, & Lortie, 1997). While sex role stereotyping begins at birth if not before (as in blue is for boys, pink is for girls), it is in middle childhood that boys and girls visibly incorporate sex-typed behavior into their self-concept. Culturally specific and often rigidly held values and behaviors are apportioned to each gender category which then internalizes a set of socially appropriate responses. These responses are played out later in work life: occupational choice, success and failure, sense of competence, risk-taking and decision-making behaviors, are just a few of the factors strongly influenced by sex role stereotyping. In her pioneering studies of school age children, the Harvard psychologist Carol Gilligan (1993) explored the differences in moral development between boys and girls. To resolve conflict, she found, boys set up hierarchical ordering while girls are concerned with functioning within a network of relationships. Later, as adults, women in the workplace continue to "self delineate through connection," relationships, and caretaking. In contrast, American men in the workplace use a "self defined through separation," rules and achievement of goals through competition. Like theories of infant development, psychological progress in childhood sets patterns for later work life which, if conformed to, will make for a well-adjusted individual. Thus, whether in school or later in the workplace, if girls play by boys' rules and achieve status through competition, they are violating stereotyped sex role behavior, are non-conforming, and poorly adjusted. It is in schools that the child finds the "culture of structure" (Chestang, 1982). This structure of schedules, regulations, and compromises has much in common with the culture of the workplace. It prepares children to adapt to workplace requirements and also to adapt to work roles by relying on their own creativity and productivity.

Adolescence

The relationship between adolescence and work, as we know it, has a history of its own. The view of adolescence as an institution in itself emerged during and after the Industrial Revolution (Kett, 1977). Educated middle-class families in 17th century Europe sent both boys and girls to work as servants or apprentices between the ages of 13 and 15 (Shorter, 1977). The lower and middle classes required their children to stay home, either to work on the farm or to continue with school after age 14 in order to secure employment more prestigious than mere "casual labor and dead end jobs." But the concept of adolescence as the awkward age, eccentric and moody, was "invented" between 1910 and 1920 with the development of psychology and child studies. The fact that today's late-modern society is driven more by market choices and less by the state will affect the role and structure of teen employment (France & Wiles, 1997).

Indeed, today adolescence is essentially viewed as the gateway to the world of work. To ease the transition from school to work, the adolescent needs a range of coping and adaptation strategies. The adolescent should to be able to contain the distress within tolerable limits; maintain self-esteem; preserve interpersonal relationships; and meet the conditions of the new environment (Enrich, 1982). The period of search, for both work and self, is impeded by the lack of correspondence between external expectations (the teenager is expected to be motivated, hardworking, punctual, ambitious, etc.) and the realities of the youth labor market (marginal, unskilled, frequently unstable, and low-grade jobs). This is of particular concern for minorities in the United States. Adolescent African American females, for example, have found that the reality of the workplace contrasts significantly with their aspirations and expectations and, though some are increasingly confidant about their careers, many suffer from the lack of role models in the labor force (Brown, 1996). Fortunately, researchers have found that early employment is not essential to the self-esteem and psychological health of adolescents. Moreover, adolescents tolerate the complex relationship between unemployment and expectation of success, commitment to work, motivation, and self-esteem better than adults (Patterson, 1997; Rodriguez, 1997). Statistically, teen unemployment did decrease by a dramatic 1.5% from 1998 to 1999 even among African American and Latino populations, affecting minority adolescents whose unemployment rate rarely goes below 50% and who have traditionally had significantly lower employment expectations (Quane & Rankin, 1998).

Adulthood

Adulthood in American culture is virtually synonymous with work. Adults are expected to work autonomously, to produce goods and services in exchange for wages, and to model for children how to be a contributing member of civic society. Adulthood, generally defined as the broad span of years between 21 and 65, can be divided into young adulthood (education and family development), stable adulthood (work and family expansion), and mid-life. Interestingly, adulthood covers the period of human development which is least investigated as an actual life stage probably because the ability to work and the duty to do so is a social given. Work problems that emerge in this life stage are attributed to personal inadequacy, moral lack, or environmental constraint, but are not viewed as developmental issues per se. Yet each stage of adulthood has developmental complexities of its own. Young adults are learning how to shift from part-time to full-time work, how to use income and to balance expectations, responsibilities, and resources. The experience of first jobs, including the socioeconomic factors that shape that experience, influences future attitudes and beliefs about work (Barling & Kelloway, 1999). Middle adulthood is often a time of generativity and high career satisfaction: education is completed (and student loans paid), careers are well underway, and family relationships are established. Secular and spiritual life are balanced. Yet this is also called the "sandwich generation," a time of conflicting responsibilities when adults are caring simultaneously for their children and their own aging parents. Between the ages of 35 and 55, employed women may suffer from the competing demands of work and family. Women experience heightened stress in their role as parental caregivers, especially if the parents live with the middle adult family and are single themselves, are in failing health, or are very old (Anastas, Gibeau, & Larson, 1990; Barnes, Given, & Given, 1995; Lee & Dwyer,

1996). Some of the stress stems from the conflict between two dominant moral imperatives: the value of work and the significance of family. Still, in a recent series of path-breaking studies on the middle years of the life span (Lachman & James, 1997), researchers found that many of the stereotyped roles of mid-life, especially for women, are changing. Mid-life no longer announces the waning of life, menopause, depression, and loss of home-making identity. Today mid-life conveys peak experiences, self-discovery, high productivity, and either found or renewed self-identity. Following mid-life, later adulthood ranges from mid or late 50s until perhaps the early 70s. While employment peaks in middle adulthood, later adulthood presents a career "fork" for many: they can either move into a period of increased individualism and creativity often with even greater productivity than in middle adulthood, or they can decrease their work-related energy and make a transition into forms of retirement. Much of this is, of course, predicated on social class and health status.

Early and Middle Old Age

When does an individual become an elderly person, and how does that affect the relationship to work? From a social policy and economic perspective, the Social Security Act of 1935 established 65 as the official retirement age. In terms of social value, 65 is the age when a person is eligible to receive government benefits, and can accept them without stigma. As a consequence of these universal benefits (Social Security indexed to inflation and Medicare), this demographic group has experienced the lowest overall poverty rate since the 1960s. Economic security for elderly people also serves as family support, since it decreases the "sandwich" pressure on young families to support their parents or grandparents. And indeed, the majority of elderly Americans are active, competent, and productive and are engaged in paid or unpaid employment despite their increasing need to maintain health care (Kahn, 1983). Computer technology has had a particularly positive effect on the employment status, home environment, and health care maintenance of elderly people (Czaja, 1996).

The function of work in later life is highly charged. For one, people whose personal and social identity was intertwined with their work for, let's say, 70 years continue to be identified with work. Many do continue to work, perhaps changing occupational status from employed to volunteer or full-time to part-time. On the other hand, changes in health status, income, and family situation may influence adjustment to the post-working, or retirement, stage of life. "The impact of psychological factors on retirement relates to the person's evaluation of the meaning of his contribution during the working years and the extent to which he harbors lingering doubts about his own value" (Chestang, 1982, p. 87). However, this perspective has been called the "male model" of retirement. Indeed, while today's workplace is changing, people who are now in the position to retire generally spent their work lives in a traditional, patriarchical structure. Men tend to experience a higher degree of life satisfaction in retirement since the pre-retirement employment experience also followed the male model (Calasanti, 1996).

ROLE OF EMPLOYMENT IN INDIVIDUAL PSYCHOLOGY

Since our understanding of our personal worth is organized around the core concept of work, American adults find their life's "meaning" in their jobs: the teacher, the stockbroker, the nun, the astronaut, the psychoanalyst, the cook. Conversely, people without work, or without what they believe is enough work, have difficulty finding meaning for their lives in other contexts. Women, people of color, and people with physical or mental disabilities who routinely encounter discrimination in hiring practices, internalize this discrimination and can find that their lives lack substantive meaning. The "person-in-environment" paradigm necessarily forms the basis of any examination of human psychology because environment and culture must be included in our understanding of how individuals process the meaning of work.

Positive Mental Health

What is psychological health and who is healthy? Are people with the "healthiest" psychological dispositions simply conforming to dominant cultural norms? We have far more information on ill health than on good health, including extensive scholarly and literary productions describing illness, the opposite of health. *The Diagnostic and Statistical Manual of Mental Disorders* (American Psychiatric Association, 1996) categorizes psychological disturbances and specifies criteria for observing and treating them. Yet, as we can see in Table 2-2, contrasting the *DSM-IV* with all its scientific apparatus to far earlier work reveals that we have made little progress in our understanding of, for example, the diagnosis of "Depression."

Nevertheless, positive mental health does exist. In Western culture it is largely an individual experience and is composed of life satisfaction, self-esteem, purpose in life, and sense of hope. And, as we have seen, most of these variables are inextricably bound up with work. Remarkably, employment status (part-time and full-time) is more significantly related to self-esteem than to education level, family configuration, and marital status especially among women (Sinacore-Guinn, 1998). The longer a person is jobless, the lower his or her self-esteem (Goldsmith, Weum, & Darity, 1997). However, gender does mitigate the damage done by joblessness young women are affected more deeply than young men but, for both, this can be reversed by one or two years of stable employment.

Identity

While work is an essential component of personal identity, pre-existing identity structure, also known as self-identity or sense of self, affects how we relate to work and the workplace. Identity formation is a characteristic task of adolescents whose early search for career choice is fraught with questions regarding personal and moral beliefs, sexuality, spirituality, quality of

TABLE 2-2. Diagnosis of Depression, 1917 and 1996

1996: Criteria for Major Depressive Episode, DSM-IV
"depressed mood (e.g., feels sad and empty, appears tearful); markedly diminished interest in all activities; significant weight loss or gain; insomnia or hypersomnia; fatigue or loss of energy; feelings of worthlessness or excessive or inappropriate guilt; diminished ability to think or concentrate; recurrent thoughts of death."

1917: *Mourning and Melancholia,* Sigmund Freud
"a state of grief [with] profoundly painful dejection, abrogation of interest in the outside world, loss of the capacity to love, inhibition of all activity, self-reproaches and self-revilings."

life, community, and family goals. An identity solidly forged in adolescence becomes in later life an important mediator between work stress and psychological well-being. Among adolescents, identity and self-efficacy are closely associated with vocational interests and occupational prestige (Vondracek & Skorikov, 1997). Among adults, a weaker identity structure and weaker work identity falls to unemployed people, whereas the employed exhibit a fairly high level of psychological well-being (Meeus, Dekovic, & Ledema, 1997). Gender identity is a large factor in the workplace, both in traditionally structured systems and in more contemporary environments that emphasize inclusiveness and nondiscrimination. Gender identity is also a determinant of an individual worker's self-efficacy and self-actualization, and has a significant impact on his or her productivity and overall participation in the life of the work organization (Ellis & Riggle, 1996).

Independence and Autonomy

The task of becoming an independent person involves three spheres: the emotional (separation from the family), the social (becoming more other-directed than self-directed), and the economic (earning enough money to meet one's financial needs) (Zastrow & Kirst-Ashman, 1997). Work gives us this independence. We value independence and we devalue dependence. Our favorite holiday is the 4th of July, known as "Independence Day." Culturally, we believe that we are all born autonomous individuals who, by virtue of our free will, naturally become adults responsible for our personal successes and failures. We dislike welfare recipients because they are considered "dependent," a lifestyle attribute that carries the weight of stigma (Goffman, 1963) equivalent to not working. Conversely, we admire wealthy people, more for the independence wealth represents than for the affluence itself. We also value initiative, self-starters, and entrepreneurs, people who take risks to become independent. What does this say about individual mental health? The psychologist David Shapiro (1981) developed a vivid new picture of human autonomy and its dynamic meaning in psychology and psychopathology. Autonomy does indeed develop from infancy onward but this self-direction can go awry, he said, and can result in forms of neurosis or "rigid character." Autonomy can become derailed, obsessive, and, in its extreme form, lead to paranoia. Thus, the psychological attribute we value the most in our culture can be used to further our personal development or it can turn against us.

Personal and Family Development

We know that work has a tremendous impact on individual personal development. And today more than ever, work organizations are asking new employees for a new focus on personal development, to be as well prepared in communication and interpersonal skills as they are in mathematics or social studies (Cassel, 1998). But individuals are not only primed by schools. They emerge from within a family context and some experts, for example the pioneering family therapist Virginia Satir, believe that families are the matrix of growth. The family is perhaps the most powerful institution is our society, more powerful than government, education, and even religion. The traditional family model (patriarchal, heterosexual, and nuclear) continues to hold a normative and forceful image in our society. This is changing in part because the generally conservative "family values" image is related to work—and the nature of the workforce is changing. Yet gender roles, and their concurrent prejudices, remain deeply embedded in our understanding of the relationship between family and work.

Even among self-employed people family intrudes more on work among women, whereas work encroaches more on family among men (Loscocco, 1997). Interestingly, men's degree of self-esteem (and individual vocational identity) influences their attitude toward gender roles: the lower men's self-esteem, the more they tend to oppose women's employment (Valentine, 1998). Women who work adjust to marriage better that non-working women (Vasudeva & Chaudhary, 1998), presumably because work provides them with a foundational identity. Change in families and in society is ideologically difficult and still today, as we have seen, only income-producing work is considered "healthy." The more we work, the more we earn, and the "healthier" or more normal we feel. In other words, both families and the individuals within them rely on work for their development.

WORK: WHEN IT WORKS AND
WHEN IT DOESN'T

Despite the expanding economy and the almost daily increase in jobs, many people do lack work. Yet American society continues to be what the economist John Kenneth Galbraith (1958) called an "affluent society." We thrive on an economics of opulence where success is measured incrementally and the "haves" are demarcated quite literally from the "have nots" by private property and moral condescension. Property, both physical and moral, is acquired through work. But what happens when human beings do not work, cannot find work, become or remain unemployed, or just give up? Are they lazy, psychologically disturbed, or immoral—characteristics frequently attributed to poor people and public assistance recipients? The sociologist William Julius Wilson (1996) vividly describes how this situation of joblessness is distinct from poverty. "A neighborhood in which people are poor but employed is different from a neighborhood in which people are poor and jobless. Many of today's problems in the inner-city ghetto neighborhoods—crime, family dissolution, welfare, low levels of social organization, and so on—are fundamentally a consequence of the disappearance of work." It is important to see that Wilson is not describing poverty alone: he is describing joblessness. Joblessness is a particularly painful form of poverty because of the cultural and psycho-social significance we attach to work. In a culture that believes that individuals are largely responsible for their own economic success or failure, almost any job is better than no job.

Does the idea of "work at any cost" help or harm the individual worker? For all its benefits, the workplace is often fraught with stress, occupational hazards, and other forces that detract from individual well-being. Work-related stress may lead to injuries and psychological disorders (Landy, Quick, & Kasl, 1994). According to the National Institute for the Occupational Safety and Health Administration (OSHA), psychological disorders ranked as one of the 10 leading work-related diseases and injuries during the 1980s. A key theme that emerged from OSHA's 1994 Priority Planning Committee was the very broad support for its workplace safety and health program. The Federal government has recognized the need to address workplace violence, especially violence against employees (Tyler, 1993). The experience of American workers also includes harassment (gender, race, and age) in its wide range of conditions that create workplace stress. Interestingly, despite these considerations and fairly radical upheavals in the contemporary work force, employees continue to be deeply identified with the social systems and the structure of the work organization (Rousseau, 1998). We can conclude that having a job is more important than liking one's job.

If holding a job is, in itself, at least morally more important than income and non-wage benefits, we can see why joblessness ranks so high among the social problems. Is the individual or the society at large responsible for causing this problem? Who is, ultimately, responsible for solving it? As with most social problems, the individual is challenged to solve "his/her" problem faster than the society will address larger structural issues. For example, though the definition of the family continues to evolve from a conventional model to many non-traditional forms, most employers continue to base their social policies regarding workers on the nuclear family structure (Akabas, 1985). Furthermore, "family-friendly" workplace policies designed to help employees balance work and family responsibilities, such as eldercare, tend to be underutilized largely because such policies continue to rate organizational productivity over employee well-being (Medjuck, Keefe, & Fancey, 1998). Mothers of children with special needs delay their entry or re-entry into the workforce (Booth & Kelly, 1998).

Thus, work organizations, though evolving, have been slow in making the structural changes needed by workers in an increasingly skilled society. Have individuals changed? Does the decreasing unemployment rate (and its corollary decreasing crime rate) reflect an upsurge in personal work motivation, or simply an increase in work availability? A recent analysis of the 1979–1992 National Longitudinal Survey of Youth data showed that, despite the "churning" labor market, the link between early, stable job experience and better employment in young adulthood is modest at best (Gardecki & Neumark, 1998). In the end, family support and individual psychology do have an effect on an individual's experience at work—whether or not the worker is disabled.

WORKING AMERICANS WITH DISABILITIES

> Slightly stooped with thick glasses and a frowning demeanor, a 30-something white man was mumbling to himself while filling up the supermarket shelves with paper towels and napkins. "Things are changing," he muttered, "K-mart isn't what it used to be. Too much stress. Now I need to go upstairs to get refills. Too much stress." A nearby customer, thinking he might be talking to her, asked him about it. "No," he answered politely, "I was only talking to myself."

Here is an adult with a developmental disability working under the types of workplace constraints that most anybody would find stressful: repetitive work, enclosed space, close supervision, pressured customers, deadlines, and quotas. For a person with a disability, however, the challenge is two-fold. On the one hand, the job is a source of prideful independence and a means of joining mainstream society. On the other hand, it demands a degree of competence and adaptive behavior—often learned skills—high enough to tolerate internal and external pressures largely invisible to the non-disabled world. Despite participation in vocational rehabilitation programs, post-participation employment, work training, and other educational activities, people with disabilities and mental health needs encounter multiple organizational deterrents to employment. These obstacles to personal achievement and social integration include attitudinal barriers, stereotypes, and assumptions about what they can and cannot do. When asked about their personal experience, individuals with disabilities contend that they are treated by professionals and the public alike as though they have explicitly fewer aspirations, abilities, and maybe even fundamental rights than non-disabled people (Gilson, Bricout, & Baskind, 1998). Perhaps most insidious, people with mental retardation or psychiatric impairment are devalued as "unpredictable" because they perceive and respond to stress differently (though some highly structured jobs are better performed by people with cognitive impairments than non-disabled people). Individuals with psychiatric disabilities have a lower chance for job placement than either those with learning disabilities or those with mental retardation (Rimmerman, Botuck, & Levy, 1995). These barriers are compounded by institutionalized racism, sexism, and ageism. Rimmerman and colleagues (1995) found that within each of the disability categories, the age by gender interaction led to differences in job placement: among early adults, men were more widely employed than women, but this finding reversed after age 35. The U.S. Census Bureau's 1994–1995 data show that 72.2% of African Americans with disabilities and 51.9% of Hispanics with disabilities are not working. The overrepresentation of minorities among unemployed disabled people stems from the nation's employment policy and overarching economic and political structure.

Because it is experienced both environmentally and psychologically, discrimination is the most powerful barrier preventing people with disabilities from full participation in society. As we have seen, the social structure of discrimination is upheld by an ideology that values work pre-emptively. If, as a culture, we value work above all else, disabled people will share in the prejudices held by their fellow citizens. The harm of self-stereotyping results from this internalized oppression and is compounded by internalized discrimination based on race, age, and sex. So too do feelings of self-rejection and behaviors such as isolation or aggression. Disabled people are hardly exempt from low self-esteem and heightened distress levels, some of the negative psychological effects associated with prolonged unemployment. Employment, found Petrovski and Gleason (1997), reduces the disabled individual's experience of stigma and loneliness without decreasing other measures of psychological health, including self-esteem and personal aspirations. Having internalized the social value of "work at any cost," people with intellectual disabilities are both satisfied with their jobs and aware of their low occupational status.

CONCLUSIONS

The American workplace has occupied the historical role of providing physical and moral sustenance to its employees, their families, and to retirees seeking post-employment support through traditional channels. In fact, employers have typically seen themselves as socially sanctioned providers of services, often as paternalistic overseers but also in the sense that their endeavors have been upheld by conventional 19th and 20th century norms. Yet few studies attribute to the idea of "work" either its rightful place in human development, or adequately describe its role in shaping mental health care. Accommodative workplaces are hardly well-respected in the general economy. They are minimally acknowledged in the business and management literature even though the Equal Employment Opportunity Commission reports that psychiatric disability is one of the foremost workplace discrimination complaints (Pardeck, 1999) and that employers do have a successful—and profitable—role in job maintenance (Gates, Akabas, & Kantrowitz, 1996). Fortunately, as we have seen in this chapter, a range of researchers and practitioners have explored the policy and practice implications of Title I, the employment provisions of the Americans with Disabilities Act (ADA), and its effects in the area of psychiatric disabilities on both worker and employer. Reviewing these sources, in the larger context of linking the American workplace to issues of access to mental health services, has formed the basis of a preliminary sketch of the place of work in human development.

This linkage between our cultural understanding of work and of the life cycle is significant for several reasons. First, the cost of health and mental health care is paramount today in the media, among providers (psychotherapists, psychoanalysts, physicians), and social welfare policy-makers. The universal dimension of access to health care—and of the place of mental health services within a universal framework—is being debated on every level of government today. Do citizens have a social right to mental health care regardless of their ability to pay? Pointing to the themes in the success or failure of workplace support for people with disabilities contains challenging implications for this public policy issue. Secondly, the number of "free-standing" outpatient clinics has decreased dramatically in the last three decades, from 51.4% of all outpatient services in 1970 to 25.3% in 1988 (Manderscheid & Sonnenschein, 1992). The press for affordability is an increasingly dominant political issue among organized providers of mental health services. Thus, it is important to ascertain if consumers/clients as well as providers have historically found the workplace experience adequate, effective, and equitable. Finally, this chapter represents an initial effort at providing a version of the human life cycle from the standpoint of the shifting role of work and its implications for health, mental health, and rehabilitation. As such, it is hoped that it will contribute a new facet to the work of mental health professionals, clinical and policy analysts alike. Exploring why, for example, the American workplace of the 1980s often chose not to develop worker-centered environments—as mandated by Federal law—should shed light on the development of, and obstacles to, universalism for people with disabilities.

REFERENCES

Akabas, S. H. (1985). Workers are parents, too. *Child Welfare, 63*(5), 387–399.

American Psychiatric Association (1996). *Diagnostic and statistical manual of mental disorders* (4th ed.). Washington, DC: Author.

Anastas, J. W., Gibeau, J. L., & Larson, P. J. (1990). Working families and eldercare: A national perspective in an aging America. *Social Work, 35*(5), 405–411.

Ashford, J. B., Lecroy, C. W., & Lortie, K. L. (1997). *Human behavior in the social environment—a multidimensional perspective*. Pacific Grove, CA: Brooks/Cole.

Barling, J., & Kelloway, E. K. (Eds.) (1999). *Young workers: Varieties of experience*. Washington, DC: American Psychological Association.

Barnes, C. L., Given, B. A., & Given, C.W. (1995). Parent caregivers: A comparison of employed and not employed daughters. *Social Work, 40*(3), 375–381.

Booth, C. L., & Kelly, J. F. (1998). Child-care characteristics of infants with and without special needs: Comparisons and concerns. *Early Childhood Research Quarterly, 13*(4), 603–621.

Brown, S. P. (1996). Black female adolescents' career aspirations and expectations: Rising to the challenge of the American occupational structure. *Western Journal of Black Studies, 20*(2), 89–95.

Bureau of Labor Statistics (2002). *ftp.bis.gov/pub/newsrelease/History/empsrt.0404.2003.*

Calasanti, T. M. (1996). Gender and life satisfaction in retirement: An assessment of the male model. *Journal of Gerontology, 51B*(1), S18–S29.

Cassel, R. N. (1998). Career readiness for the communication age based on Fortune 500 job-skill needs. *Journal of Instructional Psychology, 25*(4), 222–225.

Champlin, D. (1995). Understanding job quality in an era of structural change: What can economics learn from industrial relations? *Journal of Economic Issues, 29*(3), 829–841.

Chestang, L. (1982). Work, personal change and human development. In S. H. Akabas & P. A. Kurzman (Eds.), *Work, workers and work organizations: A view from social work*. Englewood Cliffs, NJ: Prentice Hall.

Czaja, S. J. (1996). *Aging and the acquisition of computer skills*. Mahwah, NJ: Lawrence Erlbaum.

Ellis, A. L., & Riggle, E. D. (Eds.) (1996). *Sexual identity on the job: Issues and services*. New York, NY: Harrington Park Press/Haworth Press.

Enrich, A. C. (Ed.) (1982). *Major transitions in the human life cycle*. Lexington, MA: D.C. Heath.

France, A., & Wiles, P. (1997). Dangerous futures: Social exclusion and youth work in late modernity. *Social Policy and Administration, 31*(5), 59–78.

Freud, S. (1917). Mourning and melancholia. In *The Standard Editors of the Complete Psychological Works of Sgmund Freud*, ed. James Strachey, 24 vols. (London, 1981), 14: 245.

Galatzer-Levy, R. M., & Cohler, B. J. (1993). *The essential other—a developmental psychology of the self*. New York, NY: Basic Books.

Galbraith, John Kenneth (1958). *The Affluent Society*. Boston, Houghton Mifflin & Co.

Gardecki, R., & Neumark, D. (1998). Order from chaos? The effects of early labor market experiences on adult labor market outcomes. *Industrial and Labor Relations Review, 51*(2), 299–322.

Gates, L. B., Akabas, S. H., & Kantrowitz, W. (1996). Supervisor's role in successful job maintenance: A target for rehabilitation counselor efforts. *Journal of Applied Rehabilitation Counseling, 27*(3), 60–66.

Gilligan, C. (1993). *In a different voice—psychological theory and women's development*. Cambridge, MA: Harvard University Press.

Gilson, S. F., Bricout, J. C., & Baskind, F. R. (1998). Listening to the voices of individuals with disabilities. *Families in Society, 79*(2), 188–196.

Goffman, E. (1963). *Stigma—notes on the management of spoiled identity*. New York, NY: Simon & Schuster.

Goldsmith, A. H., Weum, J. R., & Darity, W. (1997). Unemployment, joblessness, psychological well-being and self-esteem: Theory and evidence. *Journal of Socio-Economics, 26*(2), 133–158.

Kahn, R. L. (1983). Productive behavior: Assessment, determinants and effects. *Journal of the American Geriatrics Society, 31*(12), 750–757.

Kett, J. (1977). *Rites of passage—adolescence in America 1790 to the present*. New York, NY: Basic Books.

Kroeber, A. L., & Kluckhohn, C. (1955). *Culture—a critical review of concepts and definitions*. New York, NY: Random House.

Kurzman, P. A., & Akabas, S. H. (Eds.) (1993). *Work and well-being—the occupational social work advantage*. Washington, DC: NASW Press.

Lachman, M. E., & James, J. B. (Eds.) (1997). *Multiple paths of midlife development*. MacArthur Foundation Series on Mental Health and Development. Chicago, IL: University of Chicago Press.

Landy, F., Quick, J. C., & Kasl, S. (1994). Work, stress and well-being. *International Journal of Stress Management, 1*(1), 33–73.

Lee, G. R., & Dwyer, J. W. (1996). Aging parents–adult child coresidence: Further evidence on the role of parental characteristics. *Journal of Family Issues, 17*(1), 46–59.

Loscocco, K. A. (1997). Work–family linkages among self-employed women and men. *Journal of Vocational Behavior, 53*(2), 279–297.

Mahler, M., Pine, F., & Bergman, A. (1975). *The psychological birth of the human infant*. New York, NY: Basic Books.

Manderscheid, R. W., & Sonnenschein, M. A. (Eds.) (1992). *Mental health, United States 1992* (Center for Mental Health Services and National Institute of Mental Health, DHHS Publication No. (SMA) 92-1942). Washington, DC: U.S. Government Printing Office, Superintendent of Documents.

Medjuck, S., Keefe, J. M., & Fancey, P. J. (1998). Available but not accessible: An examination of the use of workplace policies for caregivers of elderly kin. *Journal of Family Issues, 19*(3), 274–299.

Meeus, W., Dekovic, M., & Ledema, J. (1997). Unemployment and identity in adolescence: A social comparison perspective. *Career Development Quarterly, 45*(40), 369–380.

Noor Al-Deen, H. S. (Ed.) (1997). *Cross-cultural communication and aging in the United States*. Mahwah, NJ: Lawrence Erlbaum.

Pardeck, J. T. (1999). Psychiatric disabilities and the Americans with Disabilities Act: Implications for policy and practice. *Journal of Health and Social Policy, 10*(3), 1–12.

Patterson, L. J. (1997). Long-term unemployment amongst adolescents: A longitudinal study. *Journal of Adolescence, 20*(3), 261–280.

Petrovski, P., & Gleeson, G. (1997). The relationship between job satisfaction and psychological health in people with an intellectual disability in competitive employment. *Journal of Intellectual and Developmental Disability, 22*(3), 199–211.

Quane, J. M., & Rankin, B. H. (1998). Neighborhood poverty, family characteristics and commitment to mainstream goals: The case of African–American adolescents in the inner city. *Journal of Family Issues, 19*(6), 769–794.

Rimmerman, A., Botuck, S., & Levy, J. M. (1995). Job placement for individuals with psychiatric disabilities in supported employment. *Psychiatric Rehabilitation Journal, 19*(2), 37–43.

Rodriguez, Y. G. (1997). Learned helplessness or expectancy value? A psychological model for describing the experiences of different categories of unemployed people. *Journal of Adolescence, 20*(3), 321–332.

Rousseau, D. M. (1998). Why workers still identify with organizations. *Journal of Organizational Behavior, 19*(3), 217–233.

Shapiro, D. (1981). *Autonomy and rigid character*. New York, NY: Basic Books.

Shorter, E. (1977). *The making of the modern family*. New York, NY: Basic Books.

Sidel, R. (1998). *Keeping women and children last—America's war on the poor* (Rev. ed.). Harmondsworth, U.K.: Penguin Books.

Sinacore-Guinn, A. L. (1998). Employed mothers: Job satisfaction and self-esteem. *Canadian Journal of Counseling, 32*(3), 242–258.

Stern, D. (1985). *The interpersonal world of the infant*. New York, NY: Basic Books.

Swick, K. J., & Rotter, M. F. (1981). The workplace as a family support system. *Day care and early education, 9*(2), 7–11.

Tyler, M. P. (1993). *A manager's guide: Traumatic incidents at the workplace*. Washington, DC: U.S. Office of Personnel Management.

Valentine, S. (1998). Self-esteem and men's negative stereotypes of women who work. *Psychological Reports, 83*(3, Pt. 1), 920–922.

Vasudeva, P., & Chaudhary, M. (1998). A study of marital adjustment amongst working and non-working women. *Journal of the Behavioral Sciences, 9*(1–2), 5–12.

Vondracek, F. W., & Skorikov, V. B. (1997). Leisure, school and work activity preferences and their role in vocational identity development. *Career Development Quarterly, 45*(4), 322–340.

Wilson, W. J. (1996). *When work disappears—the world of the new urban poor*. New York, NY: Random House.

Zastrow, C., & Kirst-Ashman, K. K. (1997). *Understanding human behavior and the social environment* (4th ed.). Chicago, IL: Nelson Hall.

CHAPTER 3

Employment and Empowerment of People with Disabilities

A Social Development Perspective

CREIGS BEVERLY AND ANN ROSEGRANT ALVAREZ

INTRODUCTION

Since time immemorial, people with disabilities, whether mental or physical, have been the subject of scorn, ridicule, fear, demonization, intolerance, ostracism, social and economic marginalization, and, all too often, outright indifference. These practices have been universal and no nation on earth is guilt free.

Writing on disability as an emerging global challenge Seipel (1994) points out that owing to stereotypes and problems beyond their control, persons with disabilities have often been isolated or segregated, and relegated to a second-class position in society. Despite some advances in recent years to mainstream those with disabilities in all societal activities, patterns of prejudice are not much changed. People with disabilities still face discrimination, restrictions, and maltreatment. They encounter architectural barriers, transportation problems, communication barriers, and restrictions in other services that can affect jobs and social opportunities (Nagler, 1990). Indeed, various polls show that people with disabilities as a group are socially, economically, vocationally, and educationally disadvantaged (Social Legislation, 1990; U.N., 1986).

Seipel (1994) goes on to state that as a result of discrimination against disabled persons in education and in the labor market, society receives few benefits from the talents of disabled individuals. Many disabled persons are able to work and live in independent settings, yet they are often directed to welfare systems rather than to labor markets. As a case in point, in the United States alone, about 170 billion dollars per year are spent to maintain disabled persons, although 66% of the non-working disabled persons would be willing to give up disability benefits for full-time employment (Social Legislation, 1990).

CREIGS BEVERLY AND ANN ROSEGRANT ALVAREZ • Wayne State University School of Social Work, Detroit, Michigan.

Because of these factors, people with disabilities experience disproportionately higher levels of poverty when compared with the general population, have difficulty in finding and sustaining gainful employment, and have a general decline in their overall quality of life (Kopels, 1995). When gender and race or ethnicity enter the equation, results are particularly drastic. Driedger (1996) explains that women "... must confront the problems of access, housing and transportation that are faced by every disabled person. These barriers, coupled with the unique challenges faced by women with disabilities—negative attitudes, lack of role models, lack of education and many forms of violence—prevent them from taking their rightful place in society" (Driedger, 1996, p. 19). Furthermore, "In developing countries, women with disabilities face triple jeopardy: discrimination due to disability, gender and developing world status" (Driedger, 1996, p.10).

When the social status and social significance of those with disabilities are devalued, human disenfranchisement invariably follows. Condeluci (1995) states that, although disenfranchisement can be self-oriented, more often than not it is a distantiation levied by society toward the individual. In most cases, the disenfranchisement is caused by some difference or distinction of the individual that is alien or misunderstood by society. As such, disability becomes not only a physical or mental status, but also a social definition (Mechanic, 1989).

As stated previously, these differences and distinctions have an adverse effect on the opportunities and options for gainful employment among persons with disabilities and yet work is one of the primary means through which social value is assigned. The value of work to individuals, families, corporations, businesses, or society in general is accepted as valid and useful personally, economically, and socially. People with disabilities should not have their opportunities for work—whether in sheltered workshops because of their degree of disability, or in America's *Fortune* 500 companies—denied because of myths, stereotypes, misunderstandings, and outright discrimination (Mechanic, 1989). In the final analysis, the gross human capital product (GHCP)—i.e., the productive output resulting from maximizing the potential of all societal cohorts—is lessened considerably due to the underutilization and therefore underproduction of persons with disabilities. This is wasteful for both the individuals concerned and for society.

DISABILITY DEFINED

Clearly, disability can be physical as well as mental. It is, however, imperative to understand that although disabilities are broken down into physical types or mental types, there is an inseparability between the mental and the physical. Every mental event has some corresponding physical correlate (Levy, 1994).

Asch and Mudrick (1995) point out that individuals, organizations, and government agencies define disability in various ways. For some, disability refers exclusively to a chronic medical condition or physical or mental impairment; for others, disability is the functional consequence of chronic mental or physical conditions; and for still others, disability is the by-product of social and physical environments that do not accommodate people with different functional abilities. Despite these various definitions of disability, there appears to be some consensus that a person with a disability can have either a permanent physical or mental impairment or a chronic health or mental health condition. The health condition or impairment may be visible or invisible to others, and it may be present at birth or begin at any age. Disabilities vary in severity; some people find it extremely difficult to participate in a wide range of employment and recreational activities, especially when the social and physical environment is inaccessible or discriminates against them, whereas others' lives are affected in a single area.

Bickenbach (1993) posits that when the overt behavior of an individual, viewed as an integrated whole rather than a collection of parts, is restricted because of the presence of one or more impairments, the health experience has become objectified. This signals the presence of a disability, defined in the International Classification of Impairment, Disability, and Handicap (ICIDH) as "any restriction or lack (resulting from an impairment) of ability to perform an activity in the manner or within the range considered normal for a human being ... ." Disability involves a limitation upon one (or more) integrated activity, ability, or behavior generally accepted as a component of everyday living or else part of a repertoire of skills and other specialized abilities associated with a specific talent, profession, job, or other social role. Disabilities may be temporary or permanent, reversible or irreversible, progressive or regressive, serious or minor; and, like impairments, they can be the product of the normal and natural, but none the less debilitating, processes of aging.

For a long time, researchers faced significant difficulties in obtaining any meaningful data on disabilities. One of the main difficulties has been divergent terminologies and concepts used by various governments, professional organizations, and researchers. The ICIDH unifies some of the conceptual problems in defining disabilities. To facilitate better data collection and management, ICIDH further defines disabilities in the following three categories (Bickenbach, 1993):

1. Impairment: any loss of or abnormality in psychological, physiological, or anatomical structure or function. Examples include blindness, deafness, loss of sight in an eye, paralysis of limb, and mental retardation.
2. Disability: any restriction or lack of ability to perform an activity in the manner within the range considered normal for human beings. Examples of disability include difficulty seeing, speaking, hearing, moving, reaching, and eating.
3. Handicapped: disability that limits or prevents the fulfillment of a role that would otherwise be normal for that individual. Examples include being bedridden, confined to home, unable to use public transportation, unable to work, and socially isolated.

However ultimately conceptualized and defined, disability is not synonymous with inability. One's body is not the totality of who one is. If treated effectively, people who experience mental illness can live long and productive lives. For some, in fact, disability is the doorway through which ability is realized.

SCOPE OF THE PROBLEM

Until fairly recently, it has been difficult—if not impossible—to determine the precise numbers of persons with disabilities in the United States, not to mention the world. Before the twenty-fourth session of the United Nations Commission for Social Development, in 1975, there was limited interest in the worldwide disability problem (Seipel, 1994). As a result of U.N. leadership and support, more useful statistics on disability were collected during the early 1980s. These were collected from the census figures of 66 nations, sample surveys, and the disability registration system of 55 nations. The statistics were then compiled and stored in the U.N. Disability Statistics Data Base (DISTAT). Based on the nations' statistics found in DISTAT, the statistical department of the United Nations published the *Disability Statistics Compendium* (1990). This publication contains data on various socioeconomic and demographic statistics. For the purpose of standardizing raw data, these data were coded and organized according to the World Health Organization's (1980) taxonomy, known as the ICIDH (Seipel, 1994).

According to Shapiro (1993), there are some 35 million to 43 million disabled Americans, depending on who does the counting and what disabilities are included. In 1991, the Institute of Medicine, using Federal health survey data, came up with the figure that 35 million—one of every seven—Americans have one or more disability that interferes with daily activities such as working or keeping a household. "Disability ranks as the nation's largest public health problem, affecting not only individuals with disabling conditions and their immediate families, but also society at large," the report concludes.

Shapiro (1993) points out, however, that during debate on the American with Disabilities Act, lawmakers, President Bush, advocates, and members of the media freely used the higher figure of 43 million. That number came from other Federal data. But even this figure did not include people with learning disabilities, some mental illness, those with AIDS, or people who are HIV positive and have other conditions covered under civil rights legislation. A 1994 census report counted 49 million. Researchers cannot agree on the size of the disability population because, as previously described, there is no consensus on what constitutes disability.

Reports from the National Institute of Mental Health (NIMH) state that those with mental illnesses are often feared, misunderstood, and still stigmatized (NIMH, 1997). The most severe mental illnesses affect some five million American adults, causing inestimable suffering to these individuals and their families. However, these severely ill persons—suffering from schizophrenia, manic-depressive illness, major depression, panic disorder, and obsessive–compulsive disorder—represent only a part of a broader problem from which few families are immune, for mental disorders can and do occur from childhood to old age, irrespective of gender or race. Overall, *one in 10 Americans experiences some disability from a diagnosable mental illness* in the course of any given year. The social, human, economic, family, and medical toll this takes is staggering.

While numbers cannot convey the distress accompanying mental disorders, the economic impact can be calculated. Mental disorders cost the United States more than $150 billion each year for treatment, for the costs of social service and disability payments made to patients, and for lost productivity and premature mortality. Schizophrenia alone costs the nation some $30 billion annually (NIMH, 1997).

If we estimate that international figures are remotely close to U.S. data, then it is absolutely clear that disability is not only a national public health problem, but an international problem, as well. The international dimensions of the problem are exacerbated by the ongoing existence of territorial wars, ethnic, religious, and regional conflicts. For example, unexploded land mines in Africa, Asia, the Balkans, and other parts of the world account not only for deaths, but for an untold number of injuries—including subsequent disabilities—annually.

Perhaps partially in recognition of this, at the conclusion of the World Summit for Social Development—held March 6–12, 1995, in Copenhagen, Denmark—governments adopted a Declaration and Programme of Action that represents a new consensus on the need to put people at the center of development. At this gathering—the largest yet of world leaders—117 heads of state or government pledged to make the conquest of poverty, the goal of full employment, and the fostering of stable, safe, and just societies their overriding objectives. Among the ground-breaking agreements made by the world's leaders in the Declaration are 10 commitments that will directly affect the nature and quality of life of disabled persons:

1. eradicate absolute poverty by a target date to be set by each country;
2. support full employment as a basic policy goal;

3. promote social integration based on the enhancement and protection of all human rights;
4. achieve equality and equity between women and men;
5. accelerate the development of Africa and the least developed countries;
6. ensure that structural adjustment programs include social development goals;
7. increase resources allocated to social development;
8. create "an economic, political, social, cultural, and legal environment that will enable people to achieve social development";
9. attain universal and equitable access to education and primary health care; and
10. strengthen cooperation for social development through the United Nations.

THE SOCIAL DEVELOPMENT ALTERNATIVE

To move away from myths, misunderstandings, misconceptions, and outright discrimination regarding people with disabilities, and to initiate movement for them toward greater democratization, enfranchisement, and empowerment in society, will require a radical reordering—perhaps even a radical restructuring—of values and priorities. It will require no less than a paradigm shift and a completely different view of human capital. This radically different perspective may be found in the social development alternative.

Midgley (1994, p. 8) states that:

> The roots of the social development perspective can be traced back to colonial times. The term was first used in the context of British colonial welfare administration in Africa in the 1950s, when social workers sought to transcend their conventional remedial roles. Apart from providing remedial services for the disabled, children, and elderly, the mentally ill, and young offenders, these administrators sought to foster social programs such as mass literacy and community development that would enhance levels of welfare for the community as whole.

Midgley (1994, p. 9) further articulates three distinctive features of social development:

> The social development perspective has several distinctive features. First, social development is inclusive. It requires the mobilization of all social institutions for the promotion of human welfare. Development is viewed as a comprehensive process, which encompasses all citizens and fosters social solidarity. Unlike approaches which rely on *treatment* interventions, social development does not delegate the responsibility for human welfare to the individual. Instead, collective mechanisms are used to include all sections of the population and promote the *general* rather than individual welfare.
>
> Second, social development seeks to integrate the economic and social aspects of the development process. Unlike approaches which emphasize the delivery of social welfare services to poor people, it views social programs as an essential ingredient of an overall growth strategy designed to promote human well-being. It reflects Titmuss's view that social policy should not serve as a *handmaiden* to the economic sector but as an equal partner in promoting welfare (1974).
>
> Third, social development offers a broad, eclectic, and pragmatic set of prescriptions. In its more recent formulations, social development theory is seeking to synthesize statist, communitarian, and even individualist notions into an inclusive, pragmatic conception (Midgley, 1993).
>
> Today, the populist ideas underlying community participation coexist with the statist collectivism, which characterized earlier social development thinking. Similarly, in keeping with the current ideological climate, notions of individual responsibility and effort are not derided as they often were in statist thought. Current social development theory does not denigrate markets but seeks rather to direct the market and harness its power for the general welfare. Today, social development theory attempts to reconcile the diverse orientations contained in approaches to poverty alleviation.

The ultimate goal of the social development movement, like that of the social work profession, is to secure for people everywhere the satisfaction of at least their basic social and material needs (Estes, 1992, 1993). Social development theory thus embodies the values of human dignity, equality, social justice, sustainable development, distributive justice, and self-determination (Elliott, 1993; Falk, 1984; Lowe, 1995).

Some scholars, most notably Gott, Kilpartick, and Nackerud (1998), posit that social development theory is partly the result of the questioning of social work's prevailing emphasis on individualistic, psychotherapeutic approaches; the re-examining of its roots in community development and the alleviation of poverty; and the influence of economic development approaches in developing countries. Clearly, it represents a radical break from both residential and institutional ideologies of social work practice.

DEVELOPMENTAL SOCIAL WORK AND REHABILITATION

The application of social development theory within the field of social work has been called developmental social work practice. Estes (1997) frames its nature, quality and intent in clear and concise terms.

> First, developmental social work practice includes the provision of personal social services to people in distress, but especially to victims of war, refugees, orphaned children. Second, developmental social workers engage in organization efforts directed at helping poor and other powerless people remove the sources of their oppression (e.g. corrupt landlords, unjust employers, colonial administrators, racism). Third, developmental social workers seek both to establish new social institutions (e.g. for credit unions, mutual aid societies, community welfare centers, seed banks, social security schemes) and to reform existing institutions so as to make them more accessible and responsive to the needs of those for whom the institutions were designed. And developmental social workers also seek to accelerate the pace of social development in local communities, states and provinces, nations, regions and, ultimately, the world itself.

Examples of this kind of work are numerous. One model is that of the Grameen Bank, originally developed in Bangladesh by Muhammed Yunus. A creative approach to the alleviation of poverty, "Grameen-style banking is characterized by providing credit without collateral through peer lending groups, and by taking the bank to the poor" (Jansen & Pippard, 1998, p. 110). Loans have typically been used for capital to establish and maintain micro-enterprise efforts. Opportunities for people with disabilities to benefit from such an approach are numerous, particularly since reports have described the successful application of the model in such countries as the Philippines, Ethiopia, Kenya, and Malaysia (Kamaluddin, 1993), as well as in the United States (Clark & Huston, 1993; Raheim, 1996).

Inherent in the principles of developmental social work is a fundamental respect for, and observance of, human rights. These rights are not selective, and not relative, but encompass universal respect, observance, and protection (Ayton-Shenker, 1995). Everyone is entitled to human rights without discrimination of any kind. The non-discrimination principle is a fundamental rule of international law that protects individuals and groups against the denial and violation of their human rights. This means that human rights are for all human beings, regardless of "race, colour, sex, language, religion, political or other opinion, national or social origin, property, birth or other status to include persons with disabilities." To deny human rights on the grounds of cultural distinction is discriminatory, since human rights are intended for everyone, in every culture (Ayton-Shenker, 1995).

POLICY DILEMMAS

Social development theory argues that the most appropriate paradigm for the development of human habitats, global villages, and human settlements is to place people (human beings) at the center of all development activities. The centrality of this belief is vested in the notion that all development decisions, before enacted, must pass the "What impact?" test. This asks: If enacted, what impact will this practice have on the nature and quality of human life?

Examples of the kinds of dilemmas created by placing people at the center of all development decisions are as follows:

1. To what extent will modernization disrupt traditional social relations and what does this mean for the culture?
2. What will be the societal impact of freeing women from traditional roles of underdevelopment?
3. Is it better to pursue a policy of full-employment for persons with disabilities or to subsidize their existence through transfer payments and social services?
4. Is it true that people are equal in their humanity, but different in their experiences and therefore in their abilities?
5. In order to maximize the benefits to the many, is it necessary to neglect the needs of the few?

This list could be expanded further. It is clear, however, that to operationalize social development theory, practitioners must be willing to accept diversity and pluralism, value differences, and above all else, maintain respect for and observance of human rights. They must also be willing to address the challenging issues outlined above, among others.

Even democratic sacred cows such as "the majority rules" must be re-examined in the context of protecting the rights of the minority with the recognition that perhaps the only way to guarantee the rights of the majority is to protect the rights of the minority. Social development theory argues for both/and, rather than either/or; it argues for win/win, rather than win/lose; it argues for peace rather than war; provisions for meeting basic needs, rather than the pursuit of materialistic excesses; it argues for freedom, rather than oppression; and it argues for maximization of all creative human capital (potential) rather than social exclusion and disenfranchisement.

The development and implementation of policies that support this perspective will help to create opportunities for people with disabilities. Existing policies can also be evaluated for their potential to contribute to these opportunities. For example, Individual Development Account (IDA) (Sherraden, 1991) legislation, passed in many states, makes it possible for low-income families and individuals to build assets through a program of savings accounts matched by governments, private sector organizations, or individuals. An important aspect of such legislation will be to ensure that people with disabilities are included in its benefits through a program of active identification and recruitment.

PRACTICE IMPLICATIONS

In the wake of the development of the U.N. principles of civil and human development in the international arena; the enactment of the Americans with Disabilities Act on July 26, 1990, in the United States; and the development of pertinent case law; practitioners working to enfranchise and empower persons with disabilities must understand that never has the world of those with disabilities changed so fast (Shapiro, 1994). Shapiro (1994) states that rapid advances in technology, new civil rights protections, a generation of better-educated disabled students out of "mainstreamed" classrooms, a new group consciousness, and political activism mean more disabled people are seeking jobs and greater daily participation in American life. But prejudice, society's low expectations, and an antiquated welfare and social service system frustrate these burgeoning attempts at independence. As a result, the new aspirations of people with disabilities have gone unnoticed and misunderstood by mainstream America.

Given these trends and realities, there is a need for practitioners to position themselves as advocates within the disability rights movement. They must be unequivocal in their belief that there is no pity or unredeemable tragedy in disability, and that it is society's myths, fears, and stereotypes that most make it difficult to have disabilities (Shapiro, 1994). Practitioners working with those with disabilities must also be thoroughly familiar with all provisions in the American with Disabilities Act. This is especially true for Title I of the Act, which prohibits discrimination in employment. While cooperation and equitable accommodations are desirable ends with employers, practitioners should not disregard the potential of litigation as a compensatory remedy when persons with disabilities, all other factors being equal, are denied opportunities for gainful employment.

Gainful employment for persons with disabilities is tied directly to educational access and educational attainment. Data are clear that people with disabilities are statistically the poorest, least educated, and largest minority population in the United States (Kopels, 1995; U.S. House of Representatives, 1990). Practitioners, therefore, also must learn to monitor and evaluate educational systems, K-12 and beyond, to ensure accessibility, availability, and effective usability for persons with disabilities. Given the level of educational underdevelopment experienced by far too many, an affirmative action plan similar to those that have been used to compensate racial minority groups for years of discrimination against them is a possible option. Practitioners should also make maximum use of media to educate the public and use every means available to them to influence the movie industry to make more films such as *Mask*, *My Left Foot*, *Rain Man*, and *Elephant Man*. These movies have had and continue to have an enormous impact on building positive public perceptions of people with mental and physical disabilities (Skarnulis, 1999).

Social workers in schools, in medical settings, in family service agencies, and elsewhere have innumerable opportunities to put forward an agenda that includes ethical treatment of people with disabilities. By serving as role models for others, advocating for the full civil rights of all people, and taking a stand in favor of the full inclusion of people with disabilities in every aspect of life, social workers can make this group of citizens a part of everyone's community (Skarnulis, 1999). Professionals concerned about the rights of people with disabilities ought to begin their practice each day with the same basic question: How can we move toward a world that values the essential humanity of all people, including those of us who have disabilities (Skarnulis, 1999)?

Regarding educational preparation, proactive practitioners must encourage schools of social work to do a much better job of training people to work with persons with disabilities. Some models for doing this are already available. For example, Kopels (1995) provides an excellent model for training future practitioners that covers the relevant domains of social work preparation, including values, ethics, diversity, social and economic justice, at-risk populations, human behavior and the social environment, social welfare policies and services, social work practice, and the field practicum.

Practitioners must also become aware of the many strong and successful self-help efforts that are already underway, and determine how they can support and facilitate these efforts without dominating or undermining them. These efforts include the Self-Help Factory, in Soweto, South Africa, specializing in electronics; training offered and businesses started by the Disabled Women's Network, in Trinidad and Tobago; the Uganda Disabled Women's Association, which runs a store through which it distributes its own products, as well as managing a revolving loan fund; and the DisAbled Women's Network (DAWN) Canada, which has affected policies to both protect and expand the rights of women with disabilities (Driedger, 1996).

CONCLUSION

In conclusion, it is clear that people who are physically and mentally challenged in the United States and the world in general—people with disabilities—continue to experience the effects of discrimination, stigmatization, and oppression (Cole, Christ, & Light, 1995; Kopels, 1995). These effects persist in the United States even after the passage of the Rehabilitation Act of 1973, the Americans with Disabilities Act of 1990, and the case law that has resulted from these statutes (Cole et al., 1995). Globally, they persist in contradiction to principles expressed and espoused by world leaders in many contexts.

The result diminishes the potential and the lives of those with and without disabilities, through literal expenditures and through egregious waste of human capital. A social development approach has much to offer, both in terms of a perspective and by providing concrete examples of how employment opportunities, education, and social services can be combined to create options for those who have been challenged by disabilities, and limited and oppressed by others' perceptions of them.

REFERENCES

Asch, A., & Mudrick, N. (1995). Disability. In *Encyclopedia of social work* (19th ed., pp. 752–761). Washington, DC: NASW Press.

Ayton-Shenker, D. (1995, March). *The challenge of human rights and cultural diversity* (pp. 4–5). New York, NY: United Nations National Department of Public Information.

Bickenbach, J. (1993). *Physical disability and social policy* (pp. 36–37). Toronto, Canada: University of Toronto Press.

Clark, P., & Huston, T. (1993). *Assisting the smallest businesses: Assessing micro-enterprise development as a strategy for boosting poor communities, an interim report.* Washington, DC: Aspen Institute.

Cole, B. S., Christ, C. C., & Light, T. R. (1995). Social work education and students with disabilities: Implications of Section 504 and the ADA. *Journal of Social Work Education, 31(2),* 261–268.

Condeluci, A. (1995). *Interdependence: The route to community* (p. XIX). Winter Park, FL: GPO Press.

Driedger, D. (1996). Emerging from the shadows: Women with disabilities organize. In D. Driedger, I. Feika, & E. G. Batres (Eds.), *Across borders: Women with disabilities working together.* Charlottetown, PEI: Gynergy Books.

Elliott, D. (1993). Social work and social development: Towards an integrative model for social work practice. *International Social Work, 36,* 21–36.

Estes, R. J. (1992). *Internationalizing social work education: A guide to resources for a new century.* Philadelphia, PA: University of Pennsylvania School of Social Work.

Estes, R. J. (1993). Toward sustainable development: From theory to practice. *Social Development Issues, 15(3),* 1–29.

Estes, R. J. (1997). Social work, social development and community welfare enters in international perspective. *International Social Work, 40(1),* 43–55.

Falk, D. (1984). The social development paradigm. *Social Development Issues, 8(3),* 4–14.

Gott, W., Kilpartick, A., & Nackerud, L. (1998). Social development and social constructionism: Strangers or bedfellows? *Social Development Issues, 20(1),* 17–19.

Jansen, G. G., & Pippard, J. L. (1998). The Grameen Bank in Bangladesh: Helping poor women with credit for self-employment. *Journal of Community Practice, 5(1/2),* 103–123.

Kamaluddin, S. (1993, March 18). Lender with a mission. Bangladesh's Grameen bank targets poorest of the poor. *Far Eastern Economic Review, 156*(11), 38–40.

Kopels, S. (1995). The Americans with Disabilities Act: A tool to combat poverty. *Journal of Social Work Education, 31*(3), 337–346.

Levy, D. (1994). Conceptual objections. Errors in understanding. In Kirk & Einbinders (Eds.), *Controversial issues in mental health*. Boston, MA: Allyn & Bacon.

Lowe, G. R. (1995). Social development. In *Encyclopedia of social work* (19th ed., pp. 2168–2173). Washington, DC: NASW Press.

Mechanic, D. (1989). Mental health and social policy (pp. 125, 204–206). Englewood Cliffs, NJ: Prentice Hall.

Midgley, J. (1993). Ideological roots of social development strategies. *Social Development Issues, 15*(1), 1–13.

Midgley, J. (1994). The challenge of social development: Their third world and ours—1993 Daniel S. Sanders Peace and Social Justice Lecture. *Social Development Issues, 16*(2), 1–12.

Nagler, M. (Ed.) (1990). *Perspective on disability*. Palo Alto, CA: Health Markets Research.

National Institute of Mental Health (1997). Mental illness in America. The National Institute of Mental Health Agenda. MD: Author.

Raheim, S. (1996). Micro-enterprise as an approach for promoting economic development in social work: Lessons from the self-employment investment demonstration. *International Social Work, 39*, 69–82.

Seipel, M. O. (1994). Disability: An emerging global challenge. *International Social Work, 37*(2), 165.

Shapiro, J. (1993). *No pity* (pp. 36–37). New York, NY: Random House.

Sherraden, M. (1991). *Assets and the poor: A new American welfare policy*. Armonk, NY: M. E. Sharpe.

Skarnulis (Ed) (1999). Who shall survive? Ethical decision making with people who have disabilities. In Ramanathan & Link (Eds.), *All other futures: Principles and resources for social work practice in a global era* (pp. 84–87). Belmont, CA: Brooks/Cole/Wadsworth.

Social Legislation (1990). The Americans with Disability Act of 1990. *Washington. Social Legislation Bulletin, 31*(40), 157–160.

Stroud, J. (1999, June 11). Mental illness is not at last. *Detroit Free Press*, p. A11.

United Nations (1986). *Disability situation, strategy and policies*. New York, NY: Author.

United Nations (1990). *Disability statistics compendium*. New York, NY: Author.

U.S. House of Representatives Committee on Education and Labor (1990, May 1). (House Report No. 101–485 (11), to accompany House Report No. 2273 (101st) (Congress, 2nd Session)). Washington, DC: U.S. Government Printing Office.

World Summit for Social Development (1996, June 12). Report of the World Summit for Social Development: Copenhagen, 6–12 March 1995. New York, NY: United Nations.

CHAPTER 4

The Recovery Framework in Rehabilitation and Mental Health[1]

LeRoy Spaniol, Cheryl Gagne, and
Martin Koehler

INTRODUCTION

For most of the past century people with mental illnesses were thought to have irreversible illnesses with increasing disability over time. There was little hope for people with these disabilities. They were often institutionalized, provided very little treatment, and forgotten by professionals and even their family members. Mental health program planning, policies, and practices had been developed and implemented to support this uncompromisingly negative view of the predicted outcome for people with mental illnesses. However, recent research on long-term outcomes for people with mental illnesses describes quite a different picture. Seven major retrospective studies carried out in Japan, Germany, Switzerland, and the United States show recovery rates of from 46% to 68% for those with the most severe forms of mental illnesses (Harding, 1989; Harding & Zahniser, 1994; Harding, Zubin, & Strauss, 1992). By recovery these studies mean that people with a history of mental illnesses were working, living in independent housing, had meaningful relationships, and were contributing to their communities in a variety of ways. This new view of the recovery potential for people with mental illnesses requires a major shift in attitudes and in mental health and rehabilitation policy and practice. If the potential for recovery is there, how can we as professional mental health and rehabilitation practitioners best help people in their recovery process? What have we learned about what is helpful and how can we implement these new attitudes and practices? In this chapter we present a series of questions and responses regarding recovery from mental illnesses. We describe what recovery is, what people are recovering from, how people are impacted by what they are recovering from, and how to assist people in their recovery process.

---

[1]A new and expanded paper based on an article published in Continuum, 4(4), 1997, 3–15 and reprinted in R. P. Marinelli & A. E. Dell Orto (eds.). (1999) *The psychological and social impact of disabiliy* (fourth edition). New York: Springer Publishing.

LeRoy Spaniol • Senior Director of the Boston University Center for Psychiatric Rehabilitation, Boston, Massachusetts.   Cheryl Gagne and Martin Koehler • Boston University Center for Psychiatric Rehabilitation, Boston, Massachusetts.

In our experience we have found that rehabilitation and mental health professionals are frequently unaware of the traumatic impact of mental illness, its treatment, and stigma on the person with a mental illness. They are also frequently unaware of the process of recovery for the person who experiences these traumas, and how they can assist the person in his or her recovery. We have written this chapter in order to increase professional awareness about how people with mental illnesses are impacted by the illness, its treatment, and stigma and discrimination, and to provide some suggestions for how professionals can assist people in their recovery.

There are four questions that we want to raise. An understanding of these four questions and our responses to them have been helpful to us in working more effectively with people with serious mental illnesses. These four questions are:

1. What is recovery?
2. What are people recovering from?
3. What is the "impact" of "what" people are recovering from?
4. How can professionals assist people in their recovery?

WHAT IS RECOVERY?

Recovery is a process, an outcome, and a vision. As a process, recovery is a common human experience. We all experience recovery at some point in our lives from injury, from illnesses, from loss, or from trauma. Recovery is a process of healing physically and emotionally, of adjusting one's attitudes, feelings, perceptions, beliefs, roles, and goals in life. It is a painful process, yet, often a process of self-discovery, self-renewal, and transformation. Recovery is a deeply emotional process. Recovery involves creating a new personal vision for oneself.

As an outcome, recovery is the ability to return to work, to live in housing of one's choice, to have friends and an intimate relationship, and to become a contributing member of one's community. Yet, historically, schizophrenia has been viewed as an irreversible illness with increasing disability over time—hopeless and intractable. While the impact of severe mental illnesses is devastating to those who experience it and to their families, it does not appear that schizophrenia is a disease of slow and progressive deterioration as was once widely believed (Bleuler, 1950; Kraepelin, 1902). People with schizophrenia can achieve partial or full recovery from the illness at any point during its course, even in the later stages of their life (Harding, Strauss, Hafez, & Liberman, 1987; Huber, Gross, Schuttler, & Linz, 1980). As Harding has said:

> … the course of severe psychiatric disorder is a complex, dynamic, and heterogeneous process which is non-linear in its patterns moving toward significant improvement over time and helped along by an active, developing person in interaction with his or her environment (Harding, 1986).

Numerous current studies have demonstrated that one half to two thirds of people with severe mental illnesses significantly recover over time (Harding & Keller, 1998; Harding & Zahniser, 1994; Harding, Zubin, & Strauss, 1987, 1992). The evidence for a specific, inflexible natural history of every disorder is simply not there.

As a vision, recovery is the organizing construct that can guide the planning and implementation of mental health services because recovery is the purpose and the goal of all the programs and services that combine to assist the person with a psychiatric disability (Anthony, 1993). The goal of recovery is to become more deeply human, in all of our uniqueness. The goal of recovery is to become part of the human stream, in all of our individuality (Deegan, 1988, 1995).

One of the main benefits of utilizing recovery as the key organizing concept in our work with people with psychiatric disability is that it allows us to look at the whole person, in all of their humanity, instead of just at their illness (Deegan, 1995). If all human beings experience recovery, then people with serious mental illnesses, who are also human, also experience recovery.

WHAT ARE PEOPLE RECOVERING FROM?

It is important to be clear about "what" people are recovering from. From a psychosocial perspective people are recovering from the catastrophe of mental illness and from multiple and recurring traumas. Trauma from the illness, the medical treatment of the illness, negative professional attitudes, lack of appropriate assisting skills of professionals, devaluing and disempowering programs, practices and environments, lack of enriching opportunities, and stigma and discrimination in society. Professionals need to acknowledge the multiple sources of trauma experienced by people with mental illnesses. People with mental illnesses are well aware of these many sources of trauma. It is important that people who provide services validate these experiences and assist people with mental illnesses to cope with them. Because of the stereotypes prevalent in the training of many mental health professionals, the "illness" has historically been the focal point of interventions (Minkoff, 1987). And the symptoms and behavior of the person have been primarily associated with the "illness" while the other sources of impact on the person have been rarely acknowledged. This has left many people with mental illnesses feeling devalued and ignored and has resulted in mistrust in and alienation from the rehabilitation and mental health system.

WHAT IS THE IMPACT OF WHAT PEOPLE
ARE RECOVERING FROM?

It is important to understand the "impact" of "what" people are recovering from; that is, "how" people are affected by the catastrophe of the illness and the multiple traumas they are recovering from. We know that multiple and recurring traumas have a devastating impact on the lives of people who experience them. They are devastating because people are left profoundly disconnected from themselves, from others, from their environments, and from meaning or purpose in life. While the illness itself causes people to feel disconnected, stigma and discrimination (negative personal, professional, and societal values, attitudes, and practices) further disconnect people and represent serious barriers to building a new life. There are five types of impact; we discuss each one in the following subsections.

Loss of Sense of Self

People with mental illnesses experience severe trauma to their sense of self. While an enduring and developing core of meaning and knowing has been acquired over time by the person prior to the disorder, the illness and its treatment severely fragment and traumatize the self (Estroff, 1989). While the self is directly and deeply affected, it continues as an enduring, personal core that precedes, transcends, outlasts and is more than an illness. Within every person with a mental illness there continues to be a persisting, healthy, trying-to-survive self and personhood, with a self-acknowledged history (Estroff, 1989).

As Estroff (1989) has reported, sickness in our culture alters the self (e.g., I am not myself today). We reject the dysfunctional self of sickness as "not me." Yet if the illness persists, what is the implication for the self?

There are a number of dilemmas confronting the person as the illness persists (Estroff, 1989):

1. When being "not myself" is my self, i.e., the illness persists.
2. When the most self-seeing, self-knowing, self-confirming others lose, alter, or put away the person's prior, not-sick self so it is unverifiable to and with them.
3. When the core self is no longer validated by others. People become identified with their illness.
4. I "am" or I "have" an illness. How does the person integrate the illness, its treatment, and self? What are the implications for the various options? For example, is there a continuum of joining versus separating from the illness? What is the experience of the person?

It is important to acknowledge the mediating function of the self. The self is a central and mediating factor among our various areas of functioning such as vocational, intellectual, emotional, social, and spiritual (Davidson & Strauss, 1992). When the self is less functional, our overall functioning will be impaired. When the self is functional, each area of functioning benefits synergistically. The self is the agent of recovery. Disconnection from the self results in an inability to move forward with one's life.

The self also has a social function. So when the self is not functioning well the person becomes more easily isolated and alienated from others. The isolation that people with psychiatric disability feel has many other causes such as stigmatizing attitudes of some professionals and family members, unemployment and poverty, hypersensitivity to stimulation and affect, impairments in attention, concentration and communication, and disorientation and confusion (Davidson & Stayner, 1997). The inability to share these barriers with others further alienates and isolates people with mental illnesses.

Chronicity, as a characteristic of the self, and from a psychosocial perspective, is a transformation of a prior, enduring, known, and valued self into a less known and knowable, devalued, and dysfunctional self (Estroff, 1989). This occurs both within the person and in the eyes of family, peers, and professionals (Estroff, 1989). Chronicity, passivity, and dependence are fostered by an internal or external environment that undermines the functional self (Davidson & Strauss, 1992). Chronicity from this perspective is a form of learned hopelessness and helplessness that continues to be supported by uninformed knowledge, attitudes, and practices.

Loss of Connectedness

Personal stories of people with mental illnesses reveal a pervasive loss of interpersonal connectedness, loneliness, and isolation, yet a profound longing to be connected in meaningful ways to others (Davidson, Stayner, & Haglund, 1998). Yet people become so shocked by the illness, stigma, and discrimination that they feel they cannot act on their own desires for contact (Davidson et al., 1998).

Davidson et al. (1998) describe many barriers to finding, building, and maintaining relationships.

1. Stigma and discrimination are major barriers. Attitudes on the part of professionals, family members, and other people in society often make it difficult to feel accepted as an equal in relationships. This feeling is further buttressed when important others see the person as a mental patient rather than as an individual with his or her own unique blend of strengths and weaknesses (Davidson et al., 1998).
2. Some people with mental illnesses may have a heightened sensitivity to sensory stimulation or to interpersonal contact. Their sensitivity may result in their picking up on subtle cues in a relationship, particularly when they involve strong feelings and emotions in oneself or in others. This heightened sensitivity, coupled with confusion over how to respond, can lead some people to be cautious about entering relationships, or even avoiding them altogether (Davidson et al., 1998).
3. Some people with mental illnesses may experience difficulty in focusing their attention or filtering out distracting internal or external experiences. Cognitive or emotional associative connections can leave people pulled in numerous directions at once (Frese, 1993).
4. Hallucinations or delusions may leave people feeling unable to focus.
5. People may feel not in control of their own feelings, thoughts, and emotions. They may wonder who is really in charge of themselves. This can form the basis for feeling that maybe others are in charge (e.g., the FBI).
6. Finally, poverty and unemployment leave people feeling disconnected.

Loss of Power

This is a loss of one's ability to act in one's own interest. This is a loss of belief in oneself. This is the loss of one's sense of agency—oneself as an active agent. People with mental illnesses may experience themselves as having no power, no real choices. Power is lost through the severing of our connections. When our connections are broken, we feel powerless. There are a variety of forms of power (Mack, 1994). The power that is healing, that is more than oneself, that can move another person, is acquired through our relationships. It is power with people not over people. It is a power acquired through reconnecting with oneself, others, our larger environment, and larger meanings in life. It is a power acquired through a deepening of our capacity to experience life fully and directly without being overwhelmed or intimidated (Mack, 1994). It is a power acquired by coming alive.

Loss of Valued Roles

Meaning in life is intimately connected to the various roles we play. Unfortunately, the onset of mental illness frequently interrupts the valued roles of people, namely wife, husband, mother, father, worker, student, son, daughter, and sibling. People with mental illnesses are still frequently assumed not to be capable of fulfilling these roles. And, people with mental illnesses often come to believe this themselves. One of the most frustrating experiences of people with mental illnesses is the awareness of the life course of friends and siblings they grew up with who have gone on to college, have acquired a career, have married, and have a house. People with mental illnesses have learned that these natural life events may never be available to them and they mourn them deeply.

Loss of Hope

The accumulation of traumatizing, devaluing experiences wears people down over time, and leads to the giving up of hope. Hopelessness, apathy, and indifference are best seen not as problems but as learned solutions. They are strategies that desperate people adopt in order to stay alive (Deegan, 1995). They are strategies desperate people adopt in order to manage an inequality in the balance of power (Mack, 1994). Without hope it is hard to cope. People just barely survive. But they do not really feel alive or a part of life. We also certainly know of many examples where hope has been taken away; where someone has been told there is no hope. This is especially devastating to people with mental illnesses. And, if it comes from a mental health or rehabilitation professional, it is doubly disabling.

HOW CAN PROFESSIONALS ASSIST PEOPLE IN THEIR RECOVERY?

It is important for professionals to understand "how" people can be assisted in their recovery; that is, in recovering from the impact of multiple and recurring traumas. Recovery is a process by which people with psychiatric disability rebuild and further develop their personal, social, environmental, and spiritual connections, and confront the devastating effects of stigma through personal empowerment. It is never too late to begin the recovery process. Understanding the recovery process and one's own recovery experience are important first steps in returning to a life that is personally fulfilling and a life that contributes to others. Recovery is ultimately a journey of the heart—a choice for life, a choice to live and to have a life (Deegan, 1996).

Reclaiming the Sense of Self

The onset of mental illness and the stigma and discrimination associated with it causes "self-shock." The sense of self is traumatized. It needs to heal and to recover. Recovery, in one sense, is recovery from "self-shock." Professionals can assist people who are in "self-shock" by being present in a gentle, caring, and non-invasive way. People who are in shock are vulnerable. They need to be listened to, attended to, and supported as any person who is in shock.

The importance of rediscovering and reconstructing an enduring sense of the self as an active and responsible agent provides an important, and perhaps crucial source of improvement for the person with a mental illness. The sense of self provides a key theoretical construct in the understanding and treatment of the person (Davidson & Strauss, 1992).

Some authors have noted the way an enhanced sense of self, such as a sense of self-efficacy, self-esteem, and an internal locus of control, can help to ameliorate various aspects of a disorder and encourage efforts at coping in the face of traumatic life events (Davidson & Strauss, 1992). For example, a positive relationship among self-esteem, fitness, and recovery from depression has been found. Yet the impact of these various life events has not been extensively looked at for people with mental illnesses (Davidson & Strauss, 1992; Skrinar, Hutchinson, & Williams, 1992). Strauss (1992) describes four key aspects of the recovery of a functional self in the following ways.

1. *Discovering a more active self.* This is a process of gradually realizing that one can act in one's own interest. That one can do things that work, that make one's life work, that influence one's life. This is a critical awareness in the recovery process. How the person does this can seem quite minimal to others (e.g., get up on time, keep an appointment, cook a meal), but the discovery that one can influence one's life through one's own incremental actions can have a profound impact on the sense of self. This initial awareness of personal efficacy will recur at different times and build up momentum. It is a fragile awareness and may be easily bruised by negative experiences. It is clear that professionals can be helpful in this process by providing opportunities for it and by acknowledging success when it occurs.

2. *Taking stock of self.* Through additional positive experiences of acting in one's own interest a person begins to feel more grounded in his or her new self. While it may continue to feel fragile, the person deliberately tests out newfound strengths. Confidence builds that one's new functional self exists and is available when needed. Supportive feedback from professionals is important during this testing period.

3. *Putting self into action.* As one's level of confidence in one's new functional self grows one continues to build one's self through personal action and feedback. This is a process of gradually enhancing and further grounding one's new functional self. It is felt as real and available. Gradually reclaiming one's living, learning, and working life and confronting negative personal, professional, and societal values, attitudes, and practices are important ways of "putting one's self into action" and, thereby, further building one's functional self. Professionals can support this process by actively helping the person to explore living, learning, or working goals, developing the steps to achieve them, and providing the support to maintain the person in the implementation of his or her goal.

4. *Appealing to self.* As one's level of confidence grows one begins to acknowledge more deeply the presence of this stronger functional self and to call upon it as needed. It becomes a readily available resource for the person. While vulnerabilities may continue to exist, one is not so easily bruised by negative life experiences. One feels empowered. As one feels more empowered one will rely less on professional help and more on family and peers.

Reclaiming Connectedness

Most people continue to make efforts to connect, whether succeeding or failing, being disappointed, retreating to heal, and trying to connect again (Davidson et al., 1998). The drive to connect is very strong. One important way that people connect is through telling their personal stories of the onset of their mental illness and what their experience of dealing with this trauma has been. This is an important way of communicating with another human being. Issues relating to the illness, its treatment, and the impact of stigma are the most difficult, yet the most important, to share. Failure to articulate one's experience can leave one especially alone and isolated (Davidson et al., 1998). Failure to communicate results in a further burying of one's feelings inside oneself.

Those people with mental illnesses who succeed in building satisfying relationships are able to come out of their isolation. They can use their relationships to further build their social, emotional, vocational, and spiritual lives. In addition, they are able to develop a variety of coping mechanisms to prevent the reoccurrence of the illness, to combat stigma, and to build their lives. Not all of these coping mechanisms are verbal. Some involve just being with others in activities such as a walk or watching TV. Even acquaintances such as the mailman or the clerk at the corner store can provide a friendly and stable environment with which to connect. For some people, detachment from the "normal" culture may actually be more adaptive. Their most meaningful relationships may be with other people with mental illnesses.

What is helpful in building relationships is what is helpful to people in general. Some of these include (Davidson et al., 1998):

1. Support from important others.
2. The opportunity to give and receive love. This is what makes life worthwhile for most people.
3. Having someone to care about increases our sense of self-esteem.
4. Tolerance and acceptance of differences.
5. Understanding and compassion.
6. Clarity in communication and expectations.
7. Focus on strengths and competencies.
8. Mutual respect for one another as unique and valuable people.
9. Validation for who one is and what one does. Validation provides fundamental affirmation.

What gets in the way in building relationships includes:

1. Negative attitudes.
2. Boundaries between people that assume one is OK and the other is Not OK. When this happens there is no room to be a normal person with feelings, desires, ambitions, and hopes. It is extremely difficult to be other than crazy.

Reclaiming Power

Power is reclaimed by rebuilding the broken connections. There are a number of strategies that professionals can support in assisting people to reclaim their power.

ACCEPTANCE.   Acceptance is one of the harder tasks in the recovery process. Acceptance means seeing and acknowledging all the various aspects of oneself without devaluing oneself. Negative judgments and evaluations are barriers to acceptance. They lead to disbelief or even denial because it is hard to accept what one devalues. Yet, acceptance does not mean approval, or even disapproval. Acceptance means seeing and acknowledging what is.

Seeing and acknowledging what is seems like a simple task at first. Don't we all do this, all the time? Unfortunately, even an introductory exposure to psychology shows us that acceptance is not so easy at all. We all have a tendency to "color" our perceptions with our past learnings, or to project feelings and meanings on what we see. Not surprisingly, certain meditative and focusing approaches require a lengthy practice in "seeing what is," because a person's personal history has often left his or her perceptions somewhat contaminated. People with mental illnesses can learn to be sensitive to their vulnerabilities in perceiving. They can learn to know themselves well enough to recognize when they are most likely to override "what is" with their own learned ideas, feelings, and sensations. They can learn how to be open to "what is" without being overwhelmed or intimidated by their history or their fears.

One of the problems with acceptance is that the mind can fool us. The experiences of a person with a mental illness can seem so real. Why deny his or her own reality, to accept what others say is not real. A frontal assault on someone's denial is usually not helpful. If a person with a mental illness knows that others view him or her as misperceiving reality, then this can help, especially if he or she trusts the person. Loosening belief takes time and trust in others. Acceptance is so hard when a person with a mental illness perceives as true what others see as a misperception. People with mental illnesses have to come to see that their perception can be colored by the illness and by their history with stigma and discrimination.

Acceptance is a process and not an event. It involves both emotional as well as cognitive aspects of oneself. It is not simply a matter of making a decision. It involves working out this decision emotionally and through one's actions. The emotions tend to lag behind one's decisions. Yet actions help to deepen the emotional commitment to one's decision. A professional can help a person with a mental illness deepen his or her confidence in acceptance through assisting the person to face the feelings acceptance brings up and through supporting the actions that concretize acceptance in his or her life.

The content of what people with mental illnesses need to accept includes their strengths as well as their deficits. They need to accept all of themselves. Acceptance is difficult because it builds on hope. Without the foundation of hope, acceptance can be too terrifying. As Pat Deegan has said, "How can we accept the illness when we have no hope? Why should one pile despair on top of hopelessness? The combination could be fatal. So perhaps people are wise in not accepting the illness until they have the resources to deal with it" (Deegan, 1996). Professionals can learn to communicate realistic hope by becoming familiar with the literature supporting recovery and by actively collaborating with a person with a mental illness in rebuilding his or her life.

Acceptance also means dealing with loss. The dreams of what could have been, the loss of who the person was before the illness, and the knowledge that peers have gone on to have a life. This is very painful. Family members know this pain also. Dealing with loss is not an easy task. Yet acceptance means seeing oneself directly, without judging. One's bottom line. People with mental illnesses need to begin their recovery from where they are.

Effective coping builds on acceptance. It builds on reality. And that reality is not only the illness. The reality also includes stigma, abusive treatments, negative professional attitudes and practices, programs that are often unappealing, and lack of opportunity in the community. Also, as people feel more confidence in themselves, they begin to acknowledge aspects of themselves that are also part of their reality. These include their many talents and strengths, their inner wisdom, and their relationships with family, friends, and helpers (Davidson & Strauss, 1992). They gradually begin to identify with these other aspects of themselves and to realize that they can call upon them as needed. Gradually, the illness becomes less dominating and all-encompassing.

Acceptance reduces unnecessary pain and anguish. Acceptance can bring on a sense of relief. People with mental illnesses are able to stop struggling with what they do not want to see or acknowledge. Anguish is replaced with the ordinary suffering that comes with dealing directly with the often-uncomfortable realities of one's life.

Acceptance for people with mental illnesses means acknowledging their own agency, their own ability to act in their own interest. It means moving from being acted upon, to assuming responsibility for their life. Acceptance helps people to find new solutions to replace the apathy, indifference, and hopelessness that have helped them survive up to now (Deegan, 1996). Acceptance is empowering. Acceptance helps people with mental illnesses to deal with the real barriers that exist within themselves and within their environment. The person influences the process of recovery. People are active participants whose feelings, meanings, and interpretations of the illness impact on the course of the illness. The individual can call upon coping and regulatory mechanisms to modify, adapt, and adjust to the illness and to actively confront the many barriers in the environment (Strauss, 1992).

Acceptance is courageous. Courage can be defined as the ability to make a commitment to an imperfect or unknown process. This is what people with psychiatric disability do. Their commitment comes from their hope. They begin to believe hope is possible. As that hope takes root, they can make a commitment to themselves and to their recovery and to do whatever is necessary to bring it about, knowing that it is not a perfect process. There are risks, there are dangers, there are failures, and there are successes. And this is OK. This is courageous.

Acceptance requires support. When others accept one, it is easier to accept oneself. When others express hope for one, it is easier for one to have hope. People with mental illnesses are not islands. They live in relation to people, places, and events. They influence and they are influenced. Their self develops in relationship (Estroff, 1989). There is a partnership in this process with people and events. They are not alone in how they experience and respond to their life.

Acceptance can lead to compassion—compassion for oneself and compassion for others. People with mental illnesses become less judging of themselves and others. They become more focused on what they need to have a life and how to get those resources. They begin to be interested in how to help other people with psychiatric disability. People who are involved in their own recovery are important sources of support and mentoring to other consumers. It is helpful to see other people making it.

Acceptance is complex. It is a process that may take a long time. It involves all of a person, the mind, the body, the emotions, and behavior. It is a courageous process. It is a journey of the heart (Deegan, 1996).

SELF-WILL/SELF-MONITORING.   Behind hopelessness is often helplessness. Doing things that are helpful to oneself creates hopefulness, often in small ways that are nevertheless very important, for example exercising, reading something we like, spending time with a friend, and completing a task that is valued. These incremental steps build a person's power and establish a new sense of who he or she is and what his or her world is all about. These steps empower people. They help people with mental illnesses to feel their "agency" and their ability to bring about a change. They gradually build a new identity and new meanings. These steps also build an important relationship with another person—someone who believes in the person with a mental illness. This gives a person with a mental illness the mirroring, feedback, and validation he or she needs.

We often hear the expression, "If there is a will there is a way." We sometimes think it is more helpful the other way around: "If there is a way there is a will." If people are given opportunities, they will be more likely to feel hopeful. If you want people to feel motivated, give them options that are appealing. The will and the motivation to have a life come out of a person's experience, often from a professional, a person, or program that is hopeful for him or her.

MUTUAL AID GROUPS/SUPPORTIVE FRIENDS.   Numerous authors have written about the profound importance that self-help and mutual aid groups can have in supporting individuals with disabilities (Gartner & Reissman, 1982; Killilea, 1976). Criticism and negative comments can undermine one's developing sense of self. Social support can facilitate a positive sense of self and a sense of empowerment (Davidson & Strauss, 1992). Professionals and families should encourage the person with a disability to join a self-help group. The risk is that the professional and family will lose a part of the person as he/she gains more independence and self-care. The benefit is that the person will find important parts of him/herself.

SPIRITUALITY.   Spirituality can be looked at as a path and a journey that leads to a deepening awareness of our connectedness to ourself, to others, to our roles in life, and to larger meaning and purpose. While the tendency to travel this path is a natural part of most of our lives, an *urgency* to "make meaning" and to "rebuild connections" is felt when we experience a crisis, trauma, loss, injury, or illness in ourself or in someone close to us.

The onset of mental illness is one such experience. It often is experienced in the person as a profound *disconnection* from him or herself, from others, from roles in life, and from larger meaning and purpose. In addition, recurring traumas from the treatment system, negative attitudes, stigma and discrimination, the pathologizing of the experience, and the absence of knowledge, skills, and supports to integrate the experience further disconnect the person. The uniqueness of this particular experience as a spiritual crisis lies in its ongoing impact on almost every aspect of a person's life. Therefore, recovery, as a spiritual journey, is a process of building or rebuilding our connectedness to ourself, to others, to our roles in life, and to larger meaning and purpose.

To be connected is a natural way of being. It is how we begin our life and represents the underlying nature of how we are in this world. Disconnectedness is something that we learn—often as a way of surviving or coping with an internal or external experience. Because connectedness is a natural way of being, it is one of our deepest yearnings and most satisfying experiences. When we are most deeply connected we are often unaware of time and even space—we are simply in the moment. Connectedness, therefore, is not simply a technique, or a way of manipulating ourself or others. Connectedness is what is authentic for us—what is natural and spontaneous; that is, to be an integrated, mutual, contributing partner in this world we live in.

Spirituality also provides solace, companionship, and meaning to a person's struggles. People with mental illness often find belonging to a particular religion helpful both spiritually and socially. And if they can find ways to connect to their church or synagogue in a volunteer capacity they can also feel needed and valued.

A SIGNIFICANT OTHER.   Relationships and biology are intimately related. If one's relationships are healthy and intimate, then one's body will respond positively, and healing will be more likely. Intimacy is an important aspect of most people's lives. Intimacy is a state of closeness that can make a person feel authentic, whole, and intensely alive. Yet, at times, closeness brings up very intense feelings in people with mental illnesses. These feelings come from real experiences in one's past where the person was at risk or hurt—often by mental health professionals. Exploring these feelings can help to understand them and possibly even where they come from. The more people with mental illnesses can become aware of their learned feelings the less likely they will be to project them onto another person. And it is usually in an intimate relationship that people with mental illnesses learn about themselves, confront their learned images and feelings, and learn how to be open to the real "other person" they are connected with.

TEMPORAL PERSPECTIVE.   Understanding recovery as a process helps people with mental illnesses to cope more effectively with specific stressful events in their life. They can come to know that the stressful events will not last forever. While it often seems like a specific crisis will last forever, it will have a beginning, middle, and an end. The knowledge that the person is in this process can bring some relief. It can help the person to focus on developing more effective coping strategies rather than "over-dramatizing" a particular distressful event.

The person can know he or she has been through this before and survived. They can come to trust their increasing ability to deal with their symptoms, their attitudes and perceptions, and the real barriers in their life.

One important aspect of the process of recovery is the tendency to be more symptomatic as a person becomes more active in his or her own behalf, and to be more vulnerable to frustration as he or she becomes more successful. New experiences can bring on new challenges that the person may not yet be prepared for. When the professional can recognize this as a normal process and not as a sign of increasing illness, it can be calming and grounding to the person struggling to build a life for himself or herself.

Reclaiming Valued Roles

There is a great deal of evidence that rehabilitation works—that people can reclaim valued roles in life and enhance their personal sense of meaning (Harding & Zahniser, 1994; Harding et al., 1987). Some of the strategies for helping people with mental illnesses reclaim valued roles include the following.

VOCATIONAL TRAINING AND WORK.   There is ample evidence from both consumer self-reports and from the research literature that work strengthens a person's self-esteem and helps that person to feel a part of the larger community. Work has many benefits for people with mental illnesses (Kirsh, 2000). Work can be a distraction from the worries and anxieties of life. Work can help one to feel normal like other people. Work can challenge a person and contribute to a sense of self-worth. Work makes people with mental illnesses feel good about themselves and connects them socially to other people (DeSisto et al., 1995; Harding et al., 1987; Rogers, 1995). Work builds on the competencies and strengths of people and builds up their pride in their accomplishments.

SUPPORTED EDUCATION.   Supported education helps people to choose, get, and maintain themselves in an academic environment. For many people their illnesses began when they were in college or trade school. Returning to this environment is especially satisfying as people again begin to think in terms of a career for themselves (Sullivan, Nicolellis, Danley, & MacDonald-Wilson, 1993).

MENTORS.   The support of other people who are in recovery is a crucial aspect of the recovery process. Peer support provides a level and quality of support that cannot be reproduced by professional or even family support. The support of someone who is in recovery and rebuilding his or her life can be especially helpful. They can provide the hope that is so often lacking to people who are beginning their recovery journey.

MODELS.   The presence of people with psychiatric disability achieving in their chosen fields is another important aspect of recovery. The presence of people with psychiatric disability in all types of work and all levels of position is critically needed so that people with psychiatric disability can have models of people who are making it.

Reclaiming Hope

Deegan (1996) made perhaps the most useful distinction between optimism and hope. She describes optimism as like a cheerleader, there for a brief period of time, and then gone.

Hope is the belief in one's self; a willingness to "hang-in there" with one's self over the long haul—to pick oneself up again when one is knocked down and to persevere. Hope is helped by people in one's environment who have this same kind of hope for one. Hope is helped by an active and enduring presence of at least one other person.

Hope is an important aspect of recovery. Hopelessness is hard to deal with directly. Helping people to be helpful to themselves leads people to feel more hopeful. Knowing that they can act in their own interest, that they are not helpless, makes them feel more hopeful. So we deal with hopelessness by dealing with helplessness; by helping people to act in their own interest—initially by taking better care of themselves. And then, by gradually helping them to acquire the knowledge, skills, and support to build a life for themselves.

Hope for people with mental illnesses frequently comes from the caring and concern of another person, often a professional. Someone who has hope in one. Someone who gives one hope. Having someone believe in one helps one to believe in oneself.

Hope motivates. It makes one want to do what one should do. Hope transcends the illness. It has to do with the person, and how he or she feels about him or herself.

Restoring hope, or rejoining the human stream, is a risky journey of the heart for a person who has withdrawn and given up hope to protect him or herself (Deegan, 1996). It should not be surprising that a person can be quite angry at professional efforts to help, can distrust the professional, or seem to sabotage our efforts at restoring hope. Giving up the learned solution and safety of hopelessness for the risk of trusting and building a life can be asking a lot. Professionals need to understand what they are asking people to do. While people with psychiatric disability deeply want to re-enter the human stream, they are also deeply aware of the potential for additional hurt and trauma (Deegan, 1996).

MEDICATION. Medication is an important aspect of recovery and reclaiming hope for many people with psychiatric disability (Francell, 1994; Sullivan, 1994). While many people struggle with medication because of its negative side-effects and the profound meanings attached to medication, it can be an important resource in the recovery process and in the reclaiming of hope.

CONCLUSION

We have raised and responded to four basic questions about recovery. Because we are still uncovering this important process we need to acknowledge with sincere humility that there is still a long way to go and much to learn. But what we have learned is that people grow emotionally, physically, and intellectually as part of this process we call recovery. They grow emotionally through enhanced self-esteem, self-efficacy, self-respect, meaningful connections to others, meaningful work, a sense of hope, and personal empowerment. They grow physically through increased fitness, improved nutrition, and better health care. They grow intellectually through a better understanding of their disability, effective coping mechanisms, and the development and implementation of personal goals. It is through our connections with people who are experiencing mental illnesses that we will continue to learn and to grow in our knowledge about recovery.

REFERENCES

Anthony, W. A. (1993). Recovery from mental illness: The guiding vision of the mental health service system in the 1990's. *Innovations and Research, 2*(3), 17–24.

Bleuler, E. (1950). *Dementia praecox or the group of schizophrenias* (J. Zinkin, Trans.). New York, NY: International Universities Press.

Davidson, L., & Stayner, D. (1997). Loss, loneliness, and the desire for love: Perspectives on the social lives of people with schizophrenia. *Psychiatric Rehabilitation Journal, 20*(3), 3–12.

Davidson, L., Stayner, D., & Haglund, K. E. (1998). *Phenomenological perspectives on the social functioning of people with schizophrenia.* In K. T. Mueser & N. Tarrier (Eds.), *Handbook of social functioning in schizophrenia.* Boston, MA: Allyn & Bacon.

Davidson, L., & Strauss, J. S. (1992). Sense of self in recovery from severe mental illness. *British Journal of Medical Psychology, 65*, 131–145.

Deegan, P. (1988). Recovery: The lived experience of rehabilitation. *Psychosocial Rehabilitation Journal, 11*(4), 11–19.

Deegan, P. (1995). *Recovery from psychiatric disability.* Presentation at AMI of Massachusetts Curriculum and Training Committee Conference, Boston State House, Boston, MA.

Deegan, P. (1996). Recovery as a journey of the heart. *Psychiatric Rehabilitation Journal, 19*(3), 91–98.

DeSisto, M. J. et al. (1995). The Maine and Vermont three-decade studies of serious mental Illness I. Matched comparison of cross-sectional outcome. *British Journal of Psychiatry, 167*, 331–338.

Estroff, S. E. (1989). Self, identity, and subjective experiences of schizophrenia: In search of the subject. *Schizophrenia Bulletin, 15*(2), 189–196.

Francell, Jr., E. G. (1994). Medication: The foundation of recovery. *Innovations and Research, 3*(4), 31–40.

Frese, F. (1993). Twelve aspects of coping skills for people with serious and persistent mental illness. *Innovations and Research, 2*(3), 39–46.

Gartner, A. J., & Reissman, F. (1982). Self-help and mental health. *Hospital and Community Psychiatry, 33*(8), 631–635.

Harding, C. M. (1986). Speculations on the measurement of recovery from severe psychiatric disorder and the human condition. *Psychiatric Journal of the University of Ottawa, 11*(4), 19–204.

Harding, C. M. (1989). Long-term follow-up studies of schizophrenia: Recent findings and surprising implications. *Yale Psychiatric Quarterly, 11*(3), 3–5.

Harding, C. M., & Keller, A. B. (1998). Long-term outcome of social functioning. In K. T. Mueser & N. Tarrrier (Eds.), *Handbook of social functioning in schizophrenia.* Boston, MA: Allyn & Bacon.

Harding, C. M., Strauss, J. S., Hafez, H., & Liberman, P. (1987). Work and mental illness. I. Toward an integration of the rehabilitation process. *Journal of Nervous and Mental Disease, 175*(6), 317–327.

Harding, C. M., & Zahniser, J. H. (1994). Empirical correction of seven myths about schizophrenia with implications for treatment. *Acta Psychiatrica Scandinavica, 90*(Suppl. 384), 140–146.

Harding, C. M., Zubin, J., & Strauss, J. S. (1987). Chronicity in schizophrenia: Fact, partial fact, or artifact. *Hospital and Community Psychiatry, 38*(5), 477–486.

Harding, C. M., Zubin, J., & Strauss, J. S. (1992). Chronicity in schizophrenia: Revisited. *British Journal of Psychiatry, 161*(Suppl. 18), 27–37.

Huber, G., Gross, G., Schuttler, R., & Linz, M. (1980). Longitudinal studies of schizophrenic patients. *Schizophrenia Bulletin, 6*, 592–605.

Killilea, M. (1976). Mutual help organizations: Interpretations in the literature. In G. Kapplan & M. Killilea (Eds.), *Support systems and mutual help.* New York, NY: Grune & Stratton.

Kirsh, B. (2000). Work, workers, and workplaces: A qualitative analysis of narratives of mental health consumers. *Journal of Rehabilitation, October/November/December*, 24–30.

Kraeplin, E. (1902). *Dementia praecox, in clinical psychiatry: A textbook for students and physicians* (6th ed.). New York, NY: Macmillan.

Mack, J. E. (1994). Power, powerlessness, and empowerment in psychotherapy. *Psychiatry, 57*, 178–198.

Minkoff, K. (1987). Resistance of mental health professionals to working with the chronic mentally ill. In A.T. Meyerson (Ed.), *Barriers to treating the chronic mentally ill.* San Francisco, CA: Jossey–Bass.

Rogers, J. (1995). Work is key to recovery. *Psychosocial Rehabilitation Journal, 18*(4), 5–10.

Skrinar, G. S., Hutchinson, D. S., & Williams, N. (1992). Exercise: An adjunct therapy for persons with psychiatric disabilities. *Medical Science and Sports Exercise, 24*(5) (Suppl. 536).

Strauss, J. S. (1992). The person—key to understanding mental illness: Towards a new dynamic psychiatry, III. *British Journal of Psychiatry, 161*(Suppl. 18), 19–26.

Sullivan, W. P. (1994). A long and winding road: The process of recovery from severe mental illness. *Innovations and Research, 3*(3), 11–19.

Sullivan, A., Nicolellis, D. L., Danley, K. S., & MacDonald-Wilson, K. (1993). Choose-get-keep: A psychiatric rehabilitation approach to supported education. *Psychosocial Rehabilitation Journal, 17*(1), 55–68.

CHAPTER 5

Business and Legal Conditions Supporting the Employment of Individuals with Disabilities

ROBERT ERLANDSON

The conundrum: Today's social, political, business, and technological environments support the employment of individuals with various types of disabilities and yet the employment rate of individuals with disabilities remains dismally low. Seventy-five percent of working-age people with disabilities who want to work are unemployed (U.S. Department of Labor, 1999). One can speculate as to the reasons for this high unemployment rate. However, any positive initiatives that might follow such speculation will require a deeper understanding of the social, political, business, and technological environments within which we all function.

The health of an economy determines the overall need for workers. Today's global market place has created the need for businesses to be more cost-effective and provide higher quality products and services, with greater variety than ever before (Crow, 1989; Deming, 1982; U.S. Department of Labor, 1999). Dominant forces emerging from these global pressures are the quality assurance, quality control, and *kaizen* (continuous improvement) initiatives exemplified by ISO 9000 and QS 9000 quality standards and certification processes. Superimposed on these fundamental market dynamics are worker demographics and a collection of laws, rules, and regulations that govern employment practices. The positive effects of worker demographics, *kaizen* techniques, legislation, and technological advances can all be discounted if public opinion and perceptions, including those of the vocational rehabilitation and job placement specialists, see no opportunities or potential. The purpose of this chapter, and the next, is to expand the reader's vision of what is possible with respect to job creation, performance improvement, employment opportunities, and job retention for individuals with disabilities. This chapter will discuss social, political, business, and technological environments and how they combine to support the employment of individuals with disabilities through the use of accessible design techniques.

ROBERT ERLANDSON • Wayne State University College of Engineering, Detroit, Michigan.

WORKER DEMOGRAPHICS

The U.S. Department of Labor has recently published a major study of trends and challenges for work in the 21st century (U.S. Department of Labor, 1999). The study projects the U.S. population to grow by 50% in the next 50 years. As our population grows, it also becomes more diverse. Immigration will account for about two thirds of this expected growth. This large influx of immigrant workers presents challenges with respect to training, literacy, and communications in the workplace.

America's workforce is also aging. The Ford Motor Company conducted a study that found that its North American workforce has an average age of 47 (Jimmeerson, Jacobs, & Fischer, 1993). The American workforce has a growing number of individuals who are disabled and who are living longer with more severely disabling conditions (U.S. Department of Labor, 1999). Ergonomic experts at Ford Motor Company have estimated that about 60% of its North American workforce is working under some form of medical restriction(Jimmeerson et al., 1993).

These factors present a very complex situation: an aging workforce, a workforce with growing problems in literacy and communication skills, coupled with severe global competitive economic pressures. In many respects, the existing and projected workforce is drawing closer in terms of physical abilities, sensory/motor skills, and reading/communication skills to patterns that have been traditionally associated with persons who have cognitive disabilities.

Therefore, from several perspectives, business and vocational rehabilitation service concerns have considerable overlap. It is in the best interest of both groups to collaborate on cost-effective procedures to address mutual concerns.

INDUSTRY TRENDS

Lean Production

American industry is moving closer to what is called *lean production* (Womack, Jones, & Roos, 1990). This evolution has profound implications for individuals with disabilities. Lean production systems will be discussed in comparison with two other productions systems: *craft production* and *mass production*. Craft production is exemplified by the use of highly skilled workers using relatively simple, but flexible tools to make high quality, customized products one item at a time (Womack et al., 1990). This is an expensive method of production and does not support high volume production. These shortcomings along with increased consumer demand and technological advances such as steam power and electricity led, at the beginning of the 20th century, to mass production as an alternative.

Mass production is exemplified by the use of narrowly skilled professionals designing products made by unskilled or semi-skilled workers using expensive single-purpose machines (Womack et al., 1990). These machines produce a high volume of standardized products. With mass production the consumer gets a narrow choice of products, but at relatively low prices (Womack et al., 1990).

In contrast, the lean producer is exemplified by the use of teams of multi-skilled workers at all levels of the organization (Womack et al., 1990). The workers use flexible, increasingly automated machines to produce a large variety of products at relatively high volumes. The intent is to combine the advantages of craft and mass production while avoiding

**TABLE 5-1. Characteristics of Craft, Mass, and Lean Production
(Summarized from Womack et al., 1990)**

	Craft production	Mass production	Lean production
Worker	Highly skilled, with an apprenticeship	Interchangeable, largely unskilled	Problem-solver, team member, cross-trained, rotation of jobs
Organization	Decentralized	Centralized	Between craft and mass
Tool	General purpose machine tools	Specialized tools	Agile, flexible
Production	Low volume, customized, high quality products, low inventory	Sequenced, high volume, standardized products, acceptable level of defects, high inventory	Higher than mass, lower costs than mass, higher quality than mass—approaching craft, more variety than mass or craft

their respective disadvantages, which include high costs of the former and production rigidity of the latter (Womack et al., 1990). From the employee perspective, the trends are toward more job rotation, more cross-training, fewer job classifications, more team work. Table 5-1 summarizes some of the characteristics of craft, mass, and lean production systems.

From a production perspective the trends are toward lower costs, more variety, faster delivery times, and higher quality. Lean production uses less of everything when compared with mass production, space, tools, and human effort. There is a difference in the production objectives of mass and lean producers. According to Womack et al. (1990), "mass producers set a limited goal for themselves—'good enough,' which translates into an acceptable number of defects, a maximum acceptable level of inventories, a narrow range of standardized products." On the other hand, lean producers "set their sights explicitly on perfection: continually declining costs, zero defects, zero inventories, and endless product variety" (Imai, 1997; Womack et al., 1990). These objectives are an ideal, but they are at the heart of quality improvement processes, such as QS 9000 (Hoyle, 1997) and ISO 9000 (Randal, 1995).

ISO 9000 and QS 9000

Without the establishment of the ISO and QS quality standards and certification processes there would not be as much attention on the implementation of quality assurance and quality control procedures in American industry. It is the quality control tools and techniques that embody accessible design principles and it is the application of these accessible design principles that lead to improved job performance and job creation for individuals with disabilities.

The International Organization for Standardization (ISO) is a Geneva-based worldwide federation, founded in 1946 to promote the development of international standards for world trade. International standards are prepared through Technical Committees (Randal, 1995). The U.S. representative to ISO is the American National Standards Institute (ANSI).

ISO 9000 is a collection of quality standards written to be widely applicable to a wide range of industries and products. The collection is organized into models and guidelines. The models define specific minimum requirements for external suppliers and the guidelines are specified for development of internal quality systems (Randal, 1995). In order to ensure the uniform application of these standards, a rigorous certification process was implemented.

Initially, many American companies did not believe there were any advantages to ISO 9000 certification. That was the case until they realized that to trade with Europe, they had to demonstrate compliance with ISO 9000 standards. The automotive industry quickly realized that ISO 9000 compliance was necessary and soon other industries followed suit. ISO 9000 covers a wide range of products and services (Randal, 1995). Many members of the service sector have published their own interpretative guides. Since the launch of ISO 9000 over 95,000 certificates have been awarded (Hoyle, 1997).

In 1992 the Ford Motor Company, Chrysler, and General Motors moved to harmonize their supplier system by the creation of QS 9000 quality standards. This initiative was in response to the ISO movement, but also as part of a conscious movement toward a leaner production model (Hoyle, 1997). QS 9000 moves more toward a total quality management (TQM) standard than ISO 9001 (Hoyle, 1997). The requirements for simultaneous engineering, continuous improvement (covering quality, delivery, and price), zero defects, business plans, failure mode analysis, and many more important aspects make QS 9000 a much more stringent standard than ISO 9000 (Hoyle, 1997).

The implications for job creation, employment, and retention of individuals with disabilities are significant. The ISO and QS standards require the implementation of quality assurance and quality control procedures, such as *kaizen* or continuous improvement techniques. These techniques embody accessible design principles.

ACCESSIBLE DESIGN

Accessible design means to design processes, products, and services so that as many people, with as broad a spectrum of abilities as possible, can access and use the processes, products, or services. The cost of implementing accessible design features is a constraint. Hence, there is a dynamic tension between the objective of increasing accessibility through the use of accessible design techniques and the cost of implementing such techniques.

The movement towards leaner production and service systems and the advent of ISO and QS quality standards requirements have changed the cost–benefit relationship for the utilization of accessible design techniques through the implementation of quality control procedures. It is now cost-effective to more consciously focus on accessibility concerns while concurrently addressing quality control issues. An interesting win–win scenario is feasible. One can introduce quality control procedures in compliance with QS and ISO requirements, receiving the business benefits of improved quality and lower costs, while concurrently improving the job performance and creating jobs for individuals with disabilities. Thus, accessible design is not only about creating a place in industry for people with disabilities, it is about improving the performance of able-bodied workers as well.

Kaizen—Continuous Improvement

As an accessible design tool, quality control procedures can be considered part of a larger collection of continuous improvement tools and techniques. *Kaizen*, a Japanese term meaning "continuous improvement" (Imai, 1986), has come to signify a collection of productivity enhancement techniques that include quality control procedures. Research has shown that the application of *kaizen* techniques tends to reduce both the physical and cognitive demands of tasks (Erlandson, Noblet, & Phelps, 1998; Erlandson & Phelps, 1995).

Kaizen applications, then, hold the potential of a win–win scenario: while providing quality and economic benefits to businesses, they can also eliminate or remove job-related barriers for individuals with disabilities.

Kaizen procedures were not originally developed to create options for individuals with disabilities; rather, they were developed by industry to make business more competitive and cost-effective in today's world market economy. The fact that these design approaches might concurrently be cost-effective and be reasonable job accommodations for individuals with disabilities is not generally recognized.

Chapter 19 deals explicitly with the applications of *kaizen* techniques, the accessible design principles employed, and the resultant impact on worker productivity and job creation.

LEGAL IMPERATIVES

In addition to OSHA ergonomic standards (Occupational Safety and Health Administration, U.S. Department of Labor), four laws exist that, together, are having a dramatic impact on worksite and job accessibility. The first is the Architectural Barriers Act of 1968 (ABA), as amended, "which requires buildings or other facilities financed with certain Federal funds to be accessible to persons with disabilities" (Access Board, 1998). This law laid the groundwork for the Americans with Disabilities Act of 1990 (ADA), which prohibits discrimination against the employment of individuals with disabilities because of their disability (Access Board, 1999). The Workforce Investment Act of 1998, with amendments to the Rehabilitation Act of 1973, particularly Section 508, requires electronic and information technology purchased by the Federal government to be accessible (Advisory Board, 1999). Finally, the Telecommunications Act of 1996 requires the accessibility of telecommunications and customer premises equipment (Federal Communications Commission, 1999b).

OSHA, U.S. Department of Labor

OSHA, which is part of the U.S. Department of Labor, is charged with the responsibility of overseeing the health and safety of American workers. Recently, OSHA published its proposed ergonomics program standards to address work-related musculoskeletal disorders (MSDs) (OSHA, 1999). Work-related MSDs are currently the leading cause of lost-workday injuries and workers' compensation costs (OSHA, 1999). The ergonomic standards are intended to reduce worker exposure to ergonomic risk factors.

The OSHA standards define *ergonomics* as the science of fitting jobs to people (OSHA, 1999). Ergonomists have an extensive collection of tools and techniques for identifying ergonomic risk factors and for creating ergonomically sound work environments. Ergonomic risk factors include forceful exertions, dynamic motions, repetition, awkward postures, static postures, contact stress, vibration, and excessive temperatures (hot or cold) (OSHA, 1999). *Engineering controls* and *administrative controls* are two broad categories of intervention techniques. The term "engineering controls," as applied to the elimination or reduction of work-related MSD hazards, includes changing, modifying, or redesigning workstations, tools, facilities, equipment, materials, and processes (OSHA, 1999). The engineering controls should impact ergonomic risk factors. Administrative controls can be used to reduce the magnitude, frequency, or duration of exposure to ergonomic risk factors (OSHA, 1999).

Administrative controls include employee rotation, job task enlargement, alternative tasks, and employer-authorized changes in workplace (OSHA, 1999).

At this time it is not clear what elements of the proposed OSHA standards will be implemented. Whatever the fate of these standards, the fundamental industrial engineering ergonomic approach to MSDs and worker safety will persist. This perspective differs from the traditional approach of vocational rehabilitation and job placement specialists who typically attempt to fit the person with a disability to the job. Such retrofitting includes the use of assistive technology, customized jigs, intensive on-the-job training, and job coaches (Gold, 1972; Hagner, Rogan, & Murphy, 1992). The newly evolving OSHA standards create an opportunity for vocational rehabilitation and job placement specialists to work with businesses on OSHA-identified problems to redesign jobs using accessible design principles. Such a job redesign process has the potential not only to create more ergonomically sound work environments for able-bodied workers, but also to create positions for people with disabilities that, before the redesign, may have been unavailable.

OSHA's proposed standards provide both an opportunity and a challenge. Reducing the ergonomic demands of jobs will make the jobs more accessible. However, administrative controls such as job rotation, task enlargement, and alternative tasks present challenges to the education, training, and employment of individuals with cognitive impairments. However, as will be discussed in Chapter 19, *kaizen* techniques have the potential to facilitate on-the-job training and reduce worker errors by creating job processes that provide considerable feedback to the workers (Erlandson & Sant, 1998; Erlandson et al., 1998).

The powerful combination of OSHA, ISO, and QS quality standards are pushing worldwide industries toward more lean operations. The common ground that is pushing these initiatives in the same direction is that all of them embody the principles of accessible design. The application of accessible design principles, regardless of the driving force (OSHA, ISO, QS) creates jobs that are more accessible to individuals with a wider range of abilities. This is a secondary effect not targeted by the original driving forces, but one rehabilitation job placement professionals need to be aware of in order to better serve their clients.

The ABA and ADA

The ABA (Access Board, 1998) brought to national attention a growing pressure to recognize and address the needs of individuals with disabilities. This law in particular reflects the moral and ethical drives present in society at that time, as it mandated that Federal buildings and facilities be accessible to individuals with disabilities. This physical accessibility made possible social, educational, and economic accessibility to the affairs conducted within these buildings and facilities. The ABA laid the ground work for the ADA.

The ADA covers a number of accessibility issues (Access Board, 1999). With respect to employment, it prohibits employment discrimination against qualified individuals who have a disability. The ADA defines "a qualified individual with a disability" as one able to meet legitimate skill, experience, education, or other requirements of employment and who can perform the "essential functions" of the job with or without a reasonable accommodation (National Institute on Disability and Rehabilitation Research, 1992). The law goes on to define "a reasonable accommodation" as any modification or adjustment to a job or the work environment that will enable a qualified applicant or employee with a disability to perform the essential functions of the job (National Institute on Disability and Rehabilitation Research, 1992).

A reasonable accommodation might be assistive technology and the associated assistive technology service. An *assistive technology device* is defined as "any item, piece of equipment, or product system ... that is used to increase, maintain, or improve functional capabilities of individuals with disabilities" (National Institute on Disability and Rehabilitation Research, 1992). An *assistive technology service* is defined as "any service that directly assists an individual with a disability in the selection, acquisition, or use of an assistive technology device" (National Institute on Disability and Rehabilitation Research, 1992).

The application of accessible design principles through quality control strategies or OSHA engineering control strategies typically redefines the essential functions of a job and reduces the physical and cognitive demands of the job. In this scenario, the ADA provides a legal imperative for employment as the essential functions of jobs are redefined. However, vocational rehabilitation or job placement specialists must be aware of these trends to take full advantage of the potentials they offer.

Technology-Related Legislation

The Workforce Investment Act of 1998 contains amendments to the Rehabilitation Act of 1973. The changes to Section 508 of the 1998 amendments specify accessibility requirements for Federal departments and agencies that use electronic and information technology (Advisory Board, 1999). Section 508 defines electronic and information technology (E&IT) as electronic technology that is used in carrying out information activities, involving any form of information (Advisory Board, 1999).

It is understood that E&IT addresses a broader spectrum than information technology alone and includes the full breadth of the information environment of the future (Advisory Board, 1999). The intent of Section 508 is to ensure that government employees and the public have access to the government's information environment as it evolves. As specified, information activities include, but are not limited to, "the creation, translation, duplication, serving, acquisition, manipulation, storage, management, movement, control, display, switching, interchange, transmission, or reception of data or information" (Advisory Board, 1999). Furthermore, the evolving regulations would require the documentation (instructions, service, etc.) associated with E&IT also be accessible and useable. Lastly, the E&IT should not interfere with the assistive technology used daily by people with disabilities (Advisory Board, 1999).

The Telecommunication Act of 1996, Section 255, mandates that all telecommunications products and services be accessible and usable by persons with disabilities, to the extent that it is readily achievable (Federal Communications Commission, 1999b). This law introduces the requirement of usability as well as accessibility and requires the use of accessible design principles in the design of the products and services and the inclusion of people with disabilities on product development activities, such as inclusion on focus groups and product trials (Federal Communications Commission, 1999a, 1999b).

While Section 508 deals explicitly with Federal departments and agencies, it is reasonable to assume that provisions of the law will eventually be expanded to include broader segments of society. Traditionally laws and regulations start with Federal government requirements for Federal property, products, and services, and evolve to include broader segments of society. For example, the ABA of 1968 evolved to the ADA of 1990, the Telecommunication Act of 1996 evolved from the ADA and Rehabilitation Act of 1973. Hence, one can realistically anticipate that the mandates of Section 508 will follow a similar path. Furthermore, the Federal government is such a large customer that it makes business sense to offer enhancements made for the Federal government to the general public.

The mandates and guidelines discussed above, which focus on the accessibility and usability of telecommunication products and services as well as E&IT and facilities, mean that jobs that utilize such technologies are becoming more accessible. In turn, the essential functions of jobs that involve the affected technologies need to be re-examined and possibly redefined. This redefinition of essential functions could lead to more job opportunities for individuals with disabilities.

IMPLICATIONS FOR INDIVIDUALS WITH DISABILITIES

A conundrum was originally presented: Today's social, political, business, and technological environments support the employment of individuals with various types of disabilities and yet the employment rate of individuals with disabilities remains dismally low. Heightened awareness and increased knowledge of the potential win–win scenario offered by the advance of QS and ISO quality requirements, OSHA ergonomic standards, industry's movement toward leaner operations, worker demographics, and a host of legal mandates, rules, and regulations provide options and insights as to how one might approach this conundrum.

Quality tools, *kaizen* tools, and the OSHA engineering controls all employ accessible design principles in their implementation. Application of these principles concurrently bring about the quality, cost, and performance improvements industry is seeking and, because they reduce the physical and cognitive demands of the jobs, they improve the job performance and create job opportunities for individuals with physical and cognitive disabilities. While the former results are what industry is explicitly seeking, the later results are not generally recognized.

Industry and business have their own agendas. It is the vocational rehabilitation and job placement professionals' responsibility to recognize the potentials being presented and take advantage of them to benefit both their clients and employers. This is difficult because potential employers typically see the vocational and job placement professionals as only interested in placing their clients and not really interested the employers' business needs. This perception of placement professionals does not leave them with a great deal of credibility in the eyes of the employers when it comes to business affairs.

An understanding of the employer's business and the environment within which the business operates is essential to establishing credibility. Understanding the potential win–win scenarios offered by enhancing the current environment through the application of accessible design and being able to communicate the benefits of such an enhancement to an employer is essential for successful placement. However, in the end, it is the individual's performance on the job that determines the prospects of his/her employment. Worker productivity is the key, and this is the topic of Chapter 19.

As people with mental health concerns increasingly enter the workforce, accessible design will emerge as an important interdisciplinary approach to rehabilitation practice. Job design and job carving currently stand as important approaches to supporting the employment of people with disabilities in the workplace. Accessible design holds promise as a strategy to tailoring work to specific cognitive requirements for people with mental health challenges.

ACKNOWLEDGMENTS.   The work presented was supported by grants from the National Science Foundation (BSE-9707720 and DUE-9972403), and contracts from the Region IV Assistive Technology Consortium. I would also like to acknowledge the editorial support provided by Ms. Kristine Bradow.

REFERENCES

Access Board (1998). *Laws concerning the Access Board.* Washington, DC: Author.

Access Board (1999). *Americans with Disabilities Act accessibility requirements.* Washington, DC: Author.

Advisory Board (1999). *Final report of the EITAAC.* Washington, DC: Author.

Crow, K. A. (1989). *Design for manufacturability: Its role in world class manufacturing.* Palos Verdes Estates, CA: Defense Resource Management Associates.

Deming, W. E. (1982). *Out of crisis* (15th ed.). Cambridge, MA: Massachusetts Institute of Technology.

Erlandson, R. F., & Phelps, J. A. (1995, June 11–16). *Simplification of essential functions using design for assembly techniques.* Paper presented at the RESNA '95 Annual Conference, Vancouver, BC.

Erlandson, R. F., Noblet, M. J., & Phelps, J. A. (1998). Impact of Poka-Yoke device on job performance of individuals with cognitive impairments. *IEEE Transactions on Rehabilitation Engineering, 6*(3), 269–276.

Erlandson, R. F., & Sant, D. (1998). Poka-Yoke process controller designed for individuals with cognitive impairments. *Assistive Technology 10,* 102–112.

Federal Communications Commission (1999a, July 14). *Implementation of Sections 255 and 251(a)(2) of the Communications Act of 1994, as enacted by the Telecommunications Act of 1996* (WT Docket No. 96-198). Washington, DC: Author.

Federal Communications Commission (1999b, November 19). Access to telecommunications service, telecommunications equipment and customer premises equipment by persons with disabilities. *Federal Register, 64*(223), 63235–63258.

Gold, M. (1972). Stimulus factors in skill training of the retarded on a complex assembly task: Acquisition, transfer, and retention. *American Journal of Mental Deficiency, 76,* 517–526.

Hagner, D., Rogan, P., & Murphy, S. (1992, January/February/March). Facilitating natural supports in the workplace: Strategies for support consultants. *Journal of Rehabilitation,* 29–34.

Hoyle, D. (1997). *QS 9000 quality systems handbook.* Newton, MA: Butterworth-Heinemann.

Imai, M. (1986). *Kaizen* (1st ed.). New York, NY: McGraw-Hill.

Imai, M. (1997). *Gemba Kaizen* (1st ed.). New York, NY: McGraw-Hill.

Jimmeerson, G. D., Jacobs, C. J., & Fischer, D. S. (1993). *Design for ergonomics in manufacturing* (White Paper). Ann Arbor, MI: National Center for Manufacturing Sciences.

National Institute on Disability and Rehabilitation Research (1992). *ADA; Q&A—The Americans with Disabilities Act: Questions and answers.* Washington, DC: U.S. Department of Justice Civil Rights Division, U.S. Equal Employment Opportunity Commission.

Occupational Safety and Health Administration (1999). Ergonomics program: Proposed rule. *Federal Register, 64*(225), 65768–66078.

Randal, R. C. (1995). *Randall's practical guide to ISO 9000: Implementation, registration, and beyond.* Reading, MA: Addison-Wesley.

U.S. Department of Labor (1999, December 12). *Futurework: Trends and challenges for work in the 21st century.* Available: www.dol.gov/dol/asp.public/futurework/report.htm

Womack, J. P., Jones, D. T., & Roos, D. (1990). *The machine that changed the world.* New York, NY: Harper–Collins.

CHAPTER 6

Reasonable Job Accommodations for People with Psychiatric Disabilities

JERRY OLSHESKI AND RICHARD SCHELAT

Work continues to be the single characteristic used most often to define a person's citizenship, resources, and community participation (Carling, 1994; Mancuso, 1990). It provides the framework for a person's identity, self-esteem, daily schedule, socioeconomic status, and participation as a consumer in the community. Work also provides social contacts and a sense of belonging in the community. But people with psychiatric disabilities have rates of unemployment as high as 85% (Anthony, Kennard, O'Brien, & Forbes, 1989. Research findings also suggest there is no direct or simple relationship between a psychiatric diagnosis and a person's specific functioning deficits (Jordan et al., 1996) or a person's ability to work. Anthony et al., 1989; Gordon, Eisler, Gutman, & Gordon, 1991). So other factors, in addition to a person's specific psychiatric disability, must contribute toward high unemployment rates for people with psychiatric disabilities.

The stigma created by attitudinal barriers affects all people with disabilities, but the general public has had a long-standing and significant discomfort with people who have psychiatric disabilities (Asch, 1984; Goffman, 1963; Link, Cullen, Mirotzink, & Streuning, 1992; Noe, 1997; U.S. Congress, 1994). Not surprisingly, stigma against people with psychiatric disabilities may be the most poignant in the world of work. Many employers continue to engage in behaviors and practices in the hiring process that devalue and discriminate against workers with psychiatric disabilities (Roberts, 1995).

Although many employers have implemented disability management programs designed to prevent and accommodate physical disabilities in the workplace, similar success has not been realized in the realm of psychiatric impairments (Akabas, Gates, & Galvin, 1992; Olsheski & Breslin, 1996). Employers only now are becoming aware of the work disruptions, lost time, and increased costs associated with emotional impairments among their employees.

JERRY OLSHESKI • Department of Counseling and Higher Education, Ohio University, Athens, Ohio.
RICHARD SCHELAT • Ohio Bureau of Vocational Rehabilitation, Athens, Ohio.

Many employers find it difficult to make accommodations for employees with psychiatric disabilities. In a recent survey of 375 employers conducted by Watson Wyatt and the Washington Business Group on Health, 58% of the respondents indicated that mental health issues are a rising concern in non-occupational disability, and one third of the respondents expressed great difficulty in managing mental illness in the workplace (Watson Wyatt Worldwide, 1997). Another survey of medical and personnel directors of *Fortune* 1000 firms indicated that more than 70% of respondents rated mental health problems as fairly to very pervasive in the workplace (Warshaw, 1990).

Information from a variety of sources indicates that mental health disorders have a significant vocational and economic impact in our society. It has been estimated that over half of the 550 million lost work days due to absenteeism each year in American industry are in some ways related to psychological stress (Elkin & Rosch, 1990). Data reported by the National Institute of Occupational Safety and Health (NIOSH) indicated that the number of workers' compensation claims resulting from mental disorders increased from 1980 to 1990, and approximately one in 10 workers suffers from depression, costing society nearly $27 billion annually (Millar, 1992). Social Security Administration data show that social security awards for mental disorders are now more common than any other type of disability, and that workers below the age of 50 experience as much as two to four times the disability for mental disorders than for musculoskeletal or circulatory problems (Sauter, 1992).

In light of these findings, this chapter provides information that rehabilitation professionals and employers may find useful in hiring, accommodating, and retaining individuals with psychiatric disabilities.

Individuals who have severe psychiatric disabilities are legally protected from discrimination in the world of work. The next section provides an overview of two key pieces of Federal legislation that prohibit discrimination and mandate reasonable accommodations for people with disabilities in the world of work: the Rehabilitation Act of 1973; and the Americans with Disabilities Act (ADA).

FEDERAL LEGISLATIVE REMEDIES TO DISCRIMINATION

The Rehabilitation Act of 1973

The Rehabilitation Act of 1973 was the first Federal legislation designed to prohibit discriminatory practices against "otherwise qualified handicapped individuals" in both the public and private sectors (Wright, 1980). The law defined handicapped individuals as persons who have a physical or mental impairment that substantially limits one or more major life activity; or have a record of such impairment; or are regarded by others as being handicapped.

The second prong of the definition was included to rule out the possibility of people being discriminated against because of past impairments that may not affect a current situation. The third prong of the definition was included to rule out the impact of others' attitudes and prejudices toward a disability even without evidence that the disability currently impacts a major life activity. The scope of the law was considered to be broad at the time.

The 1973 Act covered all employers or programs receiving funds from the Federal government, and it was directed toward program accessibility, services, and employment opportunities (Wright, 1980). Specifically, Section 504 prohibited discriminatory employer practices in hiring, placement, employee classification, or advancement. This section also required employers to make reasonable accommodations for the limitations of an otherwise qualified handicapped individual unless the employer could demonstrate that to do so would constitute an undue hardship for the employer. In addition, pre-employment medical exams as well as disclosure of a handicap as a condition of employment were prohibited.

Under the Rehabilitation Act, the employee could establish a prima facie case of employment discrimination by demonstrating four criteria: the person was an individual with a handicap; the person was qualified for a job but for the disability; the person was denied the job, promotion, or raise for which the person applied; and the person was excluded solely because of the disability (Pollett, 1995). After the person or plaintiff established a prima facie case, the burden shifted to the employer to demonstrate that either the person was not otherwise qualified or that any possible accommodation would cause the employer undue hardship.

Bowe (1990) reported that the real impact of the Rehabilitation Act has been limited, and that the law had little effect on employment of people with disabilities. The Rehabilitation Act applied to only 10% of American employers, and only 200,000 of the 34 million people entering the workforce since 1970 reported having disabilities, suggesting little change in employment practices. These facts set the stage for increased pressure to correct the disparities in employment rights for people with disabilities and led to the passage of the ADA.

The Americans with Disabilities Act (ADA)

The ADA was signed into law by President George Bush on July 26, 1990, with bipartisan support, and it was described as "a watershed in the history of disability rights" (U.S. Congress, 1994, p. 1) and "the most significant piece of civil rights legislation since the passage of the 1964 Civil Right Act" (O'Keeffe, 1994, p. 1). The ADA complements and extends the benefits of the Rehabilitation Act of 1973, and in no way reduces the scope, coverage, or standards applied under the Rehabilitation Act of 1973 (Turley & Beck, 1991). The ADA includes provisions that: apply to nearly all public and private entities; differentiate the concepts of disability and handicap; and include accessibility requirements in all aspects of public life activities.

A most notable change in the coverage of the ADA is that it covers all public and private employers with 15 or more employees, leaving far fewer employment situations untouched by the law. The wider scope of the law combined with increased media attention and education about the ADA is reflected in the rising number of complaints filed with the Equal Employment Opportunity Commission (EEOC). West (1996) reported that from July 26, 1992, to May 31, 1994, approximately 28,000 complaints were filed with the EEOC under Title I alone, of which only 34% were closed for no cause.

Although the ADA is broad in its scope, the information contained in this chapter focuses on the definitions, terms, and applications of Title I which prohibits discrimination against people with disabilities in all aspects of employment. Title I provides that no covered entity shall discriminate against a qualified individual with a disability because of the disability in regard to job application procedures, hiring, advancement, employee compensation, job training, and other privileges of employment. However, there are some psychiatric disabilities that are excluded from coverage under the ADA, including continued alcohol or drug abuse, use of illegal drugs, several types of sexual disorders, compulsive gambling, and kleptomania. In addition, people who pose what is called a "direct threat" to the health and safety of others are not covered under the ADA. Campbell (1994) cautioned that the "direct threat" aspect of the ADA regulations is most sensitive to stereotypical and prejudiced views of a person with a psychiatric disability and may be used to terminate rather than accommodate the employee. However, Parry (1993) reported court findings that require a direct connection between the person's actual behaviors and violence.

More recent EEOC guidelines about pre-employment questioning do allow employers to ask if the applicant or employee will need a reasonable accommodation if: (1) the employer reasonably believes a person will need a reasonable accommodation because of an obvious disability, or (2) the employer reasonably believes a person will need a reasonable accommodation after a person voluntarily discloses a hidden disability (Barlow, Hatch, & Murphy, 1995; Brady, 1996; Ravid, 1992).

As previously noted, the presence of a psychiatric disability, which may or may not be noticeable, does not equate with an inability to perform work or prevent a person from meeting the essential job functions. Reasonable accommodations can be very important for persons with psychiatric disabilities and can allow them the opportunity to continue to meet the essential functions of their current jobs or the essential functions of positions they are seeking.

Job accommodations are considered reasonable, however, only if they do not impose an "undue hardship" on the employer (Job Accommodation Network, 1991). Defining what constitutes an "undue hardship" may be more subjective than identifying the essential functions of a job, but it is still the concept that is used to differentiate between reasonable and unreasonable accommodations.

Parry (1993) reported that although the undue hardship regulations do not directly affect the rights of individuals with disabilities they do affect the analysis of what is considered reasonable. Unreasonable cost is often an employer's primary line of defense for not providing a requested accommodation. In those cases, employees would have the opportunity to contribute toward that expense or bring in personal or other resources such as vocational rehabilitation services to lower the cost into a range that would be reasonable for the employer. However, costs may not be the most immediate concern of employers when it comes to accommodating individuals having only psychiatric disabilities because extensive modifications to the physical work setting may not be necessary. When job accommodations for persons with psychiatric disabilities are needed, the employer's main concern related to "undue hardship" may well be the potential impact that the accommodation has on the ability of other workers to perform their job duties and the impact on the establishment's ability to conduct business. In order for the job accommodation process to be successful, the employer has to understand the impact of the person's mental functional limitations, not only in terms of performing the essential functions of the job, but also the potential impact that such limitations may have in disrupting the job performance of coworkers and business operations.

It is apparent that the ADA regulations are written in a way that allows considerable subjective interpretation. And it is not surprising that employers continue to be confused about what constitutes reasonable accommodations, especially for people with psychiatric disabilities (Milite, 1994). The ADA does provide parameters that relate to personal, job, and employer functions and capacities. Each of these three areas of function and capacity must be defined before applying ADA regulations. But people with psychiatric disabilities are likely to have functional limitations unique to their own condition, and the individuals with the disabilities may be the best people to ask about their strengths, weaknesses, and functional capacities (Mancuso, 1995).

The ADA also recognizes that a person's behavior or functional capacity is a product of the interaction between the person and the work environment (Hantula & Reilly, 1996). Individuals bring their own unique characteristics, behaviors, and "environment" to the interaction. Effective reasonable accommodations require an understanding of the interaction between the unique traits of the individual and the physical and mental requirements of the work environment. The next section addresses the reasonable accommodation process.

THE REASONABLE ACCOMMODATION PROCESS

Reasonable accommodations as mandated by the ADA cannot be implemented by unilateral actions of either the employer or the employee. Successful accommodations require the involvement of all key parties in the work environment. These other significant parties may include supervisors, coworkers, union officials, health care personnel, occupational and physical therapists, ergonomists, and rehabilitation professionals, among others, that may have a relationship to the person with a disability as well as the specific setting in which accommodations are needed (Blanck, Anderson, Wallach, & Tenney, 1994; Crist & Stoffel, 1992; Drake, McHugo, Becker, Anthony, & Clark, 1996; Mancuso, 1995; Olsheski & Breslin, 1996; Zuckerman, 1993).

Reasonable accommodations require an accurate assessment of the individual's functional capacities as well as an accurate evaluation of the job requirements and work environment (Breslin & Olsheski, 1996). Austin and Green (1998) concluded that reasonable accommodations for individuals with psychiatric disabilities should not be treated substantially different from those pertaining to physical disabilities. Both approaches require a functional understanding of the individual's capacities and the job requirements.

Psychosocial Job Analysis

In the accommodation of physical disabilities, job analysis methods have been fairly effective in quantifying the physical demands and environmental factors associated with specific jobs (Field & Field, 1998). Job analysis assessments for people with psychiatric disabilities also must include psychosocial information that describes the mental demands associated with the essential functions of the job.

According to Austin and Green (1998), the successful implementation of job accommodations for individuals with psychiatric disabilities requires answering a series of important questions: What are the essential duties? What particular duties are impeded by the conditions? Within those duties, what particular tasks pose difficulty? Are these impeded tasks related to the condition? How will the proposed accommodations compensate for deficiencies caused by the psychiatric condition(s)? Are alternative modes of accommodation feasible? What will be the impact of the accommodation in the person's work group? How will the accommodation best be integrated and still be confidential? (pp. 8, 9).

Answers to these questions require a synthesis of the job analysis and functional capacity information to identify the vocational impact of the person's limitations and to develop reasonable accommodation strategies. Employers can take a number of steps in the evaluation and implementation of job accommodations for people with psychiatric disabilities including using the *DSM-IV* to identify functional limitations of disorders, maintaining a relationship with a local mental health professional for possible consultation, developing profiles of more common psychiatric disabilities, describing the mental demands or requirements of jobs, and providing training to supervisors and managers (Austin & Green, 1998).

Useful information concerning the functional limitations of specific psychiatric disorders, the likely range of limitations, and typical job accommodations is now evolving (Fischler & Booth, 1999; Job Accommodation Network, 1991). These models rate the degree that the disorder impairs certain (mental) vocational abilities. Recommendations for job accommodations for each disorder are also provided. The impact of the disorder on cognition, pace, persistence, reliability, motivation, interpersonal functioning, honesty, stress tolerance, and other job-specific requirements is described in terms of their effect on such work performance abilities as understanding and memory, concentration, social interaction, and adaptation (Fischler & Booth, 1999).

Another valuable source of psychosocial job analysis information is the Occupational Information Network (ONET) developed by the U.S. Department of Labor (Peterson et al., 1997). The content model of ONET contains six domains of information, including worker characteristics, worker requirements, experience requirements, occupational requirements, occupation-specific requirements, and occupation characteristics.

Some of the information contained in the ONET model is directly related to the mental requirements of various occupations. For example, the "worker characteristics" domain describes the basic skills the worker needs in such areas as active listening and critical thinking to perform a specific job. Social skill requirements, also included in the "worker characteristics" domain, describes the level of social skills required of the worker to perform a particular occupation. Social skills include social perceptiveness, persuasion, and instructing. Additional information contained in the "worker characteristics" domain that is relevant to psychiatric disabilities is the descriptions of "work styles" that are required for certain jobs. Work styles include characteristics of the employee that influence typical performance as well as the individual's ongoing adaptation to and performance of work. For example, some jobs require an achievement-oriented work style which emphasizes such traits as effort, persistence, and initiative; other jobs may require an interpersonal-oriented work style which demands abilities related to cooperation and concern for others.

Information concerning work conditions is contained in the "occupational requirements" domain of ONET. Work conditions describe the physical, structural, and interpersonal environment in which a particular occupation is conducted (Isaacson & Brown, 2000). Employers and rehabilitation professionals can use ONET to help identify the vocational impact of an individual's psychiatric condition and to develop a strategy for making reasonable accommodations.

In summary, supervisors and other involved parties need to be educated about the individual's strengths, limitations, and the nature of accommodations. In making accommodations for physical disabilities an accurate understanding of the physical demands of the job and the individual's physical capacities are required. Likewise, reasonable accommodations for psychiatric disabilities require an accurate understanding of the mental demands of the job and the individual's psychological capacities. By understanding the capacities of the individual and the functional requirements of the job, accommodations may be implemented in a manner that does not adversely affect the performance of other employees or business operations.

Blanck et al. (1994) summarized the following guidelines for assessing reasonable accommodations: (1) get the facts regarding essential job functions and the capacities of the employee with a disability; (2) identify what specific disability-related limitations need accommodating; (3) assess the need for expertise and objective review; (4) assess costs and undue hardship; (5) engage in a problem-solving dialogue; (6) develop an accommodation plan; and (7) evaluate the accommodation plan.

The next section provides a review of the most common psychiatric disabilities that impact employment: affective disorders and personality disorders.

DIFFERENTIAL ACCOMMODATIONS BASED ON DIAGNOSTIC CONSIDERATION

Affective Disorders

Affective disorders are the most prevalent psychiatric disorders and therefore the most likely to be found in employees and new applicants for employment (Klerman, 1988; Regier, Narrow, & Rae, 1993; Seligman, 1990; Seligman & Moore, 1995). It is estimated that up to 30% of the population experiences depressive episodes and other affective disorders, but only a minority of those people seek professional attention for the disorder regardless of the intensity of the person's discomfort.

The severity of symptoms varies with each individual, and it is important to distinguish normal mood swings of sadness, frustration, or excitement from diagnosable affective disorders. The diagnosis of an affective disorder usually is made on the basis of the intensity and duration of normal emotions (Klerman, 1988). Although no single characteristic can be used to describe a person with a mood disorder, Gotlib and Colby (1987) and D. W. Sue, D. Sue, and S. Sue (1994) have described the following general emotional, behavioral, cognitive, and physiological characteristics that typically accompany people with mood disorders: *emotional*—anxiety, guilt, anger/hostility, irritability, social distress; *behavioral*—neglect of appearance, lethargy, slow motor movements, reduced activity levels; *cognitive*—difficulty with decision-making, reduced concentration, and distortion of the size of tasks; *physiological*—sleep disturbances with increased fatigue, and multiple somatic complaints.

Anxiety disorders have more pervasive effects for the individual that impact most every system in the body. Like mood disorders, they also present some of the following typical or general characteristics that are worthwhile noting (Gotlib & Colby, 1987; Sue et al., 1994): *emotional characteristics*—anxiety, social distress, possible panic, vigilance in scanning for potential feared objects or situations; *behavioral characteristics*—restlessness, general withdrawal, avoidance of feared activities; *cognitive characteristics*—feeling on edge, difficulty concentrating, fear of unknown or projected dangers, fear of losing control; and *physiological characteristics*—muscle tension, sleep disturbance, autonomic hyperactivity, dizziness or lightheadedness, flushes or chills, and frequent urination.

The *DSM-IV* (American Psychiatric Association, 1994) delineates the symptoms of affective disorders more explicitly. These symptoms may be used by employers, employees, and rehabilitation professionals to assess the functional implications of a condition and evaluate the need for job accommodations (see Table 6-1).

The most effective treatment interventions for affective disorders have included medications and counseling (Seligman, 1990). Symptom reduction, stabilization, and the development of counseling strategies to reduce the severity or frequency of future symptoms are central to successful treatment and satisfactory work performance.

The degree of impact that certain disorders have on specific vocational abilities differs among the various mood and anxiety disorders. For example, the limitations related to Major Depression may cause significant impairments in the individual's ability to meet such mental job demands as maintaining attention and concentration for extended periods, completing a normal work week without interruptions due to symptoms, and working at a consistent pace.

TABLE 6-1. Mood and Anxiety Disorders

Disorder	Symptoms
Major depressive disorder	At least two weeks of depressed mood or loss of interest accompanied by at least four other symptoms of depressions which may include: weight loss or weight gain; insomnia or hypersomnia nearly every day; psychomotor agitation or retardation; fatigue of loss of energy nearly every day, feelings of worthlessness; excessive or inappropriate guilt; decreased ability to think or concentrate nearly every day; indecisiveness nearly every day; recurrent thoughts of death or suicidal ideation with or without an attempt or a specific plan
Dysthymic disorder	At least two years of depressed mood for more days than not accompanied by other depressive symptoms that do not meet criteria for a major depressive episode
Manic episode	A distinct period of abnormally and persistently elevated, expansive or elevated mood lasting at least one week with three or more other symptoms that may include: inflated self-esteem or grandiosity; decreased need for sleep; more talkative than usual; flight of ideas; distractibility; increase in goal-directed behaviors or psychomotor agitation; excessive involvement in pleasurable behaviors
Bipolar I disorder	One or more manic episodes usually accompanied by a major depressive episode
Bipolar II disorder	One or more major depressive episodes accompanied by at least one hypomanic episode
Cyclothymic disorder	At least two years of numerous periods of hypomanic episodes that do not meet the criteria for a manic episode and numerous periods of depressive symptoms that do not meet the criteria for a major depressive episode
Panic attack	A discrete period in which there is sudden onset of intense apprehension, fearfulness, or terror. During the attack other symptoms may include: shortness of breath; palpitations; chest pain; choking or smothering sensations; or fear of losing control
Agoraphobia	Anxiety about or avoidance of places or situations from which escape might be difficult or help may not be available in the event of a panic attack
Specific phobia	Clinically significant anxiety provoked by exposure to a feared object or situation often leading to avoidance behaviors
Post-traumatic stress disorder	For at least one month, reexperiencing an extremely traumatic event accompanied by symptoms of increased arousal and avoidance of stimuli associated with the trauma. Other behavioral symptoms may include: difficulty sleeping or staying asleep; irritability or outbursts of anger; difficulty concentrating; hypervigilance; and exaggerated startle response
Generalized anxiety disorder	At least six months of persistent and excessive anxiety and worry that may include three or more of the following symptoms: restlessness or feeling on edge; easily fatigued; difficulty concentrating or the mind going blank; irritability; muscle tension; and sleep disturbance

Adapted from American Psychiatric Association (1994). *Diagnostic and statistical manual of mental disorders* (4th ed.). Washington, DC: Author.

Potential accommodations for this disorder may include assigning simple, straightforward tasks to aid memory and concentration as well as flexible work hours to accommodate the effects of medication and changes in energy level (Fischler & Booth, 1999).

Although an affective disorder may be an employee's presenting or acute problem, it also is possible that the problem may be related to a more long-standing condition such as a maladaptive personality (Fong, 1995). The American Psychiatric Association (1994), Millon (1981), and Seligman (1990) have indicated that it is not unusual for people with affective disorders to have a comorbid diagnosis of a personality disorder. By understanding the

constructs of personality and personality disorders, employers and rehabilitation professionals can recognize the functional implications of these problems and more accurately assess
the resulting vocational impact and need for accommodations.

Personality Disorders

Stone (1993, p. 4) refers to personality as "the individual, typical, and enduring manner
each of us evokes for conveying our emotions, gestures, and behavior to those around us."
Both healthy personalities and personality disorders are enduring, stable patterns of behavior
that begin early in one's life. When specific traits cluster together they are referred to as a personality style (Sperry & Mosak, 1993). If these styles become inflexible and maladaptive,
causing significant impairment in occupational or social functioning, then the diagnosis of a
personality disorder may be indicated.

It is important to note the primary differences between a "healthy" personality and the
pathological aspects of a personality disorder. One difference concerns the degree to which
the personality traits deviate from the expectations of the culture in which the individual
interacts and functions. Traits associated with a personality disorder markedly depart from
what is considered normal and appropriate in the individual's cultural context (Phillips &
Gunderson, 1994). Cultural relevance should be considered because what may be considered
to be a disadvantage in one culture or environment may be beneficial in another. For
example, aggressiveness, ruthlessness, and self-centered determination may be admired in
one environment or culture and considered antisocial in another.

A second differentiating factor is the degree to which the personality leads to significant
distress or impairment in social, occupational, or other important areas of functioning. The
behaviors and attitudes related to a personality disorder may result in significant distress or
impairment in one's daily living including problems in getting along with others and in
maintaining employment.

Finally, individuals with personality disorders have ineffective coping strategies owing
to their inflexible behavioral schema (Freeman & Leaf, 1989). That is, people with personality
disorders are very reluctant to give up or modify a perception of the world or a behavioral rule
(their schema) regardless of its consequence(s). They are different from people with "normal"
personalities who have non-compelling schema, are able to surrender particular views of the
world, and can use different behavioral strategies to influence positive long-term outcomes
for themselves. People with personality disorders find ways to adjust to and extract short-term
benefits from a fundamentally biased schema that restricts or burdens their long-term
capacity to deal with the challenges of life.

Another characteristic of personality, in general, as well as personality disorders is that
many people are unaware of their traits, and they may not perceive the traits as problematic;
that is, the traits are transparent or ego-syntonic to the individual (Millon, 1981).

This particular characteristic and the long-standing nature of the personality traits makes
treatment and modification of personality disorders very challenging (Seligman, 1990; Sperry &
Mosak, 1993). A listing of the personality disorder categories in the DSM-IV are provided in
Table 6-2.

The vocational impact of personality disorders varies as suggested by the different types
of symptoms associated with each disorder and the severity of the disorder. Individuals
with a paranoid personality disorder, for example, may have serious limitations in social interactions required on the job. Potential accommodations for this type of disorder may include

TABLE 6-2. Personality Disorders

Disorder	Symptoms
Paranoid personality disorder	A pattern of distrust and suspiciousness such that others' motives are interpreted as malevolent
Schizoid personality disorder	A pattern of detachment from social relationships and a restricted range of emotional response
Schizotypal personality disorder	A pattern of acute discomfort in close relationships, cognitive or perceptual distortions, and eccentricities of behavior
Antisocial personality disorder	A pattern of disregard for, and violation of, the rights of others
Borderline personality disorder	A pattern of instability in interpersonal relationships, self-image, and affects, and marked impulsivity
Histrionic personality disorder	A pattern of excessive emotionality and attention seeking
Narcissistic personality disorder	A pattern of grandiosity, need for admiration, and lack of empathy
Avoidant personality disorder	A pattern of social inhibition, feelings of inadequacy, and hypersensitivity to negative evaluation
Dependent personality disorder	A pattern of submissive and clinging behavior related to an excessive need to be taken care of
Obsessive–compulsive personality disorder	A pattern of preoccupation with orderliness, perfectionism, and control

Adapted from American Psychiatric Association (1994). *Diagnostic and statistical manual of mental disorders* (4th ed.). Washington, DC: Author.

having the person work alone or as independently as possible to reduce suspiciousness and anxiety. Individuals diagnosed with an antisocial personality may have problems maintaining socially accepted behaviors on the job. Possible accommodations for the person having an antisocial personality include close and persistent supervision to prevent undesired behavior, plus frequent reminders about limits, expectations, and job requirements to ensure compliance with workplace procedures (Fishler & Booth, 1999).

EXAMPLES OF REASONABLE ACCOMMODATIONS

Reasonable accommodations for a person with a psychiatric disability are likely to be unique for that individual's limitations, job tasks, and work environment. However, there are various accommodations that are worthy of consideration which address the different behavioral limitations identified in the previous sections on affective and personality disorders. Some examples of potential reasonable accommodations for people with psychiatric disabilities are summarized below.

1. *Modifications to the physical environment.* Install room or work site dividers to reduce distractions and increase concentration; arrange for an enclosed office to reduce a person's anxiety about noise or interpersonal interactions; and allow work at home as necessary.

2. *Schedule modifications.* Modify arrival and departure times to take advantage of an employee's most productive times; allow additional rest periods or breaks through the work

day; allow time to leave work for treatment to maintain stability and reduce the likelihood of relapse; and allow time off for recuperation using assorted types of leave.

3. *Work procedure modifications.* Assign non-essential job tasks to other employees; assign back-up coverage in the event of an acute episode, and transfer the employee to a vacant position.

4. *Job restructuring.* Change the time of day at which a task normally is completed; and create part-time and reduced work hours opportunities for returning to work.

5. *Changes in interpersonal communication.* Provide work-related supervisory requests or responses in writing for those who may be anxious and forgetful in direct interpersonal interactions; provide positive along with any negative feedback to balance the supervision; promote self-appraisals that complement and contrast supervisory appraisals; educate coworkers about appropriate and effective interpersonal communication styles.

APPLYING DISABILITY MANAGEMENT PRINCIPLES

Disability management has been defined as "a workplace prevention and remediation strategy that seeks to prevent disability from occurring, or lacking that, to intervene early following the onset of disability, using coordinated, cost-conscious, quality rehabilitation services that reflect an organizational commitment to continued employment of those experiencing functional work limitations" (Akabas et al., 1992, p. 2). Employer-based disability management programs developed in response to the rising costs associated with work-related disability, primarily in the workers' compensation arena. A number of employers are now reporting substantial financial savings and better vocational outcomes as a result of implementing various types of disability management interventions. These programs ordinarily include formal policies and procedures, transitional work return programs, and on-site physical and occupational therapy services (Breslin & Olsheski, 1996; Habeck, 1996; Olsheski & Breslin, 1996; Shrey & Olsheski, 1992).

Disability management represents a departure from traditional vocational rehabilitation services that are viewed as reactive, clinical, and applied late after the onset of the condition (Habeck, 1996). In contrast, disability management represents a systematic approach to managing disability at the organizational level and involves the active participation of employers and employees in the design, implementation, operation, and evaluation of various disability management program functions.

Employers may find certain disability management principles, which have proven to be successful in managing physical disabilities, to also be effective in managing and accommodating psychiatric disabilities at the work place. Traditionally, employee assistance programs (EAPs) that deal with mental health problems among workers have not been integrated with the company's disability management initiatives. Consequently, EAP services may focus on the treatment of symptoms but fail to address job retention or return to work issues. More holistic disability management programs are being developed which include the integration of psychiatric rehabilitation and physical rehabilitation interventions (Watson Wyatt Worldwide, 1997). Disability management and psychiatric rehabilitation are complimentary because both approaches share the common goals of continued employment of the person with a disability.

Employers and rehabilitation professionals may find the following disability management strategies to be helpful in accommodating psychiatric disabilities at the work place.

Development of a Joint Union/Management Steering Committee

An essential component of disability management program development involves the use of a steering committee as the organizational vehicle charged with developing program policies and procedures. This committee is composed of a cross-section of key players within the company including management, supervisors, department heads, employees, and union officials. If mental health problems are included in the disability management program, then it is important that the EAP coordinator or a mental health consultant be involved in committee deliberations and policy development. The committee may also serve as a group that meets to discuss the feasibility and implementation of specific job accommodations. Policies and procedures concerning the accommodation of psychiatric disorders can be developed and shared with all staff, supervisors, and workers.

Staff Development

Successful disability management programs require the commitment of all levels of the organization to the program's mission, goals, and objectives. Management and union officials, as well as employees, should be trained in program policies and procedures to ensure that the role they play in the process is effective. In addition to internal staff development efforts, all external service providers must be oriented to the goals and objectives of the program. It is important that mental health service providers adopt and support the return-to-work philosophy of the disability management program. These professionals need to understand policies and procedures that address the job accommodation process and they must have established patterns of communication with internal personnel who are directly involved with accommodation and return-to-work decisions.

Transitional Work Return Programs

Transitional work is defined as "any job or combination of tasks and functions that may be performed safely and with remuneration by an employee whose physical capacity to perform functional job demands has been compromised" (Shrey & Olsheski, 1992, pp. 307–308). This definition can be broadened to include employees who have impaired mental capacities that cause difficulty in meeting the functional demands of the job. Like supported employment interventions, transitional work programs also involve the use of real work activities as therapeutic modalities to condition, readjust, and accommodate employees with functional limitations.

Transitional work programs have a unique set of features that differentiate them from traditional light duty programs. These unique features include: established program time parameters to avoid open-ended periods of light duty; the use of clinical rehabilitation services at the work site to provide expertise on accommodations and to monitor the functional recovery or task progression of the employee; the use of on-site functional assessments and job analysis data to develop individualized transitional work plans; and formal policies and procedures governing the role of all key players and program operations (Olsheski & Breslin, 1996).

Employers may find that, with some adaptations, the transitional work approach can be as effective in the accommodation and job retention of employees with psychiatric disabilities as it has been for those with physical disabilities. For example, just as physical and occupational therapists are used in a "job coaching" role to provide on-site assessment and support of employees with physical problems, qualified mental health professionals could assume a similar role for those with psychological problems. Similar to the role of the physical therapist, the mental health professional could evaluate the functional limitations of the employee's psychological impairment, analyze the mental demands of the job, and recommend specific accommodations that are incorporated in the individual's transitional work plan. Issues pertaining to confidentiality should be addressed in program policies with input from EAP coordinators and mental health service providers.

Developing Transitional Work Plans for Employees with Psychiatric Disabilities

The development of individualized transitional work plans involves a number of essential components. These components are summarized below:

1. *Program referral*: Employees who experience work disruptions or absences due to psychiatric conditions are typically referred for transitional work services by their EAP coordinator/counselor, their treating therapist, or attending physician. It is important that measures are taken to protect the employee's confidentiality. The employee must authorize the release of confidential information before this information is given to any party involved in the transitional work program, including work supervisors, coworkers, or other treatment professionals. Usually, referrals are directed to the internal staff member who coordinates the transitional work program.

2. *Assessment*: Two types of assessment are necessary in the development of the employee's transitional work plan. First, an assessment of the employee's mental residual functional capacities is needed. This assessment describes the symptoms and functional limitations associated with the employee's psychiatric condition. For example, an employee who has a depressive condition might have problems with work pace, reliability, interpersonal functioning, etc. By understanding how the employee's psychiatric symptoms impact the performance of essential job functions, the need for specific accommodations can be identified. Secondly, a psycho-social job analysis must be completed to determine the mental, psychological, and social requirements of the job. The job analysis should also evaluate the physical demands of the job if the employee has physical limitations or if the physical demands of the job interact with the psychiatric condition. Job analysis information is essential in evaluating the degree of congruency between the employee's mental capacities and specific job requirements.

3. *Case staffing*: After completion of the assessment phase, key individuals who are involved in making job accommodation decisions meet to discuss the case and determine the feasibility of the employee's participation in the transitional work program. Results from the employee's functional assessment and the job analysis are analyzed, and this information is used in the development of the individualized transitional work return plan. Supervisors, treating therapists, case managers, and program coordinators are the usual participants at the case staff meeting.

4. *Development and implementation of the transitional work plan*: The transitional work plan is the document that synthesizes assessment data generated by the functional evaluation of the employee and the job analysis. This information is used to identify specific job accommodations, the nature and frequency of on-site clinical supervision sessions, and

the duration of the transitional work program. This written plan is signed by the treating therapist, the employee, and the employee's work supervisor.

5. *Program supervision, discharge, and follow-up*:   The treating therapist provides clinical supervision of the employee during the course of his/her participation in transitional work. Supervision may include helping the employee with accommodations, resolving problems with supervisors and coworkers, recommending additional accommodations, or responding to other work performance issues. Upon completion of the transitional work program as specified in the employee's plan, a staff meeting is conducted to determine if the employee needs additional accommodations or if the employee can return to full-duty status without accommodations. In addition, an evaluation of the reasonableness of permanent accommodations may also take place at the discharge staffing. The discharge staffing is usually attended by the same parties who were involved in the design of the employee's transitional work plan.

SUMMARY

Court rulings have been inconsistent about the reasonable nature of changes in the interpersonal work environment (Lindsey, 1995), but education of workers about the ADA and psychiatric disabilities seems to be imperative for a successful accommodation. It is apparent that most accommodations include little direct cost, and the relatively lower costs reduce the likelihood of an undue hardship defense based on financial criteria. The application of disability management principles may also provide employers with an organizational framework that promotes the successful job retention and accommodation of employees with psychiatric disabilities.

To accomplish more effective job accommodation methods for people with psychiatric disabilities, it is important that employers and rehabilitation professionals understand the relationships among symptoms, functional limitations, and the impact the psychiatric disability has on an individual's vocational performance. Through a better understanding of these relationships, more individuals with psychiatric disabilities will be able to secure and maintain meaningful employment.

REFERENCES

Akabas, S., Gates, L., & Galvin, D. (1992). *Disability management: A complete system to reduce costs, increase productivity, meet employee needs, and ensure legal compliance.* New York, NY: AMACON.

American Psychiatric Association (1994). *Diagnostic and statistical manual of mental disorders* (4th ed.). Washington, DC: Author.

Anthony, W. A., Kennard, W. A., O'Brien, W. F., & Forbes, R. (1989). Psychiatric rehabilitation: Past myths and current realities. *Community Mental Health Journal, 22*(4), 249–264.

Asch, A. (1984). The experience of disability: A challenge for psychologists. *American Psychologist, 39*(5), 529–536.

Austin, B., & Green, D. (1998). Recommendations to employers on implementing EEOC's enforcement guidance on the ADA and psychiatric disabilities. *Employment in the Mainstream, 23*(3), 5–9.

Barlow, W. E., Hatch, D. D., & Murphy, B. S. (1995). Recent legal decisions affect you. *Personnel Journal, 74*(12), 105.

Blanck, P. D., Anderson, J. H., Wallach, E. J., & Tenney, J. P. (1994). Implementing reasonable accommodations using ADR under the ADA: The case of a white-collar employee with bipolar mental illness. *Mental and Physical Disability Law Review, 18*(4), 458–464.

Bowe, F. (1990). Into the private sector: Rights and people with disabilities. *Journal of Disability Policy Studies, 1*(1), 89–101.

Brady, R. L. (1996). The ADA and job interviews. *HR Focus, 73*(4), 20.

Breslin, R., & Olsheski, J. (1996). The impact of a transitional work return program on lost time: Preliminary data from the Minster Machine Company. *NARPPS Journal, 11*(2), 35–40.

Campbell, J. (1994). Unintended consequences in public policy: Persons with psychiatric disabilities and the Americans with Disabilities Act. *Policy Studies Journal, 22*(1), 133–145.

Carling, P. J. (1994). Reasonable accommodations in the workplace for individuals with psychiatric disabilities. In S. M. Bruyere & J. O'Keeffe (Eds.), *Implications of the Americans with Disabilities Act for psychology* (pp. 103–136). New York, NY: Springer.

Crist, P. A., & Stoffel, V. C. (1991). The Americans with Disabilities Act of 1990 and employees with mental impairments: Personal efficacy and the environment. *American Journal of Occupational Therapy, 46*(4), 434–443.

Drake, R. E., McHugo, G. J., Becker, D. R., Anthony, W. A., & Clark, R. E. (1996). The New Hampshire study of supported employment for people with mental illness. *Journal of Consulting and Clinical Psychology, 64*(2), 391–399.

Elkin, A., & Rosch, P. (1990). Promoting mental health at work. *Occupational Medicine* (5), 739–754.

Field, T., & Field, J. (1998). *Classification of jobs*. Athens, GA: Elliott & Fitzpatrick.

Fischler, G., & Booth, N. (1999). *Vocational impact of psychiatric disorders: A guide for rehabilitation professionals*. Gaithersburg, MD: Aspen.

Fong, M. (1995). Assessment and *DSM–IV* diagnosis of personality disorders: A primer for counselors. *Journal of Counseling and Development, 73*(6), 635–639.

Freeman, A., & Leaf, R. C. (1989). Cognitive therapy applied to personality disorders. In A. Freeman, K. Simon, L. E. Beutler, & H. Arkowitz (Eds.), *Comprehensive handbook of cognitive therapy* (pp. 403–434). New York, NY: Plenum Press.

Goffman, E. (1963). *Stigma: Notes on the management of spoiled identity*. Englewood Cliffs, NJ: Prentice-Hall.

Gordon, R. E., Eisler, R. L., Gutman, E. M., & Gordon, K. K. (1991). Predicting prognosis by means of the DSM–III multiaxial diagnoses. *Canadian Journal of Psychiatry, 36*, 218–221.

Gotlib, I. H., & Colby, C. A. (1987). *Treatment of depression*. Elmsford, NY: Pergamon Press.

Habeck, R. (1996). Differentiating disability management and rehabilitation. *NARPPS Journal, 11*(2), 8–20.

Hantula, D. A., & Reilly, N. A. (1996). Reasonable accommodation for employees with mental disabilities: A mandate for effective supervision. *Behavioral Sciences and the Law, 14*(1), 107–120.

Isaacson, L., & Brown, D. (2000). *Career information, career counseling, and career development* (7th ed.). Boston, MA: Allyn & Bacon.

Job Accommodation Network (1991). *Regulations for title I of the Americans with Disabilities Act*. Morgantown, WV: Author.

Jordan, L. C., Luke, D. A., Mowbray, C. T., Herman, S. E., Davidson, W. S., & Conklin, C. (1996). Correlates of functioning in a population with dual diagnoses: An examination of diagnosis and problem history. *Journal of Mental Health Administration, 23*(3), 260–271.

Klerman, G. L. (1988). Depression and related disorders of mood (affective disorders). In A. M. Nicholi (Ed.), *The new Harvard guide to psychiatry* (pp. 309–336). Cambridge, MA: Belknap Press.

Lindsey, D. (1995). Workplace psychological disabilities and the ADA. *Behavioral Health Management, 17*(3), 34–36.

Link, B., Cullen, F., Mirotzink, J., & Streuning, E. (1992). The consequences of stigma for people with mental illness: Evidence from the social sciences. In P. Fink & A. Tasman (Eds.), *Stigma and mental illness*. Washington, DC: American Psychiatric Press.

Mancuso, L. L. (1990). Reasonable accommodation for workers with psychiatric disabilities. *Psychosocial Rehabilitation Bulletin, 14*(2), 3–19.

Mancuso, L. L. (1995). Achieving reasonable accommodation for workers with psychiatric disabilities: Understanding the employer's perspective. *American Rehabilitation, 22*(1), 2–8.

Milite, G. (1994). Understanding reasonable accommodations. *Supervisory Management, 39*(2), 1–2.

Millar, J. (1992). Public enlightenment and mental health in the workplace. In G. Keita & S. Sauter (Eds.), *Work and well-being: An agenda for the 1990's*. Washington, DC: American Psychological Association.

Millon, T. (1981). *Disorders of personality*. New York, NY: Wiley.

Noe, S. R. (1997). Discrimination against people with mental illness. *Journal of Rehabilitation, 63*(1), 20–26.

O'Keeffe, J. (1994). Disability, discrimination, and the Americans with Disabilities Act. In S. M. Bruyere & J. O'Keeffe (Eds.), *Implications of the Americans with Disabilities Act for psychology*. New York, NY: Springer.

Olsheski, J., & Breslin, R. (1996). The Americans with Disabilities Act: Implications for the use of ergonomics in rehabilitation. In A. Bhattacharya & J. McGlothlin (Eds.), *Occupational ergonomics: Theory and practice.* New York, NY: Marcel Dekker.

Parry, J. W. (1993). Mental disabilities under the ADA: A difficult path to follow. *Mental and Physical Disability Law Reporter, 17*(1), 100–112.

Peterson, N., Mumford, M., Borman, W., Jeanneret, P., Fleishman, E., and Levin, K. (Eds.) (1997). *ONET final technical report, Vol II.* Salt Lake City, UT: Utah Department of Workforce Services.

Phillips, K. A., & Gunderson, J. G. (1994). Personality disorders. In R. E. Hales, S. C. Yudofsky, & J. A. Talbott (Eds.), *The American psychiatric press textbook of psychiatry* (pp. 701–728). Washington, DC: American Psychiatric Press.

Pollett, S. L. (1995). Mental illness in the workplace: The tension between productivity and reasonable accommodation. *Journal of Psychiatry and Law, 23*(1), 155–184.

Ravid, R. (1992). Disclosure of mental illness to employers: Legal recourses and ramifications. *The Journal of Psychiatry and Law, 20*(1), 85–102.

Regier, D. A., Narrow, W. E., & Rae, D. S. (1993). The de facto U.S. mental health and addictive disorders service system: Epidemiological catchment area prospective 1-year prevalence rates of disorders and services. *General Archives of Psychiatry, 5*, 85–94.

Roberts, M. (1995). Mental health consumers as professionals: Disclosure in the workplace. *American Rehabilitation, 21*(1), 20–23.

Sauter, S. (1992). Introduction to the NIOSH proposed strategy. In G. Keita & S. Sauter (Eds.), *Work and well-being: A strategy for the 1990's.* Washington, DC: American Psychological Association.

Seligman, L. (1990). *Selecting effective treatments.* San Francisco, CA: Jossey-Bass.

Seligman, L., & Moore, B. M. (1995). Diagnosis of mood disorders. *Journal of Counseling and Development, 74*(1), 65–69.

Shrey, D., & Olsheski, J. (1992). Disability management and industry-based work return transition programs. *Physical Medicine and Rehabilitation, 6*(2), 303–314.

Sperry, L., & Mosak, H. H. (1993). Personality disorders. In L. Sperry & J. Carlson (Eds.), *Psychopathology and psychotherapy* (pp. 299–368). Muncie, IN: Accelerated Development.

Stone, M. H. (1993). *Abnormalities of personality.* New York, NY: Norton.

Sue, D., Sue, D., & Sue, S. (1994). *Understanding abnormal behavior.* Geneva, IL: Houghton Mifflin.

Turley, L., & Beck, R. (1991). *Americans with Disabilities Act: Manual for counselors, employers, and consumers.* Carbondale, IL: Southern Illinois University.

U.S. Congress (1994). *Psychiatric disabilities, employment, and the Americans with Disabilities Act.* Washington, DC: U.S. Government Printing Office.

Warshaw, L. (1990). *Stress, anxiety, and depression in the workplace: A report of the NYGBH/Gallup survey.* New York, NY: New York Business Group on Health.

Watson Wyatt Worldwide (1997, May). Staying at work: Productivity through integrated disability management. *Watson Wyatt Insider.*

West, J. (1996). Introduction. In J. West (Ed.), *Implementing the Americans with Disabilities Act* (pp. 5–28). Cambridge, MA: Blackwell.

Wright, G. N. (1980). *Total Rehabilitation.* Boston MA: Little, Brown.

Zuckerman, D. (1993). Reasonable accommodations for people with mental illness under the ADA. *Mental and Physical Disability Law Review, 17*(3), 311–319.

CHAPTER 7

Strategic Career Development for People with Disabilities

David P. Moxley, John R. Finch, James Tripp, and Stuart Forman

INTRODUCTION

A viable career may be one of the most important assets a person can possess in American society. Not only is a viable career linked to economic success but also perhaps, more importantly, a career influences one's personal happiness and quality of life (Sears, 1982; Sharf, 1997). Career influences one's sense of self and it defines a person in relation to others. It is common in American society for people meeting for the first time to inquire what the other does for a living and the ensuing explanation often involves stories of employment or career. Explaining to another person "what I do" is an important interactional ritual that frames conversation, fosters social relatedness, smooths social interaction, and helps people to understand and know one another. Within American culture, such conversations are almost essential to the portrayal of oneself as someone who is to be taken seriously. The centrality of employment and career within such interactional rituals indicates that career is both important to defining oneself and to interpreting oneself to others. Culturally, work and career are central to personal identity.

It is not surprising that Sharf (1997) emphasizes the centrality of career to self-concept by noting that people come to see themselves in relation to their work, jobs, or career lines. Sears (1982) offers a more encompassing idea of career. From Sears' perspective career encompasses the scope of people's lives—their work, leisure, and avocational activities that define them personally and that they chose, enact and even abandon over their life span. Sears reminds us that career is an expression of what we come to value and what makes us distinctive. From this more encompassing perspective, career is not only what a person does now but also it involves those experiences people accumulate over their life spans.

For people with disabilities having a career may be one of the most important life assets given the cultural importance of work in adult life. Increasing the involvement of people with

David P. Moxley • Wayne State University School of Social Work, Detroit, Michigan.   John R. Finch • Rehabilitation Consultant, Columbus, Ohio.   James Tripp • Wayne State University School of Social Work, Detroit, Michigan. Stuart Forman • Wayne State University, Detroit, Michigan.

disabilities in the American workforce has been one of the most significant challenges facing rehabilitation and mental health practice. Indeed, despite the implementation of the Americans with Disabilities Act, people with disabilities represent one of the most under-represented groups in the American workforce. Work and career have been opportunity struc-tures difficult to open for people with disabilities, particularly people coping with serious mental illness and psychiatric disabilities. Despite efforts to offer incentives to employers and to facilitate employment of people with disabilities through flexible benefits, workplace participation has not risen substantially over the past decade.

People with disabilities prioritize work and career as important life outcomes of reha-bilitation, but workplaces themselves may not readily accept or welcome these potential workers. Stigma, fear, and lack of understanding continue to create barriers to workforce par-ticipation making traditional employment difficult to achieve as an outcome. Nonetheless, there are many promising alternatives to traditional employment. People with disabilities are experimenting with the creation of their own work, following a growing national trend to engage in contract work, home-based work, and self-employment (Liptak, 2001). In addition, people with disabilities are finding career options within human services and exploring ways of offering services to other people with disabilities. The emergence of community-based and nonprofit enterprises, whether in the form of cooperative employment, social enterprises, or arts and cultural collectives, offers people with disabilities promising alternative careers.

Rehabilitation and mental health professionals can offer people with disabilities services that facilitate their career awareness and career development. These services can be easily integrated into their existing work roles so that these professionals need not identify them-selves as specialists in career development. Given the integral relationship between career and personal fulfillment and development, career development undertaken by rehabilitation and mental health professionals can be seen as an augmentation of the other personal services they offer to their recipients (Liptak, 2001). Almost any service rehabilitation and mental health professionals offer to recipients can incorporate strategies to facilitate the development of career assets. It is an aim of this chapter to outline strategic career development based on the career issues and needs people with disabilities experience and to illuminate how rehabilita-tion and mental health professionals can use them to assist people with disabilities to focus strategically on career development.

CONTEMPORARY CHALLENGES TO DEFINING CAREER

Many theories of career development focus on how individuals come to define them-selves vocationally and how they choose work. Few theories place the vocationally develop-ing individual into the context of work and examine how careers themselves, opportunities for career, and social forces creating careers influence career development. Many of these theo-ries treat careers as static and relatively unchanging. But increasingly it is becoming difficult to define career. The modern workplace has changed substantially with the introduction of new technologies that have influenced how work is undertaken and performed, and the skills and abilities workers now need to meet heightening expectations of performance have changed considerably over the past two decades (Appelbaum & Batt, 1994).

The guarantee of work itself has changed as part-time, temporary, and contracted out employment become more dominant in the workplace. Declines in wages and restructuring of benefits have altered incentive structures. The availability of work in many communities has become uncertain. Major employers may quickly relocate plants and offices, and industrial, financial, and service institutions move to geographic locales to take advantage of lower wage structures. Still other companies may streamline operations to intentionally downsize by reducing the number of jobs and accompanying overhead.

Given the changing context of work, career cannot be equated with one's job or even with one's professional role. As Liptak (2001) emphasizes, career must be viewed holistically, as encompassing those factors that combine sociologically, psychologically, economically, and educationally to form a career that unfolds over the life span. Given the dynamic nature of contemporary work and the potential of new careers yet undefined or fully appreciated, the concept of career is as dynamic as the societal and organizational contexts in which it unfolds.

Nonetheless, even though career is difficult to define, people certainly view careers as an asset. A career offers numerous benefits, whether personal, economic, or interpersonal. It is not surprising, therefore, that career is a critical element of a person's social capital and the absence of a career, at least in American society, can seriously impede social involvement or even isolate people who are without careers from the mainstream of community life. The wholesale absence of careers can isolate entire communities from society, set in motion a process of community decline, and degrade quality of life (Wilson, 1996).

Yet, the future of careers is not necessarily negative. Emergent social issues can create new careers and nascent technologies can create new work roles and jobs that anticipate the emergence of new career lines. Changes in social forces, such as the reframing of aging from a negative disease state to a period of productive growth and development, can bring about new patterns of work and career. The extension of the productive years of career between the ages of 70 and 100 suggest that careers and career patterns are now changing. The idea of productive aging indicates that work and career remain vital even into later life, a time when former paradigms of aging suggested that people must leave the workforce.

Octogenarians who have successfully negotiated personal and social crises and have witnessed and mastered paradigmatic changes to their own work may bring a sense of wisdom to the workplace. Career-oriented aged individuals may take new work roles as teachers, mentors, and consultants. They may become leaders of those future organizations that understand the importance of conserving traditions while facilitating change.

No longer does career only mean a specific track or a specific line of work. It no longer means lifelong or even long-term employment with one organization or the execution of a specific or singular role over a life span. Career is certainly encompassing of social change itself and perhaps now must be appreciated from the perspectives of individuals who define and create their own careers. As new forms of employment take root in American society, such as cooperative employment, itinerant employment, and portfolio-based employment, people increasingly will invent their own careers by accommodating to social change, which may be the ultimate driver of career change. Yet even though there is considerable ambiguity surrounding the definition of career at this time there is little ambiguity around its social meaning. Career will continue to be a central source of self-definition for many people given the considerable importance society apportions to work.

THE CONTRIBUTIONS OF TRADITIONAL CAREER DEVELOPMENT THEORIES TO THINKING ABOUT CAREER ASSETS

Even though there are numerous theories of career development, and variations in overarching explanations of the sequence and stages of careers, these theories share one commonality: they all emphasize the centrality of career within people's lives and within the human life span. According to these theories career is something one acquires through developmental experiences that interact with child-rearing, biological or genetic endowment, and learning experiences. Lent, Brown, and Hackett (1994) and Lent, Hackett, and Brown (1996) identify how influential career-relevant learning experiences shape career choices and decisions. The early work of Ginzberg, Ginsburg, Axelrod, and Herma (1951) suggests a movement through three distinct phases including childhood fantasy about careers, a tentative decision period during late childhood and adolescence, and a realistic period of adulthood when crystallization of a career takes place.

The developmental self-concept theory of Super (1963, 1990, 1994) emphasizes the process by which people come to view themselves. According to Super's theory, people develop a subjective sense of career as a product of role-playing, exploration, and reality testing that results in differentiation of the person's sense of self. Career, according to Super, is a form of self-expression but one that is a product of biology, social role-playing, and the appraisal of how others react to the person's career choice and performance. Career satisfaction, according to Super (1963), is an outcome of the extent to which people can express their self-concepts.

Holland's (1959, 1973) theory of vocational choice focuses on the development of personality, which he assumes is a product of the interaction between heredity and social opportunity influenced by parents, teachers, social class, culture, and the physical environment. According to Holland, the manner in which people come to choose how they interact with the environment influences career choice. The choice of occupation reflects motivation, knowledge, ability, and personality and Holland identifies six domains in which individuals express their choices. The selection of one of these six domains is an outcome of the confluence of these many factors and influences.

Roe's (1957) theory of career choice is grounded in the early experiences of childhood and the influence of family or home life. According to Roe, occupational choice is a product of the childhood environment, the satisfaction of needs, and the development of personality. Parental reaction to the child's personality—whether in the form of emotional preoccupation with the child, avoidance of the child, or acceptance of the child as an individual—can influence career choice in different ways. Parental reaction, according to Roe, shapes career choice and influences a person's subsequent selection of careers from a broad array of potential choices ranging from the arts and entertainment to science or service.

Rather than focusing specifically on the individual, Tiedeman (1961) notes that career development is a series of decisions as people move toward maturity and that are influenced by school, work experiences, life experiences, and interaction with other people. Each career choice, according to Tiedeman, is important to subsequent entry into a career since choices stimulate anticipation of a career, implementation of a career, and subsequent adjustment. Opportunities to exercise career choice and engage in this sequence stimulate changes to a person's self-concept, which in turn influence subsequent career decisions. Career development is personal development, a product of choosing, entering, and progressing in a particular career experience. Thus, career development is truly developmental. Career experiences build on one another, as the person's self concept evolves and matures and illuminates still other career alternatives (Miller-Tiedeman & Tiedeman, 1990; Tiedeman, 1961).

Krumboltz (1994) offers a social learning theory of career development and notes that four factors interact in the selection of a career: genetic endowment, environmental conditions, learning experiences, and task-approach skills. Environmental conditions influence opportunities and the range of work roles and career ladders available to people, and the number, nature, and consequences of learning experiences influence the emergence of career preferences. Task-approach skills incorporate the setting of goals, the clarification of values, generating potential alternatives, and obtaining the knowledge and information one needs to make choices from an array of alternatives. The development of careers occurs in a complex matrix of personal and social forces that combine to influence choice. But, according to Krumboltz, people can learn to master career choice through opportunities for education and decision-making, direct experience with career alternatives, and vicarious exposure to specific work situations.

Each of these career development theories suggests practical approaches to helping people with disabilities to acquire career assets. The idea that one matures from a career perspective is invaluable in thinking about the early experiences people with disabilities need to gain an understanding of work and to gain insight into themselves as workers (Benz & Halpern, 1993). Certainly those theories that underscore the influential role of parents and significant adults highlight the important roles they serve in fostering awareness of work and career, in modeling their own career commitments, in implementing career discussions, and in fostering the emergence of career-oriented self-efficacy (Ochs & Roessler, 2001). The availability of parents or significant adults who will interact with young people with disabilities about career is certainly an important asset.

Helping people to assess their career experiences, to reflect on the meaning they derive from these experiences, and to consider how they influence their life satisfaction and career direction are important assets. The idea that career awareness, choice, and decision unfold within focused dialogues about work and career is a simple but powerful tool (Ochs & Roessler, 2001). The provision of direct experiences with the world of work and with specific jobs may increase the readiness of young people with disabilities to explore work and may strengthen career self concept, particularly if these young people have access to a variety of career-oriented learning experiences. Increasing the number and diversity of opportunities people have within the world of work can serve to clarify career direction, another important asset for people to possess.

CAREER DEVELOPMENT AS STRATEGY

These theories suggest that career development is an orderly process through which people move to achieve career outcomes. And, these theories suggest that career development is a patterned process that unfolds as people progress in their maturity and gain insight into their preferences and aims. However, career development is complex and a host of factors can influence a person's development of a career, their movement along a particular pathway, or their transfer of the knowledge, skills, competencies, and networks they obtain in one career line to another (Mamo & Mueller, 2000).

Becker and Strauss (1956) propose a career contingency theory in which a number of factors intersect to foster career entry, development, and success. These factors are personal (e.g., motivation and needs), contextual (e.g., formal and informal relations with people who can facilitate career entry), and societal (e.g., creation of new occupational pathways). For Becker and Strauss, career is contingent on a host of factors and it is contingent on local and societal change. External environmental factors that lead to new technologies can create new domains of work (Abbott, 1988). According to Wiener (1991), who uses HIV/AIDS as an example, changes in laws and patient care practices within the health domain have fostered new work roles, the emergence of new specializations, and new career pathways in patient care. People may cross over from one career line such as nursing to assume a new career such as patient advocacy within an emerging area of care that may not have existed when the person first entered his or her career.

Career, according to contingency theory, may be as much dependent on local opportunities and social change as it is on a person's preferences, goals, and learning experiences. According to this perspective, personal development is, in part, a function of social development. Careers are social opportunities people actuate based on a strategy to achieve something they value using emergent opportunities to enter new careers and to create new definitions of self. On a local level, social movements may emerge that offer new ideologies regarding these identities. The movements themselves can open up opportunities that were once closed, create new definitions of how work can be undertaken, and select those who should perform this new work (Mamo & Mueller, 2000).

An important exemplar of this theory lies in the disability rights movement, which has sought to create new social roles and statuses for people with disabilities in the greater society. The disability rights movement has created rights that emphasize the legitimacy of career and the importance of work opportunities. And the movement has created its own service institutions involving centers of independent living, self-help organizations, and mutual support initiatives. The movement discounts dominance by well-meaning professionals and identifies the distinctiveness of self-help and mutual support.

The movement itself has fostered new thinking within established institutions about the contributions people with disabilities can make to human service organizations and as providers of human services. In this sense, possessing a disability may serve as a life experience or credential that can certify one for entry into positions once regulated by formal credentials. The movement and the new role opportunities it has opened within local communities literally have introduced new models of service provision. In some states new markets for the provision of personal assistance have emerged, and people with disabilities can use public benefits to purchase services from vendors who employ people with disabilities to offer personal assistance. The disability rights movement has the potential to introduce a broader array of service options as alternatives to systems of care dominated by professionals who are not themselves disabled or who lack first-hand knowledge of disability (Mowbray, Moxley, Jasper, & Howell, 1997).

It is too early to say whether these alternative systems of support will create numerous job opportunities for people with disabilities or even if established human service organizations will develop viable career lines for people who are recipients but who hold potential as members of the professional staff. There is some research evidence to suggest that human service organizations create career lines for recipients only when it serves their interest or earns them recognition in the professional community (Mowbray, Moxley, & Collins, 1998).

The kind of social change the disability rights movement has introduced is an example of how career contingency theory may operate in local communities. It suggests how career opportunities emerge from social change and social movements, which in turn can facilitate changes to career pathways within organizations.

Career contingency theory suggests that career development does not only involve direct experience with work roles, social learning, and personal awareness and information. From the perspective of contingency theory, career development is perhaps more the actuation of personal and conscious strategy than it is the facilitation of a normative and patterned process of development that unfolds in a linear manner. The formulation of career strategy requires individuals to understand their environments and to appraise opportunities that are emerging within their communities and societies as a function of change. Then the formulation of career strategy requires individuals to appraise their personal interests and determine the investments they are willing to make to take advantage of a changing environment. From the perspective of contingency theory, career development involves the accumulation of assets that are portable and can be used in changing social contexts to cross over to other careers. In this sense, career development is dynamic, and one of the most important assets a person can possess is flexibility.

Career strategy must take into consideration organizational pathways that offer opportunities to individuals. Initially, career development strategy may not involve the person thinking through a specific career line but in identifying the assets they want to acquire in preparation for moving either to another career or to enhance their career as they move from one organization to another. In this sense, career comes to mean the person's chosen pathway through life and the assets they develop that converge on the formation of a career identity that is robust enough to facilitate the person's flexibility in a world that is increasingly dynamic (Dubois, 2000).

The acquisition and documentation of assets may be one of the most important outcomes of strategic career development. The accumulation of these assets may prepare people with disabilities to take advantage of emergent opportunities, to interpret and make sense of these opportunities, and to increase their readiness to take advantage of them.

THE SERENDIPITY OF CAREER DEVELOPMENT

The meaning of career has broadened in a changing and unpredictable world and changes in the substance and availability of work have made commitment to a singular career somewhat precarious. Career development and planning, as a result, has had to become more encompassing of issues earlier approaches have not factored into the service process (Liptak, 2001) precisely because the nature of work and career has undergone considerable change. The idea that career development and planning is a process of individual strategy formulation involves the challenge of helping people to find careers in a world characterized by unpredictability and serendipity (Mitchell, Krumboltz, & Levin, 1999).

Rather than being a totally rational process guided by technical considerations of testing, focusing, and matching, career development also may need to encompass sensitivity to transforming unplanned events into career opportunities. Chance encounters may open up unexpected opportunities or ones the emergence of which could not have been predicted earlier. The authors have witnessed chance encounters between students with disabilities and practicing professionals who are willing to become sponsors or mentors of the students in tutorials, supervision, and internships. Chance encounters spark relationships that can then lead to the deepening of relationships between student and professional and then result in employment opportunities through networks, organizations, or activities the professional opens to the student.

Extensive social contact with others can set in motion opportunities to interact with people from a broad range of careers and can create opportunities to explore careers. So, it is not surprising that many theorists of career development factor into their theoretical perspectives the importance of thinking about career as involving the accumulation of individual experiences that unfold over the life span and that come to define the identity of the person (Sears, 1982; Super, 1951).

Sensitivity to chance and serendipity and the career development opportunities uncertainty can reveal suggests that purposeful engagement in career development can be reframed. Most importantly, career development personnel can interact with their clients in a manner that grooms the core qualities of curiosity, persistence, flexibility, optimism, and risk-taking (Mitchell et al., 1999). These qualities suggest that the individual is willing to tolerate ambiguity in the pursuit of a career, to examine life events and activities to identify their career implications, and to pay attention to unplanned events or chance encounters with others for what they suggest about potential career ideas or direction. Confusion about career identity can be reframed as a period of self-exploration. Indecision about career can be reframed as the development of open-mindedness about career possibilities or freedom to engage in what Ginzberg et al. (1951) referred to as fantasy (Mitchell et al., 1999). Leaving a job after a short tenure can be seen as on-the-job assessment and appraisal, which, in turn, can result in opportunities for reflection, self-evaluation, and future choice.

Unfortunately, given changes to rehabilitation and mental health practice, the process-orientation that Mitchell et al. refer to as "planned happenstance" may be structured out of practice in the name of accountability-driven efficiency. And, focusing on the strategic use of happenstance may require a more psychotherapeutic approach to career development than what traditionally oriented counselors may feel competent to undertake (Crites, 1981).

A form of career development counseling that uses serendipity, chance, and unexpected events may need to focus on all the social roles an individual undertakes or performs and, in this sense, career counseling becomes synonymous with personal counseling (Yost & Corbishley, 1987). Work life and personal life are not separate. They influence one another and can create positive and negative consequences for one another. In this sense, a strategic approach to career development will encompass many of the individual's life domains (Liptak, 2001) and requires mental health or rehabilitation practitioners to examine career holistically from the perspective of these multiple domains since career assets may emerge in many different areas of a person's life.

Combining traditional career development theories and contingency theory can illuminate two principal qualities of career development with people coping with disabilities. First, career development is a planned intervention that facilitates formal assessment and appraisal, goal planning, service provision, work experience, and the direct support of work alternatives. Second, career development can take on an improvisational quality as the mental health or rehabilitation practitioner and recipient work with happenstance as it unfolds during the course of the counseling relationship. These two qualities can make career development work somewhat paradoxical—it can be planned, orderly, and intentional and it can possess a contingent, opportunistic, and fluid quality.

CAREER DEVELOPMENT NEEDS OF PEOPLE WITH DISABILITIES

Many students with disabilities manifest lower levels of career maturity compared with nondisabled students. Herr (1993) frames career maturity as personal flexibility, one of the principal career assets a person can possess in a changing and unpredictable environment. Herr's concept of personal flexibility involves the acquisition of self-knowledge in relation to career interests, self-confidence, and interpersonal skills that support effective interaction with others. These core skills or attributes, according to Herr, prepare people to engage their environment and do so with the belief that they can influence their career situation and progress in the world of work. An underlying factor in the achievement of personal flexibility is self-efficacy—the basic belief that individuals can influence their environment to bring about outcomes they desire or value.

Research on youth with disabilities indicates that they have limited knowledge of the world of work and of specific jobs (Rojewski, 1993) and that involvement in decisions about career can provoke considerable anxiety leading to the avoidance of situations in which these decisions are explored or made (Wehmeyer, 1993). Since career exploration and decision-making can provoke anxiety, young people with disabilities may look to others to make career decisions for them (Wehmeyer, 1993) and this can result in excessive dependence on others, particularly adults to whom they are close. Contributing to heightened anxiety is the possibility that young people with disabilities can face real difficulties in appraising their abilities, even though they have many of the same career aspirations as non-disabled youth.

Ochs and Roessler (2001) suggest that lowered career maturity among young people with disabilities reflects a developmental lag. Such a lag can diminish abilities to address effectively the demands young people with disabilities face in making a transition to the world of work. Research that compared special education students with general education students indicated that students with disabilities scored lower on measures of career decision-making, self-efficacy, career outcome expectations, career exploration intentions, and vocational identity (Ochs & Roessler, 2001).

This portrait suggests that people with disabilities can benefit from efforts to foster general self-efficacy, social self-efficacy, and specific self-efficacy in the areas of career and employment. Lowered self-efficacy suggests that people with disabilities may experience weak intentions to explore careers and to experiment with various work roles in an effort to discover a career direction that best fits them. They may believe that they cannot bring about the career outcomes they come to value.

A developmental lag in career maturity or personal flexibility is largely a result of a limited exposure to the world of work combined with lowered expectations that people with disabilities internalize about their prospects for successful work and career. Expanding exposure to the world of work and facilitating reflection on the part of people with disabilities about their career expectancies and intentions may contribute important outcomes to fostering career maturity and increasing personal flexibility. Helping people with disabilities to learn about themselves within the world of work may be one of the most fundamental strategies for clarifying vocational identity (Lent et al., 1994, 1996), building confidence (Super, 1990), and fostering positive intentions for career exploration (Ochs & Roessler, 2001).

SPECIFIC CAREER DEVELOPMENT STRATEGIES

The idea that career development unfolds in a normative manner and can be influenced by happenstance suggests that the development of personal flexibility based on increased self-efficacy may be important strategic outcomes in working with people with disabilities. Of course, the authors assume that the issues previously outlined pertain to those individuals whose disabilities are serious and long-term, and which had an early onset. Certainly the career development issues of those individuals who acquired disabilities after launching their careers are likely to be quite different.

Bandura (1977, 1997) identifies four sources of self-efficacy involving the (1) provision of vicarious experiences; (2) identification and appreciation of performance accomplishments;

(3) verbal persuasion to support appropriate risk-taking; and (4) emotional arousal that facilitates awareness of feelings and motivation to act. Mental health and rehabilitation professionals can use these sources of self-efficacy to strengthen the intentions, expectations, and actions of people with disabilities in relationship to finding and entering careers that they chose.

Vicarious Experiences

The exposure of people with disabilities to vicarious experiences can facilitate their acquisition of positive beliefs of themselves as efficacious individuals. These vicarious experiences come in the form of exposure to role models and opportunities for people with disabilities to compare themselves with actual people who engage in valued roles. Vicarious experiences in relation to career development not only mean that people with disabilities have opportunities to observe actual work situations, but they also have opportunities to interact with people who actually engage in career and work roles that hold potential interest for them. Interacting with these individuals through conversation, job shadowing, and informal interactions can help people with disabilities to compare themselves with these role models and they can come to understand important characteristics they may share with these role models.

Supplementing this kind of interaction with role models can be symbolic comparison. Washington and Moxley (2001c) report on the successful use of photographs of successful Black women to stimulate the self-reflection about work and career among African American women recovering from chemical dependency. The women in recovery were able to contemplate how these successful women came to their positions of success by overcoming barriers created by social disadvantage, racism, and sexism. But mere exposure to successful role models is not sufficient to enhance self-efficacy. It is important to offer opportunities for people with disabilities to reflect on the lives of these role models and to identify how these people inspire them to action. Inspiration can instill hope and motivation. And, contemplating how people who faced immense odds overcame challenging barriers can be a practical source of instruction to individuals who must overcome serious barriers if they are to develop careers.

Performance Accomplishments

A second source of self-efficacy involves the illumination of performance accomplishments by mustering evidence of personal ability, competence, interest, passion, and achievement. People with disabilities can face many issues that can increase learned helplessness and despair. One natural consequence of these issues is that people with disabilities may come to view themselves as inept or as unable to perform effectively within particular roles and, as a result, they likely lower their expectations for success. In terms of career development strategy, it is important to assess from a strengths perspective the accomplishments of people with disabilities across many life domains amplifying what individuals do well and noting what activities they invest time and energy in. This process of appraisal and appreciation is important given the idea that careers are holistic and encompass a range of life domains. Some important activities that a narrow focus on work and employment can overlook involve performance accomplishments in caring for others, caring for animals, investing time in understanding music, cultural and ethnic interests, culinary activity, singing, involvement in social action campaigns, and artistic expression with paint, textiles, clay, or other media.

A former client of one of the authors expressed a strong interest in acrylic painting but possessed no formal art education. Indeed, he felt that formal training would merely dampen his enthusiasm for his artwork. Nonetheless, he invested considerable effort in his artistic expression, converted his apartment into a studio, studied the lives of artists such as Pollack, and experimented with different ways of expressing his childhood memories. Since he had few friends and no family members the client was unable to share this activity with others who could potentially mentor him. One day he revealed his portfolio to a psychiatrist after she noted that his disability prevented him from entering a viable career.

What was interesting about this client is that he was unaware of the cultural movement in which he was engaged. When he discovered the world of "outsider art" he found an affinity group of other artists who were not formally trained. He discovered that his paintings on cardboard, particle board, and bark reflected a genre of contemporary art that was expanding nationally and within many localities.

The author worked with the client as an aspiring artist. The client assembled specific products that served as evidence of his performance accomplishments and prepared written narratives for each artistic product. With the assistance of a university student, he prepared a video of his apartment studio and workshop in which he served as the narrator of his collected works.

It was happenstance that brought this client into the world of art. But he came to view it as a career and wisely he separated his career intentions and expectations from his strategy to secure income. He was able to put together a minimal but adequate income from several different sources and did not look to his art as a source of income. Instead, he viewed his art as his career, and as an expression of his personal journey through life.

Identification of performance accomplishments can begin with an exploration of what occurs in a person's life and how a person spends his or her time during the course of a day. It can incorporate an inventory of tangible evidence of performances and accomplishments that the individual values and result in a collection of this evidence into the format of a portfolio (Washington & Moxley, 2001b).

The portfolio itself is a compendium of performance accomplishments and offers people a tool useful in defining themselves using interests, accomplishments, and/or social role (e.g., artist). The mental health or rehabilitation professional can work with the person to identify overarching narratives or themes that infuse this collection with personal meaning. Themes can be creatively cast to help the person to find career relevance in what they may have once taken for granted. Portfolios can help people to define themselves as, for example, artists, poets, cooks, childcare workers, scholars, entertainers, or social activists.

Verbal Persuasion

The third source of self-efficacy is designed to facilitate movement or action in the clarification of career identity, intentions, and expectations. The use of verbal persuasion can counteract diminished motivation to engage new experiences, to approach people for fear of rejection, and to think about new possibilities. Verbal persuasion is important because people may settle for their current circumstances even though their situations may be unproductive, produce little personal satisfaction, or even create serious harm. Most people find change to be anxiety-provoking and may resist undertaking any activity that can threaten the status quo.

The mental health or rehabilitation professional that engages in verbal persuasion is not telling a person what to do. The professional does not seek to diminish the person's autonomy or lower his or her self-determination. Verbal persuasion involves encouragement, support, and perhaps even specific suggestions for action. The professional may suggest that a person move forward in enrolling in an adult education course on, for example, commercial meal preparation. Verbal persuasion that follows from vicarious experiences and an appreciation of performance accomplishments can set the stage for a person to consider acting on a direction he or she chooses that may prove quite relevant to a subsequent career path.

The client who identified with outsider art was reluctant to undertake actions that would help him come to understand his artistic activity as a potential career. He was reluctant initially to explore outsider art, but the author worked with him to identify relevant role models and to catalog the work of these role models in a scrapbook. The mental health worker suggested that he then locate studios within the city that featured the work of outsider artists and to visit these. At first the client was reluctant to engage in this activity. He was concerned that they would find his work lacking. The mental health professional brought information about these studios into the career development sessions and after exploring this material the client/artist decided to visit three studios to explore the work of other artists. Subsequent sessions were devoted to persuading the client/artist to introduce himself to the gallery owners, to share his portfolio with them, and to ask them to introduce him to other artists. These activities provoked considerable anxiety but as the client/artist resolved each challenge a new identity slowly took root.

Emotional Arousal

The fourth source of self-efficacy is reflected in the narrative of the client/artist. Emotional arousal involves helping people to become aware of their feelings, which can move them to act. The client/artist confronted considerable anxiety but at the same time he experienced considerable excitement about defining himself as an outsider artist and sharing his work and new found sense of self with others. These two feeling states interacted early in the individual's process of career development. The motivation to avoid the new situation and its career potential was simply stronger than the motivation to approach the new situation.

Although he found the prospect of sharing his work with others exciting, the idea of following through with this action was frightening, resulting in his unwillingness to take reasonable risk to define himself as an outsider artist. Exploration of these feelings and the excitement and fears they generated enabled the client/artist to reduce his anxiety about moving forward on a career path as an outsider artist. The positive emotional arousal became dominant and he chose to undertake those actions that would enable him to actuate an identity as an artist. In other words, the feeling of excitement and the anticipation it created helped him to internalize new intentions—for example, he was willing to visit art studios. New intentions then came to the fore, such as introducing himself to studio owners and sharing his portfolio with these owners. All of his actions aroused positive and negative feelings and fostered some ambivalence, something the client learned to avoid since in the past he often experienced failure.

Emotional arousal often involves approach and avoidance and positive and negative feelings. The negative feelings can be used as signals for a coming change in career intentions and expectations. Washington and Moxley (2001a), for example, show how African American women in recovery from chemical dependency use prayers as a means to reconcile positive and negative feelings. One theme that dominated the prayers of these women involved the return of their children from foster care and subsequent engagement in positive and nurturing parenting of their children. The vision of a "good parent" was embedded in the prayer among many negative feelings about having lost their children as a result of their addictions, anger toward the child welfare system for taking away their children, and grief at having lost their parenting roles. Exploring these prayers enabled the women to reconcile these feelings and to begin to focus on their vision of themselves as good parents.

Emotional arousal can involve the awareness of how negative and positive feelings coincide in many situations, reconciliation of the negative feelings, and emergence of the positive feelings as dominant ones in the awareness of the individual. It is likely that as positive feelings become more dominant emotional arousal leads to action in relation to forward movement in the process of career development.

CONCLUSION

The incorporation of these four sources of self-efficacy into the process of career development does not occur in a linear fashion. Indeed, they likely are used together at different times to facilitate planned career development through career exploration, the formation of career intentions, the execution of these intentions, and the formation of self-knowledge relevant to strengthening vocational identity. They can be used during the process of career development counseling to increase readiness to engage in career exploration and during later stages of counseling to sustain career development activities.

These four sources also serve as a heuristic relevant to addressing the happenstance and serendipity of career development. Mental health or rehabilitation professionals working with their clients on career development can assess whether there are imbedded in novel events vicarious experiences or role models to which clients can compare themselves productively. They can reflect on the extent to which novel situations arouse the emotions of clients and move them to act, and create opportunities for supportive persuasion. And they can reflect on whether seemingly novel events are relevant to clients' previous performance accomplishments and to the themes and scope of their portfolios.

These four sources of self-efficacy are undertaken as specific strategies relevant to resolving a number of the career issues people with disabilities face. Practitioners should evaluate the extent to which these strategies influence the formation of maturity and contribute to personal flexibility. These are the assets rehabilitation and mental health professionals want to help their clients acquire so that they are resilient in the face of changing and dynamic careers.

The idea that career development is strategic suggests that the mental health or rehabilitation counselor and client are working jointly on a set of projects that reveal career as the integration of the client's vocational identity, intrinsic motivation, purpose, and search for meaning (Young, Valach, & Collin, 1996). It is appropriate then that a portfolio serves as the integrative tool of strategic career development. The portfolio offers an opportunity to the client to construct his or her own sense of vocation in conjunction with the practitioner and to assemble and interpret in narrative form those accomplishments, performances, products, and artifacts that taken together form the meaning of career or vocation to the client. So, the purpose of the portfolio is integrative because strategic career development is integrative. Ultimately, strategic career development is measured by the extent to which it enables people with disabilities to find meaning and purpose in their lives and is not measured by the extent to which people accomplish goals, undertake activities, or fulfill career development plans.

REFERENCES

Abbott, A. (1988). *The system of professions: An essay on the division of expert labor.* Chicago, IL: University of Chicago Press.

Appelbaum, E., & Batt, R. (1994). *The new American workplace: Transforming work systems in the United States.* Ithaca, NY: Cornell University Press.

Bandura, A. (1977). Self-efficacy: Toward a unifying theory of behavioral change. *Psychological Review, 84,* 191–215.

Bandura, A. (1997). *Self-efficacy: The exercise of control.* New York, NY: W. H. Freeman.

Becker, H. S., & Strauss, A. L. (1956). Careers, personality, and adult socialization. *American Journal of Sociology, 57,* 470–477.

Benz, N. R., & Halpern, A. S. (1993). Vocational and transition services needed and received by students with disabilities during their last year of high school. *Career Development for Exceptional Individuals, 16,* 197–211.

Crites, J. O. (1981). *Career counseling: Models, methods, and materials.* New York, NY: McGraw-Hill.

Dubois, D. D. (2000). The seven stages of one's career. *Training & Development, 54,* 45.

Ginzberg, E., Ginsburg, S., Axelrod, S., & Herma, J. (1951). *Occupational choice: An approach to a general theory.* New York, NY: Columbia University Press.

Herr, E. L. (1993). Contexts of and influences on the need for personal flexibility for the 21st century, Part II. *Canadian Journal of Counselling, 27,* 219–235.

Holland, J. L. (1959). A theory of vocational choice. *Journal of Counseling Psychology, 6,* 35–44.

Holland, J. L. (1973). *Making vocational choices: A theory of careers.* Englewood Cliffs, NJ: Prentice-Hall.

Krumboltz, J. D. (1994). Improving career development theory from a social learning perspective. In M. L. Savickas & R. W. Lent (Eds.), *Convergence in career development theories* (pp. 9–32). Palo Alto, CA: Consulting Psychologists Press.

Lent, R., Brown, S., & Hackett, G. (1994). Toward a unifying social cognitive theory of career and academic interest, choice, and performance. *Journal of Vocational Behavior, 45,* 79–122.

Lent, R., Hackett, G., & Brown, S. (1996). A social cognitive framework for studying career choice and transition to work. *Journal of Vocational Education Research, 21,* 3–31.

Liptak, J. (2001). *Treatment planning in career counseling.* Belmont, CA: Wadsworth.

Mamo, L., & Mueller, M. (2000). Changes in medicine, changes in nursing: Career contingencies and the movement of nurses into clinical trial coordination. *Sociological Perspectives, 43*(4), S43.

Miller-Tiedeman, A. L., & Tiedeman, D. V. (1990). Career decision making: Individualistic perspective. In D. Brown, L. Brooks, & Associates (Eds.), *Career choice and development* (2nd ed., pp. 308–337). San Francisco, CA: Jossey-Bass.

Mitchell, K., Krumboltz, J., & Levin, A. (1999). Planned happenstance: Constructing unexpected career opportunities. *Journal of Counseling and Development, 77,* 115–122.

Mowbray, C., Moxley, D., & Collins, M. E. (1998). Consumers as mental health providers: First person accounts of benefits and limitations. *The Journal of Behavioral Health Services and Research, 25*(4), 397–411.

Mowbray, C., Moxley, D., Jasper, C., & Howell, L. (Eds.) (1997, April). *Consumers as providers in psychiatric rehabilitation.* Baltimore, MD: International Association of Psychosocial Rehabilitation Services.

Ochs, L. A., & Roessler, R. T. (2001). Students with disabilities: How ready are they for the 21st century? *Rehabilitation Counseling Bulletin, 44,* 170.

Roe, A. (1957). Early determinants of vocational choice. *Journal of Counseling Psychology, 4,* 212–221.

Rojewski, J. W. (1993). Theoretical structure of career maturity for rural adolescents with learning disabilities. *Career Development for Exceptional Individuals, 16,* 39–52.

Sears, S. (1982). A definition of career guidance terms: A National Vocational Guidance Association perspective. *Vocational Guidance Quarterly, 31*(2), 137–143.

Sharf, R. S. (1997). *Applying career development theory to counseling.* Pacific Grove, CA: Brooks/Cole.

Super, D. E. (1951). Vocational adjustment: Implementing a self-concept. *Occupations, 10,* 88–92.

Super, D. E. (1963). *Career development: Self concept theory.* New York, NY: The College Entrance Examination Board.

Super, D. E. (1990). A life-span, life-space approach to career development. In D. Brown, L. Brooks, & Associates (Eds.), *Career choice and development* (2nd ed., pp. 197–261). San Francisco, CA: Jossey-Bass.

Super, D. E. (1994). A life-span, life-space perspective on convergence. In M. L. Savickas & R. W. Lent (Eds.), *Convergence in career development theories* (pp. 63–71). Palo Alto, CA: Consulting Psychologists Press.

Tiedeman, D. V. (1961). Decision and vocational development: A paradigm and its implications. *Personnel and Guidance Journal, 40,* 15–21.

Washington, O. G. M., & Moxley, D. P. (2001a). The use of prayer in group work with African American women recovering from chemical dependency. *Families in Society, 82*, 49–59.

Washington, O. G. M., & Moxley, D. P. (2001b). The use of scrapbooks and portfolios in recovery-based group work with chemically dependent women. Manuscript submitted for publication.

Washington, O. G. M., & Moxley, D. P. (2001c). Promising group work practices to empower women coping with chemical dependency. *American Journal of Orthopsychiatry, 73*(1), 109–121.

Wehmeyer, M. L. (1993). Perceptual and psychological factors in career decision-making of adolescents with and without cognitive disabilities. *Career Development for Exceptional Individuals, 16*, 135–146.

Wiener, C. (1991). Arenas and careers: The complex interweaving of personal and organizational destiny. In D. Maines (Ed.), *Social organization and social process: Essays in honor of Anselm Strauss* (pp. 175–187). New York, NY: Aldine de Gruyter.

Wilson, J. (1996). *When work disappears: The world of the new urban poor*. New York, NY: Knopf.

Yost, E. B., & Corbishley, M. (1987). *Career counseling: A psychological approach*. San Francisco, CA: Jossey-Bass.

Young, R. A., Valach, L., & Collin, A. (1996). A contextual evaluation of career. In D. Brown, L. Brooks, and Associates (Eds.), *Career choice and development* (3rd ed., pp. 477–512). San Francisco, CA: Jossey-Bass.

SERVICE ROLES AND CONTEXTS IN REHABILITATION AND MENTAL HEALTH PRACTICE

A number of institutional roles and contexts are involved in both rehabilitation and mental health in facilitating the vocational development and subsequent employment of persons coping with a range of disabilities. The four chapters comprising this section focus on these roles and contexts and how they influence the vocational development and employment of service recipients. Taken together these chapters make a statement about how contemporary human service systems are focusing on the employment of the people they serve.

In Chapter 8 entitled "The Role of Vocational Rehabilitation Counselors in Mental Health Services," Garske examines the role of the rehabilitation counselor in the provision of services to people coping with serious mental illness. The author's rich and extensive background in this area makes him well qualified to consider the kinds of attitudes, knowledge, and skills rehabilitation counselors require to facilitate the employment success of people dealing with psychiatric disabilities. He underscores how vocational rehabilitation counselors, with their focus on employment, can make significant contributions to the advancement of mental health service delivery. Within the subtext of Garske's chapter is the idea that work serves a fundamental role in a person's achievement of sound mental health and, as a consequence, the involvement of rehabilitation counselors in mental health service delivery cannot be ignored or discounted.

The authors of Chapter 9, "The Role of Mental Health Professionals in Responding to Employment Needs," underscore how mental health professionals can respond to the employment needs of the people they serve. Thus, we learn from this chapter that employment is not isolated to the domain of rehabilitation. Chapters 8 and 9 suggest that mental health professionals and rehabilitation personnel constitute "two sides of the coin." Joseph and Margaret Walsh help us to understand how the various professionals involved in the provision of mental health services can address work and the consequences it creates for people who receive these services. They show how mental health professionals can help people to sustain employment through seven strategies that facilitate the achievement of employment outcomes by the people they serve.

Chapters 10 and 11 focus on two major service systems: state rehabilitation authorities, and state and local mental health authorities. Both systems focus on the facilitation of employment among people coping with disabilities, yet they likely vary in their motivations to address employment. State rehabilitation authorities have a specific Federal mandate in this area under the Rehabilitation Act, while local mental health authorities increasingly address the facilitation of vocational development and employment for at least two reasons. First, because employment is essential to the mental health of people who are coping with serious mental illness and, second, because advocates, recipients, and enlightened professionals are concerned with the relative low rates of participation of people with psychiatric disabilities in employment. Ultimately, rehabilitation and mental health providers, and recipients and their advocates, understand that employment is a fundamental aspect of, if not an essential contributor to, anyone's quality of life.

In Chapter 10, Fabian and her colleagues offer specific ideas about how state rehabilitation authorities are seeking to improve employment outcomes among people with psychiatric disabilities and the authors give readers a sense of the strategies and tools these systems can use to improve these outcomes. In Chapter 11, Knisley and her colleagues address how state and local mental health authorities are trying a variety of strategies to create vocational development and employment opportunities.

Together the chapters of Section II can foster the reader's reflection on how to integrate rehabilitation and mental health services within the roles of various professionals and within state and local service systems. Ultimately, it is rehabilitation and mental health professionals working together with recipients that will make the achievement of employment outcomes not only a possibility but also a reality.

CHAPTER 8

The Role of Vocational Rehabilitation Counselors in Mental Health Services

Gregory G. Garske

The 1992 amendments to the Rehabilitation Act called for the state–federal vocational rehabilitation system to give emphasis to individuals with the most severe disabilities, that is, disabilities that significantly limit one or more life functions. Within this group of persons with severe disabilities are persons who have a psychiatric disability that impairs their functioning in obtaining employment (Finch & Wheaton, 1999). While this legislation is welcome, the mandate is not necessarily new. The Vocational Rehabilitation Amendments of 1943, referred to as the Barden–LaFollette Act, extended state vocational rehabilitation services from serving only persons with physical disabilities to serving persons with mental retardation and mental illness. Unfortunately, when compared with persons with other disabilities, persons with severe mental illness (SMI) have extremely low rehabilitation success rates (Marshak, Bostick, & Turton, 1990).

Around the turn of the century, an estimated 4 to 5 million adults in the United States were considered to have a serious mental illness. Although some gains have been made in service provision for individuals with SMI, the increasing number of individuals with severe and life-long psychiatric disabilities continues to challenge rehabilitation professionals (Garske, 1999). The public vocational rehabilitation (VR) program provides services to an estimated 175,000 persons a year who are identified as seriously and persistently mentally ill (Kaye, 1998). According to MacDonald-Wilson, Revell, Jr, Nguyen, and Peterson (1991), vocational rehabilitation programs have demonstrated limited success for people with psychiatric disability, considering that this population represents the next-to-the-largest category of disability served by the state–federal VR system.

Individuals with severe mental illness may experience deficits in social skills and interpersonal situations, personal management, symptom management, cognition, and coping with stress (Bond, 1995; Corrigan, Rao, & Lam, 1999). While such individuals may possess the necessary functional competencies, educational qualifications, and have a strong desire to

Gregory G. Garske • Division of Intervention Services, Bowling Green State University, Bowling Green, Ohio.

work, many have not been successful in the labor market (Garske, 1999). While there appears to be a consensus among rehabilitation professionals that employment is an important part of life for persons with mental illness (VandenBoom & Lustig, 1997), estimates of unemployment for the working-age members of this population are at a rate of around 85% (National Institute on Disability and Rehabilitation Services, 1993). Even when persons with serious psychiatric disability seek vocational services, they have success rates of only about half of those with physical disabilities (Marshak et al., 1990).

SIGNIFICANCE OF WORK

The pursuit of meaningful work is increasingly a goal for persons with severe mental illness. Like other Americans, people with psychiatric impairments wish to lead normal lives and view work as a signifier of normal adult life (Becker & Drake, 1994). In Western culture, work is highly valued and is considered a socially integrating force. However, many persons with severe psychiatric disabilities are excluded from the world of work (Ahrens, Frey, & Burke, 1999).

Employment can be a normalizing factor. Individuals who are unemployed and lack alternative societal roles are often stigmatized. Through work, individuals can obtain daily structure and may also develop a network of interpersonal contacts (Bond, Drake, & Becker, 1998). Involvement in work can help combat negative symptoms by providing a constructive alternative to a passive lifestyle. It may also facilitate a higher self-esteem and perceived quality of life (VanDongen, 1996). According to Rogers (1951), an individual's self-concept, values, feelings, and self-worth guide his or her behavior.

Treadgold (1999) reminded us that prominent personality theorists have endorsed the importance of meaningful work in relation to personal growth and development. For example, Sigmund Freud suggested that a person's capacity to love and work can greatly influence healthy ego development and feeling of normalcy. According to Freud, work gives a person a secure place in a portion of reality, in the human community. Abraham Maslow believed that one's work could be considered a tangible expression of facilitating one's drive toward self-actualization. Similarly, Erik Erikson discussed work as a possible means of finding meaning in our lives. It is toward this end that we progress, as adults, through several stages of development. First, we gain a sense of identity, then intimacy, generativity, and finally integrity. Consequently, persons with SMI, who either did not have critical developmental opportunities as children, or for whom the developmental tasks of their childhood and youth may no longer be relevant, need to be exposed to similar opportunities to develop or redevelop a vocational personality (Fabian, 1999).

OBSTACLES TO EMPLOYMENT

People with severe psychiatric disabilities face a multitude of barriers to vocational rehabilitation and meaningful employment. The movement to integrate people with SMI is still a relatively new vocational rehabilitation initiative. Vocational rehabilitation for people with serious mental disorders was not an issue prior to deinstitutionalization. People with mental illness spent much of their lives on back wards in state hospitals or in back rooms at home, and the concept or possibility of rehabilitation was never considered. It was not until antipsychotic medications became available to control some of the symptoms of these illnesses, and patients were emptied out of the hospitals, that it became apparent that many people with even very serious mental illnesses can learn work skills and seek and retain jobs (Torrey, Erdman, Wolfe, & Flynn, 1990). Even with these major treatment breakthroughs, barriers continue to exist. Issues of dysfunction, disability, and disadvantage are more often more difficult than the actual impairments. An inability to perform valued tasks and roles, and the resultant loss of self-esteem, remain as significant barriers to recovery. The barriers caused by being categorized as "mentally ill" can be overwhelming (Anthony, Cohen, & Farkas, 1990). The barriers to employment for people with severe mental disorders include societal stigmatic attitudes of professionals, family members, consumers, and employers; economic incentives of social insurance programs (e.g., Supplemental Security Income, Social Security Disability Insurance, Medicaid, and Medicare); lack of access to vocational services; and services that emphasize assessment and prevocational goals rather than competitive employment and following supports (Bond & McDonel, 1991).

Stigmatization appears to play a major role in limiting the vocational success rates of persons with severe mental illness. At the heart of the problem is the old belief that severe impacts of mental illness limit the employment prospects of people with psychiatric disabilities (National Institute on Disability and Rehabilitation Services, 1993). According to Mechanic (1996), stigmatization of people with mental illness has been a pervasive problem. In resource-constrained programs, staff often prefer to work with those less ill and those who seem to offer greater promise of substantial improvement. There is a long legacy of neglect of those most in need, in part because they were devalued. In fact, mental health and vocational rehabilitation workers often unwittingly reinforce stigma through their interactions with clients by holding faulty ideas about the nature of the disability, by perpetuating negative stereotypes by expecting clients to conform to dictated treatment and dependency roles, and by using unskilled jobs inappropriately (Garske & Stewart, 1999). For example, vocational workers often limit vocational placements to the so-called four F's: food, flowers, folding, and filth (referring to the stereotypical entry-level positions often offered to clients with long-term mental illness: food service, gardening, laundry or clerical work, and janitorial services). The handicapping effects of stigma may often be more powerful than the disability itself (National Institute on Disability and Rehabilitation Services, 1993). Hence, stigma can produce discrimination, loneliness, and loss of hope. Unlike persons with less stigmatizing physical disabilities, persons with psychiatric disabilities are often treated as less-than-human and incompetent. This maltreatment, combined with the effects of the illness, can lead to disconnectedness, spiritual crises, and disempowerment (Deegan, 1990).

Besides coping with the effects of stigmatic barriers, people with severe psychiatric disabilities experience a variety of psychosocial obstacles in every day functioning. Some common limitations are: (1) difficulties with interpersonal situations, including the most basic ones (greeting a friend on the street, paying for a purchase in a store); (2) problems coping with stress (including minor hassles, such as finding an item in a store); and (3) difficulty concentrating, and lack of energy or initiative (Bond, 1995).

To help people with severe mental illnesses become and remain contributing members of society, rehabilitation, vocational training, and assistance in work settings are essential. Major obstacles to employment of individuals with severe mental illnesses result from the individual's lack of currently marketable skills. Additional problems may stem from negative interactions with coworkers and supervisors who may lack information about the nature of mental illnesses and the person's strengths and limitations (Task Force on the Homeless and Severe Mental Illness, 1992). It may be that the VR agency is attempting to achieve results with clients with severe psychiatric disabilities by using methods that do not compensate for their clients' unique characteristics. For this reason, clients with severe psychiatric disabilities may create havoc within the structure of the agency and increase daily pressures on the rehabilitation counselor. Still, while the involvement of rehabilitation counselors in psychiatric rehabilitation may prove to be stressful, their involvement seems both appropriate and necessary (Garske, 1992).

PSYCHIATRIC REHABILITATION APPROACH

Definitions of rehabilitation essentially converge around the idea that the client should achieve the best life adjustment in his or her environment. It appears that rehabilitation professionals have little difficulty in understanding this concept in relation to physical disability, yet many rehabilitationists do not understand what is involved in the principles and practices of psychiatric rehabilitation (Anthony, 1991). While there are obvious differences between the two treatment approaches, the psychiatric rehabilitation approach is based on a rehabilitation model, the same model of impairment–disability–handicap that underlies the field of physical rehabilitation (Rogers, Anthony, & Jansen, 1991). According to Bond (1995), psychiatric rehabilitation provides individuals with psychiatric disabilities the opportunity to work, live in the community, and enjoy a social life, at their own pace, through planned experiences in a respectful, supportive, and realistic atmosphere. Psychiatric rehabilitation typically involves helping individuals gain or improve the skills and obtain the resources and support they require to attain their goals. The mission of psychiatric rehabilitation as defined by Anthony et al. (1990) is to assist persons with long-term psychiatric disabilities to increase their functioning so that they are successful and satisfied in the environments of their choice with the least amount of ongoing professional intervention. The process by which this mission can be achieved includes developing individuals' skills and/or developing more supports in their environments; in other words, helping people to change and/or change their living, learning, or working environments (Anthony, 1991). Psychiatric rehabilitation practice is guided by the basic philosophy of rehabilitation in that people with disabilities require skills and environmental supports to fulfill the role demands of their living, learning, social, and working environments (Anthony et al., 1990). According to Lamb (1988), no part of this work is more important than giving these clients a source of mastery over their internal drives, their symptoms, and the demands of their environment.

Traditionally, medication and psychotherapy were the two major treatment approaches, with little attention given to preventing or reducing functional limitations or handicaps to social performance. According to the Task Force on the Homeless and Severe Mental Illness (1992), community treatment of the person who is severely psychiatrically impaired should focus on the teaching of those coping skills necessary to live as independently as possible in his or her community. It is the presence or absence of such skills, rather than symptoms, that is the determining factor related to rehabilitation outcome. Psychosocial programs must encompass the development or relearning of skills and competencies required for successful interpersonal and social functioning as well as those needed for specific vocational pursuits. Psychosocial programs may provide training in activities of daily living, such as cooking, shopping, housekeeping, and budgeting. Whatever diagnostic category these individuals may fit into, or whatever specific mental symptom they manifest, they are all characterized by a relative inability to master age-appropriate tasks. Therefore, the individual's functional impairment may result in the inability to live independently and to sustain gainful employment and the neglect of personal hygiene and health needs. Consequently, individuals may experience a breakdown in social support systems, and, in extreme cases, even an inability to provide for basic nutrition and emergent medical problems.

According to Anthony et al. (1990), the preferred method of increasing a client's skills or abilities is a skills-training approach. In such an approach, the intent of the rehabilitation diagnosis, as opposed to the traditional psychiatric diagnosis, is to identify those specific client skill deficits that are preventing the person from functioning more effectively in his or her living, learning, and/or work community. For clients with skill deficits, despite a high degree of motivation for employment, a referral to traditional vocational rehabilitation programs may contribute to a negative experience and may reduce their motivation for future work. Therefore, a thorough assessment of individual client needs may be necessary in order to make a successful work referral (Braitman et al., 1995).

Two primary strategies emphasized in state-of-the-art rehabilitation efforts with people who have mental illness include the strengthening of client skills and competencies and strengthening environmental supports. Psychiatric rehabilitation practice should be guided by the basic philosophy of rehabilitation; that is, persons with disabilities require skills and environmental supports to fulfill the role demands of various living, learning, and working environments (Rogers et al., 1991). Highly endorsed client skill strengthening approaches involve social and independent living skills training, symptom management, and job-finding clubs. Environmental support strengthening approaches identified as critical include family behavior management and the use of peer groups in the transition to community living. Finally, supported employment was cited as a critical service component which places equal emphasis on both the strengthening of client skills and competencies and environmental supports.

From a rehabilitation counselor's point of view, it is understandable that a major focus of rehabilitation may be primarily on improving vocational outcomes for people with severe psychiatric disabilities. However, clients who have poor social skills and no peer relationships and who are unable to adjust to community living need more than vocational counseling services. Many clients require comprehensive services dealing with a variety of psychosocial and emotional issues before they can focus effectively on vocational issues.

PSYCHIATRIC REHABILITATION MODELS

A possible misconception about psychiatric rehabilitation services is that they are provided through highly structured procedures within mental health centers, sheltered workshops, group homes, hospitals, and other such settings. While some services may fit this description, the locations where rehabilitation may take place are endless. Community settings may include clients' homes, places of employment, grocery stores, laundromats, and parks (Bond, 1995).

Among the many psychiatric rehabilitation models in current practice, the clubhouse model and the community support system (CSS) model deserve special attention. According to Bond (1995), the clubhouse model is a comprehensive group approach that focuses on practical issues in informal settings. Clubhouses offer vocational opportunities, housing, problem-solving groups, case management, recreational activities, and academic preparation. The centerpiece of the clubhouse model is transitional employment (TE). Developed at the Fountain House in New York, TE was originally developed as an integral part of the clubhouse approach. Clubhouse programs address the basic needs of members for housing, recreation, and social support (Bond & McDonel, 1991). Clients, or members, as they are

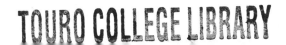

called, are placed in part-time, entry-level positions, usually for three to nine months and are supervised by the psychosocial rehabilitation center. A TE program is designed to develop a client's self-confidence, job references, and work habits necessary to secure permanent employment (Anthony et al., 1990). The clubhouse model is a well-defined model with a strong national network. According to Bond, only a few studies have evaluated the effectiveness of clubhouse approaches, especially for individuals who are motivated to pursue community employment and who enjoy group activities.

The CSS initiative was begun in 1977 by the National Institute of Mental Health (NIMH). The intent was to assist states and communities in developing the broad array of services that comprise the CSS. This initiative eventually became known as the NIMH Community Support Program (CSP) with case management as one of the essential CSS services (Anthony et al., 1990). One of the leading models of case management is the assertive community treatment (ACT) approach that works with clients on an individual basis, mostly in clients' homes and neighborhoods rather than in offices. According to Bond (1995), the ACT programs are staffed by a group of professionals who work as a treatment team in the community. ACT was first developed in Madison, Wisconsin, and has spread throughout the United States, especially in the Midwest (Bond & McDonel, 1991). The ACT team keeps in frequent contact with clients and helps with things such as budgeting money, shopping, finding housing, taking medication, finding jobs, and problem-solving difficulties on the job. Community treatment of persons with severe mental disabilities focuses primarily on the teaching of basic coping skills necessary to live and function as autonomously as possible in the community. These coping skills consist of activities of daily living skills, vocational skills, leisure time skills, and social or interpersonal skills (Bond, 1995). The emphasis on social skills and social skills training has received considerable attention in the field of psychiatric rehabilitation in the past two decades. For example, Tsang and Pearson (1996) noted how psychiatric patients, especially those with schizophrenia, have significant deficits in social skills and social performance. They are often unable to find competitive work, or if they secure a job, may lose it because of poor interpersonal skills (Corrigan, Reedy, Thadani, & Ganet, 1995). Characteristics of the ACT approach make it distinctive. The first characteristic is assertive outreach in which staff initiate contacts rather than depending on clients to keep appointments. A second characteristic of ACT is its emphasis on continuity and consistency. Finally, ACT programs combine treatment and rehabilitation in a comprehensive and interdisciplinary approach (Bond, 1995). According to Fischler and Booth (1999), an interdisciplinary team approach, including a vocational rehabilitation professional, a psychologist, a workplace supervisor or human resources representative, and perhaps a social worker, psychiatric nurse, psychiatrist, or other helping professional familiar with the situation, is invaluable.

VR COUNSELOR'S ROLE AND DILEMMA

Regardless of disability population, it can be concluded that the role of the rehabilitation counselor can be described as encompassing the following functions: client assessment; affective counseling; vocational counseling; case management; and job placement (Walker, 1995). The primary role of a qualified rehabilitation counselor is to work with clients who have various disabilities in order to help them develop or enhance the vocational skills required to secure gainful employment, the coping skills needed to achieve increased independence, or the other skills necessary to function in the community (The Foundation for Rehabilitation Education and Research, 1997).

For people experiencing physical disabilities, the methodology of the public rehabilitation agency is usually quite effective. The counselor collects information related to the client's disability and assesses his or her vocational goal. With the participation of the client, the services are smoothly coordinated, and the client often enters the labor force with a renewed sense of self-worth. However, this practice is too cursory to achieve rehabilitation with many clients who have severe psychiatric disabilities (Rogan, 1980). VR clients with severe mental illness present a variety of problematic challenges for the VR counselors. For example, unlike physical illnesses, severe mental illness presents no clear pattern of symptomology, etiology, diagnosis, treatment, cause, and prognosis. Fischler and Booth (1999) indicated that psychological and psychiatric disorders involving emotion, behavior, cognitive ability, and interpersonal skills present a unique set of challenges for employees, employers, and for professionals who work in the field of VR. According to Rutman (1994), the disabilities engendered by mental illness tend to produce symptoms affecting many major areas of functioning. As a result, persons with psychiatric disabilities interested in employment opportunities often require a broader range of services and supports than do persons with other disabilities.

The 1992 amendments to the Rehabilitation Act emphasized the primary of consumer choice and self-determination in the areas of selecting a job (Fabian, 1999). As people with disabilities are increasingly expected to assume control of the rehabilitation process, the role of the rehabilitation counselor must broaden to include educating clients, facilitating choice, and assisting in negotiations for needed services (Ford & Swett, 1999). The shared partnership with persons with SMI may become problematic due to motivation problems associated with their illness. Some individuals with psychiatric disabilities experience impairments (such as apathy/abolition and asocialty/anhedonia) as a result of their mental illness and subsequent medication (Braitman et al., 1995). Indeed, making vocational choices requiresa level of self-awareness and self-understanding that some persons with SMI may not have acquired or may have lost as a result of the effects of their illness (Fabian, 1999). Motivation may also be affected by poor vocational history (e.g., job loss, unsuccessful outcomes in vocational rehabilitation programs), social anxiety, or a fear of losing entitlements.

Counselors often express having inadequate resources and flexibility to serve clients with severe mental illness. One of the most difficult phases is the process of placement and vocational stability (Thomas, Thomas, & Joiner, 1993). For the public VR program, system barriers for effectively addressing the needs of individuals with SMI include the time-limited nature of service provision, the inflexibility of the system to respond to the cyclical nature of the disability, and the lack of collaborative strategies designed to ensure a partnership between community-based agencies and the VR counselor (Fabian, 1999).

While there are differences in state services, the VR system is defined in federal regulations, and every state's program follows the same basic service process. Across all state agencies the system is defined in terms of "statuses," or steps of the service process (McGurrin, 1994). A client is considered to be rehabilitated if he or she has maintained a vocational placement for 90 days. Clients who do succeed in retaining employment for 90 days and are assessed as no longer feasible for rehabilitation may also be closed. For many clients with physical disabilities, this system of VR counselor productivity and accountability may be practical. However, this goal-oriented and time-limited system seems inappropriate when used with persons with SMI. Hu and Jerrell (1998) noted that the primary hindrance to the effective and efficacious service delivery to consumers with mental illness is the conceptualization that consumers with mental illness should have their cases successfully closed. More specifically, this hindrance is based within the rubric that successful rehabilitation is determined by closing a case. Many counselors believe there should be a re-evaluation of program expectations regarding "successful closures" given the array of difficulties encountered by this unique client population. Given the opportunity, VR counselors would rather spend more counseling and support time with clients and job development than with employers (Thomas et al., 1993).

FUTURE CHALLENGES

Today, rehabilitation counselors are not only working in state VR agencies, but many are working in community mental health centers, psychiatric hospitals, community residential programs, supported employment programs, and community support programs. It is encouraging that the paradigm is changing and rehabilitation counselors are becoming proactive and learning to work with people with severe and life-long psychiatric disabilities. VR interventions have now become an integral part of the history and evolution of the psychiatric rehabilitation field (Anthony et al., 1990). However, while gains have been made in psychiatric rehabilitation programming, it appears that major challenges still exist (Garske, 1999). Based on current trends, it appears that qualified rehabilitation counselors will continue to be in demand to work with persons with severe psychiatric disabilities. In this case, it is recommended that graduate level rehabilitation counselor training programs assess the adequacy of their curricula regarding this specialized preparation (McReynolds, Garske, & Turpin, 1999). Psychiatric rehabilitation can be a complex and formidable task for the rehabilitation counselor. Individuals with SMI often struggle with a wide variety of challenges and needs which likewise challenge the rehabilitation counselor. Such challenges and needs can include assisting the person to learn social skills, interpersonal skills, coping skills, personal hygiene and self-care, as well as symptom and medication management (Corrigan et al., 1999). For a rehabilitation counselor, the task can seem daunting, especially if adequate training in the complexities and nuances of working with individuals with SMI has not been provided. Psychiatric rehabilitation professionals must have advanced training in an array of knowledge areas, including psychopathology, psychopharmacology, medical and psychosocial aspects of disabilities, vocational aspects of disabilities, assessment, intervention techniques, and community resource utilization (Chan et al., 1998). In agreement with Farkas and Anthony (1980), the goal of training rehabilitation professionals must flow from the goal of rehabilitation. In other words, the goal of training would be to have the potential psychiatric rehabilitation practitioner learn the knowledge, skills, and values necessary to effect positive client outcomes. The mastery of various conceptual components (knowledge), performance components (skills), and affective components (attitudes and values) is critical to the professional's efforts to increase client functioning and to reduce the client's dependence on the mental health system.

Regardless of the types of services provided to people with severe mental illness, a consensus exists among policy-makers, providers, clients and their families, and researchers that one of the most serious contemporary problems in the mental health field is the widespread fragmentation of mental health services (National Institute of Mental Health, 1991). Over the years, attempts have been made to make the service system for persons with SMI more rational, systematic, and integrated, but the service system remains largely a patchwork of settings, providers, policies, administrative sponsors, and founders. Despite the seeming plethora of care providers, the service system still suffers from severe problems of fragmentation, accessibility, and appropriateness (Torrey et al., 1990). Nationally, about one third of all VR offices are reported to have formal inter-agency collaboration agreements with one or more local mental health agencies (Katz, 1991). In response to this problem, vocational rehabilitation and mental health agencies are beginning to make progress. It was generally accepted in the late 1980s that the needs of persons with chronic and severe psychiatric disabilities extend well beyond the boundaries of any one system and require coordinated efforts with an array of health and human service agencies. According to Bybee, Mowbray, and McCrohan (1996), maintaining a separation between vocational and non-vocational services continues to foster a perception that the staff at VR and mental health agencies are working at cross-purposes. Owing to the complexities of severe mental illness, it would seem appropriate that future collaboration efforts be pursued.

REFERENCES

Ahrens, C. S., Frey, J. L., & Burke, S. C. (1999). An individualized job engagement and placement approach for persons with the most serious mental illness. *Journal of Rehabilitation, 65*(4), 17–23.

Anthony, W. A. (1991). Psychiatric rehabilitation. In R. P. Marinelli and A. E. Dell Orto (Eds.), *The psychological and social impact of disability*. New York, NY: Springer.

Anthony, W. A., Cohen, M., & Farkas, M. (1990). *Psychiatric rehabilitation*. Boston, MA: Center for Psychiatric Rehabilitation.

Becker, D. R., & Drake, R. E. (1994). Individual placement and support: A community mental health center approach to vocational rehabilitation. *Community Mental Health Journal, 30*, 193–206.

Bond, G. R. (1995). Psychiatric rehabilitation. In A. E. Dell Orto & R. P. Marinelli (Eds.), *Encyclopedia of Disability and Rehabilitation*. New York, NY: Macmillan.

Bond, G. R., Drake, R. E., & Becker, D. R. (1998). The role of social functioning in vocational rehabilitation. In K. T. Mueser & N. Tavrier (Eds.), *Handbook of social functioning in schizophrenia*. Needham Heights, MA: Allyn & Bacon.

Bond, G., & McDonel, E. (1991). Vocational rehabilitation outcomes for persons with psychiatric disabilities: An update. *Journal of Vocational Rehabilitation, 1*, 9–20.

Braitman, A., Counts, P., Avenport, R., Zurlinden, B., Roger, M., Clauss, J., Kulkami, A., Kymla, J., & Montgomery, L. (1995). Comparison of barriers to employment for unemployed and employed clients in a case management program: An exploratory study. *Psychiatric Rehabilitation Journal, 19*(1), 3–8.

Bybee, D., Mowbray, C. T., & McCrohan, N. M. (1996). Toward zero exclusion in vocational opportunities for persons with psychiatric disabilities: Prediction of service receipt in a hybrid vocational/case management service program. *Psychiatric Rehabilitation, 19*(4), 15–28.

Chan, F., Leahy, M. J., Chan, C., Lam, C., Hilburger, J., Jones, J., & Kamnetz, B. (1998). Training needs of rehabilitation counselors in the emerging mental health/managed care environment. *Rehabilitation Education, 12*, 333–345.

Corrigan, P. W., Rao, D., & Lam, C. (1999). Psychiatric rehabilitation. In F. Chan & M. Leahy (Eds.), *Health care and disability case management* (pp. 527–564). Lake Zurich, IL: Vocational Consultants Press.

Corrigan, P. W., Reedy, P., Thadani, D., & Ganet, M. (1995). Correlates of participation and completion in a job club for clients with psychiatric disability. *Rehabilitation Counseling Bulletin, 39*, 42–53.

Deegan, P. (1990). Spirit breaking: When the helping professions hurt. *The Humanistic Psychologist, 18*, 301–313.

Fabian, E. S. (1999). Rethinking work: The examples of consumers with serious mental health disorders. *Rehabilitation Counseling Bulletin, 41*(4), 302–316.

Farkas, M., & Anthony, W. A. (1980). Training rehabilitation counselors to work in state agencies, rehabilitation and mental health facilities. *Rehabilitation Counseling Bulletin, 24*, 128–1144.

Finch, J. R., & Wheaton, J. E. (1999). Patterns of services to vocational rehabilitation consumers with serious mental illness. *Rehabilitation Counseling Bulletin, 42*, 214–227.

Fischler, G., & Booth, N. (1999). *Vocational impact of psychiatric disorders: A guide for rehabilitation professionals*. Gaithersburg, MD: Aspen.

Ford, L. H., & Swett, E. A. (1999). Job placement and rehabilitation counselors in the state-federal system. *Rehabilitation Counseling Bulletin, 42*, 354–365.

Garske, G. G. (1992). Working with people who have severe psychiatric disabilities. *American Rehabilitation, 18*, 23–24, 36–37.

Garske, G. G. (1999). The challenge of rehabilitation counselors: Working with people with psychiatric disabilities. *Journal of Rehabilitation, 65,* 21–25.

Garske, G. G., & Stewart, J. R. (1999). Stigmatic and mythical thinking: Barriers to vocational rehabilitation services for persons with severe mental illness. *Journal of Rehabilitation, 65,* 4–8.

Hu, T. W., & Jerrell, J. M. (1998). Estimating the cost impact of three case management programmes for treating people with severe mental illness. *British Journal of Psychiatry, 173*(Suppl. 36), 26–32.

Katz, L. (1991). Interagency collaboration in rehabilitation of persons with psychiatric disabilities. *Journal of Vocational Rehabilitation, 1,* 45–57.

Kaye, H. S. (1998). *Vocational rehabilitation in the United States* (Disability statistics abstract No. 20). Washington, DC: Department of Education National Institute on Disability and Rehabilitation Research.

Lamb, H. R. (1988). One-to-one relationship with the long-term mentally ill: Issues in training professionals. *Community Mental Health Journal, 24,* 328–337.

MacDonald-Wilson, K. L., Revell, W. G., Nguyen, N., & Peterson, M. E. (1991). Supported employment outcomes for people with psychiatric disability: A comparative analysis. *Journal of Vocational Rehabilitation, 1,* 30–44.

Marshak, L. E., Bostick, D., & Turton, L. (1990). Closure outcomes for clients with psychiatric disabilities served by the vocational rehabilitation system. *Rehabilitation Counseling Bulletin, 33,* 247–250.

McGurrin, M. C. (1994). An overview of the effectiveness of traditional vocational rehabilitation services in the treatment of long-term mental illness. *Psychosocial Rehabilitation, 17*(3), 37–54.

McReynolds, C. J., Garske, G. G., & Turpin, J. D. (1999). Psychiatric rehabilitation: A survey of rehabilitation counseling education programs. *Journal of Rehabilitation, 65,* 45–49.

Mechanic, D. S. (1996). Key policy considerations for mental health in the managed care era. In R. W. Manderscheid & M. A. Sonnenschein (Eds.), *Mental health, United States, 1996* (Publication No. (SMA) 96-3098). Washington, DC: U.S. Government Printing Office, Superintendent of Documents.

National Institute of Mental Health (1991). *Caring for people with severe mental disorders: A national plan for research to improve services.* DHHS Pub. No. ADM 91–1762. Washington, DC: U.S. Government Printing Office.

National Institute on Disability and Rehabilitation Services (1993). Rehab brief: *Strategies to secure and maintain employment for people with long-term mental illnesses, 15*(10), 1–4.

Rogan, D. (1980). Implementing the rehabilitation approach in a state rehabilitation agency. *Rehabilitation Counseling Bulletin, 24,* 49–60.

Rogers, C. R. (1951). *Client-centered therapy: Its current practice, implications, and theory.* Boston, MA: Houghton Mifflin.

Rogers, E. A., Anthony, W., & Jansen, M. A. (1991). Psychiatric rehabilitation as the preferred response to the needs of individuals with severe psychiatric disability. In M. G. Eisenberg & R. L. Glueckauf (Eds.), *Empirical approaches to the psychosocial aspects of disability.* New York, NY: Springer.

Rutman, I. D. (1994). How psychiatric disability expresses itself as a barrier to employment. *Psychosocial Rehabilitation Journal, 17,* 15–35.

Task Force on the Homeless and Severe Mental Illness (1992). *Outcasts on Main Street* (DHHS Publication No. ADM 92-1904). Washington, DC: U.S. Government Printing Office.

The Foundation for Rehabilitation Education and Research (1997). *Rehabilitation counseling: The profession and standards of practice.* Rolling Meadows, IL: Author.

Thomas, T. D., Thomas, G., & Joiner, J. G. (1993). Issues in the vocational rehabilitation of persons with serious and persistent mental illness: A national survey of counselor insights. *Psychosocial Rehabilitation Journal, 16,* 129–134.

Torrey, E. F., Erdman, K., Wolfe, S. M., & Flynn, L. M. (1990). *Care of the seriously mentally ill: A rating of state programs* (3rd ed.). Washington, DC: Public Citizen Health Research and the Alliance for the Mentally Ill.

Treadgold, R. (1999). Transcendent vocations: Their relationship to stress, depression, and clarity of self-concept. *The Journal of Humanistic Psychology, 39,* 81–105.

Tsang, W. H., & Pearson, V. (1996). A conceptual framework for work-related social skills in psychiatric rehabilitation. *Journal of Rehabilitation, 62,* 61–67.

VandenBoom, D. C., & Lustig, D. C. (1997). The relationship between employment status and quality of life for individuals with severe and persistent mental illness. *Journal of Applied Rehabilitation Counseling, 28,* 4–8.

VanDongen, C. D. (1996). Quality of life and self-esteem in working and nonworking persons with mental illness. *Community Mental Health Journal, 32,* 535–548.

Walker, M. L. (1995). Rehabilitation counseling. In A. Dell Orto and R. P. Marinelli (Eds.), *The encyclopedia of disability and rehabilitation* (pp. 618–623). New York, NY: Macmillan.

CHAPTER 9

The Role of Mental Health Professionals in Responding to Employment Needs

JOSEPH WALSH AND MARGARET S. WALSH

In this chapter we present a set of assets that mental health professionals can offer in responding to the employment needs of the people they serve. These assets are presented as a framework that can guide practice and sensitize practitioners to their involvement in addressing the mental health consequences employment and work create, consequences created by the demands or absence of work. The authors consider the following seven topics: (1) developing the worker–client relationship; (2) assessing interpersonal problems that emerge on the job; (3) supporting vocational development and exploration in anticipation of establishing new career directions; (4) facilitating role transitions relating to employment; (5) fostering the management of stressors that are created through employment and work; (6) addressing the personal consequences of social and economic change; and (7) fostering personal development with implications for employment and work. For each of these topics, we include treatment approaches mental health professionals often use in practice.

The assets that mental health professionals provide derive from their holistic, bio-psychosocial approach to assessment and intervention with persons who face serious psychiatric challenges. This approach requires an appreciation of the recipient's functional status, conscious and unconscious motivations, latent capabilities, conflicted strivings for dependence and independence, and environments for living, learning, work, and playing (Kanter, 1989). With this clinical information mental health professionals provide interventions that will support the recipient's vocational activities and the work of the vocational counselor. We focus on what Roessler and Rubin (1992) call "affective counseling," which is directed at helping recipients deal with feelings about their disabilities and their concerns about participating in employment.

JOSEPH WALSH • Virginia Commonwealth University School of Social Work, Richmond, Virginia.
MARGARET S. WALSH • State Human Rights Director, Commonwealth of Virginia Department of Mental Health, Mental Retardation, and Substance Abuse Services, Richmond, Virginia.

PREDICTORS OF CLIENT SUCCESS

The deficits imposed by cognitive impairments related to serious psychiatric disability are well known. They include a slower processing of sensory information, difficulty selecting appropriate environmental stimuli for response, short-term memory problems, the inability to generalize from one situation to others, concentration problems, impairment of insight and judgment, and difficulty organizing and planning actions (Gerhart, 1990). The assets that mental health practitioners can provide must be framed in a context of known predictors of vocational success. Several recent studies have identified a variety of predictors.

Mowbray, Bybee, Harris, and McCrohan (1995) investigated the relationship of current work status and expectations for work to a variety of factors for 269 recipients in two case management agencies in Michigan. Predictors of work status included diagnosis (schizophrenia was a negative predictor), functional level, number of hospitalizations, and residential stability. Recipients' expectations for work were predicted by functional level, attitude toward work, and age. Bybee, Mowbray, and McCrohan (1996) studied another case management program in Michigan that included vocational specialists. The predictors of job placement among these 2,790 clients included age, education, employment history, work expectations, and the sense of work pride.

Braitman et al. (1995) studied still another case management program in Michigan to compare barriers to employment experienced by 129 unemployed and 50 employed recipients. They determined that motivation was essential to success, operationalized as positive attitudes, punctuality, the ability to accept criticism, being a self-starter, and the ability to concentrate. They added that barriers to motivation included adverse effects of medication, health problems, and fears of losing entitlements. In an exploratory study of 86 persons in a supported employment program in Baltimore, Regenold, Sherman, and Fenzel (1999) identified the importance of self-efficacy to vocational success, defined as the capacity to organize and execute a course of action.

Okpaku, Anderson, Sibulkin, Butler, and Bickman (1997) conducted an experimental study of the effects of case management on the job status of 152 social security applicants and beneficiaries in two states. They found that some recipients did not succeed in job placements because of fears of benefits losses, attitudes of dependency, self-esteem problems, aversion to risk-taking, and fears of failure. An ethnographic study of 13 recipients in one New Hampshire supported employment program identified predictors of work search and retention (Alverson, Alverson, Drake, & Becker, 1998). These factors included the valuing and maintaining of mental and physical functioning, participation in social groups (including family, friends, and groups in the volunteer setting or workplace), and an absence of material poverty.

In summary, the predictors of employment placement success that can be directly impacted by the work of mental health professionals include residential stability, overcoming fears about benefits losses, attitudes toward work, work expectations, a sense of work pride, habits of punctuality, self-esteem and self-efficacy, the ability and willingness to take risks, the ability to accept criticism, being a self-starter, proper management of medications, the valuing of mental and physical functioning, and participation in social groups.

DEVELOPING THE WORKER–CLIENT RELATIONSHIP

Persons with mental illness experience a process of social disengagement (Lantz & Belcher, 1988). With the onset of symptoms, the person becomes disassociated from others, as he or she can no longer interpret the external world as before. Careful efforts by others, including mental health professionals, to negotiate shared meanings of social and vocational situations with the client can increase the person's motivation and capacity to reconnect with the social world. As Scheff (1984) notes, people who receive the negative social label of mental illness may become frustrated in their attempts to return to conventional social roles when others (friends, family, employers, and even practitioners) are reluctant to relinquish negative stereotypes. The labeling of a person as having mental illness also is limiting if it denies the person's need to maintain a view of reality which, however distorted, represents his or her personal experience. Methods of intervention, which run counter to the recipient's view of the world, detract from the potential for professionals to deal constructively with his or her essential concerns.

The worker–client relationship provides a context for positive outcomes in all clinical situations (Sexton & Whiston, 1994). The working alliance, ideally established within the first three meetings, consists of a positive emotional bond between the parties, mutual comfort in their interactions, and an agreement on a course of action that will guide treatment and service provision. It develops in unpredictable ways from the expectations, beliefs, and knowledge that each person brings to the relationship. Horvath's (1994) literature review concluded that the quality of the working alliance was more predictive of positive outcomes in mental health counseling than any other variable.

A primary asset that mental health professionals can offer recipients is an empathy that characterizes all rehabilitative activities, vocational and otherwise. This goes beyond an attitude of caring to include an articulation of the expected roles of the recipient and significant others in all life situations. So, for example, a symptomatic person who begins a job may define the situation primarily as one in which he or she must manage the anxiety associated with hostile, intrusive hallucinatory voices he believes comes from coworkers, rather than one where certain levels of productivity through cooperation with coworkers must be maintained. If these differences are not explored, accepted, and mediated by the professional, that job opportunity is likely to fail.

The articulation of worker–client roles provides a framework in which the recipient's assumptions about the nature and extent of intervention can be understood. A lack of congruence between the client's and the worker's understanding of their mutual roles has been shown to be a significant factor in premature termination of treatment by recipients (Maluccio, 1979). Several authors have independently affirmed that positive clinical outcomes are enhanced when initial client–worker contacts are focused on a clear structuring of their mutual expectations and the client's orientation to the process of intervention (Fischer, 1978; Frank & Frank, 1993; Thomlinson, 1984). The importance of this procedure supports the integration of educational activities about the process of intervention in the early work stage (Germain & Gitterman, 1996). The mental health professional, through his or her involvement in all aspects of the client's life, can help the person understand the roles of the vocational counselor as well.

ASSESSING INTERPERSONAL PROBLEMS

Interpersonal problems on the job should be predictable for each recipient, as they will be similar to those that have been present in other areas of the person's life. The common symptoms of mental illness that give rise to interpersonal problems at work include alienation from one's feelings, a need for social isolation to ensure comfort, bizarre behaviors and thoughts, negative personality traits, poor hygiene, and suspiciousness or paranoia

(Blankertz & Robinson, 1996). Worksite characteristics that may affect the client's interpersonal behavior include the number of coworkers, amount of requisite public contact, physical and mental demands of the work, the gender of coworkers, and noise levels. The mental health professional must assess these characteristics prior to job placement, and advocate for an alternative placement if they appear severe enough to impede performance and jeopardize job success.

Before focusing on intervention with interpersonal problems that clients may experience in work settings, we present the concept of social support, defined as the interactions and relationships that provide a person with assistance or feelings of attachment to others (Hobfoll, Freedy, Lane, & Geller, 1990). Social support enhances physical health, mental health, and stress-coping capability (Bloom, 1990). It reinforces one's sense of identity, promotes an ordered worldview, ensures proper communication channels with the outside world, provides material help, and contains distress through reassurance (Caplan, 1990). Support may be material and emotional. The mental health professional's first responsibility to the client who embarks on employment activities is to plan for adequate social support in the workplace and elsewhere, as these will minimize the negative effects of interpersonal conflict.

The mental health professional must structure social supports for persons with psychiatric disabilities in unique ways. Their social networks, or people with whom they routinely interact, tend to include only from 5 to 15 people, or half the number found in general populations (Walsh, 1994). Smaller network sizes are partly the result of social skills deficits but also reflect a protective distancing, as many persons with mental illness function comfortably with comparatively low levels of stimulation. Additionally, interaction with a broad range of social network clusters (categories of persons such as family, friends, neighbors, school peers, coworkers, and church members) is adaptive. A range of clusters provides clients with a series of different social connections, some of which can provide assistance when others are not available.

Blankertz and Keller (1997) have outlined four types of supports, which all persons need for vocational success. These include intrapersonal supports (self-esteem and self-efficacy), interpersonal supports (the availability of supportive others), a range of network clusters, and person–worksite support. Marrone, Balzell, and Gold (1995) have articulated five elements of interpersonal support primarily in the workplace, including coworker support, training support, self-management support, organizational support, and personal network support (i.e., support away from the workplace).

Once an appropriate job match is obtained in conjunction with a vocational counselor, the mental health professional must anticipate interpersonal challenges that might occur at work and help the client plan for them. Examples include whom to interact and talk with (developing support networks), what to talk about, how much to say, whether to talk about the mental illness, how to manage disruptive thoughts, and how to solve interpersonal problems that can disrupt work performance. Frequently the recipient does not understand the culture of the work environment and so the professional can also address this through educational means.

The recipient's inability to generate, evaluate, and implement solutions on the job contributes to the occurrence and persistence of interpersonal problems. Problem-solving is a systematic intervention strategy provided by the mental health professional in which the client is helped to become a better problem-solver, particularly on the job (Hepworth, Rooney, & Larsen, 2002). The recipient expands his or her repertoire of problem-solving skills by increasing the number of alternatives for resolving a problem, and increasing the probability that an effective response will be selected from a pool of alternatives. The five steps of the procedure include an orientation of the recipient to the process, interpersonal problem formulation in concrete terms, compiling a list of alternatives for resolving a given problem, evaluating response alternatives, implementing a preferred alternative, and evaluating the outcome of the application.

Problem-solving can incorporate social skills training activities to help recipients develop and strengthen social behaviors for effective functioning in the workplace. Recipients with good social skills achieve higher self-esteem, form satisfactory social relationships, and are able to perform roles effectively to prevent or minimize vocational dysfunction. This skills-training process includes a series of steps similar to problem-solving. The worker presents the rationale for intervention, describes the skill to be mastered, identifies the components of the skill, models the skill, role-plays each component of the skill with the client, evaluates the role-play, and combines the elements of the skill into additional role-plays. The client applies the skill in real-life work situations, and later reviews outcomes with the professional. The worker should incorporate training in both the cognitive (knowledge about relationships and perceptual skills) and the behavioral aspects of relationships in skill training (self-presentation, social initiatives, conversational skills, maintenance skills, and conflict resolution skills).

SUPPORTING VOCATIONAL DEVELOPMENT AND EXPLORATION

Vocational intervention should not be pursued as a distinct activity. It is part of a holistic process of approach to a person's life goals which may include recovery from mental illness, reducing social isolation, managing depression, reducing boredom, and establishing a life structure (Torrey et al., 1990). Vocational development is maximized when the recipient's general interests are assessed, work is integrated into overall goals, professional supports are flexible, and assistance is rapid (Ridgway & Rapp, 1999). Immediate attention to the recipient's vocational interests is often indicated—in one study of 86 recipients, accelerated entry into vocational activities was more effective in securing job acquisition than gradual support employment activities (Bond, Dietzen, McGrew, & Miller, 1995).

Donegan (1999) wrote that in supporting vocational development recipients must receive assistance in acquiring basic living and social skills, and just as importantly family and significant others' needs for support and education must be addressed. With recipients who belong to minority groups, mental health professionals must encourage their exploration of preferences within the cultural group, encourage choices, promote an overall sense of identity, support family and cultural values, and help them learn to relate positively to persons within and outside their primary group, overcome any victim attitudes, and develop positive role models and goals (Arnold & Granger, 1999).

The mental health professional needs to be knowledgeable about vocational resources in the local community and have contacts that can assist recipients in these ways. Linkages must be established for a comprehensive vocational assessment to determine appropriate career directions for the client. For example, one of the authors referred a client (John) to a reputable clubhouse program, which included a vocational component. He was given a comprehensive vocational evaluation, which included interest inventories, work sample assessments, and interviewing and functional assessments. After John narrowed his potential vocational choices, he participated in several situational assessments in the community arranged by the vocational rehabilitation counselor, and a job-seeking skills class held at the clubhouse.

The mental health professional can work with the vocational counselor to make appropriate client referrals to local employment services, community colleges, and adult education programs. The recipient should also be helped to become comfortable using libraries and Internet services. Based on the assessment, the mental health professional must support only realistic and attainable vocational goals for both the short and long term. If the recipient is determined to pursue a type of work that is unlikely to be successful, then the professional should support alternatives that have some similar characteristics to that job.

In addition to working with individuals, the professional can promote the development of clients through vocational exploration groups. Diamond (1998) describes success with one eight-week psychoeducational group for up to 10 recipients, which is open-ended and focused on vocational decision-making. The group leaders facilitate an informal, unstructured process of discussion and exploration of vocational options. Members are able to help each other consider their strengths, limitations, and potential for various types of vocational activity prior to taking specific actions.

Family support and education is imperative in supporting vocational development. Families consistently request help from professionals to understand mental illness and medications, learn to motivate the client member to change, acquire realistic expectations for the client member, resolve crisis situations, and reduce their own anxieties (Garson, 1986; Hatfield, 1990; Mermier, 1993). Families often cite vocational services as their greatest concern. In one study of 1,400 members of the National Alliance for the Mentally Ill, 45% of families reported that their ill relative was not engaged in productive activity (Lefley, 1996).

As part of a comprehensive service plan, mental health professionals can provide educational interventions to help families toward the above goals. Family educational interventions, focused on vocational and other issues, can be carried out in psychoeducational groups, single family sessions, or both. Groups can provide families with an opportunity to learn from experiences of others. Single-family work, however, ensures that all topics will be relevant to that family's unique situation. Five topic areas that should be included in any family educational intervention plan include diagnosis, medication, community resources (including vocational resources), professional roles and intervention techniques, and strategies for managing an unmotivated client relative.

FACILITATING ROLE TRANSITIONS
RELATING TO EMPLOYMENT

Life transitions, which include major changes in primary social roles, are stressful for all persons. New roles involve new sets of expectations from others, and sometimes a new sense of identity (Davis, 1996). The unknown may be perceived as threatening, however, and some persons who move into employment fail to make a successful adjustment because they do not understand or feel competent to adjust to new role expectations. A person, for example, who has functioned as a homemaker for many years will experience a great role disruption, both on the job and elsewhere, when becoming a part-time computer programmer.

Mental health professionals can attend to their clients' need for gradual role transitions through long-range planning and helping them through a series of small steps culminating in job acquisition. Initial goals should be low-stress and low-risk in nature so that that person can experience success and grow in confidence. Two examples of this strategy are helping a person acquire suitable volunteer experiences for a few hours each week, and encouraging a person to take a course at the local community college. The mental health professional can make unique contributions to this process by helping recipients understand and respond to role changes in other areas of life brought on by vocational activity. These may include gains and losses in personal acquaintances and leisure time; increased responsibility for self-care; and new social possibilities employment opens up in the lives of people receiving mental health services.

Several examples of attention to role changes have been articulated. Ramon (1989–1990) wrote about discharge from a psychiatric hospital as a type of transition. The professional can view this experience as a transitional crisis; a time in which a person's relationships to others and sense of self are disrupted. In managing this transition, the worker can attend to the client's loss of old roles (that were based on controlled social interaction) and help develop a new sense of self and purpose through guided interactions. With regard to employment, the client can be introduced to people who have recently begun working, or who are involved in similar job activities. In this way the person can be linked with role models on which to pattern new behaviors. The professional can help recipients understand the changing role expectations of others so that they will be prepared to meet and perhaps exceed these requirements in their own work.

Another strategy for individual and group intervention with clients in transition is the worker's incorporation of status elevation ceremonies (Rouse, 1996). These involve the implementation of formal and informal rituals, organized celebrations demarking important milestones such as graduation, rites of passage, framed in positive terms, as a means of preparing recipients for new social positions and advancing social integration. These positive rituals should celebrate the accomplishments of people that have led to the achievement of new statuses, for example, becoming a worker. Significant others can participate in these ceremonies as a means of affirming the social support that is available to recipients.

FOSTERING THE MANAGEMENT OF STRESSORS

The acquisition of new employment can be assumed to be stressful for a client and may arise at any time. Hoffman and Kupper (1996) found in a study of 31 clients that there was a critical period for stress and coping 9–12 weeks after the job begins, as many people experience a decrease in work performance and failure in coping with stress after an initial adjustment. Stress may be related to the performance and interpersonal demands of the job but also to such challenges as keeping appointments with the mental health professional, getting enough rest, maintaining stamina, and managing issues of time and how much and how often the person engages in work.

It is likely that mental health professionals will need to increase the amount of time they spend with recipients during the initial adjustment to work. Pernell-Arnold and Granger (1999) recommend that mental health professionals utilize specific intervention activities to help recipients combat work-related stress, including the teaching of stress management skills, cognitive restructuring, family support, social support development, and social skills development. Additionally, the professional needs to monitor the use of psychotropic medications and their adverse effects during the adjustment process as the person reacts to stress in the workplace and in their lives outside of employment.

Stress management is a process of enhancing the recipients' job functioning by guiding their exposure to and mastery of situations that evoke stress (Shannon, 1994). It includes teaching clients about relaxation, nutrition, physical fitness, and stress inoculation training. This last of these elements is a process of identifying the stress-provoking stimulus, enhancing the person's motivation to confront the situation, and jointly planning a problem-solving sequence. Intervention principles include isolating the stress-evoking stimulus, developing a hierarchy of graduated tasks toward mastery of the stressor, beginning work on a task that the client selects, and the provision of ongoing support as the recipient confronts the situation. Davis, Eshelman, and McKay (1988) provide a set of instruments with which the mental health professional can help the recipient identify symptoms, sources, and type responses to job stress, and then devise exercises for goal attainment.

In cognitive restructuring, an individual's pattern of thinking is evaluated and adjusted to allow more flexibility and creativity in responding to stress (Granvold, 1994). The goals of cognitive restructuring are to eliminate cognitive distortions, or false beliefs about oneself and the environment that mediate behavior and mood problems. It is an empirical effort undertaken collaboratively between the recipient and mental health professional. The steps include education in the logic of cognitive theory, an assessment of the person's unrealistic assumptions regarding a problem issue, determining how these can be most efficiently replaced (through tasks that provide behavioral reinforcement), implementing tasks, and evaluating outcomes. A variant of this process is self-instruction training, which increases the client's control over his or her behavior by improving the quality of internal, self-directed speech.

Changing client stressors, which accompany work or volunteer activities, make medication management particularly important tools for mental health professionals. Bentley and Walsh (1996) have outlined roles for professionals with regard to clients using psychotropic medications, which apply to vocational settings. In the role of physician's assistant, the professional supports the recommendations of the recipient's physician regarding how medication is to be used. The collaborator performs preliminary screenings to determine the recipient's needs for medication, makes referrals to physicians, and regularly consults with the physician and client. The advocate supports the recipient's expressed wishes regarding medication and presents them to others in the service milieu. As an advocate, the mental health professional may assist clients and family members to relate to physicians and others in obtaining services. The professional also is a monitor of the positive and negative physical, psychological, and social effects of medication. The educator provides recipients and significant others (including other professionals, such as the vocational counselor) with information about issues relevant to the person's medication usage, including actions, benefits, risks, and side-effects.

ADDRESSING THE PERSONAL CONSEQUENCES OF SOCIAL AND ECONOMIC CHANGE

We have noted earlier that two barriers to employment are the recipient's general reluctance to take risks and the specific fear of losing benefits. While many recipients are eager to work, the mental health professional must never underestimate the extent to which such a change presents multiple new demands on the person's time, energy, and lifestyle. Even the person with high work motivation may be overwhelmed by these demands and decide that the risks are not worth the stress involved. Among the client's potential financial losses are social security benefits, housing subsidies, and health insurance. Social changes include such issues as learning to dress appropriately and shop for clothes, fulfilling responsibilities to other persons at the worksite, using public transport, structuring the workday, and budgeting income on a daily basis.

In addressing the economic consequences of work the professional must be knowledgeable about federal, state, and local benefits systems (e.g., social security and Medicaid). Mental health professionals do not need to be experts in entitlements but must be able to make appropriate linkages so that recipients have access to a network of experts, including advocates. In these linkage activities the mental health professional must demonstrate a willingness and ability to function as a member of a rehabilitative team. Clinical skills are important, as mental health professionals must make decisions about timeliness, relevance, and scope of referrals. Other major roles include mediation and advocacy, so that recipients obtain ready access to services for which they are entitled. Through ongoing clinical assessment the professional must determine those situations in which recipients can function as their own mediator or advocate, and those in which the professional's active intervention is required to effect change.

Regarding social consequences, the mental health professional must provide quality supportive counseling, and perhaps temporarily serve as the primary support for the person who begins an employment experience. Ego supportive counseling techniques (ventilation, exploration, reflection) are particularly appropriate for helping the person come to terms with personal and social changes (Goldstein & Noonan, 1999). These interventions are less focused and directive than those described earlier as the mental health professional provides recipients with adequate time and an environment of acceptance to encourage their reflections about social changes employment induces. The professional supports an ongoing process of self-exploration so that recipients can decide what new social behaviors seem most consistent with their personal goals.

FOSTERING PERSONAL DEVELOPMENT WITH IMPLICATIONS FOR EMPLOYMENT AND WORK

Work is an important element of one's general thrust to find meaning in life. We might think of enhanced quality of life as the ultimate goal in working with recipients coping with serious mental health issues. Wolf (1997) describes this as an emergent condition, including a person's overall satisfaction with his or her living situation, daily activities, family and social relations, financial status, occupation, safety, physical status, and mental health status. Indeed, the concept of quality of life is broad in scope and influenced by numerous factors.

Counseling can serve to place the recipient's vocational activities into a context of existential concerns. These include all decisions the person makes which reflect ultimate meanings, purposes, and commitments (Krill, 1996). Five categories of meaning include: religious or secular belief systems, social concerns, creative pursuits, hope, and relationships (Frankl, 1987). Existential concerns arise from, or help to manage, anxieties inevitably produced by thoughts about death, the possibility of social isolation, freedom inherent in making choices and responsibility for these choices, and concerns about one's place in the world (Yalom, 1980). While not necessarily confronted on a daily basis these issues have major influence on how all people organize their lives.

Mental health professionals can foster their clients' personal development by encouraging their exploration of these issues with the ego-supportive techniques we described earlier in the chapter. Existential concerns may be inappropriate to raise with recipients who are absorbed by immediate problem situations, but they may be relevant when clients demonstrate an inclination to look beyond the self and the immediate situation in understanding personal dilemmas (May & Yalom, 1995). Any intervention may be considered to support the recipient's personal development when it engages the person more fully in life activity, encourages the recipient to look externally for solutions to problems rather than focus exclusively on the self, and encourages the person to care about events and issues outside their own inner world.

SUMMARY

Mental health professionals are rarely experts in vocational rehabilitation, although they likely invest considerable effort in addressing the work and employment issues recipients bring to sessions. With their attention to broad psychological and social aspects of behavior, they can bring much to the process of helping recipients coping with serious mental health challenges secure worthwhile employment. Mental health professionals can support the work of the vocational counselor, integrate vocational experiences into the case management or treatment process, and assist recipients adjust to the realities of employment and help them address the consequences of going to work. Mental health professionals must be collaborative team members in all of these processes, understanding the nature and boundaries of their work and role as well as appreciating the contributions others make to the vocational development of recipients.

REFERENCES

Alverson, H., Alverson, M., Drake, R. E., & Becker, D. R. (1998). Social correlates of competitive employment among people with severe mental illness. *Psychosocial Rehabilitation Journal, 22*(1), 34–40.

Bentley, K. J., & Walsh, J. (1996). *The social worker and psychotropic medication: Toward effective collaboration with mental health clients, families, and providers*. Pacific Grove, CA: Brooks/Cole.

Blankertz, L., & Keller, C. (1997). The provision of long-term vocational supports for individuals with severe mental illness. *Continuum, 4*(1), 51–63.

Blankertz, L., & Robinson, S. (1996). Adding a vocational focus to mental health rehabilitation. *Psychiatric Services, 47*(11), 1216–1222.

Bloom, J. (1990). The relationship between social support and health. *Social Science and Medicine, 30*, 635–637.

Bond, G. R., Dietzen, L. L., McGrew, J. H., & Miller, L. D. (1995). Accelerating entry into supported employment for persons with severe psychiatric disabilities. *Rehabilitation Psychology, 40*(2), 75–94.

Braitman, A., Counts, P., Avenport, R., Zurlinden, B., Rogers, M., Clauss, J., Kulkami, A., Kymla, J., & Montgomery, L. (1995). Comparison of barriers to employment in unemployed and employed clients in a case management program: An exploratory study. *Psychiatric Rehabilitation Journal, 19*(1), 3–8.

Bybee, D., Mowbray, C. T., & McCrohan, N. (1996). Towards zero exclusion in vocational opportunities for persons with psychiatric disabilities: Predictors of service receipt in a hybrid vocational/case management program. *Psychiatric Rehabilitation Journal, 19*(4), 15–27.

Caplan, G. (1990). Loss, stress, and mental health. *Community Mental Health Journal, 26*(1), 27–48.

Davis, L. V. (1996). Role theory and social work treatment. In F. J. Turner (Ed.), *Social work treatment* (4th ed., pp. 581–600). New York, NY: Free Press.

Davis, M., Eshelman, E. R., & McKay, M. (1988). *The relaxation and stress workbook* (3rd ed.). Oakland, CA: New Harbinger.

Diamond, H. (1998). Vocational decision making in a psychiatric outpatient program. *Occupational therapy in mental health, 14*(3), 67–80.

Donegan, K. R. (1999). Youth with serious emotional disturbances (SED) and the transition to work. *Employment of people with psychiatric disabilities*, 1–27.

Fischer, J. (1978). *Effective casework practice: An eclectic approach*. New York, NY: McGraw Hill.

Frank, J. D., & Frank, J. B. (1993). *Persuasion and healing: A comparative study of psychotherapy* (3rd ed.). Baltimore, MD: Johns Hopkins University Press.

Frankl, V. E. (1988). *The will to meaning: Foundations and applications of logotherapy*. New York, NY: Meridian.

Garson, S. (1986). *Out of our minds*. Buffalo, NY: Prometheus.

Gerhart, U. C. (1990). *Caring for the chronic mentally ill*. Itasca, IL: F. E. Peacock.

Germain, C. B., & Gitterman, A. (1996). *The life model of social work practice: Advances in theory and practice* (2nd ed.). New York, NY: Columbia University Press.

Goldstein, E. G., & Noonan, M. (1999). *Short-term treatment and social work practice: An integrative perspective.* New York, NY: Free Press.

Granvold, D. K. (1994). Concepts and methods of cognitive treatment. In D. K. Granvold (Ed.), *Cognitive and behavioral treatment: Methods and applications* (pp. 3–31). Pacific Grove, CA: Brooks/Cole.

Hatfield, A. B. (1990). *Family education in mental illness.* New York, NY: Guilford.

Hepworth, D., Rooney, R., & Larsen, J. (2002). *Direct social work practice: Theory and skills* (6th ed.). Belmont, CA: Brooks/Cole.

Hobfoll, S., Freedy, R., Lane, C., & Geller, P. (1990). Conservation of social resources: Social support resource theory. *Journal of Social and Personal Relationships, 7,* 465–478.

Hoffman, H., & Kupper, Z. (1996). Patient dynamics in early stages of vocational rehabilitation: A pilot study. *Comprehensive Psychiatry, 37*(3), 216–221.

Horvath, A. O. (1994). Research on the alliance. In A. O. Horvath & L. S. Greenberg (Eds.), *The working alliance: Theory, research and practice* (pp. 259–286). New York, NY: Wiley.

Kanter, J. (1989). Clinical case management: Definition, principles, components. *Hospital and Community Psychiatry, 40,* 361–368.

Krill, D. F. (1996). Existential social work. In F. J. Turner (Ed.), *Social work treatment* (4th ed., pp. 250–281). New York, NY: Free Press.

Lantz, J., & Belcher, J. (1988). Schizophrenia and the existential vacuum. *International Forum for Logotherapy, 11*(1), 16–21.

Lefley, H. P. (1996). *Family caregiving in mental illness.* Thousand Oaks, CA: Sage.

Maluccio, A. N. (1979). *Learning from clients.* New York, NY: Free Press.

Marrone, J., Balzell, A., & Gold, M. (1995). Employment supports for people with mental illness. *Psychiatric Services, 46*(7), 707–711.

May, R., & Yalom, I. (1995). Existential psychotherapy. In R. J. Corsini & D. Wedding (Eds.), *Current psychotherapies* (5th ed., pp. 262–292). Itasca, IL: F. E. Peacock.

Mermier, M. B. (1993). *Coping with severe mental illness: Families speak out.* Lewiston, ID: Edwin Mellen Press.

Mowbray, C. T., Bybee, D., Harris, S. A., & McCrohan, N. (1995). Predictors of work status and future work orientation in people with a psychiatric disability. *Psychiatric Rehabilitation Journal, 19*(2), 15–28.

Okpaku, S. O., Anderson, K. H., Sibulkin, A. E., Butler, J. S., & Bickman, L. (1997). The effectiveness of a multidisciplinary case management intervention on the employment of SSA applicants and beneficiaries. *Psychiatric Rehabilitation Journal, 20*(3), 34–41.

Pernell-Arnold, A., & Granger, B. (1999). Culturally competent employment services for people with psychiatric disabilities. In L. L. Mancuso & J. D. Kotler (Eds.), *Employment for people with psychiatric disabilities* (pp. 89–112). Alexandria, VA: National Association of State Mental Health Program Directors.

Ramon, S. (1989–1990). The relevance of symbolic interactionism perspectives to the conceptual and practice construction of leaving a psychiatric hospital. *Social Work and Social Sciences Review, 1*(3), 163–176.

Regenold, M., Sherman, M. F., & Fenzel, M. (1999). Getting back to work: Self-efficacy as a predictor of employment outcome. *Psychiatric Rehabilitation Journal, 22*(4), 361–367.

Ridgway, P., & Rapp, C. Active ingredients in achieving competitive employment for people with psychiatric disabilities: A research synthesis. In L. L. Mancuso & J. D. Kotler (Eds.), Employment for people with psychiatric disabilities (pp. 61–88). Alexandria. VA: National Association of State Mental Health Program Directors.

Roessler, R. T., & Rubin, S. E. (1992). *Case management and rehabilitation counseling: Procedures and techniques* (2nd ed.). Austin, TX: Pro-ed.

Rouse, T. P. (1996). Conditions for successful status elevation ceremony. *Deviant Behavior, 17*(1), 21–42.

Scheff, T. J. (1984). *Being mentally ill: A sociological theory* (2nd ed.). New York, NY: Aldine.

Sexton, T. L., & Whiston, S. C. (1994). The status of the counseling relationship: An empirical review, theoretical implications, and research direction. *The Counseling Psychologist, 22*(1), 6–78.

Shannon, C. (1994). Stress management. In D. K. Granvold (Ed.), *Cognitive and behavioral treatment: Methods and applications* (pp. 339–352). Pacific Grove, CA: Brooks/Cole.

Thomlinson, R. J. (1984). Something works: Evidence from practice effectiveness studies. *Social Work, 29,* 51–57.

Torrey, W. C., Bebout, R., Kline, J., Becher, D. R., Alverson, M., & Drake, R. E. (1990). Practice guidelines for clinicians working in programs providing integrated vocational and clinical services for persons with severe mental disorders. *Psychiatric Rehabilitation Journal, 21*(4), 388–393.

Walsh, J. (1994). The social networks of seriously mentally ill persons receiving case management services. *Journal of Case Management, 3,* 27–35.

Wolf, J. (1997). Client needs and quality of life. *Psychiatric Rehabilitation Journal, 20*(4), 16–24.

Yalom, I. D. (1980). *Existential psychotherapy.* New York, NY: Basic.

CHAPTER 10

State Rehabilitation Authorities and Their Role in Responding to the Employment Needs of People with Serious Mental Illness

ELLEN FABIAN, LARRY ABRAMSON, AND SHARI WILLIS

Work holds a central importance in an individual's life, providing direct economic and social benefits and contributing to self-esteem and quality of life. For the three to four million people whose functioning is impaired by significant mental disorders (SMDs), employment remains an important but often elusive goal. Although the data on labor force participation rates among persons with SMDs do vary, periodic studies reported in the literature suggest that only from 15% to 50% of these individuals are employed competitively (Anthony, 1994; National Institute on Disability and Rehabilitation Research, 1999). For more than 50 years, the public vocational rehabilitation (VR) program has been actively involved in helping people with significant mental health disorders to enter or re-enter competitive employment. The purpose of this chapter is to describe the role of the public VR program in facilitating employment for people with SMDs, and to provide examples of collaborative solutions and recommendations through case illustrations.

THE PUBLIC VR PROGRAM

The federally funded public VR program helps individuals with disabilities to prepare for and secure competitive employment, and thus become more independent and integrated into the community. Since its inception in 1920, the program has represented a state–federal partnership, with the federal government contributing approximately 80% of the share of implementing the program in each of the 50 states and the District of Columbia. The VR

ELLEN FABIAN AND SHARI WILLIS • CAPS Department, University of Maryland, College Park, Maryland.
LARRY ABRAMSON • Director of the Back to Work Program, St. Luke's House, Bethesda, Maryland.

program is administered through the Rehabilitation Services Administration (RSA) in the U.S. Department of Education.

The majority of program funds are used by state VR offices to provide services such as counseling, job development, and placement, and to purchase services such as skills training and supported employment from other providers. Services are arranged through joint determination by the VR counselor and the consumer, and implemented through an Individual Employment Plan (IEP). By design, VR services are time-limited and outcome-oriented.

The program has historically been viewed as a good investment by Congress and its supporters, with evidence pointing to its effectiveness in terms of cost–benefit studies that demonstrate gains in benefits by service recipients compared with service costs (Rubin & Roessler, 1996). However, critics of the program have raised a number of questions over the past decade or so, including whether service benefits persist over time, whether the program can serve all eligible individuals, and whether services are flexible enough to meet the varied needs of consumers (Noble, Honberg, Hall, & Flynn, 1997). These and other criticisms should not obscure the fact that the basic intent of the program is consistent with the values of American society, based as it is on the principle of maximizing an individual's potential and independence. Indeed, recent advances in biomedical research coupled with equal employment legislation such as the Americans with Disabilities Act (ADA) suggest that now more than ever, a public VR program is necessary in order to help persons with disabilities become more productive and independent.

The VR program has always operated within a philosophy of providing an individualized plan of services matched to client needs. The system's highly standardized service delivery process consists of a continuum of service stages or statuses, beginning with eligibility determination and proceeding through evaluation, plan development, provision of services, job placement, and case closure. Services offered to help the client achieve his or her employment goal might include counseling and guidance, vocational training, supported employment, work adjustment, and job-seeking skills training. The VR counselor either directly provides or purchases the necessary services from eligible vendors, educational institutions, and rehabilitation facilities. Federal regulations designate timelines for certain case statuses, so that, for example, eligibility determination must be completed within 60 days, evaluation cannot exceed 18 months, and cases cannot be closed successfully until the individual has been working for 90 days. The program's outcome-oriented focus has facilitated Congressional measure of its effectiveness through annual tracking of the number of cases closed as "successfully rehabilitated." Recent program data indicate that more than 230,000 individuals were successfully rehabilitated in 2001, 17% of whom were people with SMDs (RTI International, 2002).

Although the early focus of the VR program was on providing services to people with disabilities who were not severely functionally impaired, the Rehabilitation Act of 1973 and its subsequent amendments shifted priority for VR services toward those persons whose impairments meet federal criteria of a "severe disability." A severe disability is generally defined as a physical or mental impairment serious enough to affect or preclude functioning in a major life area, such as living or working. More recent amendments to the Rehabilitation Act have added new provisions regarding such important areas as consumer involvement in IEP development; reducing the time allowed for eligibility determination; and eliminating the previous eligibility requirement of "employment feasibility" in favor of a standard of "presumption of benefit," meaning that any individual who expresses a desire to work may benefit from VR services.

VR SERVICES TO INDIVIDUALS WITH
SIGNIFICANT MENTAL ILLNESS
LEGISLATION

The Bardon–Lafollette Act of 1943 extended the provision of VR services to persons with serious mental illness for the first time. Although a small number of individuals with SMDs received services during the first decade or so of this expansion, the number grew considerably over the years. This rise was in part a reflection of the rapid expansion of community-based programs such as rehabilitation facilities and sheltered workshops. First authorized by the Vocational Rehabilitation Act Amendments of 1954, these workshops and facilities proliferated, serving over 55,000 individuals with SMDs by 1969 (Parker, Thoreson, Haugen, & Pfeifer, 1970). The focus of many of these facilities was on assisting people with severe disabilities to acquire the work behaviors and vocational skills that would enable them eventually to work competitively in the community. These "train and place" models were, unfortunately, more aspirational than real. For example, studies examining the rate at which individuals moved from sheltered workshops to competitive employment indicated that fewer than 15% of people in these facilities transitioned into community jobs (Parent, Hill, & Wehman, 1989).

In response to these poor data, supported employment programs, or "place and train" approaches, were authorized and funded through Title VI-C of the Rehabilitation Act Amendments of 1986. Supported employment is predicated on a value system that endorses the capacity of any individual, no matter how severe his or her disabilities, to work when given appropriate services and supports. The outcome literature on the effectiveness of sup-ported employment in sustaining long-term employment outcomes for persons with SMDs is not as positive as it is for other groups of individuals with severe disabilities (Fabian, 1992). However, there is evidence suggesting that these programs, particularly the individual place-ment and support model, are the most effective vocational rehabilitation intervention for those persons with SMDs who demonstrate employment gains as a result of participation in them (Drake, McHugo, Becker, Anthony, & Clark, 1996).

Another legislative change that directly benefited consumers with SMDs was the cre-ation of a Client Assistance Program (CAP) in each state, as mandated by the Rehabilitation Act of 1973. This program serves applicants and clients of programs funded under the Act by advising them of available benefits and helping them resolve any difficulties they may encounter when attempting to get services. CAPs assist clients by providing information on services and benefits available under both the Rehabilitation Act and Title I of the ADA; providing advice on and interpretation of the Act and its accompanying regulations; negotiat-ing with service providers to resolve problems; and representing and advocating for clients at mediation sessions, informal reviews, formal hearings, and in court. The majority of CAP clients need assistance from the CAP for some difficulty they have had in applying for or receiving VR services. A study of the 1996–1997 CAP data indicated that a significant proportion of CAP clients are persons with mental illness (Westat, 1999).

Finally, the Rehabilitation Act Amendments of 1992 and 1998 introduced a number of significant changes, particularly in shifting the focus of rehabilitation services to the con-sumer through a variety of regulations based on choice and self-determination. These changes represent a "recalibration" of the public VR program to more effectively and efficiently respond to the needs of consumers with severe disabilities (Noble et al., 1997). The Rehabilitation Act Amendments of 1992 also included a change in the regulations regarding supported employment programs. These Amendments specifically allowed for the provision of ongoing job coaching away from the job site under special circumstances, especially at the request of the consumer. This approach to job-coaching services was specific to the unique circumstances and needs of consumers with significant mental health disorders.

VR PROGRAM OUTCOMES

Recent national VR referral data indicate that more than 20% of persons applying for services have serious mental health disorders RTI International 2002. Although the number of persons with SMDs who applied for and received VR services has risen dramatically over the past 50 years, the public VR system's record of successful rehabilitation among clients with mental disorders has consistently lagged behind that of other disability groups (United States General Accounting Office, 1993).

There are several compelling explanations for the relatively poor outcome data for individuals with psychiatric disabilities. First and most important is the historical fact that the VR system was established to meet the rehabilitation needs of individuals with less severe, more stable, physical disabilities incurred as a result of accident or disease. For these clients, assistance with establishing new career goals and providing counseling or skills training to attain those goals within a time-limited framework made sense. But for persons with SMDs, whose impairments may be both pervasive and episodic rather than stable, there are clear challenges involved in achieving a positive outcome within a limited period of time.

A second explanation lies in the very nature of the VR program itself as a time-limited, highly structured sequence of service delivery. Many individuals with psychiatric disabilities require a flexible system of services and supports that can be adapted in response to their changing needs (Rutman, 1994). For example, an individual with bipolar disorder who does not experience frequent cycles of the symptoms of that illness might perform extremely well at a job for six months, and then begin to experience exacerbations of symptoms and stress that make it difficult to work. Within the VR system, such a client's case might have long been closed as successfully rehabilitated. For these clients, the result might be that just at the moment that they require the most supports, they have to expend the most effort to get them while still trying to maintain their jobs. Although the VR system provides a mechanism for post-employment follow-up services, this status is infrequently used by counselors (Noble et al., 1997).

A third issue is that service accountability is based on the number of cases that are successfully rehabilitated and closed, which means that the individual has achieved his or her employment goal and has maintained it for a minimum of 90 days. This accountability framework induces counselors to expend the most effort on those clients for whom they will receive the most benefit in terms of how the system evaluates their work. This tends to operate as a built-in disincentive to investing time and energy in cases of individuals with SMDs, as it is difficult for counselors to accurately predict their symptom exacerbation and their capacity to both persevere with the VR process long enough to obtain a job and to maintain that job for the requisite period of time.

Despite these difficulties, clients with SMDs also derive several benefits from the structure of services and programs offered within the VR system. One benefit is the individualized nature of the vocational rehabilitation service delivery system. Generally, decisions regarding what services an individual needs in order to achieve his or her rehabilitation goal are made jointly by the counselor and the client. This customized approach to service delivery is a positive aspect of the system, as it emphasizes devising services to meet individual needs rather than taking a cluster or generic approach to service delivery. Another positive aspect of the system is the legislative requirement that counselors attempt to ensure consumer participation in the VR process. Consumers are involved in identifying their career goal, developing a plan to meet the goal, and modifying existing plans to make them more congruent with their own preferences.

The VR program's focus on outcomes is a characteristic of the system that may be both an advantage and a disadvantage for consumers with mental illness. The fact that program effectiveness is measured by a well-defined criterion—whether the client gets and keeps a job—highlights a unique aspect of the program within the system of disability-related services. However, since the VR program is not an entitlement program, but only an option available to eligible persons with disabilities, the system has a limited capacity to provide rehabilitation services to the vast number of individuals who need them (Noble, 1998).

COLLABORATION BETWEEN THE PUBLIC VR PROGRAM AND THE PUBLIC MENTAL HEALTH PROGRAM

The need for cooperation between the public VR program and the public mental health system has been evident almost as long as the public program has been providing services to individuals with SMDs. As stated earlier in this chapter, these clients frequently present a unique and complex constellation of needs that must be addressed in order to promote successful employment. Furthermore, research has made it clear that cooperative team approaches to managing these needs present the most effective method of seamless service delivery (Katz, Geckle, & Goldstein, 1990; Noble et al., 1997). Without collaboration, mental health and vocational rehabilitation professionals may be working at "cross purposes" (Mowbray, Bybee, Harris, & McCrohan, 1995), with one group of professionals recommending treatment options or services that are not consistent with those recommended by the other group. The classic example of this inconsistency is seen when a mental health professional providing treatment to a VR client requires the client to attend therapy sessions that are scheduled during the period when the individual is supposed to be at a job (Noble et al., 1997).

Federal policy has attempted to keep pace with the need for collaboration across service providers. In 1978, a formal cooperative agreement was established between the Rehabilitation Services Administration and the National Institute of Mental Health to attempt to foster collaborative intersystem activities and services. Although implementation of the agreement has varied widely among states, it has provided a foundation for acknowledging the importance of collaborating on a state level in order to improve service delivery and service outcomes for clients with SMDs.

Since the 1978 Agreement, there have been several reports in the literature on the effect of collaborative efforts and activities on client outcomes. For example, in 1989, a study of VR and mental health system activities surveyed and reported on the efforts of VR state administrators and counselors throughout the country in order to identify best practices in promoting cooperation between agencies (Tashjian & Hayward, 1989). Best practice recommendations in this report included specialized psychiatric caseloads for VR field counselors, co-location of VR counselors at mental health programs, smaller caseload sizes to reflect some of the unique challenges presented by individuals with SMDs, collaborative and joint training programs, and increased utilization of post-employment services to aid in job retention for those clients receiving services through a mental health agency. An examination of the collaborative activities included in current VR state plans indicates that while a majority have cooperative plans in place, few states actually described comprehensive state-wide activities that appear to be consistent with these recommendations. Some of these innovative state plans are described later in this chapter.

Collaboration between VR and mental health service systems is complicated by a number of factors. One is that state mental health departments invest their resources in clinical and therapeutic services rather than in employment (Pratt, Gill, Barrett, & Roberts, 1999). For example, the National Alliance for the Mentally Ill (NAMI) in its national survey of state mental health programs conducted in 1993, found that on average state agencies invested only 3% of their annual budgets in vocational activities for public mental health clients (Noble et al., 1997). Of the funds they did invest in employment activities, agencies allocated only 0.08% of their budgets to the long-term costs associated with the VR supported employment program. This minimal investment is troubling in light of evidence suggesting that collaborative supported employment programs are among the most effective VR methods for persons with SMDs (Drake et al., 1996).

A second factor complicating collaborative activities is the lack of standardization among mental health programs. The legislation authorizing the public VR program sets national standards and regulations for practices and procedures; legislation also requires that these practices be implemented in a similar fashion across the country. In contrast, there is wide variation among state mental health authorities and departments. Practices and procedures often vary significantly depending on state needs, configurations, and available revenues. This means that collaborative or jointly funded activities that work in one state may not be applicable to another.

In addition, many of the psychosocial or psychiatric rehabilitation programs that actually deliver services to publicly funded mental health clients within a given state are also diverse, and operate with unique organizational structures, financial arrangements, funding sources, and regulatory requirements (Pratt et al., 1999; Rutman, 1994). Thus, even within a single state, a successful collaboration between a VR counselor and a mental health practitioner in one agency may not be easily duplicated in another setting. Literature suggests that the majority of psychosocial rehabilitation programs minimize VR services, and generally persist in operating from a vocational readiness model, where clinical and pre-vocational services are thought to be the necessary precursors of employment (Noble et al., 1997; Toms Barker, 1994). These practices are in contradiction to research suggesting that individuals with SMDs can move immediately into competitive employment without having to spend considerable time in work adjustment or vocational readiness activities (Blankertz & Robinson, 1996; Bond, Dietzen, McGrew, & Miller, 1995).

Finally, the different philosophies and assumptions that guide VR and mental health service delivery systems frequently interfere with seamless treatment decisions. For example, mental health professionals are concerned with symptom alleviation, and recommend decreasing environmental stresses, such as work, as a means of achieving this outcome. However, vocational rehabilitation professionals point to decades of empirical research indicating that symptoms do not necessarily interfere with vocational behavior (Neff, 1988), and suggest that work environments can be modified in a way that promotes vocationally relevant behavior while reducing environmental stresses (Rutman, 1994). Such contradictory philosophies may interfere with treatment recommendations, unless mental health and rehabilitation professionals carefully and mutually consider both treatment plans and vocational recommendations.

EXAMPLES OF COLLABORATIVE
PRACTICES

Despite the difficulties inherent in collaboration between VR and mental health counselors, successful collaborative activities do take place at the system level and at the provider level. This section provides examples of such collaborative efforts in order to illustrate how policy changes are implemented at the state and local levels.

State Level

In several states, mental health agencies have contributed to improving employment outcomes through cooperative agreements with their state VR programs, primarily in the implementation of supported employment programs. For example, in the State of Washington, the department of mental health has significantly expanded funding and availability of supported employment services for people with SMDs through its mental health centers. Similarly, the state mental health agency in Rhode Island has a cooperative agreement with the VR agency that is designed to promote supported employment and to connect psychosocial day programs to employment-driven services. These types of cooperative funding of supported employment programs help bridge the gap between the limited funding available from VR program funds, and the more substantial and long-term funding available from state mental health budgets.

Other states have focused more on developing coordination mechanisms for improving services to consumers with SMDs. In Arizona, for example, the state Rehabilitation Services Administration has entered into agreements with the Department of Behavioral Health Services to develop clinical teams to facilitate vocational rehabilitation referrals, engage in planning and coordination services, and apply jointly for grants. Idaho has developed a collaborative plan with the state mental health agency to place VR field counselors on case management teams in order to more effectively address consumer employment issues. Finally, some states, such as Maryland, Pennsylvania, and Arizona, have instituted collaborative state VR and mental health personnel training and planning practices, including regular staff development activities, specialized psychiatric rehabilitation focus groups, and regular collaborative staff meetings in order to facilitate the identification of system barriers for consumers with SMDs.

Even when states do not have strong or active cooperative agreements in place, local mental health agencies, working collaboratively with VR field counselors, can implement mutually beneficial practices that more effectively address the employment needs of their consumers. The following section of this chapter highlights these practices through case study illustrations.

Local Level

The following cases highlight how VR counselors in the public program can work closely with local mental health agencies to maximize case service efforts and dollars on behalf of clients with SMDs.

Billy had been at the state hospital for the past six months. At discharge, he indicated that he wanted a job and needed a place to live. He was referred to a local mental health agency offering housing and supported employment services. When Billy moved into his group home, he immediately referred himself to the supported employment program affiliated with the mental health agency. In turn, employment services staff referred Billy to the local VR office, where he completed an application. His discharge from the state hospital, together with his medical records collected by the supported employment service staff, accelerated his eligibility determination for VR services, and avoided a lengthy delay in evaluation and eligibility determination. The time saved allowed the supported employment program staff, the VR counselor, and the client to form a team in order to identify Billy's strengths, assess quality job matches, and develop a job retention plan. Billy found a job and started work three months after hospital discharge.

Sally had been successfully employed at a software company for the last nine months. Sally's skills did not match the requirements for a finance clerk, but the company was able to separate out three essential tasks of the position so that she was able to perform in a successful manner. In her nine months of employment, her supported employment job coach was in regular contact with Sally and her employment. During her tenure, Sally received positive evaluations, and her case was closed as "successfully rehabilitated" by the VR counselor. In Sally's tenth month of employment her company was purchased by a large technology firm who centralized all financial functions in other staff. Sally contacted her VR counselor to let her know the status of her job. The VR counselor visited the site, reviewed Sally's evaluations, and contacted another "high tech" business to locate a new job for her, which Sally was eventually able to secure. The seamless transition from one job to another was conducted through post-employment service purchase of services by her VR counselor. In addition to job development activities, the counselor also contracted for intensive initial job-coaching services at the new site. The rapid response to changes within the business community, coordination with the mental health agency, and relationship with the business community allowed the VR counselor to maximize the use of the post-employment service status to maintain a successful closure.

RECOMMENDATIONS

Although the public VR program has not experienced a great deal of success in serving job applicants with SMDs, this chapter highlights some effective system and local practices to achieve more successful outcomes. The following recommendations are drawn from the issues and illustrations in the chapter.

1. At the state level, foster collaboration and communication by cross-training of mental health and VR staff, and by instituting a team of active individuals from both systems to plan activities and discuss how state mental health policy changes will affect VR service delivery.

2. Focus on team-building and communication between state VR personnel and key psychosocial rehabilitation staff and consumers through staff training, in-service workshops, and by partnering with local universities as a vehicle for facilitating communication.

3. Ensure that key mental health agency staff are aware of the state VR program through visits to local field offices, meetings with VR counselors, and review of VR policies and procedures. Familiarizing staff with VR program structure avoids some of the misunderstandings that arise because mental health agency staff may be unaware of some of the system constraints in which their colleagues operate.

4. Work cooperatively to promote employment as a critical and valued outcome for consumers with SMDs in state mental health programs and facilities. This can be achieved through collaborative training efforts, through relationships with local universities that may offer undergraduate and graduate training programs in rehabilitation-related areas. One of the major barriers to successful consumer employment is that many mental health agencies are unfamiliar with the program technologies available to support and sustain work, and so minimize or ignore vocational program strategies and methods that can maximize independence for consumers.

5. Ensure that state mental health program staff understand the Title VI-C Supported Employment Program, and work as effective advocates within their mental health state systems to promote state funding through public mental health dollars, of long-term job supports for supported employment consumers.

The public VR program has been providing services to individuals with significant mental health disorders for more than 50 years. Although the history of success of these services has not been as optimistic as consumers and families would hope, continuing efforts to achieve better outcomes through collaborative activities and flexible services may improve the overall employment picture for these individuals.

REFERENCES

Anthony, W. A. (1994). Characteristics of people with psychiatric disabilities that are predictive of entry into the rehabilitation process and successful employment. *Psychosocial Rehabilitation Journal, 17*(3), 3–13.

Blankhertz, L., & Robinson, S. (1996). Adding a vocational focus to mental health rehabilitation. *Psychiatric Services, 47*, 1216–1222.

Bond, G. R., Dietzen, L. L., McGrew, J. H., & Miller, L. D. (1995). Accelerating entry into supported employment for persons with severe psychiatric disabilities. *Rehabilitation Psychology, 40*, 91–111.

Drake, R. E., McHugo, G. J., Becker, D. R., Anthony, W. A., & Clarke, R. I. (1996). The New Hampshire study of supported employment for people with severe mental illness. *Journal of Consulting and Clinical psychology, 64*, 391–399.

Fabian, E. S. (1992). Longitudinal outcomes in supported employment: A survival analysis. *Rehabilitation Psychology, 37*, 23–35.

Katz, L., Geckle, M., & Goldstein, G. (1990). A survey of perceptions and practice: Interagency collaboration and rehabilitation of persons with long-term mental illness. *Rehabilitation Counseling Bulletin, 37*, 290–301.

Mowbray, C. T., Bybee, D., Harris, S. N., & McCrohan, N. (1995). Predictors of work status and future work orientation in people with psychiatric disabilities. *Psychiatric Rehabilitation Journal, 19*(2), 17–28.

National Institute on Disability and Rehabilitation Research (1999). Infouse on-line at www.disabilitydata.com.

Neff, W. S. (1988). Vocational rehabilitation in perspective. In J. A. Ciardiello & M. D. Bell (Eds.), *Vocational rehabilitation of persons with prolonged psychiatric disorders* (pp. 5–18). Baltimore, MD: Johns Hopkins University Press.

Noble, J. H. (1998). Policy reform dilemmas in promoting employment of persons with severe mental illness. *Psychiatric Services, 49*, 775–781.

Noble, J. H., Honberg, R. S., Hall, L. L., & Flynn, L. M. (1997). *A legacy of failure: The inability of the federal–state vocational rehabilitation system to serve people with severe mental illnesses.* Arlington, VA: National Alliance for the Mentally Ill.

Parent, W., Hill, M., & Wehman, P. (1989). From sheltered to supported employment outcomes: Challenges for rehabilitation facilities. *Journal of Rehabilitation, 55*(4), 51–57.

Parker, R., Thoreson, R., Haugen, J., & Pfeifer, E. (1970). Vocational rehabilitation service needs of mental patients: Perceptions of psychiatric hospital staff. *Rehabilitation Counseling Bulletin, 13*, 271–279.

Pratt, C. W., Gill, K. J., Barrett, N. M., & Roberts, M. M. (1999). *Psychiatric rehabilitation.* New York, NY: Academic Press.

RTI International (2002). *Longitudinal study of the Vocational Rehabilitation Program.* (ED Contract No. HR92022001). Washington, DC: U.S. Department of Education Rehablitation Services Administration. Author.

Rubin, S. E., & Roessler, R. T. (1995). *Foundations of the vocational rehabilitation process.* Austin, TX: Pro-Ed.

Rutman, I. (1994). How psychiatric disability expresses itself as a barrier to employment. *Psychosocial Rehabilitation Journal, 17*(3), 15–35.

Tashjian, M., & Hayward, J. (1989). *Best practices study of vocational rehabilitation services to severe mentally ill persons.* Berkeley, CA: Policy Study Associates.

Toms Barker, L. (1994). Community based models of employment services for people with long term mental illness. *Psychosocial Rehabilitation Journal, 17*(3), 55–65.

United States General Accounting Office (1993). *Vocational rehabilitation: Evidence for federal program's effectiveness is mixed.* (GAO/PEMD-93-19). Washington, DC: Government Printing Office, Superintendent of Documents.

Westat (1999). *A study of the differences among types of client assistance programs.* Rockville, MD: Author.

CHAPTER 11

Involvement of State and Local Mental Health Authorities in Addressing the Employment Needs of People with Serious Mental Illness

MARTHA B. KNISLEY, PAMELA S. HYDE, AND
EVETTE JACKSON

INTRODUCTION

This chapter examines the role of state and local mental health authorities in the promotion of services to meet the employment needs of individuals with serious and persistent mental illness (SPMI). This examination focuses first on a historical overview of the roles of state and local authorities, how their roles in employment services have evolved over time, and what state and local innovations have occurred as part of that evolution. Second is a discussion of the collaborative role of the state mental health authority with the state vocational rehabilitation agency and the perceived effectiveness of that collaboration. Third is the presentation of recommendations regarding the ways state and local authorities can be more effective in creating and supporting vocational and employment opportunities for people with SPMI.

MARTHA B. KNISLEY • Director of the District of Columbia Department of Mental Health, Washington, D.C.
PAMELA S. HYDE • Secretary, New Mexico Department of Human Services, Santa Fe, New Mexico.
EVETTE JACKSON • The Technical Assistance Collaborative, Inc., Boston, Massachusetts.

ROLES OF STATE AND LOCAL MENTAL
HEALTH AUTHORITIES

Historically, the dominant purpose of state mental health authorities was to operate state psychiatric inpatient facilities. In the past 50 years, this purpose has shifted. While state mental health authorities continue to operate state psychiatric inpatient facilities and, in some cases, community-based services, they have also become planners, regulators, and funders or purchasers of complex, multi-faceted systems of care. They perform these functions as a single agency or in collaboration with other agencies that have critically related responsibilities.

During the last 50 years, state hospital census nationwide reduced dramatically from over 500,000 to just over 60,000 (Geller, 2000) and resources for community services increased substantially. In the latest national report about state expenditures for mental health, expenditures for community-based services exceeded those for state hospital services for the first time (U.S. Department of Health and Human Services, 1997). Initially, federal dollars to support community mental health services went directly to local communities. States had little or no input into how the funds were to be used. Local communities had an increasing role in mental health service planning and delivery, and local mental health authorities began to be created. This separation between state and community services changed dramatically in 1980 with the passage of the Mental Health Systems Act when states were allocated community mental health funds from the National Institute of Mental Health (NIMH) through federal block grants. As Medicaid has become an increasingly important source of funding for mental health services, many states have become purchasers of care on behalf of covered populations through behavioral health carve-outs or collaborations with Medicaid health care delivery systems.

In addition to being both a provider and a funder or purchaser of care, state and local authorities are increasingly acting as regulators. As regulators, state and local mental health authorities are charged with the responsibility of ensuring that professionally competent services are provided and that tax dollars are appropriately spent utilizing licensure, certification, quality management, and improvement processes. This combination of measures seeks to ensure that consumers'[1] lives are actually improved as a result of mental health services funded and delivered.

Likewise, planning has become a critical role of state and local authorities. With the advent of federal dollars into state systems and federal planning requirements for block grants, which stipulate target populations (e.g., homeless mentally ill persons, adults with SPMI, children with severe emotional disturbances, and persons with mental illness and substance abuse disorders), state mental health authorities began to develop plans for their systems of mental health care and for key ancillary service areas such as housing and employment. Some Governors and State Legislatures have also introduced requirements for comprehensive and/or strategic human services plans that include plans for mental health services. In turn, states with local authorities usually require these local entities to provide comprehensive needs assessments and/or plans in order to receive state and state-controlled federal funds for mental health services.

---

[1]The term "consumer" is controversial in some circles. The term is used here because many states use this term in the name or mission of the offices or units described. The term generally means current or former service recipients, especially those who have been labeled with or who have experienced serious and persistent mental illnesses. In some states, other behavioral health and developmentally disabled service recipients are included in the term, and family members are considered consumers in some states.

These changing roles of state and local authorities is reflected in the changing ways in which state and local authorities participate in meeting the employment needs of SPMI persons.

HISTORICAL PERSPECTIVE

Fifty years ago, state-operated psychiatric facilities had expansive work programs in house. Patients were a major part of the economy of state hospitals operating dairies, kitchens, and farms and filling clerical, housekeeping, maintenance, mail delivery, and other critical positions with little or no pay. Work, interestingly enough, was seen as a core and essential therapeutic activity for all able patients and as a necessary and valued part of hospital operations.

This practice of using patients to assist in hospital operations ended when hospital employment programs became subject to federal and state labor laws as a result of class action lawsuits in the mid 1960s.[2] These lawsuits resulted in decisions requiring working patients to be treated as paid employees. Patients who wanted or needed to work were shifted to occupational therapy and limited skills training activities. These activities were seen as adjunctive treatment therapies rather than the core purpose of the inpatient experience or as hospital operations.

The diminishing role of patients in the day-to-day operation of hospitals was not because the patients were not functioning properly in job roles. However, this shift to thinking of employment activities as ancillary resulted in patients having to demonstrate "readiness" in order to be referred or accepted into employment or vocational services outside of the "secure and structured" state hospital environment. This readiness prerequisite did not exist prior to vocational preparation becoming a part of the treatment process and may have had less to do with a patient's ability to work versus the institution's real or perceived liability for the actions of discharged patients in real-world job settings. Vocational testing and skills training to assist individuals to be "ready" came to be viewed as the role of vocational services rather than actual jobs for individuals with SPMI. As services began to move into the community, the idea that individuals had to demonstrate readiness and that employment and vocational services were ancillary continued. This belief has resulted in a low expectation on the part of many consumers and providers, not to mention the employing public, about the role of work in a consumer's life and his/her capacity to obtain and maintain competitive employment.

In the 1970s, the federal government began to promote the development of community support systems (CSSs) and community support programs (CSPs) as the most effective model for the delivery of services for persons with SPMI. The CSP model is based on 10 core principles (Hughes & Weinstein, 2000). These principles are derived from an examination of the full continuum of services that were originally available for persons in state hospitals, and the supports needed by individuals to survive and thrive in the community. Community support system design documents and demonstrations have focused on the development of a full array of community supports ranging from crisis services to access to vocational programs and entitlements. The principles also focused on community integration, meaning among other things that for persons with SPMI to realize his/her full employment potential, he/she should have

---

[2]*Souder v. Brennan*, 367 F.Supp. 808 (D.D.C. 1973): A class action suit holding that the use of patients to work in positions in state hospitals and other institutional settings is subject to the Fair Labor Standards Act and requiring the U.S. Department of Labor to enforce minimum wage and overtime rules for such patients/individuals.

the same access to vocational services and actual employment as other persons, together with the supports to ensure that this occurs.

Because state vocational rehabilitation agencies were able to "draw down" federal dollars for every state dollar expended, state mental health authorities were encouraged to seek the support of state vocational rehabilitation agencies. States entered into a memorandum of agreements (MOA) to transfer state dollars to vocational rehabilitation agencies to be used to match federal dollars with specific understandings about how mental health clients would be referred to the agency, and served by vocational rehabilitation counselors as stipulated in the MOA. Unfortunately, these efforts were only minimally successful in terms of the actual number of serious mentally ill individuals becoming competitively employed. For example, according to the Social Security Administration (SSA), only between 5% and 10% of the over 600,000 Supplemental Security Income (SSI) and Social Security Disability Income (SSDI) recipients in the State of New York are working.[3] SSA statistics suggest that in FY 2000, less than 0.5% of SSI and SSDI beneficiaries and recipients went to work as a result of its vocational rehabilitation agency efforts (Tishman & Martin, 1998). Some states now fund community agencies to help people gain access to services offered by state and local vocational rehabilitation agencies.

Local authorities play a role in access to these vocational services for persons with SPMI. About half the states across the country rely on local authorities to plan for and fund mental health services, to ensure services are provided in accordance with state and federal laws, and to ensure that individuals with mental illness have access to the services they need in the most effective and timely manner. Many states have strengthened the role of local authorities over the years to ensure persons leaving state psychiatric facilities get the follow-up care they need and to ensure transitions from one type of care to another. States have also asked local authorities to develop community support systems or similar "systems of care" by coordinating mental health services together with other community services and with available public benefits such as Medicaid, Social Security Income, housing, etc. This has often required that local authorities develop relationships with local vocational rehabilitation offices, local employment and small business offices, and local economic development offices to assist persons with SPMI to gain access to vocational related services and benefits. Some local authorities fund consumer operated businesses or job clubs to encourage and support consumer self-reliance and recovery.

CURRENT STATUS OF STATE AND LOCAL AUTHORITIES' RESPONSE TO EMPLOYMENT OF PEOPLE WITH SPMI

Since most state and local mental health authorities do not have a mandate to respond to employment needs of people with SPMI, they often do so only to the degree the authority has the resources and the values-base to support these services. In fact, it has been debated in some circles whether issues such as employment, housing, education, or income supports are the proper responsibilities of the mental health system. Some believe that the mental health system's primary role is treating the symptoms of the mental illnesses that prevent stable employment, housing, or participation in educational activities. This philosophy, of course,

[3]New York State Vocational and Educational Services for Individuals with Disabilities: Proposed State Plan for Vocational Rehabilitation and Supported Employment Services for Federal Fiscal Years 2001–2006.

presumes that persons with SPMI can participate in such services without special accommodation as do other individuals seeking employment, if the symptoms of the mental illness are controlled.

The recent evidence-based understanding of the impacts of mental illness on the development and lives of persons with SPMI suggest that the role of the mental health system in employment has to be more than just symptom control (Mueser, Drake, & Bond, 1997; O'Neill & Bertollo, 1998; Torrey et al., 1998). The growth of a recovery philosophy (Anthony, 1993; Markowitz et al., 1996) has led some to advocate that the mental health system's role is to assist consumers in developing job skills and employment opportunities through the use of peer support and self-help services, and that assistance in gaining normal, competitive employment (or similar meaningful activity) is fundamental to a person's recovery in addition to or in some cases in lieu of the more traditional symptom management or insight-oriented therapeutic treatments. These philosophies suggest that full participation in competitive employment by persons with SPMI will require that systems offer flexibly designed and responsive services and supports needed to provide the greatest likelihood for individual success in the workplace, regardless of whether or not symptoms are controlled, and regardless of whether or not these necessary services and supports are traditional mental health treatments.

As the debate continues, persons with SPMI often find themselves trapped, requiring services and supports from different agencies with conflicting missions, different target populations, and/or different or conflicting rules and requirements that make it difficult for an individual to be successful in his/her employment goals. Regardless of the controlling philosophy, most state and local authorities try to address the employment needs of persons with SPMI in their various roles as planner, provider, funder/purchaser, or regulator. How this might occur is described below.

Authority as Provider

State and local authorities provide direct support for consumers' employment needs in three, often limited, ways. First, they actually employ people with SPMI in their own operations. Many states have administrative units devoted to consumer services. Current or former service recipients largely staff these units. Likewise, some state or local authorities hire an ombudsperson or other prominent consumer position to assist consumers with service access and resolution of complaints as well as to model consumer involvement and employment.

Second, in states where the state or local authority directly provides community services, the authority sometimes directly operates employment or vocational services in much the same way that private (often non-profit) agencies do. Third, some states and local authorities operate (or fund) long-term residential rehabilitation programs that may include work adjustment programs (WAPs) or other vocational readiness programs. These programs may or may not be connected with community-based vocational services and do not regularly lead to or support people actually gaining competitive employment in the commercial world.

Authority as Planner and Funder

The planning and funding roles of state and local authorities with regard to employment services often blend together in a single approach that ranges from very modest to very comprehensive. State-developed initiatives often result in or stem from specially earmarked funds from the state legislature or federal block grant funds for high priority services not otherwise provided or funded by traditional mental health providers or fund sources (such as Medicaid or state treatment dollars). Some states select a particular service model and fund it exclusively, while other states strongly support providing assistance to local authorities or providers to develop a broader array of services designed to support people in meeting their vocational goals. These initiatives tend to be small in comparison with larger outpatient, inpatient, and day program allocations. There has been little or no increase in the amount of financial support provided for these initiatives over the past 15 years,[4] and there have been few documented increases in the number of persons with SPMI going to work as a result of these funds. While over 60% of persons with SPMI indicate a desire to work (Bond & Becker et al., 2000), less than 15% and often closer to 7–8% of such individuals are actually employed for pay for any significant portion of any given month (Turner & Tenhhor, 1978).

Planning and funding of employment services by state and local authorities has begun to increase in the last few years. Some states have assigned administrative staff to develop vocational or employment services. In keeping with the community support system model, state and local authorities have attempted to engage state vocational authorities in these endeavors. In the final section of this chapter, attention will be given to the relative lack of success of these ventures.

Authority as Regulator

State authorities also use their regulatory role to define services that can be paid for with mental health funds and then monitor the provision of those services to ensure fiscal and service compliance. In keeping with the trend toward quality management and improvement-driven performance indicators, and in response to the recovery movement and advocates' call for normalized housing and jobs, state and local authorities have begun to consider employment or meaningful daily activity (e.g., education or volunteering) as appropriate outcomes to track and require of the service delivery system. Efforts to develop outcomes measures now include employment as an outcome indicator for persons receiving services for mental illness (Adams et al., 2001).

INNOVATIONS IN POLICY AND PROGRAMS

In the late 1970s and early 1980s, state and local authorities began recognizing the value of rehabilitation services as an alternative to, or as a complement, more traditional medical model services designed to control or reduce symptoms. The clubhouse model (Cella, Besancon, & Zipple, 1997), an important vehicle in the recovery movement to support persons with SPMI in obtaining and maintaining jobs, began to spread and some states began to provide limited financial support for these service models. When federal CSP funds became available in 1977, mental health authorities sought to develop agreements with state vocational authorities targeted at improving access to vocational rehabilitation (VR) services for persons with SPMI. The more entrepreneurial states took advantage of potentially lapsing

[4]Personal conversation with Judith A. Cook, Ph.D., Professor and Director of the National Research and Training Center on Psychiatric Disability, University of Illinois, Department of Psychiatry, Fall 1999.

federal dollars to match those dollars with state monies to create new rehabilitation initiatives. These initiatives consisted largely of expanded work assessment and adjustment programs, service enclaves (or sheltered work), and job training, along with some competitive job placements and even a few new consumer-operated business starts. In other states, some agreements led to these expansions without federal dollars. Over the years, these agreements have remained but have not expanded tremendously, and state mental health authority officials express considerable frustration with the perceived VR bureaucracy that has limited the expansion of these needed services.

In the 1970s and 1980s the federal government made CSP grants available to states, and CSP directors were designated in every state. Through CSP conferences, publications, and research initiatives, states became much more involved in promoting rehabilitation and vocational initiatives and became more aware of program innovations and a burgeoning psychiatric rehabilitation research field. The NIMH and later the Substance Abuse and Mental Health Services Administration (SAMHSA), Center for Mental Health Services (CMHS) branch funded Research and Training Centers and some limited research and demonstration grants for rehabilitation practices. State authorities became very active in promoting vocational services even in the absence of any significant funding, and many new innovations were spurred on with very small grants.

In the late 1980s, another concept became popular. With some new federal and state funds, supported employment was implemented as a state level initiative between state vocational rehabilitation and state mental health authorities. This approach had its roots in the developmental disabilities field where it is still more widely used, but it spurred on the more recent interest in diversified placement approaches and supported employment specialists, becoming part of community treatment teams and assertive community treatment programs (Allness & Knoedler, 2001). It also spurred the development and evaluation of what is now called the individual placement and support (IPS) model of vocational services (Becker, Bond, & McCarthy, 2001; Becker & Drake, 1994). The research and principles of this model espouse that persons with SPMI do not do well with traditional vocational assessment and readiness models. Rather, they do best with a model more like the one that non-mentally ill persons use; that is, seeking employment in the traditional competitive job market and learning on the job by doing, with the extra necessary job coaching and supports needed because of the psychiatric needs or social skills deficits resulting from the mental illness (Bond, Drake, & Mueser, 1997; Drake et al., 2000).

The CMHS has not been able to continue the same level of support for vocational or employment services to states nor have state officials been able to work together in the same manner as they did in the previous decade. However, most states have continued to fund operating support and start-up of new vocational programs that provide a range of services using a range of models. Given that the vocational readiness, needs, and preferences of persons with SPMI vary widely, it may be that no one model is the most effective means of meeting the multiple needs of the variety of different individuals with serious mental illness. The soundest strategy may be the promotion of a range of options and choices that can be tailored to a person's preference and needs.

The CMHS's supported employment intervention demonstrations in eight sites (Arizona, Connecticut, Maine, Maryland, Massachusetts, Pennsylvania, South Carolina, and Texas) across the country have renewed interest and attention in the potential for employment opportunities for persons with mental illness. Additionally, the current economic climate, the emphasis on welfare-to-work in the country today, the growing emphasis on recovery rather than service delivery or even rehabilitation, and recent changes in federal law eliminating barriers to employment, are all contributing to the idea that employment is a reasonable and expected outcome for adults with mental illness. The long-term impact of these efforts remains to be seen. However, the attention to employment issues is creating a climate for change beyond the individual federal demonstrations, law changes, or isolated state or locally supported projects themselves.

Closely related to these developments has been the rapid expansion of Medicaid as a fund source for community services for persons with SPMI. Medicaid funding is only available for medically related services, and states have worked diligently to define psychiatric rehabilitation services as Medicaid eligible services under the federal Medicaid Rehabilitation Option. These services are optional; a state does not have to provide them under the current Social Security Act, Title XIX, which is the federal law that authorizes Medicaid and dictates federal Medicaid and, to some extent, Medicare policy. However, most state mental health authorities offer their own state allocations as a match for these federal dollars, thus making it possible for states to fund additional Medicaid services without expanding the state's overall Medicaid budget. It should be noted that there is much competition for state dollars for Medicaid match and optional mental health services are not often given priority for these funds.[5]

Another related policy issue that impacts employment for individuals with SPMI is the issue of consumer benefit income levels. A significant number of persons with SPMI rely on SSI and SSDI benefits as their principal source of income. These federal income supports are based on an individual's status as a person with a disability resulting in an inability to engage in gainful employment. This leaves most persons on these benefits living in poverty (O'Hara & Miller, 2001). When a person on one of these disability programs returns to work, there are provisions for "work incentive" allowances. Under certain circumstances the individual can sustain part or all of his/her Medicaid and Medicare benefits. However, the combination of wages (generally very low), lack of medical and leave benefits associated with low-wage jobs, and the allowances often still leaves the individual in or near poverty. Without critical medical benefits for needed medications and inpatient or outpatient psychiatric coverage, and long waiting periods for reinstatement of benefits should the stresses of employment or symptom reoccurrence require a return to disability status, the work incentive quickly becomes a perverse disincentive.

Recent federal legislation to improve this situation was signed into law in December 1999 (Social Security Administration, 1999). The Ticket to Work and Work Incentives Improvement Act (TWWIIA, PL 106–170) is designed to improve the employment situation for people with disabilities by removing barriers to work, requiring only partial reduction of benefits until work experience and wages warrant full reduction of benefits, allowing quick return of benefits if necessary, and offering continuing Medicaid benefits for persons returning to employment from disabled statuses. The TWWIIA will also allow individuals to use vouchers/tickets to seek their own vocational training and support services, through Employment Networks, rather than having to use the traditional services and providers funded by VR agencies. The TWWIIA is being implemented as an alternative to traditional

---

[5]At a New York Association of Psychosocial Rehabilitation Services (NYAPRS) conference in July 2001, in a presentation entitled Medicaid Coverage of Adult Services under the Rehabilitation Option, Ms. Chris Koyangi of the Bazelon Center in Washington, DC, indicated that 22 states offer some form of vocational skills training or supports as a Medicaid covered service for Medicaid eligible individuals. Not all states had reported at the time of this presentation, so the actual number may be higher.

VR efforts that have been ineffective overall for persons with disabilities, and especially for persons with SPMI. The TWWIIA will be phased in nationwide by 2004. In spite of the anticipated promise of initiatives such as TWWIIA, policy-makers and persons with disabilities are still facing an uphill battle to ensure that vocational services and job placements for persons with mental disabilities can actually yield a positive outcome for individuals who need support in order to work.

COLLABORATION BETWEEN THE STATE MENTAL HEALTH AUTHORITY AND THE STATE VR AGENCY

Although the primary purpose of this chapter is to describe the role of state and local mental health authorities, it is important to discuss the collaboration between the state (and to a lesser extent the local) mental health authority and the state (or local) VR agency to present a clear picture of mental health authorities' role in vocational services. Most state mental health authorities rely in part or in whole on programs and funding from the state VR agency to channel persons with mental illness through vocational services, employment readiness, and job placement scenarios. The federal government awards VR funds to states through the Rehabilitation Services Administration (RSA). Each state has a state-level VR agency that administers the state program and receives federal grants. Each state matches the federal awards with state funds (approximately 20% state match required). The federal funds cover case services, costs for vocational rehabilitation counselors to serve persons with qualifying disabilities, payments to vendors (agencies who provide services) for specified activities, costs of adaptive devices and other equipment, and administrative costs.

The state VR agency must comply with extensive federal regulations but has considerable latitude in the way the program is operated. As a consequence, there is "wide variation among state programs in the demographic characteristics of persons served, the types of services provided and the effectiveness of those services" (Conley, 1999). A U.S. General Accounting Office study issued in 1993 evaluated the efforts of the federal–state VR program. This study revealed that overall state VR agencies do not give priority to persons with SPMI; that average vocational rehabilitation case service expenditures were less for clients with emotional disabilities (including those with mental illness) than expenditures for persons with mental retardation, physical disabilities, or sensory disabilities; and that for a majority of clients with mental illness the annual case service expenditures were less than $500. This study found that only 12 states reported specialized caseload policies so that specialized counselors serve persons with mental illness (Noble, 1998). Likewise, Goldman and Manderscheid (1987) reported in 1987 that the expected rate of referrals from state mental health agencies and their contract providers should be 487 per 100,000 population based on the estimated number of persons who receive SSI or SSDI benefits because of their mental illness. Given the increase in persons receiving these benefits due to mental illness, this expected figure has likely increased since this report.

A recent study conducted by the National Alliance for the Mentally Ill (NAMI) reports that the "average rate of referrals by state mental health agencies to vocational rehabilitation services other than programs run by state mental health agencies themselves was only about 19.8 per 100,000 population, ranging from a high of 205.6 in South Carolina to zero in most states" (Noble et al., 1997). Noble reported that on four indicators used to measure and summarize the extent to which VR efforts are made by state mental health authorities, the states' overall scores average out to zero as 32 states ranked below zero in their efforts. Only South Carolina, New Hampshire, Ohio, Maine, Colorado, Arkansas, and Arizona scored 3 or above. The impact of the new federal legislation described earlier, especially the role of vouchers in allowing disabled individuals to choose their vocational service providers, may decrease referrals to VR authorities but increase satisfaction and effectiveness of vocational services in getting and maintaining competitive and normalized employment.

State mental health authorities began collaborating with state VR agencies when the CSP initiatives began in earnest in the early 1980s. Prior to that time the relationship was limited to one of service providers making referrals of individuals to VR authorities with the encouragement of state mental health authorities. Joint funding of small projects and grants along with state mental health authority advocacy for increased VR agency support for persons with SPMI were the most frequent strategies employed by state mental health authorities. Local authorities often participated in these efforts, with some having agreements with local VR agencies for referrals, employment or location of specialized VR counselors, and/or cross training of VR and mental health caseworkers.

But the relationship between the two state agencies has become more complicated. Both fund direct service programs, both enroll individuals as clients, both have responsibility to build a system of care that can aid people in their attempt to secure employment, and both are being asked to focus on the outcome of their interventions and allocation of resources. Still there are a number of critical differences. State VR agencies have a very broad client base with respect to disability type and level of need, and their services are designed to be time limited with a very focused outcome across all these populations, namely gainful employment within a specified period of time.

On the other hand, state and local mental health authorities are concerned with one particular disability population and with the supports this group of individuals need over time to obtain and maintain positive employment experiences, whether or not consistently employed in a particular employment situation. State VR agency mandates and rules are largely federally based, whereas state and local mental health authorities must respond to federal, state, and local mandates. These differences appear to be at the root of the problems between the two bureaucracies. The two agencies often appear to be working at cross-purposes, or at least without a common mission with regard to this population. These issues present tremendous frustration both to providers and to individuals with SPMI who want individualized and varying assistance in choosing, getting, and keeping work opportunities.

The recent NAMI report recommended that the $490 million currently being spent by the VR system for individuals with mental illness be "rechanneled into local programs that integrate vocational and psychiatric rehabilitation services on a continuous, non-time limited basis." They also recommended adding a new categorical funding authority to the Rehabilitation Act, adding to the mental health services block grant, or adding funds to the budget of the SSA for financing VR services for SSI/SSDI beneficiaries (Noble et al., 1997). The NAMI review extended to surveys of psychiatric rehabilitation programs who corroborated their concerns regarding the current VR system citing delays, lack of funding, problems within and between the two state agencies, stigma among VR counselors as well as employers, and lack of specifically trained vocational counselors (within the state VR agency) as problems (Noble, 1998). In addition, a survey conducted by the National Association of County Behavioral Healthcare Directors, released in March 2000, indicates that the most common jobs developed for consumers were either custodial, clerical, or in food services. These jobs are typically entry-level, low-wage-earning positions that offer little opportunity for advancement and growth.

Likewise, state mental health program directors have spoken out on this issue. Joseph Bevilacqua, former Mental Health Commissioner in three states, has stated that the "bureaucratic obstacles and inertia that have plagued the field of vocational rehabilitation have themselves formed patterns that are rarely identified in literature." He calls for the closure of state VR agencies, stating, "efforts to change the employment culture for individuals with SPMI have been an abysmal failure" (Bevilacqua, 1999). Others have called for a reform of the system, with closer collaboration between the two agencies. Most consumers, advocates, scholars, and mental health officials are united in their view that irrationalities and inefficiencies must be removed from both systems if this approach to the employment of persons with mental illness is to be successful. Given the vouchers possible under the Ticket to Work and Social Security Program (TTWSSP) described earlier in this chapter, increased competition may result in increased attention to the needs of persons with SPMI among providers of VR services.

RECOMMENDATIONS

State and local authorities can play a significant, if not leading role in creating more employment opportunities and helping people with SPMI secure and maintain employment. Below are four recommendations likely to increase the positive impact of vocational and employment services for persons with mental illness.

Mission, Vision, Advocacy, and Voice

State mental health authorities set the direction for the public mental health service system in their state. They often have significant impact on the state Medicaid authority and state Medicaid planning and policy. The mental health authority recommends policy and funding priorities to the Governor, the state budget office, and the state's legislative body. The state authority establishes, and the state commissioner or his/her designee sits on, a variety of commissions and task forces at both the state and federal level. The state authority influences federal legislation and priorities through the national organization, the National Association of State Mental Health Program Directors (NASMHPD), and the Governor's office on Capitol Hill. The state authority that has a clear vision that includes strong support for persons with SPMI to gain and maintain employment, can strongly influence policy and the decision-makers.

Thus, the state mental health authority's mission should include a clear and direct role for funding and supporting vocational and employment related services and strong advocacy directed toward reducing barriers for people with SPMI who seek employment. This advocacy should be directed toward ensuring that the new TTWIIP is implemented so that it fulfills its promise and so that it is possible for persons with SPMI to work and live above poverty. This advocacy should articulate the wide range of barriers that exist for consumers attempting to become employed, including: (1) the disincentives to work for individuals if jobs are low-paying and yet result in loss of needed medical benefits and eligibility for disability payments should they be needed again; (2) the widespread discrimination and stigma that exists for consumers trying to enter the workplace; (3) the extra supports needed for persons who have often not been in the workforce consistently to return to work and succeed in stressful environments; (4) the barriers within the mental health system, where work is not given as high a value as treatment to reduce or manage symptoms; and

(5) the concepts of recovery and work as important elements in quality of life are not yet well understood.

Local authorities have a special vision and advocacy role regarding employment services. They have access to local employers, the media, and community leaders, as well as to the community's general public. They can and should be a leading voice regarding the ability and the value of people with SPMI going to work. These public statements should be augmented by actions such as seeing that persons have access to jobs, that editorial positions are taken, that employers gain recognition for affirmative hiring practices, and that stigma is affirmatively combated.

State and local authorities can influence other systems as well. For example, they can promote rehabilitation curricula and educational support in both undergraduate and graduate training programs at state and locally supported universities and community colleges. They can influence federal priorities and federal legislation and give high priority to joint initiatives for increased funding and case service improvement strategies with state VR agencies. They can influence the state Medicaid Plan to expand or include the rehabilitation option to give more focus on rehabilitation services and outcomes. They can propose employment-related performance indicators for Medicaid waiver programs and advocate for service definitions flexible enough to allow financial support for vocational services.

If state and local authorities do not see it as a key part of their primary mission to promote recovery in the form of gainful employment for adults with SPMI, then the number of such individuals employed will continue to be appallingly low, and such individuals will disproportionately live in poverty, thereby hampering their ability to lead satisfying and productive lives, not because of their mental illness, but because they lack the opportunity to succeed in a key facet of community life.

Resource Allocation

Perhaps the strongest message the state authority and, to the extent possible, the local authority, can send is through resource allocations. Each state and local authority makes decisions about how funds are going to be spent. While the choices are often limited and the amount of funds available is always less than what is needed, there is discretion. To date, state and local authorities have placed a lower priority on making funds available for psychiatric rehabilitation, supported employment, and other employment-related services. State budgets are generally driven by providing funds to existing mental health service providers for inpatient care, and for a myriad of other psychiatrically oriented services. The advocacy for how funds are expended is intense and many groups compete for the funds. State and local authorities thus have to establish, sometimes without vocal and organized advocates, vocational- and employment-related services as a high priority to ensure that gains are made in helping people reach their job goals.

Another way to increase resources for vocational support for consumers is through the use of supported educational or business opportunities. Work with small business loan programs and incubators and with local community colleges is paying off for some state and local authorities and some consumer groups seeking to start and support consumer-operated businesses and services. Use of research and other educational support funds is a way some states are encouraging educational opportunities for consumers that results in better employability.

Planning, Policy-Making, and Evaluating Programs

State and local mental health authorities are major planners and regulators of services funded by state, federal, and local resources for persons with SPMI across all government programs. They have a unique opportunity to influence public policy and develop strong plans for employment-related services for persons with SPMI. Authorities can establish service, funding, and local planning requirements that emphasize employment. Authorities can have a significant influence on providers' and other funders' behavior by what they ask for and what standards they set for system performance. If vocational and employment outcomes are missing from an authority's own strategic vision and system performance indicators, then they are not likely to be a priority of, or be achieved by, providers within the system of care.

Some mental health authorities refuse to include employment as an indicator of success of mental health services, arguing that mental health authorities do not generally pay for these services and therefore they cannot hold providers to this outcome. However, funding priorities and behavior will not change until employment is an expected outcome of service delivery. Decreasing or controlling symptoms, while critical, is not enough. Returning to productive and satisfactory living that offers the same opportunities as those experienced by others in the community is the true test of mental health system effectiveness. State and local authorities have an obligation to promote this type of life success for persons receiving publicly funded services. Employment is often the key to a productive and satisfying quality of life.

Promoting and Rewarding Best Practice

States have the opportunity to promote "best practice" through publications and/or recommendations to the field, matching grant awards, sponsoring conferences, giving awards and rewards, and translating "learning" from evidenced-based practices into allocation guidelines, service requirements, performance standards, and even state certification requirements.

States are beginning to promote "best practice" in employment services for people with SPMI. For example, the Ohio Department of Mental Health is developing Centers of Excellence across the state where strong emphasis on developing employment strategies will be one of several best practices if promoted. The St. Luke's Charitable Health Trust in Phoenix, Arizona, with strong support from the state mental health agency, has created the Mental Health Dissemination Network of Arizona and recently published a report entitled "Into the Light: A Search for Excellence in the Arizona Public Behavioral Health System," highlighting support for employment as a key element of the state system. Finally, in the state of Oklahoma, the Community Rehabilitation Services Unit of the Oklahoma Department of Rehabilitation Services (DRS) has developed a Milestone Payment System that was instrumental in putting people with disabilities into the workforce. The Milestone system is a reimbursement method based on incentives and outcomes under which all of those who play a role in the service delivery process benefit (Frumkin, 2001).

As stated above, other state and local authorities have added supported employment services, clubhouses, consumer-operated businesses, job coaching, purchase of business equipment, payment of transitional employment costs such as transportation or insurance, and other cutting edge vocational wrap-around support to their list of reimbursable services. In states and localities where assertive community treatment (ACT) models are promoted, requirements for vocational counselors on ACT teams are increasing (Allness & Knoedler, 2001).

Influencing "best practice" in the VR field is also important. Recent criticism of the VR system notwithstanding, the state, and in some cases the local mental health authority, has the opportunity to influence the system by building the case for better practice. In the past, other disability groups have sought to influence this field both within state and local VR organizations as well as in the preparation of new staff and the field as a whole. This ensures that future VR leaders will be more sensitive to the needs of persons with mental illness. As it stands today, VR leadership and many mental health professionals, especially those who have been in the system for many years and who were trained in a more traditional approach to vocational training and readiness, are less inclined to support people with mental illness in new and creative ways to find and keep jobs. However, this resistance is changing.

Breaking down this resistance and introducing evidence-based best practices can be done through conferences, agreements, and building interest and competencies across the entire field. State and local authorities can work with universities to influence the number of vocational counselors who are interested in and trained to specialize in working with persons with mental illness. Encouraging and financially supporting university-based rehabilitation education and counseling training programs offers opportunities to influence the future of these fields. Supporting placements, funding stipends, or faculty development are excellent ways to shape the training of future vocational workers.

The development of best practices is intimately tied to state and local authorities' advocacy and leadership roles. Often, what authorities have to offer is voice. This spokesperson role is critical. One must believe to advocate, and one must advocate in order to create change. Change for persons with SPMI is no more critical than in their fundamental role as contributing members of the communities in which they live. While employment is not the only way to contribute, in this society employment is seen as a critical indicator of health and acceptance. Employment, then, and not just vocational activities, is critical to recovery for persons with SPMI. State and local authorities have an obligation to ensure debate, fund services, and promote best practices in employment services until no person with mental illness who wants to work and is capable of working is prevented from doing so.

CONCLUSION

In our society we define ourselves as well as others by what we do—our work. Work is an essential element of our participation and acceptance in our communities. While SPMI comes with its own stresses and challenges for those affected, the lack of vocational and employment opportunities increases the stress level significantly and impacts negatively on person with SPMI's sense of self-worth and belonging within his/her families and the community.

Local and state mental health authorities must plan and invest in services and programs that create employment opportunities for an important, yet vulnerable significant segment of our population. Without such a commitment in focus, persons with SPMI will become further marginalized and stigmatized without employment opportunities. The lack of real integration between employment and mental health services will potentially result in fewer consumers receiving services, at greater cost.

The provision of mental health services with vocational and employment opportunities should not be viewed exclusively as "the government's problem," but should be viewed as a community challenge and responsibility. State and local mental health authorities have a responsibility to set the priorities, and manage and measure the effectiveness of their efforts. It is clear that priorities that integrate mental health and vocational and employment services must be developed and delivered based upon evidence-based and promising practices and research in the field. State and local mental health authorities must become effective and vocal advocates for change in their systems. The role of state and local mental health authorities in responding to the employment needs of people with SPMI can be summed up in a familiar chant of the civil rights era of the 1960s: "If not now, when? If not us, who?"

REFERENCES

Adams, N., England, M. J., Golperud, E. et al. (2001). *A proposed consensus set of indicators for behavioral health* (Accreditation organization workgroup interim report). American College of Mental Health Administration.

Allness, D., & Knoedler, W. (2001). Recommended assertive community treatment standards for new teams (revised).

Anthony, W. A. (1993). Recovery from mental illness: The guiding vision of the mental health service system in the 1990s. *Psychosocial Rehabilitation Journal, 16*(4), 11–24.

Becker, D. R., Bond, G. R., & McCarthy, D. (2001). Converting day treatment centers to supported employment programs in Rhode Island. *Psychiatric Services, 52*(3), 351–357.

Becker, D. R., & Drake, R. E. (1994). Individual placement and support: A community mental health center approach to vocational rehabilitation. *Community Mental Health Journal, 30*, 193–206.

Bevilacqua, J. J. (1999). The state vocational rehabilitation agency: A case for closure. *Journal of Disability Policy Studies, 10*(1), 90–98.

Bond, G. R., Becker, D. R. et al. (2000). Implementing supported employment as an evidence-based practice. *Psychiatric Services, 52*(3), 317.

Bond, G. R., Drake, R. E., & Mueser, K. T. (1997). An update on supported employment for people with severe mental illness. *Psychiatric Services, 48*(3), 335–346.

Cella, E. P., Besancon, V., & Zipple, A. M. (1997). Expanding the role of clubhouses: Guidelines for establishing a system of integrated day services. *Psychiatric Rehabilitation Journal, 21*(1).

Drake, R. E., McHugo, G. J., Bebout, R. R. et al. (2000). A randomized clinical trial of supported employment for inner-city patients with severe mental disorders. *Archives of General Psychiatry, 56*, 627.

Frumkin, P. (2001). *Managing for outcomes: Milestone contracting in Oklahoma* (Innovations in Management series). Cambridge, MA: Harvard University, Kennedy School of Government.

Geller, J. L. (2000). The last half-century of psychiatric services as reflected in *Psychiatric Services. Psychiatric Services 51*(1): 41–67.

Goldman, H., & Manderscheid, R. (1987). Epidemiology of chronic mental disorder. In W. Menninger & G. Hanna (Eds.), *The chronic patient*, Vol. 2. Washington, DC: American Psychiatric Press.

Hughes, R., & Weinstein, D. (2000). Assessment in psychosocial rehabilitation. In B. Caldwell (Ed.), *Best practices in psychosocial rehabilitation*. International Association of Psychosocial Rehabilitation Services.

Markowitz, F. E., DeMasi, M. E., Carpinello, S. E., Knight, E. L. et al. (1996, February). The role of self-help in the recovery process. Paper presented at the Sixth Annual National Conference on State Mental Health Agency Services Research and Program Evaluation, Arlington, VA.

Mueser, K. T., Drake, R. E., & Bond, G. R. (1997). Recent advances in psychiatric rehabilitation for patients with severe mental illness. *Harvard Review of Psychiatry, 5*, 123–127.

Noble, Jr, J. H. (1998). Policy reform dilemmas in promoting employment of persons with severe mental illnesses. *Psychiatric Services, 49*(6), 775–781.

Noble, Jr, J. H., Honberg, R. S., Hall, L. L. et al. (1997). *A legacy of failure: The inability of the federal-state vocational rehabilitation system to serve people with severe mental illness*. Arlington, VA: The National Alliance for the Mentally Ill.

O'Hara, A., & Miller, E. (2001). Priced out in 2000: The crisis continues. Washington, DC: The Consortium for Citizens with Disabilities and The Technical Assistance Collaborative.

O'Neill, D. M., & Bertollo, D. N. (1998). Work and earnings losses due to mental illness: Perspectives from three national surveys. *Administration and Policy in Mental Health, 25*(5).

Social Security Administration (1999). *A summary guide to social security and supplemental security income work incentives for people with disabilities.* Washington, DC: Author.

Tishman, M., & Martin, E. (1998). Testimony before the subcommittee on social security of the House committee on ways and means related to hearing on the Ticket to Work and Self-Sufficiency Act of 1998.

Torrey, W. C., Bebout, R., Kline, J. et al. (1998). Practice guidelines for clinicians working in programs providing integrated vocational and clinical services for persons with severe mental disorders. *Psychiatric Rehabilitation Journal, 21*(4).

Turner, J. C., & Tenhhor, J. W. (1978). The NIMH community support program: Pilot approach to needed social reform. *Schizophrenia Bulletin, 4,* 319–348.

U.S. Department of Health and Human Services (1997). *Health care spending: National expenditures for mental health and substance abuse treatment.* Washington, DC: Author.

DEVELOPING READINESS FOR EMPLOYMENT

Even though the current policy and practice environment focuses increasingly on getting people jobs immediately, some individuals need opportunities to prepare for employment. Readiness is an important phase in any change process and, in relation to employment, it takes on added meaning as people obtain the skills, motivation, and supports to get ready to move into jobs with as many success factors in place as possible. More dated models of rehabilitation and mental health practice incorporated readiness as a criterion for acceptance or rejection from job programs. In these models, people were assessed for the extent to which they were prepared to engage in employment successfully. On face, such criterion-oriented assessments suggested good practice since these programs wanted to reach those individuals who would prove to be successful. Often, however, such practice only resulted in the rejection of people who wanted to work but perhaps did not have the experience to suggest that they would be successful and resulted in the creaming of programs—that is, the acceptance of people who likely could get work on their own.

For contemporary models of rehabilitation the development of readiness is a legitimate and important outcome of a service process in which people have as many opportunities as they wish to get ready for something as complex as work, employment, and career. There are a number of different service approaches or models of rehabilitation that facilitate readiness and that integrate the development of readiness into their program theories and structures. The six chapters that compose this section focus on the development of readiness. Collectively these chapters suggest that it is possible to develop readiness and that the development of readiness is particularly important for people who are relatively inexperienced in the world of work, who have disabilities that require the development of specific employment assets, or who have disabilities the onset of which require people to get reacquainted with the demands, expectations, and requirements of employment.

Farkas and Nicolellis offer a theory guiding the development of readiness and they show how important it is for people coping with psychiatric disabilities to progress through a period in which they prepare themselves for the world of work. The theory that the authors present is applicable to a number of different areas of disability and it possesses a relevance to the broad spectrum of employment issues the field of rehabilitation and mental health practice must address. In Chapter 13, Gwilliam, Rabold, and Corrigan outline the relevance of cognitive rehabilitation to the development of readiness and they offer specific remediation and compensatory strategies that are relevant to entry into jobs such as tracking, pattern recognition, and problem-solving, the development and/or restoration of which may prove important in the movement of a person through subsequent phases of rehabilitation and entry into a specific job. Garvin illustrates in Chapter 14 the importance of group support to readiness and how participation in job-focused and skill-oriented groups can help people to identify barriers to employment and help them acquire the resources they need to be successful.

In Chapter 15, Magaw discusses how vocational development within a supportive milieu can facilitate readiness and she focuses on the specific model of the clubhouse in psychiatric rehabilitation. This author addresses vocational development as an outcome and examines how clubhouses can facilitate such an outcome through the emphasis they place on membership, the work-ordered day, participation of members in work groups, and the offer of transitional employment. The clubhouse offers enough structure to facilitate the vocational development of its members but, perhaps more importantly, it also offers an informality that sets in motion processes to help members rekindle motivation, develop stamina, gain focus, and learn about the practical aspects of getting work completed on a daily basis.

Cusick outlines an approach to benefit advisement in Chapter 16 that facilitates the willingness of people with psychiatric disabilities to seek employment. Often the receipt of benefits is seen as a disincentive for people to enter the world of work and Cusick addresses how counseling can be provided to people who need to understand the impact of their employment decisions on the maintenance of benefits. This advisement process is particularly important for people coping with psychiatric disabilities since many recipients may need to deal with symptoms and health issues that are cyclical in nature and/or that flare up at unexpected times. Benefit advisement indicates that getting ready for employment is not merely a personal process but also can involve the modification of procedures, benefits, and supports in order to facilitate long-term participation in the workforce.

In the final chapter of this section, Moxley and his colleagues recast job development and placement as a process of workplace socialization. In this sense, getting ready for employment involves helping people to integrate into the workplace and the work group as well as helping the workplace to get ready to receive and sustain the person.

Taken as a whole the chapters that compose Section III indicate that the development of readiness is indeed an important part of the rehabilitation and mental health service process and should be a common feature of those programs that seek to help people to prepare for, enter, and sustain employment.

CHAPTER 12

Fostering Readiness For Rehabilitation and Employment

MARIANNE FARKAS AND DEBBIE NICOLELLIS

Recovery from chronic illness, and regaining or retaining work, has emerged as a topic of intense interest even in the mainstream media.

> *...about 40% of the U.S. working population has some form of chronic condition, defined as any that persists for a year or longer...employers are looking for new ways to manage and retain chronically ill employees...Remember what work represents to people... "It's mastery and control over one's life. Work brings an enormous sense of personal fulfillment and self worth"*
> *Wong, Time Magazine,* January 22, 2001, pp. B4–B6.

Despite the apparent increased desire among employers to retain people with long-term disabling conditions, surveys have consistently reported that the majority of people with long-term psychiatric conditions have been unemployed (Anthony & Blanch, 1989; Mulkern & Manderscheid, 1989; Yelin & Cisternas, 1997). The ratio of successful vocational outcomes for people with physical disabilities to those with psychiatric outcomes has been quoted as 2:1 (Marshak, Bostick, & Turton, 1990). Irrespective of the low rates of actual employment, the majority of this population does want to have competitive employment (Rogers, Walsh, Danley, & Smith, 1991). Both the field of mental health and that of rehabilitation have had an ongoing interest in identifying ways in which to help people with serious psychiatric disabilities to overcome their disabilities and take their place in the workforce. The issue of how prepared people are to enter or re-enter the workforce is a critical element in identifying relevant strategies to help people with serious psychiatric disabilities succeed in their attempts to gain or regain valued place as a worker. This chapter discusses the factors related to readiness to engage in work or in vocational rehabilitation services designed to help people gain and retain employment.

MARIANNE FARKAS AND DEBBIE NICOLELLIS • World Health Organization Collaborating Center, Boston University Center for Psychiatric Rehabilitation, Boston, Massachusetts.

RESEARCH FOUNDATION FOR
REHABILITATION READINESS

It has been estimated that in the United States 2.6% of the population have a serious psychiatric disorder (*SAMHSA*, 1993). Several definitions of severe psychiatric disability characterize this target population (Goldman, Gattozzi, & Taube, 1981; NIMH, 1987; *SAMHSA*, 1993). These definitions share common elements: a diagnosis of major mental illness, of prolonged duration, with serious functional incapacity. The definition includes those with diagnoses such as schizophrenia, bipolar disorder, and severe personality disorder.

Recovery from psychiatric experiences has recently become the leading vision for the mental health field (Anthony, 1993; Harding & Zahniser, 1994; Spaniol & Koehler, 1994). Recovery has been described as a way of living a satisfying, hopeful, and contributive life even with limitations caused by the impairment (Anthony, 1993). Unfortunately, the consistently low rates of employment among people with serious psychiatric disabilities make it difficult to envision vocational recovery. Nearly 70% of those with long-term psychiatric experiences in the United States are almost entirely dependent upon Social Security programs for financial and medical support and few ever leave the Social Security rolls to move into competitive employment (U.S. GAO, 1996). Nearly 50% of those who do obtain jobs through rehabilitation programs lose them within a one-year period (Cook & Rosenberg, 1994). No more than 30% of those who work have been able to move beyond the entry-level positions that keep people with serious psychiatric disabilities at or near the poverty level (Kirszner, Baron, & Rutman, 1992). Baron and Salzer (2000) describe a "culture of unemployment" among consumers, policy-makers, and providers that is both pervasive and persistent. In this culture, mental health professionals are accustomed to believing that work may be so stressful as to threaten the consumer's possibilities for progress. Many mental health professionals and vocational rehabilitation counselors view consumers' personal work goals as "unrealistic." Research studies of psychiatric vocational rehabilitation outcomes have focused on two empirical issues: (1) the evaluation of model vocational programs, and (2) the investigation of those consumer factors that correlate with successful vocational outcome. Comprehensive reviews of evaluation studies of vocational programs (e.g., Bond, 1992; Bond & Boyer, 1988) have concluded that time-limited vocational rehabilitation programs can have a positive effect on paid employment for as long as the program intervention is in place. Supported employment, a model of vocational rehabilitation wherein consumers are first helped to obtain competitive employment and then receive ongoing skill and support development services to maintain the job, has shown effectiveness in maintaining competitive employment over time (Bond, Drake, Mueser, & Becker, 1997; Lehman, 1995). Additionally, certain features within these vocational programs were related to measures of vocational outcome. For example, when consumers' motivation was increased by measures such as paid participation in work programs (Bell, Lysaker, & Milstein, 1996), regulation of their own work hours (Bell & Lysaker, 1996), obtaining employment consistent with their expressed job preferences (Fabian, Waterworth, & Ripke, 1993), and increased satisfaction early on in the course of employment (Xie, Dain, Becker, & Drake, 1997), job tenure increased. In summary, factors such as ongoing support, increasing commitment or motivation and increasing satisfaction in job preferences all related to vocational outcome and therefore vocational readiness. The second thrust of psychiatric vocational rehabilitation research, that is, the client factors related to vocational outcome, is also relevant to vocational rehabilitation readiness. Researchers believed that by identifying those client characteristics that predicted vocational outcome, clients who would be more difficult to place and therefore would need more services and those who were "more ready" to begin work would be more easily identified. Over the last several decades a variety of studies have examined the relationship between various client demographic and clinical factors and vocational outcome (Anthony, 1994). The individual's previous work history, his or her capacity to perform work adjustment skills, and the capacity to control his or her symptoms were the most commonly cited predictors (Anthony & Jansen, 1984; Botterbusch, 2000a, 2000b; Knight & Aucoin, 1999; Collins, Mowbray, & Bybee, 2000; Tsang, Lam, Ng, & Leung, 2000). However, predicting who is likely to benefit from vocational services or achieve vocational outcomes based on demographic and clinical variables has proven to be a somewhat illusive exercise (Anthony, Rogers, Cohen, & Davies, 1995; Rogers, Anthony, Cohen, & Davies, 1997). There is some evidence to suggest that if a person seeks, and is engaged in, a vocational program, then many of the variables thought to be related to unsuccessful vocational outcomes (e.g., poor employment history, poor work adjustment skills, more hospitalizations, being unmarried, black, receiving benefits, or being unskilled) are not related to vocational outcome (Anthony, 1994).

In summary, it may be that both programmatic factors and client factors other than clinical and demographic variables are more relevant to readiness to engage in vocational services and readiness to achieve vocational outcome. These factors seem to be "personal factors" (Anthony, 1994), associated with issues such as motivation, commitment, and satisfaction rather than traditional clinical and demographic variables. These personal variables have come to be known as readiness dimensions (Cohen, Anthony, & Farkas, 1997; Farkas, Sullivan-Soydan, and Gagne, 2000).

READINESS CONCEPTS AND ASSUMPTIONS

People vary in their willingness to confront or take action in relation to change of any kind (McConnaughy, DiClemente, Prochaska, & Velicer, 1989; Prochaska, DiClemente, & Norcross, 1992; Prochaska, Velicer, DiClemente, & Fava, 1988; Snow, Prochaska, & Rossi, 1992). Some people are more willing to stay in an unsatisfying situation and will suffer the consequences rather than risk making a change. Others have less tolerance for the discomfort experienced in an unsatisfactory situation and seek change immediately. These variations do not appear to be related to a person's symptoms. While the person's response to his symptoms may, in fact, interfere with his desire to begin an involved, growth-oriented process at a particular moment in time, assessing the level of pathology does not provide specific information about readiness. People with the same diagnosis may differ greatly in their readiness to engage in a rehabilitation process. People with exactly the same symptom patterns may also differ greatly in their readiness to engage in a rehabilitation process (Blume & Schmaling, 1997; McConnaughy et al., 1989).

The process of psychiatric vocational rehabilitation focuses on gaining or improving a valued vocational role. The process of vocational rehabilitation is designed to help individuals choose, get, and keep preferred employment (Danley, Sciarappa, & MacDonald-Wilson, 1992). The process first helps the individual to choose her preferred work goal (e.g., working part-time as a childcare provider). Second, the process helps the person to assess her own skill and support strengths and deficits that contribute to success and satisfaction in the chosen work goal. Third, it helps the person to plan to get her skill and support needs met. Lastly, it helps the individual either learn the skills the person is unable to do at all, improve the ones that are within the person's repertoire but that may not be adequate, or gain the needed supports by linking with or creating necessary resources (Anthony, Cohen, Farkas, & Gagne, 2001).

This focus may challenge people to make behavioral or lifestyle changes. A person may begin to talk about the roles he desires and discover that the desired role requires many changes that he has never even contemplated making. Changing from one role (i.e., clubhouse member) to another (i.e., history teacher) may require a person to process many changes simultaneously. For example, it may imply changes in identity, in social relationships, in the level of intellectual, physical, and/or emotional energy that the person is expected to bring to the new role, and in behavioral changes it may require. Depending upon a person's readiness for change at a particular point in time, the discovery of the reality of making a decision about what the future should bring and the challenge of finding the will to do what it takes to make that choice, can be overwhelming. Rehabilitation readiness, then, enables both the individual and the practitioner to decide if the individual is, in fact, prepared for the arduous process of change involved in choosing and achieving a vocational goal (Cohen et al., 1997; Farkas et al., 2001).

There are three general assumptions underlying the concept of vocational rehabilitation readiness: readiness describes willingness; readiness changes over time; readiness is environmentally specific.

1. *Readiness describes willingness and commitment to engage in changes related to work, it does not describe capacity for work.* Readiness for rehabilitation is based on a number of indicators that reflect the person's preparedness to become actively involved in the rehabilitation process. Readiness to enter vocational services does not depend upon the person's *capacity*, but rather his or her *willingness*. Cook and Rosenberg (1994) found that consumer skills at entry into vocational programs were not related to vocational outcomes. Assessing capacity (e.g., work adjustment skills) is less important to the notion of establishing a person's readiness than is willingness for the change contemplated. The reason for this is that the process of psychiatric vocational rehabilitation itself is designed to increase the person's capacity to make the changes necessary to achieve work. A person without work adjustment skills, in other words, may improve or learn these skills during the rehabilitation process. The individual can, therefore, be willing (ready) to engage in the process, even if the capacity to work is not present at that moment. The ability to assess and develop, or to increase a person's willingness to engage in the process of rehabilitation, depends upon the skills of the practitioner (Cohen, Forbess, & Farkas, 2001; Farkas, Cohen, McNamara, Nemec, & Cohen, 2001). These skills have also been adapted specifically for practitioners in vocational rehabilitation agencies to involve the consumer in the readiness assessment and development process (Center for Psychiatric Rehabilitation, in preparation).

2. *Readiness changes over time.* Willingness to commit to changes that can lead to work, can vary over time. Fear of failure, fear of success, and fear of the unknown consequences of change can interfere insidiously and may even prevent an ongoing commitment to either the process of rehabilitation or the work of maintaining employment over time. Such a crisis of confidence can occur at any stage of the rehabilitation or recovery process (Deegan, 1997; McCrory et al., 1980; Spaniol, Gagne, & Koehler, 1999). Readiness for work therefore does not preclude the need for continued vocational rehabilitation service involvement. Cook and Rosenberg (1994) reported that vocational rehabilitation clients who received continuous support were more likely to be found working than those for whom the rehabilitation support was terminated or interrupted.

Since readiness may change as often as every month or six weeks (Felton et al., 1995; Shern et al., 1997), readiness can be facilitated. A person who is not currently ready can be helped to become more ready. Being "unready" is not a valid label, nor a reason to exclude a person from services. Rather, the goal of the rehabilitation provider is to facilitate the person's readiness to engage in those services that can increase capacity for, and access to, preferred work environments.

3. *Readiness is environmentally specific.* Readiness varies not only over time but across domains and environments as well. The rehabilitation process focuses on one domain at a time: working (job), living (home/community), or learning (school). Readiness to take on the challenge of growth in one of those areas is unrelated to readiness to take on the challenge in another area. For example, a person may be quite willing to begin the rehabilitation process of developing an educational goal to develop his or her career in the future. That same person may be totally unwilling to contemplate changes in his or her current work situation. The assessment and development of readiness, therefore, must focus on answering the question: "Am I prepared to commit myself to the rehabilitation process at this specific time with respect to this specific domain?"

One consideration in environmentally specific readiness development is that of career maturity. Danley, Rogers, and Nevas (1989) identified several levels of career maturity. The first level is the role of a worker (or having a general worker identity). The essential question one asks of oneself in relation to worker identity is: "Do I want to become a worker?" In respect to the role of a colleague, or a member of a specific field or occupation, one asks the question, "Do I want to work as a _____?" Finally, in respect to the role of an employee, holding a specific job in a specific organization, one would ask the question, "Do I want to work as a _____ at _____?" Danley (1997) goes on to demonstrate how rehabilitation efforts vary depending upon the level of career maturity of the consumer. While a consumer may not be ready for competitive employment, she may be ready to engage in rehabilitation focused on helping her to choose the general role of worker, and find a setting to help her develop and keep that role. A consumer who has never worked and has been a patient in a residential facility for 10 years may be ready to contemplate developing a sense of himself as a worker. The consumer may do janitorial tasks at a clubhouse to get a better sense of a workday schedule and the experience of being engaged in productive activity, in order to build experience in work in general. Another consumer may have a worker identity, but may not know which occupation is of interest to her. She may be ready to engage in services to help her explore different fields of work, and/or go back to school to get the necessary credentials for a selected occupation. Someone who has a worker identity and is involved in the occupation he wants (colleague identity) may be ready to engage in services to choose, get, and keep a particular job (employee identity). Each of these consumers may be *ready* to engage in vocational rehabilitation or vocational activities as long as the question of readiness is posed with respect to a specific domain or environment commensurate with the phase of career maturity they have developed.

READINESS INDICATORS FOR ASSESSING
AND DEVELOPING READINESS

The central question in determining readiness for work is whether or not the person is willing, at a *minimum*, to successfully engage in a psychiatric vocational rehabilitation process to select a preferred work role (e.g., full-time cashier) in a specific environment (e.g., Safeway) within, or for, the next 6–24 months. Successfully engaging in goal-setting means that the consumer identifies a meaningful goal that he intends to achieve.

Readiness for rehabilitation does not require the person to *begin* by being committed to a goal. It simply requires that a person be willing to engage in a process that will enable that person to select a personally satisfying goal. Achieving work that is satisfying and corresponds to personal preferences has been linked to greater job tenure (Fabian et al., 1993; Xie et al., 1997). The presence of readiness indicators increases the likelihood that the rehabilitation process will focus on a satisfying vocational goal corresponding to personal preferences and will later engage the person in gaining the skills and supports to be successful in that role and setting.

Readiness indicators are comprised of factors that influence the willingness to be engaged in the vocational rehabilitation process. There are five indicators that influence willingness to become involved in the rehabilitation process (Farkas et al., 2000a). These include: *Need*, or the extent to which a person is either unsuccessful or dissatisfied in his/her current vocational situation; *Commitment to Change*, or the extent to which a person is committed to make changes in his/her life; *Personal Closeness/Relationship*, or the extent to which he/she is open to connecting with others; *Self-Awareness*, or the extent to which the person has some level of understanding about him/herself in relation to the world of work; and lastly, *Environmental Awareness*, or the degree to which a person has some degree of awareness of the world of work.

Need for Change

The need to change work situations arises from two possible pressures. The first is the person's own perceptions about her lack of success or sense of dissatisfaction with the current situation. The second is external pressure stemming from others' perception of the person's lack of success.

Internal pressure for change comes from some degree of dissatisfaction with the current situation. The current situation can include dissatisfaction with pressures from circumstances such as: losing Social Security benefits, increases in rent and food costs, and decreases in food stamp allocations. Botterbush (2000b), for example, studied outcomes in a consumer-run vocational program for professionals with psychiatric disabilities and found that those who did not return to work or who were marginally employed were afraid to lose Social Security benefits and health insurance. The process of Assessing Readiness (Farkas et al., 2000a) begins with a structured interview exploring the individual's degree of dissatisfaction. The exploration focuses on the person's domain of greatest dissatisfaction. If the individual is experiencing her greatest dissatisfaction in the living arena because she lives alone and feels isolated, then beginning to choose a work environment may not be appropriate. She may not "need" vocational rehabilitation at this time, and may be "unready" for a work goal.

External pressure comes from the dissatisfaction of those who are important in the current environment, or "gatekeepers" (Chase & Bell, 1990). For example, they may include work supervisors, mentors, family members, and mental health or rehabilitation professionals. Gatekeepers can fire a person, for example, or pressure him to leave the environment. Inappropriate expectations by service providers or family members can lower a person's sense of need. Practitioners who worry about the degree of stress associated with work, or feel that a particular job is "as much as he can do," can decrease that individual's perception of the potential for success and satisfaction. Evidence of low level of expectations of agency and practitioners can be seen in the fact that few programs described in the literature work with people with psychiatric disabilities who are looking to launch or advance a professional or semi-professional career as compared with the number of programs designed to help consumers gain entry-level positions or non-competitive work (Botterbusch, 2000b).

The need to become involved in rehabilitation is based on the need to improve the person's satisfaction and/or to meet an environmental demand. Need for change is specific to a point in time. While there might be no pressure for rehabilitation at one point in time, circumstances or the person's feelings might change to create the need at a different point in time. If there is no Need established, and the person has little interest in work or vocational rehabilitation, then investigating other readiness indicators has no meaning and therefore the assessment of readiness is terminated for the time being.

Commitment to Change

The *need* to engage in a change process is different from the *desire* to engage in a change process. People are often willing to endure the unhappiness they have, rather than face the unpredictable implications of making a change. Increased motivation and satisfaction have been related to increased job tenure (Becker, Drake, Farabaugh, & Bond, 1996; Ellison & Russinova, 2001; Lee, Lieh-Mak, & Spinks, 1993). In many service settings the lack of progress in a helping intervention has been attributed to the individual's "lack of motivation" or "treatment resistance," which can become a static label attached to the individual rather than a signal to investigate further (Anthony et al., 2001). The rehabilitation process makes the assumption that there are many factors that contribute to motivation. Rather than viewing motivation as a negative symptom, the rehabilitation practitioner seeks to understand the internal and external factors that may contribute to a person's motivation to participate in vocational activities.

The indicator, Commitment to Change, reflects the person's intention to make a change to improve his or her own functioning or to change the environment. The three central questions the person needs to answer in determining how much he may want change are: Does change seem possible? Does the change seem desirable? Does the change seem manageable? The answers to these questions are influenced by a person's *desire* for change, the person's *expectations* about how beneficial or positive the change might turn out to be (often based on whether the person has successfully made changes in the past), a sense of *self-efficacy*, and the person's experience of *support* for the change, both of which influence the person's view of how manageable the change might be (Farkas et al., 2000b).

Desire and a felt need for change may arise from an internal sense of dissatisfaction. Information can at times increase desire. If an individual is part of a family that has maintained generational unemployment, then there may be a sense that being unemployed is "as good as it gets," in which case there may be no internal pressure to change. Being dissatisfied, in other words, may be seen as "the way things are" and not as cause for change. In this case, information such as seeing working peers with whom the person can identify can help the individual to begin to experience a desire for a worker identity.

Positive expectations can be the legacy of past work history. Collins et al. (2000) add their voices to others who have noted that without a vocational intervention, the best predictor of future work behavior may be past and current work behavior (Anthony & Jansen, 1984). Many people mentally construct a "cost–benefit" analysis when contemplating getting a job or improving their employment situation. They ask: "Will I get more out of this change than what it will cost me to make this change?" For example, "Will I lose medical benefits if I try to get a job?" Or "Will I get more out of going back to school to get a degree in this field than it will cost me financially, mentally, emotionally, and physically?" Positive expectations occur when the benefits are seen as greater than the costs. When past experiences or lack of knowledge have left the person with negative expectations for future changes, activities such as reading personal "success" stories or engaging in productive activities from which the person can benefit immediately can be helpful in increasing positive expectations.

In addition to a cost–benefit analysis, the extent to which people feel they *can* successfully make the changes that are necessary (self-efficacy), impacts the extent to which they feel committed to change. Bandura (1997) describes self-efficacy as a belief about one's own ability to influence the environment. This belief impacts on the person's desire to try new experiences or work on new skills until mastery of these skills occurs. The desire to try to keep working until mastery occurs seems to be independent of the level of skill the person possesses. In other words, how a person understands the reasons for his success plays a larger role in sustaining a person's effort over time than that person's actual ability (Weiner, 1985). The individual's experience of how much others support the idea of work and vocational rehabilitation itself also influences how willing the individual will be to enter into rehabilitation.

Setting and achieving a work goal is a lengthy and, at times, arduous process. The support of significant others helps the individual to take the first step and to continue working with the rehabilitation process, once it has begun. First-person accounts of the recovery process indicate that consumer-survivors identify the presence of another person who is just "being there" as one of the most important factors in their success (Deegan, 1988). Bond and Boyer (1988) found that two of the elements critical to helping consumers to achieve and maintain employment over time were the positive expectations held by helpers that the consumer could succeed, and the existence of intensive and consistent supports. These findings are similar to those reviewed by Cook and Rosenberg (1994). The individual's sense of self-efficacy and support affects his or her view of the manageability of the change. Sometimes, helping practitioners and family members to read literature on vocational recovery (Mowbray, Moxley, Jasper, & Howell, 1997; Russinova, Wewiorski, Lyass, Rogers, & Massaro, 2002) and to listen to the experiences of professionals who are also consumers, can help to increase the hopefulness of significant others, so that they can be more supportive of the consumer's desire for change.

In summary, a strong desire for change, expectations that the change will be positive, a sense of self-efficacy, and the perception that others are supportive, all serve to increase the individual's commitment to making a change.

Personal Closeness/Relationship

The indicator Personal Closeness or Relationship refers to the person's willingness to form a personal connection with another. Some people in general society are content with having limited or no strong personal relationships, while others enjoy being close to people. A person's willingness to form a personal connection, therefore, can range from wanting personal closeness to welcoming isolation. A person who is open to relationships is more likely to experience support and receive general support from others and therefore, is also more likely to be willing to sustain the process of rehabilitation over time. Collins et al. (2000) found that increased contact with social networks, including state vocational rehabilitation agencies, led to an increased likelihood of engagement in productive activity such as school and work.

Studies report that the individual's perception of the relationship is a consistent predictor of improvement (Bachelor, 1995; Wasylenki, Goering, Lancee, Ballantyne, & Farkas, 1988).

Research suggests that the connection is a result of the interaction and match of the client's relationship style and the practitioner's relationship style (Cohen, Nemec, Farkas, & Forbess, 1988; Tyrrell, Dozier, Teague, & Fallot, 1999). Assessing a person's preferential style for relating to others (i.e., whether they prefer to connect through emotional, physical, intellectual, or spiritual activities) is an important clue to understanding how to proceed to find out how likely that person may be to want to engage in a close relationship during the rehabilitation process.

Awareness

Awareness of self and the environment are the next two indicators of rehabilitation readiness. Knowledge of self and the world of work, along with confidence in career decision-making and career maturity, as variables related to selecting suitable vocational goals. Awareness is a function of both the individual's self-knowledge and his or her experience in the world.

SELF-AWARENESS. Self-awareness is a complex factor that has been much discussed across several disciplines, especially as it relates to people with a psychiatric disability (Amador & David, 1998; DeHoff, 1998; Ferrari & Sternberg, 1998). People differ in terms of their level of introspection. When individuals have self-awareness, it is easier to engage them in the rehabilitation process. They are able to contribute their interests, values, and personal preferences to the goal-setting process. In terms of career maturity, clinical experience would indicate that those who have not yet formed a worker identity have less self-awareness with respect to their vocational interests, values, and preferences than those who are trying to focus on issues related to being an employee in a specific position.

The vocational rehabilitation process itself can facilitate self-awareness. While job shadowing, volunteer positions, and internship activities are often used to help people to develop new skills or to understand more about the types of work available, such activities can also be used to help people to increase their self-awareness. These types of activities can be used to help an individual who is developing a worker identity, for example, to understand more about her own interests and values in relation to the world of work. Another consumer who has developed a worker identity, but does not know what field of work she would like to pursue, may need a variety of job shadowing, volunteer work, and internship opportunities to help her understand more about what she appreciates and enjoys.

ENVIRONMENTAL AWARENESS. The entire rehabilitation process is based on the fit between the person and the environment. Environmental awareness, or having an understanding about environments, is a critical component in the rehabilitation process (Farkas, Anthony, & Cohen, 1989; Anthony et al., 2001; Segal, Silverman, & Baumhohl, 1989). Environmental awareness includes knowledge about the possible differences in the people, work activities, and physical characteristics of settings in a variety of jobs and work roles. Some familiarity with different types of vocational settings is necessary to formulate an image of a future environment. A person's ideas about possible future roles have a powerful effect on his current motivation. According to Markus and Nurius (1986), the majority of daily activities may not be linked to the current view of the self, but what may be possible in the future. Environmental awareness contributes to a person's sense of possibilities. When a person understands the variety and the nature of the roles and settings that are in the arena she is interested in or concerned about, that concrete understanding may help the person lose preconceived notions that contributed to feelings of entrapment, resignation, and defeat.

In summary, the five readiness indicators of Need, Commitment to Change, Personal Closeness, Self and Environmental Awareness can help consumers and practitioners evaluate the extent to which the person is willing to engage in rehabilitation. If the person is interested in the idea of rehabilitation and in some level of work, but is not ready to begin right away, readiness indicators can guide the planning of activities designed to give the person the knowledge or experience that will help to increase his or her willingness. A case study will be presented to illustrate the concepts of assessing and developing readiness.

CASE STUDY

Carl is an unmarried 42-year-old white male with a diagnosis of bipolar disorder. He currently takes Lithium. He lives with his mother, in an apartment for the elderly or disabled, in the suburbs of a large Northeastern city. Carl has a scattered employment history. Although he graduated from an Ivy League college in the Northeast, he has struggled to choose and get started in a career. Carl can see himself as a worker (i.e., has a worker identity), but is unsure of the occupation he wishes to be in. He has held positions such as handler and stock-clerk, off and on since his graduation from college. In his last job he worked at a major department store handling large purchases for customers.

After this job, Carl remained unemployed for 2 years before seeking assistance from Career Services, a community rehabilitation provider, on the insistence of his psychotherapist. When Carl came to the service, he stated that he wanted to go back to work in some capacity. Carl was oriented to the service and to the rehabilitation process. Carl and his counselor began Assessing Readiness, which included Assessment of Need, Commitment, Personal Closeness/Relationship, and Self and Environmental Awareness. Carl was also oriented to the fact that each indicator was rated along a 5-point scale, with Level 3 being the minimum level for readiness on any one specific indicator.

Need for Change

Assessing Need involved looking closely at Carl's current unemployment and his level of satisfaction with that status. Carl was only moderately dissatisfied with being unemployed because he had mixed feelings about spending his "work day" with his mother, felt bored by not having a workplace to go to, and wanted more to do in his day. Yet Carl enjoyed having the liberty to spend his day how he wanted, and felt disconcerted by his current lack of worker role. His mother had come to accept his unemployed status, but did express that she was dissatisfied because he was not contributing to the household expenses. This moderate level of dissatisfaction both on Carl's part and that of his mother led Carl and his counselor to rate his level of Need as moderate (Level 3, on a 5-point scale). Some need, therefore, for vocational rehabilitation was established.

Commitment to Change

DESIRE.   Not only did Carl and his mother not experience great dissatisfaction with his current status, or Need, but Carl's desire for change was also moderate. He was unsure how much he really wanted to make this change.

BELIEF THAT CHANGE IS POSITIVE. Carl and his helper investigated the perceived risks and benefits to making a vocational change at this point. Carl believed that if he could successfully make the changes needed, the benefits would be: increased income, camaraderie with co-workers, a positive feeling of contributing to society, and of having a worker role. The risks involved: the sacrifice of free time, the liberty to do what he wanted, having to answer to a supervisor once again, and the anxiety that performing in the work role would bring, with the possibility of relapse. In analyzing the intensity of each of these risks and benefits, the perceived risks outweighed his perceived benefits, indicating that he did not really expect this change to turn out positively for him.

SELF-EFFICACY. Carl had gotten jobs on his own before, consequently he felt certain that he could get a job. His concerns involved keeping a job, and more specifically his ability to feel confident in his own abilities and worth as an employee to stay on the job. His belief about himself was that when others pushed for change, things happened, but that he himself was not very effective at making things happen. His sense of self-efficacy was mixed.

SUPPORT FOR THE CHANGE. Carl felt strongly that his mother would see work as a loss for her, since he would be gone during the day. On the other hand, his mother had indeed expressed some interest in his returning to work. His therapist was very enthusiastic about his making this change. Carl also had read enough about the rehabilitation process itself to feel that his rehabilitation practitioner might be able to help him make some of the changes that he felt unable to do by himself. Thus, his perceived support for the change was mixed.

Carl's overall Commitment to Change was rated by both of them as somewhat low (Level 2) since it presented such a mixed picture.

Personal Closeness/Relationship

The next step of assessing readiness explored the extent to which Carl seemed open to connecting with others. This exploration focused on his practitioner, since she was the one who would be working with him during the rehabilitation process. By this time, Carl had connected to his counselor and had shared many challenges and personal stories. Carl had connections to other people in his life (his mother and brother, therapist, doctors, and friends), and enjoyed talking about readiness and vocational rehabilitation. It seemed clear that Carl would be open to connecting and possibly receiving support from others if they offered it. This indicator was a strength in Carl's profile and was rated as a Level 4.

Awareness

SELF-AWARENESS. Carl and his counselor felt that Carl was very insightful, and had thought very carefully about the previous aspects of Readiness Assessment. He knew his strengths and weaknesses, and was willing to explore his areas of intrapersonal difficulty that served as barriers to making changes, such as his anxiety of being in the worker role again. He was knowledgeable about his interests with respect to the world of work, but was less knowledgeable about his occupational values and less conscious about the way in which he typically made decisions. Carl and his counselor rated this indicator as a Level 3, or moderate.

ENVIRONMENTAL AWARENESS.   Although Carl had held a variety of positions since his graduation from college, his knowledge of different kinds of jobs was limited. He was not sure what non-manual labor jobs entailed or would require of him. He did not know the kinds of jobs he could look for, and continued to look at handler jobs in the newspaper, even though he declared his wish to move in a different direction. He was aware, however, of the general characteristics of the world of work (e.g., employee/employer relationships, colleague interactions, expectations about punctuality, etc). He felt that his Environmental Awareness was at a Level 3.

Readiness Development

At the end of the assessment process, Carl did express interest in rehabilitation, so that he could succeed and enjoy whatever job he chose. The results of the assessment, however (see Carl's Readiness Profile, Figure 12-1), seemed to indicate that Carl was only moderately ready. Since both Need and Commitment to Change heavily influence a person's overall readiness, and neither of these indicators was high, Carl and his counselor decided that Readiness Development would be helpful before Carl got involved in setting a specific vocational goal. After some exploration, it was decided that Carl wanted to first address his Commitment to Change. Since he was mixed about wanting change to happen, Carl, his

Rating	Need for change	Commitment to change	Personal closeness	Self-awareness	Environmental awareness
Readiness	**Moderately ready** *May begin setting a goal if interest is there*	**Not ready** *Needs to develop readiness here*	**Highly ready** *Ready to begin*	**Moderately ready** *May begin if interest is there*	**Moderately ready** *May begin if interest is there*

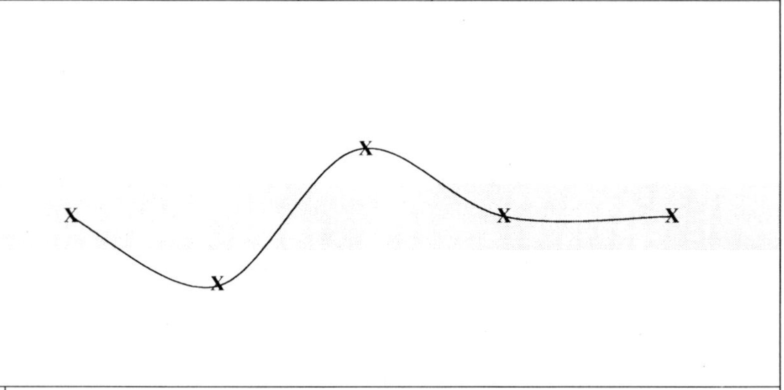

Readiness conclusion	*Carl could begin setting a vocational goal at this point, but would find it easier to do if he participated in readiness development activities first.*

FIGURE 12-1. Carl's Readiness profile. Adapted from Farkas, Cohen, McNamara, Nemec, & Cohen (2001). *Assessing Readiness: Psychiatric Rehabilitation Technology Series.* Boston, MA: Center for Psychiatric Rehabilitation.

primary therapist, and his mother decided to meet for ongoing sessions. In these sessions, they intended to work out issues such as the mother's acceptance of Carl's lack of employment and Carl's fears about his mother's loneliness, in an effort to increase Carl's need for rehabilitation and his desire for change. Carl's mother was referred to the local Alliance for the Mentally Ill chapter, a family organization, in order to provide her with more support and hope. Carl agreed to enroll in a computer skills training program to address some of the elements related to Commitment to Change. The program offered Carl a chance to have a more intellectually stimulating schedule during the day, with interactions with classmates and trainers. This could increase his desire to make a change and escape from his current boredom. Carl felt that perhaps improving his computer skills might also increase his sense of worth as an employee and his self-efficacy. In addition to this plan, Carl enrolled in a Recovery workshop (Spaniol, Koehler, & Hutchinson, 1994). A facilitator who was also a consumer discussed recovery experiences and techniques for coping. It gave Carl an opportunity to experience peer role models who were working and to share experiences and techniques that sustained them in their ongoing struggle to get and keep work worth having. Awareness would be increased by an internship which could offer him experience in another type of work (clerical or white-collar positions). And lastly, Carl's style of making changes, namely moving slowly toward them, would be accommodated by the year-long training program. Carl would not need to commit himself to computer work as his career goal; he could use this experience to later explore with his counselor to identify the career that would be meaningful and consistent with his increased understanding of himself and the world of work.

CONCLUSION

Engaging in rehabilitation and work can present individuals with a formidable prospect. From the consumer's perspective, past failures, the daunting challenge of overcoming symptoms, stigma, inertia, and lack of support can contribute to keeping many people from beginning the rehabilitation process. Perhaps even more devastatingly, these barriers keep people believing that real change, such as a move to work, is impossible (Kramer & Gagne, 1997).

Psychiatric vocational rehabilitation, delivered through a variety of program models from transitional employment programs to supported employment programs, does appear to help individuals to develop the skills, supports, and accommodations over time that they will need to succeed in either competitive employment or some form of supported employment. The modest outcomes achieved to date, however, suggest that more understanding is needed in order to boost rates of employment. While research has begun to suggest that personal factors, rather than demographics or initial capacity, are correlated with vocational outcomes, further research is needed to explore the contribution that assessing and developing readiness can make to the process of gaining or regaining meaningful work and the valued role in society that comes with it.

REFERENCES

Amador, X. F., & David, A. S. (Eds.) (1998). *Insight and psychosis*. New York, NY: Oxford University Press.

Anthony, W. A. (1993). Recovery from Mental Illness: The Guiding vision of the mental health service system in the 1990's. *Psychosocial Rehabilitation Journal, 16*, 11–23.

Anthony, W. A. (1994). Characteristics of people with psychiatric disabilities that are predictive of entry into the rehabilitation process and successful employment. *Psychosocial Rehabilitation Journal, 17*(3), 3–13.

Anthony, W. A., & Blanch, A. K. (1989). Research on community support services: What have we learned? *Psychosocial Rehabilitation Journal, 12*(3), 55–81.

Anthony, W. A., & Jansen, M. A. (1984). Predicting the vocational capacity of the chronically mentally ill: Research and policy implications. *American Psychologist, 39*(5), 537–544.

Anthony, W. A., Cohen, M. R., Farkas, M., & Gagne, C. (2001). *Psychiatric Rehabilitation*. Boston, MA: Boston University, Center for Psychiatric Rehabilitation.

Anthony, W. A., Rogers, E. S., Cohen, M., & Davies, R. R. (1995). Relationships between psychiatric symptomatology, work skills and future vocational performance. *Psychiatric Services, 46*(4), 353–358.

Bachelor, A. (1995). Clients' perception of the therapeutic alliance. *Journal of Counseling Psychology, 42*, 323–337.

Bandura, A. (1997). *Self-efficacy: The exercise of control*. New York, NY: W.H. Freeman.

Baron, R. (1997). *Hearings before the subcommittee on social security of the committee on ways and means/House of Representatives*. Washington, DC: U.S. Government Accounting Office.

Baron, R. C., & Salzer, M. S. (2000). The career patterns of persons with serious mental illness: Generating a new vision of lifetime careers for those in recovery. *Psychiatric Rehabilitation Skills, 4*(1), 136–156.

Becker, D. R., Drake, R. E., Farabaugh, A., & Bond, G. R. (1996). Job preferences among people with severe psychiatric disorders participating in supported employment. *Psychiatric Services, 47*(11), 1223–1226.

Bell, M. D., & Lysacker, P. (1996). Levels of expectation for work activity in schizophrenia: Clinical and rehabilitation outcomes. *Psychiatric Rehabilitation Journal, 19*(3), 71–76.

Bell, M. D., Lysacker, P. H., & Milstein, R. M. (1996). Clinical benefits of paid work activity in schizophrenia. *Schizophrenia Bulletin, 22*(1), 51–67.

Blume, A. W., & Schmaling, K. B. (1997). Specific classes of symptoms predict readiness to change scores among dually diagnosed patients. *Addictive Behaviors, 22*, 625–630.

Bond, G. R. (1992). Vocational rehabilitation. In R.P. Liberman (Ed.), *Handbook of psychiatric rehabilitation* (pp. 244–263). New York, NY: Macmillan.

Bond, G. R., & Boyer, S. L. (1988). Rehabilitation programs and outcomes. In J.A. Ciardiello & M.D. Bell (Eds.), *Vocational rehabilitation of persons with prolonged mental illness* (pp. 231–263). Baltimore, MD: Johns Hopkins University Press.

Bond, G. R., Drake, R., Mueser, K., & Becker, D. (1997). An update on supported employment for people with severe mental illness. *Psychiatric Services, 48*, 335.

Botterbusch, K. F. (2000a). Career development patterns among professional persons with severe psychiatric disabilities: Implications for practice. *Journal of Applied Rehabilitation Counseling, 31*(2), 24–32.

Botterbusch, K. F. (2000b). Consumer outcomes in a vocational program for professional persons with severe psychiatric disabilities. *Journal of Rehabilitation Administration, 24*(2), 25–38.

Center for Psychiatric Rehabilitation (In preparation). *Certificate program in psychiatric vocational rehabilitation: A training curriculum*. Boston, MA: Boston University, Center for Psychiatric Rehabilitation.

Chase, S. E., & Bell, C. S. (1990). Ideology, discourse, and gender: How gatekeepers talk about women school superintendents. *Social Problems, 37*, 163–177.

Cohen, M. R., Anthony, W. A., & Farkas, M. D. (1997). Assessing and developing readiness for psychiatric rehabilitation. *Psychiatric Services, 8*, 644–646.

Cohen, M. R., Forbess, R., & Farkas, M. (2001). *Rehabilitation readiness: The technology of developing readiness*. Boston, MA: Boston University, Center for Psychiatric Rehabilitation.

Cohen, M. R., Nemec, P. B., & Farkas, M. (2001). *Rehabilitation readiness: The technology of connecting*. Boston, MA: Boston University, Center for Psychiatric Rehabilitation.

Cohen, M. R., Nemec, P. B., Farkas, M. D., & Forbess, R. (1988). *Psychiatric rehabilitation training technology: Case management* (Trainer package). Boston, MA: Center for Psychiatric Rehabilitation, Boston University.

Collins, M. E., Mowbray, C. T., & Bybee, D. (2000). Characteristics predicting successful outcomes of participants with severe mental illness in supported education. *Psychiatric Services, 51*(6), 774–780.

Cook, J., & Rosenberg, H. (1994). Predicting community employment among persons with psychiatric disabilities: A logistic regression analysis. *Journal of Rehabilitation Administration, 18*, 6.

Danley, K. S. (1997). *The choose-get-keep approach to employment support: An intervention manual*. Boston, MA: Boston University, Center for Psychiatric Rehabilitation.

Danley, K. S., Rogers, E. S., & Nevas, D. B. (1989). A psychiatric rehabilitation approach to vocational rehabilitation. In M.D. Farkas & W.A. Anthony (Eds.), *Psychiatric rehabilitation outcomes: Putting theory into practice* (pp. 81–86). Baltimore, MD: Johns Hopkins University Press.

Danley, K. S., Sciarappa, K., & MacDonald-Wilson, K. (1992). Choose-get-keep: A psychiatric approach to supported employment. *New Directions in Mental Health Services, 53*, 87–96.

Deegan, P. E. (1988). Recovery: The lived experience of rehabilitation. *Psychosocial Rehabilitation Journal, 11*, 11–19.

Deegan, P. E. (1997). Recovery and empowerment for people with psychiatric disabilities. *Social Work in Health Care, 25*(3), 11–24.

DeHoff, S. L. (1998). In search of a paradigm for psychological and spiritual growth: Implications for psychotherapy and spiritual direction. *Pastoral Psychology, 46*, 333–346.

Ellison, M. L., & Russinova, Z. (2001). Survey of professionals and managers with psychiatric conditions. Unpublished manuscript. Boston, MA: Boston University, Center for Psychiatric Rehabilitation.

Fabian, E. S., Waterworth, A., & Ripke, B. (1993). Reasonable accommodations for workers with serious mental illness: Type, frequency and associated outcomes. *Psychosocial Rehabilitation Journal, 17*(2), 163–172.

Farkas, M. D., Anthony, W. A., & Cohen, M. R. (1989). An overview of psychiatric rehabilitation: The approach and its programs. In M.D. Farkas and W.A. Anthony (Eds.), *Psychiatric rehabilitation programs: Putting theory into practice* (pp. 1–27). Baltimore, MD: Johns Hopkins University Press.

Farkas, M. D., Cohen, M. R., McNamara, S., Nemec, P. B., & Cohen, B. F. (2000). *Assessing readiness: Psychiatric rehabilitation technology series.* Boston, MA: Boston University, Center for Psychiatric Rehabilitation.

Farkas, M. D., Sullivan-Soydan, A., & Gagne, C. (2000). *An introduction to rehabilitation readiness.* Boston, MA: Boston University, Center for Psychiatric Rehabilitation.

Felton, C. J., Stastny, P., Shern, D. L., Blanch, A., Donahue, Knight, & Brown. (1995). Consumers as peer specialists on intensive case management teams: Impact on client outcomes. *Psychiatric Services, 46*, 1037–1044.

Ferrari, M. D., & Sternberg, R. J. (Eds.) (1998). *Self-awareness: Its nature and development.* New York, NY: Guilford.

Goldman, H. H., Gattozzi, A. A., & Taube, C. A. (1981). Defining and counting the chronically mentally ill. *Hospital and Community Psychiatry, 32*, 21–27.

Harding, C., & Zahniser, J. (1994). Empirical correction of seven myths about schizophrenia with implications for treatment. *Acta Psychiatrica Scandinavica Supplementum, 90*(Suppl. 384), 140–146.

Kirszner, M., Baron, R., & Rutman, I. (1992). *Employer participation in supported and transitional employment for persons with long term mental illness* (Final report to the National Institute on Disability and Rehabilitation Research). Philadelphia, PA: Matrix Research Institute.

Knight, D., & Aucoin, L. (1999). Assessing job readiness skills: How students, teachers, and employers can work together to enhance on-the-job training. *The Council for Exceptional Children, 31*(5), 10–17.

Kramer, P. J., & Gagne, C.G. (1997). Barriers in recovery and empowerment for people with psychiatric disabilities. In L. Spaniol, C. Gagne, & M. Koehler (Eds.), *The psychological and social aspects of psychiatric disability* (pp. 467–476). Boston, MA: Boston University, Center for Psychiatric Rehabilitation.

Lee, P., Lieh-Mak, F., & Spinks, J. (1993). Coping strategies of people with schizophrenia. *British Journal of Psychology, 163*, 177–182.

Lehman, A. F. (1995). Vocational rehabilitation in schizophrenia. *Schizophrenia Bulletin, 21*(4), 645–656.

Markus, H., & Nurius, P. (1986). Possible selves. *American Psychologist, 41*, 954–969.

Marshak, L. E., Bostick, D., & Turton, L. J. (1990). Closure outcomes for clients with psychiatric disabilities served by the vocational rehabilitation system. *Rehabilitation Counseling Bulletin, 33*(3), 247–250.

McConnaughy, E. A., DiClemente, C. C., Prochaska, J. O., & Velicer, W. F. (1989). Stages of change in psychotherapy: A follow-up report. *Psychotherapy, 26*(4), 494–503.

McCrory, D. J., Connolly, P. S., Hanson-Meyer, T. P., Sheridan-Landolfi, J. S., Barone, F. C., Blood, A. H., & Gilson, A. M. (1980). The rehabilitation crisis: The impact of growth. *Journal of Applied Rehabilitation Counseling, 11*, 136–139.

Mowbray, C. T., Moxley, D. P., Jasper, C. A., & Howell, L. L. (1997). *Consumers as providers in psychiatric rehabilitation.* Columbia, MD: International Association of Psychosocial Rehabilitation Services.

Mulkern, V. M., & Manderscheid, R. W. (1989). Characteristics of community support program clients in 1980 and 1984. *Hospital and Community Psychiatry, 40*, 165–172.

National Institute of Mental Health (1987). *Toward a model plan for a comprehensive, community based mental health system.* Rockville, MD: Division of Education and Service Systems Liason.

Prochaska, J. O., DiClemente, C. C., & Norcross, J. C. (1992). In search of how people change: Applications to addictive behaviors. *American Psychologist, 47*, 1102–1114.

Prochaska, J. O., Velicer, W. F., DiClemente, C. C., & Fava, J. (1988). Measuring processes of change: Applications to the cessation of smoking. *Journal of Consulting and Clinical Psychology, 56*, 520–528.

Rogers, E., Martin, R., Anthony, W., Massaro, J., Lyass, A., Danley, K., & Penk, W. (2001). Assessing readiness for change among persons with severe mental illness. *Community Mental Health Journal, 37*(2), 97–112.

Rogers, E. S., Anthony, W. A., Cohen, M., & Davies, R. R. (1997). Prediction of vocational outcome based on clinical and demographic indicators among vocationally ready clients. *Community Mental Health Journal, 33*(2), 99–112.

Rogers, E. S., Walsh, D., Danley, K. S., & Smith (1991). *Massachusetts client preference assessment: Final report.* Boston, MA: Boston University, Center for Psychiatric Rehabilitation.

Russinova, Z., Wewiorski, N., Lyoss, A., Rogers, E. S., Massaro, J. (2002). Correlates of vocational recovery for persons with schizophrenia. *International Review of Psychiatry, 14*(4), 303–311.

Segal, S., Silverman, C., & Baumhohl, J. (1989). Seeking person–environment fit in community care placement. *Journal of Social Issues, 45*(3), 49–64.

Shern, D. L., Felton, C. J., Hough, R. L., Lehman, A. F., Goldfinger, S., Valencia, E., Dennis, D., Straw, R., & Wood, P. A. (1997). Housing outcomes for homeless adults with mental illness: Results from the second-round McKinney Program. *Psychiatric Services, 48*, 239–241.

Snow, M. G., Prochaska, J. O., & Rossi, J. S. (1992). Processes of change in alcoholic anonymous: Maintenance factors in long-term sobriety. *Journal of Studies on Alcohol*, 362–371.

Spaniol, L., & Koehler, M. (Eds.) (1994). *The experience of recovery.* Boston, MA: Boston University, Center for Psychiatric Rehabilitation.

Spaniol, L., Gagne, C., & Koehler, M. (1999). Recovery from serious mental illness: What it is and how to support people in their recovery. In R. P. Marinelli & A. E. Dell Orto (Eds.), *The psychological and social impact of disability (4th ed.).* New York, NY: Springer.

Spaniol, L., Koehler, M., & Hutchinson, D. (1994). *Recovery workbook: Practical coping and empowerment strategies for people with psychiatric disability.* Boston, MA: Boston University, Center for Psychiatric Rehabilitation.

Substance Abuse and Mental Health Services Administration (1993). *SAMHSA strategic plan.* Washington, DC: Department of Health and Human Services.

Tsang, H., Lam, P., Ng, B., & Leung, O. (2000). Predictors of employment outcome for people with psychiatric disabilities: A review of the literature since the mid '80s. *Journal of Rehabilitation, 66*(2), 19–31.

Tyrell, C. L., Dozier, M., Teague, G. B., & Fallot, R. D. (1999). Effective treatment relationships for persons with serious psychiatric disorders: The importance of attachment states of mind. *Journal of Counseling and Clinical Psychology, 67*(5), 725–732.

United States General Accounting Office (April 1996). *SSA disability: Program redesign necessary to encourage return to work* (Report to the Chairman, Special Committee on Aging and the US Senate). Washington, DC: General Accounting Office (GAO/HEHS 96-62).

Wasylenki, D., Goering, P., Lancee, W., Ballantyne, R., & Farkas, M. (1988). Impact of a case manager program on psychiatric aftercare. *Journal of Nervous and Mental Disease, 173*, 303–308.

Weiner, B. (1985). An attributional theory of achievement motivation and emotion. *Psychological Review, 92*, 548–573.

Won Tesoriero, H. (2001, January 22). Bearing no ill will. *Time Magazine*, pp. B4–B6.

Xie, H. Y., Dain, B. J., Becker, D. R., & Drake, R. E. (1997). Job tenure among persons with severe mental illness. *Rehabilitation Counseling Bulletin, 40*(4), 230–239.

Yelin, E. H., & Cisternas, M. G. (1997). Employment patterns among persons with and without mental conditions. In R. J. Bonnie & J. Monahan (Eds.), *Mental disorder, work disability, and the law. The John D. and Catherine T. MacArthur Foundation series on mental health and development* (pp. 25–54). Chicago, IL: University of Chicago Press.

CHAPTER 13

Cognitive Remediation for Increasing Functional Independence

LAURIE R. GWILLIAM, DENISE RABOLD, AND JOHN CORRIGAN

Cognitive performance (thinking skill) is an essential aspect of human function and minimal abilities are a necessary, though not sufficient, condition for a productive and satisfying lifestyle. We all rely on certain basic mental abilities as we make our way through daily routines. We may in a typical day, for example, use reading, writing, memory, arithmetic, trial and error, and other forms of problem-solving, and various oral language skills. Of course, these abilities are usually combined with hand and eye coordination and require minimum levels of attention and concentration. Most individuals appear to make their way through the complex mazes of work, school, and home management relatively smoothly; however, it is probably true that each individual possesses a unique pattern of strengths and weaknesses of mental ability. Impairments can exist at any level of severity. Some weaknesses may be minor annoyances, while more serious deficits may limit activities or require specific attention for effective management. The concept of impairment of cognition is certainly not new, nor is the idea of compensation for related deficits in performance. Indeed, the process of normal aging usually involves awareness of and compensation for decreases in mental abilities.

There are many causes for impairment of brain function. Cognitive deficits can result from psychiatric disorders, substance abuse, cerebral vascular accidents, traumatic brain injury, progressive degenerative diseases (e.g., multiple sclerosis), HIV, aging, and genetic and/or birth defects. Treatment interventions to ameliorate cognitive deficits have been pursued in all of these clinical populations. This chapter addresses the process of treatment and training of persons with known impairments of cognitive functioning that result in limitations in everyday activities. We will attempt to explain the process of assisting persons with cognitive impairments in their efforts to manage their problems so that they can lead more

LAURIE R. GWILLIAM AND JOHN CORRIGAN • Department of Rehabilitation and Physical Medicine, College of Medicine and Public Health, Ohio State University, Columbus, Ohio. DENISE RABOLD • NeuroRehab, Inc., Columbus, Ohio.

effective lives, and make more effective use of their personal strengths. We will focus our attention on more "molar" interventions, versus multifaceted, integrative or milieu-oriented treatment programs such as those described by Prigatano (1986) for traumatic brain injury or Brenner et al. (1994) for schizophrenia. We will use the term "cognitive remediation," and consider it synonymous with "cognitive retraining," and "cognitive rehabilitation."

OVERVIEW OF THE CONSTRUCT

The Brain Injury Special Interest Group of the American Congress of Rehabilitation Medicine (Harley et al., 1992) defined cognitive remediation as a "... systematic, functionally oriented, service of therapeutic cognitive activities, based on an assessment and understanding of a person's brain-behavioral deficits" (p. 63). Cognitive remediation is a therapeutic intervention that develops skills or trains strategies that will assist individuals to function more independently in their daily lives. Interventions are guided by objective data that depicts an individual's pattern of strengths and weaknesses in thinking skills. Cicerone et al. (2000) delineated four methods used during cognitive remediation in order to effect change:

1. reinforcing, strengthening, or re-establishing previously learned patterns of behavior;
2. establishing new patterns of cognitive activity through compensatory cognitive mechanisms for impaired neurological systems;
3. establishing new patterns of activity through external compensatory mechanisms, such as personal orthoses or environmental structuring and support; and;
4. directing efforts toward enabling persons to adapt to their cognitive functioning directly, to improve their overall levels of functioning and quality of their lives (p. 1597).

A national consensus conference conducted in 1993 concluded that cognitive remediation should be individualized, holistic, and functionally oriented (Berquist et al., 1994). Four principles were posited:

1. As the functional goal becomes more complex (for example, "using a calendar" as compared with "returning to work"), it becomes more important that cognitive remediation be part of a comprehensive, integrated approach and not conducted as an isolated modality.
2. Functional goals should be meaningful to the person treated.
3. Generalizability of skills must be explicitly addressed in treatment plans.
4. Cognitive remediation can include teaching new skills; it is not just rehabilitation of that lost or impaired.

The consensus conference guidelines clearly suggested that, to be most effective, the process of cognitive remediation must be tailored for the unique needs of the individual. Although certain techniques have been accepted, these techniques are used in different ways with each client. A major distinction in treatment approaches has been made between those intended to restore an impaired ability and those that teach strategies to compensate for its loss (Ben-Yishay & Diller, 1993; Gordon & Hibbard, 1992).

Restoration versus Compensation

In general the techniques of cognitive remediation fall into two categories: restoration and compensation. The restorative approach attempts to regain function by remediating the impaired cognitive ability (for example, selective attention, spatial perception, or memory retrieval) using systematic training. The primary technique is to engage a person in repetitive exercises designed to ameliorate the specific impairment. A compensatory approach focuses on the disability (for example, following written instructions, navigating the community, or remembering appointments) and trains a person to use strategies to again accomplish these tasks. The primary techniques include training in self-cuing and use of external "prosthetics." Some have argued that this distinction is arbitrary, because compensation or adjustment is itself a cognitive ability (Ylvisaker, cited in Carney et al., 1999). In clinical settings, any given treatment plan often incorporates aspects of both approaches.

In theory, the two approaches accomplish similar ends using quite different means. A successful restorative approach will positively affect all behaviors served by the impaired ability without specifically addressing each behavior. A compensatory approach requires training in strategies for each unique functional situation. This distinction is sometimes called the "generalizability" of the remediation. The strategies developed as part of a compensatory approach must be generalized (or applied) to specific situations in a person's life. A restorative approach does not have to be generalized to everyday activities; however, those activities will only be successfully resumed when every underlying impairment involved in the behavior is restored. In practice, there is more spontaneous generalization (to other skills and to other tasks) than either theoretical approach presumes.

Restorative approaches are thought to be most effective when the impaired cognitive function is less severe or onset was more recent. Our clinical experience has been supportive of the restorative approach when it is used for the treatment of problems involving attention, visuospatial processing, domain-specific memory, and arithmetic. The effectiveness of a compensatory approach is only limited by the ability to generalize strategies to all relevant situations. Our clinical experience suggests that a compensatory approach for problems arising from deficits in attention, visuospatial processing, language, memory, and problem-solving can be useful regardless of severity or time post-onset.

Effectiveness

There is a rapidly expanding body of published research for the effectiveness of cognitive remediation, though most studies have involved clients with acquired brain injuries, schizophrenia, or alcoholism. Carney et al. (1999) performed an evidence-based review of the effectiveness of cognitive remediation for persons with traumatic brain injuries. From 600 references, 32 items met inclusion criteria for their review. They found some evidence that cognitive remediation can positively impact memory, psychological well-being, and interpersonal skill, and that certain techniques provide effective cognitive prostheses. However, the primary finding of their review was that insufficient research evidence existed to conclude that cognitive remediation produces durable outcomes. Cicerone criticized the review and its conclusions based on a comprehensive review of the research literature conducted by the Brain Injury Special Interest Group of the American Congress of Rehabilitation Medicine (Cicerone et al., 2000). That review analyzed 171 studies, and identified 29 controlled trials (versus the five identified by Carney et al., 1999). Cicerone and colleagues reported that 20 of these 29 studies showed positive findings for the effects of cognitive remediation. While this review of research supported overall effectiveness, there was also evidence of selective efficacy due to both individual differences and types of cognitive impairments addressed.

Interest in and research on cognitive remediation for persons with schizophrenia was greatly shaped in the 1990s by two events. Brenner and colleagues published their detailed description of a multifaceted and hierarchical treatment model, Integrated Psychological Therapy, that used remediation of cognitive deficits as a prerequisite of other functional improvements (cf. Brenner et al., 1994). Second, Goldberg and colleagues at the National Institutes of Health asserted that impaired performance by schizophrenics on the Wisconsin Card Sorting Test (WCST) was immutable (Goldberg, Weinberger, Berman, Pliskin, & Podd, 1987). Numerous researchers sought to either test the tenets of Integrated Psychological Therapy or disprove the assertion that the WCST performance could not be altered. A decade later, it is clear that performance on attention tasks can be improved, as can scores on the WCST; however, it is not clear that either of these gains consistently translate to expected benefits in everyday functioning (Bellack, Gold, & Buchanan, 1999; Rund & Borg, 1999). Appropriately, this research literature appears to be shifting its focus from restorative to compensatory approaches (Bellack et al., 1999).

The criticisms of cognitive remediation research are that studies have not used experimental designs or have otherwise lacked sound methodological rationales (Ben-Yishay & Diller, 1993; Carney et al., 1999; Cicerone, 1999). Studies that tested a highly controlled treatment intervention have been criticized for lacking the flexibility of adapting techniques to the needs of the individual as practiced by experienced professionals. Studies that allow practitioners to pursue treatment in the fashion they normally would have been criticized for being too poorly controlled. Furthermore, questions as to what outcomes constitute evidence of effectiveness have complicated this research. As in research on schizophrenia, the vast majority of studies on cognitive remediation find improvement on the cognitive ability that was the direct target of training; however, generalization to other, related cognitive abilities, or transfer to higher level functional abilities, is observed less often. The history of studying the effectiveness of this intervention is reminiscent of attempts to prove the effectiveness of psychotherapy, both in difficulty and developmental history. Research in cognitive remediation is being reframed from addressing the question "is it effective?" to the more specific query, "what cognitive remediation techniques, for whom, under what conditions, with what specific goals?" Answering a similar multifaceted question became the "search for the Holy Grail" of psychotherapy research, and will likely engage cognitive remediation researchers for some time.

CLINICAL CONSIDERATIONS

The success of cognitive remediation is highly dependent on the clinician's ability to provide treatment specific to a person's impairment, while taking into account his or her unique functional situation, and generalizing the training to important, real-world uses. We will briefly describe basic considerations central to each of these qualities.

Strategies for Different Types of Cognitive Impairment

We have found it useful to categorize cognitive impairments, broadly, as disorders of attention and concentration; initiation and planning; judgement and perception; learning and memory; and speed of information processing. Disorders of attention and concentration can be further divided into types of attention such as focused, sustained, and divided. Some examples are provided below of cognitive remediation strategies that can be incorporated into a treatment plan for clients with these different types of impairments.

Attention and concentration play a fundamental role in one's ability to function independently. Some simple compensatory strategies to increase attention and concentration are adapting the environment by reducing distractions, initiating frequent breaks in activity, and use of reinforcers for maintaining behavior. The use of reauditorization, a form of self-talk, can also be trained. The individual repeats, out loud initially, what is being attended to. This strategy will frequently be trained in the therapist's office while the individual is working on a task that requires focused, sustained, or divided attention. There are several computer software packages on the market that work well as therapy stimuli.

Disorders of initiation and planning of goal-directed behavior are very common. These deficits can be functionally identified as difficulties with ordering or sequencing information, impulsivity, perseveration, and lack of integration of information. The primary compensatory approach is to give the individual structure. Time frames and cues for the passage of time assist with initiation. Listing steps, along with providing a framework for moving from identification of a problem to the solution (including benchmarks of completion), is a strategy for enhancing one's ability to sequence. Verbal mediation can also be used to train an individual to identify, label, and define a nonverbal problem.

Judgment and perception are closely related impairments. Failure to perceive a situation accurately is often the source of ineffective or inappropriate decisions to act. Impairments in this area can lead to misinterpretation of situations, unrealistic self-appraisal, and inappropriate behavior. The use of video taping and discussion of alternative methods of responding can be helpful. Making lists that contain "do's and don'ts" and rules for specific problem situations can also be a useful compensatory strategy.

Disorders of learning and memory can be positively affected by a compensatory approach. There are numerous strategies for increasing one's memory, ranging from simple habits such as maintaining a daily log or schedule, to the more sophisticated, voice-activated dictation devices. The ability to remember information is essential for new learning. There are strategies for memory such as association, chunking, and the use of mnemonics that can be trained in therapy then generalized to functional settings.

Impaired speed of information processing is evident in slowed reactions and/or psychomotor inefficiencies. Strategies, in many cases, focus on changing the environmental demands so that the individual is not confronted with the need to react quickly in any given situation. For example, in an academic setting extended time for testing is an effective adaptation, as is access to another student's notes for acquiring information presented during lectures. In a work environment, individuals with slowed information processing speed perform optimally when they work at their own pace, versus at a rate dictated by the environment. A moving assembly line is an obvious example of an externally dictated pace; less obvious are jobs that require one to handle live inquiries from the public.

Individualizing Treatment

Each human being has a unique neuropsychological make-up due to differences in personality, genetics, physiology, education, experience, and environment. Efforts to help persons with cognitive impairments must attempt to accommodate all malleable factors affecting (or limiting) an individual's behavior. Cognitive remediation should proceed only after a thorough evaluation of the individual's profile of cognitive abilities, personality and emotional make-up, motivation, and social situation. This evaluation should consist of objective assessments (such as the Luria–Nebraska Neuropsychological Battery or Halstead–Reitan Neuropsychological Test Battery), subjective functional analysis of behavior, and a clinical interview. Using data derived from this evaluation, a profile of cognitive strengths and weaknesses can be generated and a cognitive remediation treatment plan developed. Based on the aforementioned characteristics of the individual's behavior and cognitive functioning profile, decisions are made as to what approaches would be most suitable for this individual. Generally speaking, restorative techniques would be used to focus on weaknesses, while compensatory techniques are often driven by a person's strengths, which serve as the basis for developing effective strategies.

Maximizing a person's awareness of deficits is normally the first step in the remediation process. Counseling and education may be required for the individual to reach an understanding of the deficits that are limiting performance. Understanding is important for the individual to sustain motivation and enter into a therapeutic alliance with the therapist—a relationship in which there are common definitions of the problems to be addressed and goals to be attacked. Some effort should be given to providing functional examples of areas that have been identified as impaired. Once these areas are functionally identified, it is equally important to gauge, and perhaps enhance, the individual's motivation for attaining the expected benefits of amelioration.

Generalizing Learned Strategies

Much time in therapy is spent on training and refining compensatory strategies, both in the therapeutic setting and at home, school, or work. It is important that the strategies are "user friendly" and reinforcing so that the individual will want to use them, and immediately experience a positive effect. Homework is given so that strategies can be practiced in functional settings and feedback obtained. The feedback is requested in order to determine strategy effectiveness, and should be elicited from both the client and a knowledgeable individual in his/her immediate environment.

Without generalization compensatory strategies are meaningless. In almost all cases generalization does not occur spontaneously but rather must be trained. It is important to spend time implementing the learned compensatory strategies in as many different environments as possible and discussing this process with the individual so that his/her awareness is raised. Once the individual has displayed successful generalization of learned strategies to the target environments, he/she may be discharged from cognitive remediation; however, the individual is cautioned as to the need for continued vigilance about generalization from one setting to another. The extent to which the therapist has engendered the client's openness to hearing feedback from others often determines his/her success in adapting strategies to new or changing situations. Frequently, individuals return to therapy when major life transitions occur, such as vocational changes, entering a new school, marriage, birth of a child, or loss of a significant other.

Cognitive Remediation Strategies for Employment and Community Support

As noted above, utilization of cognitive remediation begins with a thorough assessment of the individual's cognitive abilities, personality and emotional make-up, motivation, and social situation. Consideration of the individual's goals, activities he/she plans to resume, settings in which they will take place, and functional abilities required to perform such activities, is also needed in order to formulate an appropriate and effective plan of cognitive remediation. When goals include a return to employment, such a consideration properly includes gathering information about the nature of the work performed, the specific tasks involved, the cognitive abilities needed for performance of those tasks, and the physical work environment (e.g., environmental factors that ameliorate and/or exacerbate cognitive limitations, and how that environment might be structured and modified).

Both restorative and compensatory approaches to cognitive remediation may play a role in return-to-work strategies. As noted earlier, restorative approaches take a "bottom-up" approach; remediation is directed towards restoring a particular area of cognitive functioning (such as attention) rather than towards developing strategies for successfully performing specific work tasks. Compensatory approaches, on the other hand, focus upon developing strategies for accomplishing specific functions. Development of compensatory strategies to help an individual successfully return to work might include determining which specific work activities are affected by the individual's cognitive impairment (for instance, keeping a schedule, organizing tasks, or sustaining effort for the entire day). Once such activities are identified, further steps would include developing specific cues, alterations to the work environment, environmental supports and/or assistive devices to enable the individual to compensate for his/her impairment and successfully perform the activities. After strategies have been identified and developed, the individual can be trained in their use. Practice with implementing these strategies in the actual work setting is most likely to result in successful performance, since difficulty may arise when an individual attempts to transfer skills learned in one environment into another. Finally, strategies can be monitored and refined as needed by obtaining feedback from the individual and others about the adequacy, effectiveness, and ease of use of each strategy.

Throughout this chapter, various examples of specific cognitive and functional impairments have been discussed, along with examples of possible cognitive remediation strategies and how they might be used in educational, employment, community, and other settings. The following case example is provided in order to further illustrate how cognitive remediation strategies might be developed and used in an employment setting

CASE STUDY

LL was a 20-year-old college student when he sustained a blunt traumatic brain injury. He was administered a neuropsychological evaluation approximately 9 months following his injury. The results of this evaluation revealed a mild impairment of functional brain ability with residual deficits in immediate and delayed memory, novel problem-solving, focused attention, and psychomotor efficiency. Generally, LL was functioning in the low average intellectual range. Cognitive remediation was recommended and subsequently initiated with focus on the following treatment goals:

1. developing and maintaining strategies for functional memory abilities;
2. developing and training skills for management and organization of personal activities;
3. increasing focused/sustained attention;
4. improving problem-solving abilities; and
5. assisting in college re-entry.

His goal was to return to college and attain a bachelor's degree. Much time and effort went into searching for the right institution that would be able to provide appropriate academic accommodations. Prior to initiation of college coursework, LL was trained to independently use the following compensatory strategies: day planner and scheduler, "to do lists," reauditorization, and verbal mediation. These strategies were trained in the therapeutic setting using various cognitive remediation software programs on a personal computer. His mother was involved and assisted in providing feedback as to the effectiveness of strategy generalization.

LL entered a small private college approximately 6 months following the initiation of cognitive remediation. This institution had a disability student services office and worked very closely with instructors and the therapist. LL took classes on a part-time basis through the first year. After evaluating his strengths, weaknesses, and interests as they related to various majors, LL decided to pursue a degree in Business Communications. On the first day of every semester LL would provide his instructors with a one-page written description of his accident, residual difficulties including cognitive impairments, a list of compensatory strategies used for coursework, and the therapist's name and phone number. The following were the compensatory strategies requested:

1. LL should initially set up weekly appointments with his instructors to review class and reading material along with any questions;
2. LL should take his tests in a distraction-free environment;
3. LL requires extra time on tests due to his delayed processing skills;
4. LL requires verbal reminders to write appointment times or other important information in his date book;
5. LL should be told directly of any tutoring or other support services available and given names or phone numbers of who to contact; and
6. LL should obtain notes from another student in his class so that he does not miss important information in lectures.

Though numerous meetings with school personnel were required, and intermittent contact with the therapist occurred throughout his undergraduate schooling (sessions were weekly during the first year of classes), 4 years later LL graduated with a BA in Business Communications.

Upon graduation from college LL was able to find a job as a sales clerk in a large bookstore and no longer felt the need for cognitive remediation. Two years later he returned to therapy requesting cognitive remediation as it related to vocational activities. He had been in and out of several jobs since his graduation. At the time of returning to therapy he was working in an unskilled labor position that he recognized had "no future career path." He wanted to use the college degree for which he had struggled so long and hard. He wanted to find a position that would allow him to use his business communications skills. After several interviews he was offered a position with a large bank as a project coordinator in their facilities management department. Several meetings occurred with his supervisors, selected coworkers, and a company vice-president to discuss LL's strengths and weaknesses and the compensatory strategies needed for successful functioning. LL was continuing to have difficulty with his memory and psychomotor efficiency. For this position the following compensatory strategies were set in place:

1. maintain a list of current projects with priorities for implementation;
2. develop written steps for each project's completion;
3. develop a summary of general responses to staff inquiries;
4. maintain an organizational flowchart;

5. maintain a planner for appointments, meetings, deadlines, and "to do" lists;
6. schedule weekly meetings with his supervisor and summarize in writing the main points discussed;
7. maximize communications via e-mail or written memos; and
8. use a set routine for daily activities (e.g., checking "in" box, e-mail, voice mail, etc.).

LL has been in this position for almost 3 years. Cognitive remediation continued intermittently for the first year, after which it was determined that he had successfully generalized compensatory strategies, and his employer was satisfied with his performance. At termination, both LL and the employer were reminded that if his position and/or responsibilities drastically change it might be necessary to reinitiate cognitive remediation.

CONCLUSION

In summary, cognitive remediation is a systematic intervention designed to help individuals strengthen and/or compensate for impaired cognitive abilities. Cognitive impairments can be categorized as involving deficits in one of the following five areas: (1) attention and concentration; (2) initiation and planning; (3) judgment and perception; (4) learning and memory; and (5) speed of information processing. Cognitive remediation strategies can be utilized to address each of these areas of impairment, and may include both strategies to strengthen and restore an existing cognitive function, or to compensate for impairments by identifying and utilizing other cognitive strengths. Determination of cognitive remediation strategies requires consideration not only of the impairment, but of the individual, as well as his/her goals, personality, motivation, and environment. Finally, cognitive remediation, while useful in a variety of settings, may play a key role in an individual's ability to resume work following cognitive impairment. By assessing the individual, the job tasks, and the employment environment, it is possible to identify strategies that enable the individual to meet the cognitive demands of his/her particular job. These strategies need to be tailored both to the individual's own unique strengths, weaknesses, and preferences and to the specific work environment. Furthermore, as demands on the individual change, cognitive remediation strategies may be updated and refined to assist the individual in adapting to new tasks and circumstances.

At the outset we indicated that the type of cognitive remediation techniques we would be discussing are the more molar therapeutic strategies, versus milieu approaches such as those described by Prigatano (1986) or Brenner et al. (1994). Of course, molar strategies are integral components of milieu programs. LL's case exemplifies another quality of molar approaches to cognitive remediation: treatment can be an integral component in the changing milieu of a person's life. For the same individual, there are different techniques for different impairments affecting differing life situations. The constants are the therapist's ability to form a therapeutic alliance as the foundation of treatment, skill in the development of an appropriate treatment plan, knowledge of cognitive remediation strategies, and the ability to sustain clients' motivation and that of key individuals in their lives. This chapter has provided a brief look at cognitive remediation theory, research, and technique. This knowledge must be combined with knowledge of brain–behavior relationships and skill in providing therapeutic relationships in order to attain the outcomes our clients desire and deserve.

REFERENCES

Bellack, A. S., Gold, J. M., & Buchanan, R. W. (1999). Cognitive rehabilitation for schizophrenia: Problems, prospects, and strategies. *Schizophrenia Bulletin, 25*(2), 257–274.

Ben-Yishay, Y., & Diller, L. (1993). Cognitive remediation in traumatic brain injury: Update and issues. *Archives of Physical Medicine and Rehabilitation, 74*, 204–213.

Berquist, T. F., Boll, T. J., Corrigan, J. D., Harley, J. P., Malec, J. F., Millis, S. R., & Schmidt, M. F. (1994). Neuropsychological rehabilitation: Proceedings of a consensus conference. *Journal of Head Trauma Rehabilitation, 9*(4), 50–61.

Brenner, H. D., Roder, V., Hodel, B., Kienzle, N., Reed, D., & Liberman, R. P. (1994). *Integrated psychological therapy for schizophrenia patients.* Seattle, WA: Hogrefe & Huber.

Carney, N., Chestnut, R. M., Maynard, H., Mann, N. C., Patterson, P., & Helfand, M. (1999). Effect of cognitive rehabilitation on outcomes for persons with traumatic brain injury: A systematic review. *Journal of Head Trauma Rehabilitation, 14*(3), 277–307.

Cicerone, K. D. (1999). Commentary: The validity of cognitive rehabilitation. *Journal of Head Trauma Rehabilitation, 14*(3), 316–321.

Cicerone, K. D., Dahlberg, C., Kalmar, K., Langenbahn, D. M., Malec, J. F., Bergquist, R. F., Felicetti, T., Giacino, J. T., Harley, J. P., Harrington, D. E., Herzog, J., Kneipp, S., Laatsch, L., & Morse, P. A. (2000). Evidence-based cognitive rehabilitation: Recommendations for clinical practice. *Archives of Physical Medicine and Rehabilitation, 81*, 1596–1615.

Goldberg, T. E., Weinberger, D. R., Berman, K. F., Pliskin, N. H., & Podd, M. H. (1987). Further evidence for dementia of the prefrontal type in schizophrenia? *Archives of General Psychiatry, 44*, 1008–1014.

Gordon, W. A., & Hibbard, M. R. (1992). Critical issues in cognitive remediation. *Neuropsychology, 6*(4), 361–370.

Harley, J. P., Allen, C., Braciszewski, T. L., Cicerone, K. D., Dahlberg, C., Evans, S., Foto, M., Gordon, W. A., Harrington, D., Levin, W., Malec, J. F., Millis, S., Morris, J., Muir, C., Richert, J., Salazar, E., Schiavone, D. A., & Smigelski, J. S. (1992). Guidelines for cognitive remediation. *NeuroRehabilitation, 2*(3), 62–67.

Levine, B., Robertson, I. H., Clare, L., Carter, G., Hong, J., Wilson, B. A., Duncan, J., & Stuss, D. T. (2000). Rehabilitation of executive functioning: An experimental–clinical validation of goal management training. *Journal of the International Neuropsychological Society, 6*, 299–312.

Prigatano, G. P. (1986). *Neuropsychological rehabilitation after brain injury.* Baltimore: Johns Hopkins University Press.

Rund, B. R., & Borg, N. E. (1999). Cognitive deficits and cognitive training in schizophrenic patients: A review. *Acta Psychiatrica Scandinavica, 100*, 85–95.

CHAPTER 14

Utilization of Group Approaches to Address Employment Issues

CHARLES GARVIN

INTRODUCTION

This chapter describes the various group approaches that are utilized to assist people requiring rehabilitation services to seek and retain employment as well as to advance their employment careers. First presented is a rationale for the use of groups in rehabilitation followed by a short overview of group work purposes and principles for the reader who is unfamiliar with these ideas. The remainder of the chapter is devoted to a discussion of the employment-related purposes relevant to group services and the specific group modalities that can be utilized to accomplish these purposes. Throughout the chapter the reader should assume that when we state that the worker will do something, we always mean that whenever possible the worker will help the members to respond to each other in these ways.

GROUP WORK IN REHABILITATION

There are many reasons why group services should be an important part of mental health rehabilitation. First, because consumers of these services face many of the same barriers and stresses and have had many similar life experiences, they can provide a great deal of empathy and support to one another as they face this new challenge. The relevant group work concept is that of "mutual aid" in which the worker's primary task is to help the group to become the kind of entity that maximizes this kind of member interaction.

A second reason is that of efficiency in the use of time. Information can be imparted, for example, to several people in the same period as it takes to provide it to one person; group members can learn vicariously from others' experiences; and several persons are likely to have more ideas and knowledge relevant to rehabilitation tasks than the worker–client dyad may possess.

A third reason is the potency of a group, compared with a single individual, to engage in social action. There are times when rehabilitation efforts are stymied because of

---

CHARLES GARVIN • University of Michigan School of Social Work, Ann Arbor, Michigan.

environmental barriers such as a lack of a needed service, discrimination in the workplace including prejudice against mental health consumers, or the absence of a resource such as childcare or transportation. The members of a group can sign a petition or form a delegation to present their case to someone in authority with greater impact than when a single individual engages in an analogous action. An understanding of how to facilitate groups can be used in the rehabilitation setting with staff or staff–consumer groups such as the teams that are created in these settings. One example of this is an agency that creates teams composed of a case manager, employment specialist, consumer advocate, and training consultant to orchestrate the services offered to consumers.

THE CONCEPT OF GROUP WORK

By the term "group work" we mean something broader than usually implied by the term "group therapy." We refer to a broad array of groups facilitated by trained practitioners, often social workers, psychologists, or counselors, but we do not exclude from this definition situations in which the facilitators are consumers who have received special training in group facilitation. We are not referring, however, to self-help groups such as Alcoholics Anonymous in which leadership functions are performed by persons who are not differentiated from other members.

The common elements of these groups are: (1) an emphasis on mutual aid; (2) a set of norms supporting member participation in group decision-making, confidentiality, and respect for member rights; and (3) a group size that allows each member to interact with all other members (less than about 15 members). There are, nevertheless, differences in the ways these groups are organized and conducted related to the specific purposes of the groups and needs of the members. These differences include the following:

1. The number of group sessions may range from a single session group to a group with no set termination.
2. The degree to which the sessions are structured may range from a group with a specific educational curriculum to a group totally governed by what members bring up at the time.
3. The degree to which membership is "open" or "closed" may range from a group with a different membership at every meeting to a group with which no new members are allowed to affiliate after the group has begun.
4. The degree to which the group interaction is verbal may range from a group exclusively devoted to "talk" to a group exclusively devoted to an activity such as crafts or music.
5. Whether the group was "created" by the group worker (a formed group) or was created by the members on their own prior to contact with a group worker (a natural group).

Group work in different circumstances will differ along all of these dimensions depending on the specific rehabilitation purposes sought.

GROUP WORK PRACTICE PRINCIPLES

Readers unfamiliar with group work should consult one of the major group work texts (e.g., Garvin, 1997; Shulman, 1999; Toseland & Rivas, 1998) as space does not permit an extensive discussion of general principles here. We will, however, present a brief summary of group work as a review for the experienced group worker and an introduction for others. We assume that in most instances in rehabilitation services the group is formed by the worker or the agency, rather than created by the members independently. Our discussion of group work practice is based on that assumption, and can be best understood in terms of the group's tasks during its beginnings, middles, and endings.

Group Beginnings

Before the group holds its first meeting, the workers have several *pre-group tasks*. These include determining the specific purposes they will propose to the members, recruiting members (such as through asking coworkers for referrals, advertising the group in the agency or community), meeting individually with prospective members (to determine their interest in being in the group and to orient them to the group), and selecting members for the group while considering what kind of member composition will best promote the group's attaining its purposes (Bertcher & Maple, 1985).

As the workers plan for their first group meeting they should engage in a process of "tuning-in" in which they imagine what it is like to be in the members' situation and how members are likely to feel about coming to the meeting (Shulman, 1999). At the first meetings the worker will introduce activities to help the members to initiate relationships with one another and with the worker (so-called "warm-up" activities). The worker will discuss the purposes of the group and help the members to understand and either accept or modify them. Examples of group purposes are "to help members learn the skills of applying for jobs" and "to help members cope with impediments to success they encounter while working." Members will be assisted to develop individual goals related to the group's purposes. Some of the activities to be utilized in later meetings that will help them attain these goals will also be planned. Workers will assist the members to establish group norms such those regarding confidentiality, meeting attendance, and supportive actions toward other members.

Some groups, especially those that meet for only a few sessions or have ever-changing memberships, do not progress past the formation stage. They can still have some purpose such as orienting members to the service or helping them attain short-term goals. Other groups progress past the formation stage but return to it when normal progress is disrupted, such as when there is a substantial addition of new members.

Middle Stages of the Group

After the tasks of the first (often referred to as "formation") stage of the group have been accomplished, the group is ready to engage primarily in activities to accomplish group purposes. Depending on the group purpose, these may consist of problem-solving discussions, educational presentations, expressive activities such as art or music projects, simulations such as role-plays, and social action to remove external barriers to the members attaining their goals. In a later section of this paper, when we describe different kinds of rehabilitation groups, we indicate in which groups these different approaches predominate.

When it is fully explained to practitioners, group work will, at first, seem complex. This is because the worker must think in terms of several system levels: individual members, subgroups composed of several members, the group as an entity, and systems outside of the group such as the agency, the community, the members' ethnic groups, and even the larger society. Workers will, in specific circumstances, intervene with any of these as well as in interactions among them. One approach to group work, in fact, sees the role of the worker to be a mediator between systems (Schwartz, 1994). Inasmuch as a major thrust of group work is to help members to help one another and to help the group become an entity that sustains this, the worker, however, will interact with the group as an entity more than with individual members. Workers' actions, as in any interpersonal helping situation, will be directed at members' cognitions, affects, or instrumental behaviors, although some worker actions will have more impact on one of these classes of behaviors than others. Actions directed primarily at cognitions include helping members to correct unreal or distorted ideas ("I will *never* succeed at work no matter how hard I try"); helping members to increase their understanding of their own behavior ("I now understand that I was fighting with my boss because I saw him as my always critical father"); and helping members to create their own solutions by going through a problem-solving process (identifying the problem and the range of possible actions to solve it, evaluating the impact of each action, selecting the optimal solution, implementing the chosen solution). This is not to imply that the worker takes on all of the above interventions. The worker's intention should be to help members help each other in these and other ways.

The worker will also pay attention to members' affects such as anxiety, depression, elation, disappointment, or anger. At times, the member will be helped to cope with the affect when the worker empathetically takes note of it ("You seemed very sad when you spoke of the difficulty you had being assigned to the training program you had requested"). At other times, workers will help members to handle their anxiety about employment-related situations by teaching them relaxation exercises (Toseland & Rivas, 1998), breathing exercises, or even meditation. At still other times, workers will help members to express their emotions in appropriate ways in the group rather than inhibiting this expression.

Workers will help members to acquire behaviors that will enable them to attain their goals. At times this is accomplished through presenting the members with a model such as through observing a film or another person in the group who role-plays the desired behavior. The member can subsequently rehearse the behavior in the group, also through role-play. At other times the worker will help the member to acquire or retain the new behavior by employing conditioning principles such as reinforcement ("You did an excellent job of showing the group how you would be more assertive in requesting a change in your job assignment") (Sundel & Sundel, 1980).

The worker may also introduce a variety of program activities including music, drama, arts and crafts, trips, and games. Employment-related skills and attitudes could often best be acquired through these means. The following are examples of this:

- A game was used to help members to become aware of how they responded to competitive situations.
- A musical activity was used to help members relax after an especially anxiety-producing discussion of the steps they had to take to search for a job.
- A craft activity was introduced to help members become aware of how they reacted when they experienced frustration while attempting to accomplish a difficult task.

Ending Stage

Groups also will have tasks related to their endings. These may vary in intensity depending on whether the group has met for a long or a short period of time and how salient the group has been in the members' lives. Nevertheless, the worker should recognize that virtually all groups have had some important meaning to the members and the members will have thoughts and feelings about the group ending. When they can express these, they will be more likely to remember what they have learned through the group experience and to proceed to other experiences that will extend this learning.

Another important concept in working with groups is *group development*. According to many authorities, groups progress through phases (Garland, Jones, & Kolodny, 1976; Sarri & Galinsky, 1985). An understanding of these phases helps the group worker to act in ways that are appropriate to the group's tasks at that phase. The first or formation phase involves helping the members with the formation tasks we noted above. The next phase often brings power and control issues into play in which members often compete for leadership and this may include challenging the authority of the worker. A work phase is likely to follow in which the members proceed to carry out goal-oriented activities. There may be subsequent power struggles in some groups, especially those that extend over time. When the group is about to end, termination issues predominate in which members deal with their feelings about ending the group, reduce their attachments to the group, and prepare for the ways they will continue to accomplish their goals after the group ends.

THE USE OF GROUP WORK IN
EMPLOYMENT AND REHABILITATION

Rehabilitation Task

Groups can be used to help clients accomplish many employment-related rehabilitation tasks. We shall describe each of these and then indicate the kinds of group approaches that help members accomplish such tasks.

1. Skill development. Groups can help members to develop the skills required for job success (social skills for relationships with fellow employees or employers) or even particular job-related skills (following work rules). In some circumstances specific job performance skills can be taught in groups.
2. Socialization to the world of work. Groups can help members to develop attitudes and goals that are required to achieve job success as well as to establish their plans for their work careers.
3. Motivation for work. Groups can help members who are poorly motivated for employment to increase their level of motivation.
4. Support in facing stresses of attaining and maintaining employment. Groups can help members to reduce their subjective stress through the support and empathy that members can provide one another.
5. Problem-solving. Members can learn in groups how to identify work problems and employ rational problem-solving processes to generate, evaluate, and apply solutions.
6. Extensive personal change. Some clients may require extensive modification in their customary ways of coping with work-related issues. A *group therapy* experience may be utilized to help members confront these ways of coping and explore alternative behavioral patterns. This may involve the development of a better understanding of these patterns, often referred to as *insight*, and an opportunity to experiment in a safe setting with alternatives.

TABLE 14-1. Group Work Technologies and Change Theories:
Their Relationship to Accomplishing Rehabilitation Tasks

Rehabilitation task	Group approaches	Relevant change theories
Skill development	Skill training, education, relationship enhancement	Cognitive–behavioral, adult learning, interpersonal learning
Socialization to the world of work	Education and experiential	Adult learning
Motivation for work	Consciousness raising, operant	Humanistic psychology, behavioral psychology
Support	Relationship enhancement	Interpersonal learning
Problem-solving	Problem-solving	Adult learning
Personal change	Group psychotherapy	Ego psychology, cognitive–behavioral
Social change	Social action	System change, conflict resolution

7. Social change. Groups can often be more effective than individuals acting alone in bringing about changes in the social environment.

The reader will be helped to grasp the range of group approaches and how these relate to rehabilitation tasks through an examination of Table 14.1.

GROUP APPROACHES

Skill Development

Group skill development approaches are derived from cognitive–behavioral and adult learning theories (Rose, 1989). These theories characterize adults as acquiring new behaviors through: (1) understanding the rationale for the behaviors; (2) observing models enacting the behaviors; (3) practicing the behaviors in a safe setting; and (4) receiving feedback in the form of coaching, reinforcement, and constructive criticism.

The specific procedures employed in groups are the following:

1. The process begins with an analysis of the specific situations to which the members must respond and the criteria for the kinds of behaviors that are required in the situation.

> Example: Clubhouse members participated in a job skills group the purpose of which was to help them cope with their first day at work. One of the problems they identified was to form a relationship with one or more coworkers with whom they were required to interact (e.g., other cooking staff in a restaurant). Criteria discussed included introducing oneself through provision of information such as one's name and job assignment and asking for similar information in a place and at a time that is appropriate.

2. The second stage is to have an opportunity to observe the performance of a model.

> Example: The group worker and an agency volunteer role-played two employees becoming acquainted on the job who provided each other with their names and described what their job assignments were.

3. The third stage is for the member seeking to acquire the skill to participate in a role-play that offers an opportunity to practice the skill.

4. The fourth stage is for the other group members to provide feedback on the member's actions in the role-play. It is important to stress that the feedback should begin with what the other members *liked* about the role-play followed by suggestions for improvements.

> Example. After John role-played initiating a relationship with a fellow employee, the group worker asked the other members to provide feedback. Sandy said that she liked the way John made eye contact. Jill added that John seemed confident of himself as shown by speaking clearly and without hesitation. Mark suggested that John not apologize for taking up the time of the other person. It would be sufficient to ask the other worker if he had time to spend a few minutes getting acquainted.

5. Finally, the group worker helps the member to create a *homework assignment* in which the member accepts a task assignment to try the skill out one or more times prior to the next meeting. It is understood that the member will report on this assignment at the next meeting. If more practice is then required, this will occur at that meeting.

Education

Group workers in rehabilitation settings often provide an educational experience to group members. Examples of such educational topics are the job opportunities in a given field, the steps to be used in obtaining knowledge about a job, the resources that can be used to choose a job career, and the kinds of skills and experience needed for a job. Group workers must use educational techniques to impart content such as the following:

1. Develop curricular units that are well organized and appropriate to the time available.
2. Use educational aids such as charts, handouts, and power-point presentations.
3. Provide an experiential element such as role-plays or other simulations.
4. Create an atmosphere in which questions and discussion are encouraged.
5. Enable carryover from one session to the next through homework assignments.
6. Stimulate retention through such devices as individual notebooks in which participants keep handouts, record homework, and preserve notes.

Relationship Enhancement

There are a number of group procedures that help members to enhance their abilities to form or improve relationships with other employees or trainees. We do not suggest that these constitute a curriculum, but rather interventions that can be used selectively in ways that are appropriate to the needs of the members and the purposes of the specific group. In a rehabilitation and employment-related group the objective is to deal with relationships with other employees and the group work experience is a very potent one for this purpose because of the multiple opportunities for feedback and for simulating work situations.

These procedures are employed when members have relationship difficulties that interfere with their work performance. Examples are members who do not work cooperatively, react to others with hostility, withhold information about their own needs (lack of assertiveness), or do not offer or elicit the kind of support employees legitimately expect from one another. We recognize, however, that people differ from one another in their degrees of sociability and we do not expect the workplace to be "one happy family" but argue that there is at least a minimum quality of interaction working with others requires for job success and retention.

The following are procedures that are used by group workers to enhance the relationship skills of members:

1. *Teach how to initiate relationships.* Many individuals have not acquired this basic skill; thus they avoid others or approach them at inopportune times in ways that repel the other person. The group worker can employ the skill development methods described earlier in this chapter. For the purpose of initiating relationships members can be taught to consider the time and place (e.g., not when the other person is busy at a task), and to begin with offering one's name and asking if it is a good time for the other person to converse.

2. *Obtaining and giving feedback.* An important skill is to be able to obtain and then think about the reactions others have to oneself and to offer the same kind of information. A direct request for such information may put the other too much "on the spot" but this is not the only way of securing it. Members can be taught non-verbal cues (e.g., a furrowed brow). At times, a more direct response may be elicited if a relationship has already been developed but members can be taught non-threatening ways of asking for this that are still direct ("I wonder how you felt about what I said").

3. *Offering and receiving positive feedback.* People tend to have positive feelings toward another person who offers them a compliment. This can be emphasized by the group worker and can be facilitated by a number of group exercises. A common one is to go around the group asking members to say something they appreciate about the person to their left. Another such "go-around" is to ask the "persons on the left" to give feedback emphasizing what they liked about the compliment and possibly adding a suggestion about strengthening the way it was delivered.

4. *Offering and receiving negative feedback.* It is difficult but sometimes necessary to criticize the work of another. The way this is done can either enhance or destroy good work relationships. Group members can be taught through role-plays and other techniques to precede criticisms they direct at others with positive statements if possible, to focus on the behavior rather than the person, and to offer to help the other person improve. When receiving criticisms from others, members can ask for specific examples and ideas on how to improve. If the person who offers the criticism only gives critical feedback, this can sometimes be pointed out.

5. *Expressing empathy.* People also tend to have positive attitudes toward others when they hear that the others have heard and understood a feeling they have expressed. Members can be trained to make empathic statements using the approach we outlined above for developing skills. An empathic statement by a listener reflects the feeling of the speaker as well as the context in which the feeling occurred.

> *Example.* Bob told the group that he was frightened of losing his job because he had not gotten up on time and was a half-hour late. Bill responded that he knew Bob was scared about getting fired, he had had a similar experience. In this situation, Bill reflected the feeling and the context *in his own words* showing that he had thought about what Bob said. The group worker commented that this was a good example of the discussion the group had had last week on empathy.

6. *Determining appropriate self-disclosure.*   Often people who require rehabilitative services have not had enough social opportunities to learn how much and what kinds of information to give about their personal lives to others. This includes information on disabilities such as mental illnesses. A major issue here is that there are no easy formulas and decisions on self-disclosure must be based on sound use of judgment. Nevertheless, members can be taught principles such as the following as bases for judgment: (1) How much does the other person need to know? (2) What are the consequences if I do not disclose the information even if it is requested and how can I phrase the refusal? (3) Do I have the kind of relationship that will continue to grow if we know more about each other and what do we need to know at this time about each other? The group members can be given vignettes to use in applying the above principles or they can present examples out of their own lives.

7. *Building trust.*   A relationship between two people requires that the individuals develop trust in one another. Trust means that they can assume they will not harm one another, will honor commitments made to one another, and will be honest in what they say to each other. Clients in rehabilitation settings are likely to have had encounters with others who were not trustworthy that may now interfere with their ability to trust people. Group work experiences can help them to learn how to determine whether people they encounter at work may be trusted. These are derived from the above definition of trustworthy relationships; namely, to ask whether there is any evidence the other person is harmful, does follow through on commitments, and speaks the truth. Members can also be reinforced for acting in a trustworthy manner in the group.

8. *Determining appropriate degrees of intimacy.*   Members can be taught that there are different categories of intimacy such as casual acquaintanceships, close friendships, and long-term commitments such as found in marriages. Relationships may progress from one to another of these levels. Group discussions can help members to determine which level of relationship they seek with fellow employees, how to determine whether the desire is reciprocated, and how to cope with problems that prevent attaining the desired level of intimacy. Members can discuss their aspirations and fears with respect to relationships, and the patience required to build a relationship. Their level of self-esteem and self-confidence is often an issue here.

Experiential Learning

By experiential learning, we do not refer in this chapter to using simulations or focusing the members' attention on group interactions. We refer, instead, to the group affording members opportunities to have experiences related to their occupational goals. Examples are trips to workplaces and training sites or the provision of actual work experiences during group sessions. When trips or work experiences are planned, the group worker should arrange for the following:

1. The experience should be clearly related to the purposes and goals of the group as well as the group's stage of development. These events should not be used to "fill time." They rarely should be used only as "fun." They should also be introduced in the middle stages of the group when relationships have been initiated and the group's purposes are well established.
2. There should be adequate planning for the experience. This includes discussing: the purpose with the members; how members are expected to behave during the experience; and what members would like to know or need to know about the experience.

3. The group worker should anticipate and plan for problematic events that might occur such as a member behaving inappropriately during a trip. The worker's response to this might be privately to coach the member on appropriate behavior or to have an arrangement for the member to be helped to return to the agency.
4. The event should be debriefed with the members. This involves reviewing what the members have observed, their reactions to the experience, their questions, and their future plans related to building on the experience.

Consciousness Raising

In the context of vocational rehabilitation, this term refers to the members becoming aware of attitudes regarding employment of which they may not be aware. These attitudes have been instilled by previous experiences as illustrated by the following examples:

1. A white member anticipated that all other coworkers would be people of color who would be antagonistic to her.
2. A member anticipated that coworkers would be superior in performance to her and her lack of abilities would cause her to be excluded from the informal work group.
3. A member, without realizing it, resents taking direction from anyone in authority.

The group worker can employ a variety of procedures to bring these beliefs to the members' awareness so that their validity can be tested and alternative beliefs derived from current realities can be developed. One procedure is to ask members about previous experiences with analogous situations, what their feelings were at the time, and whether these feelings continue into the present. Another procedure is to show members pictures about work situations and to ask them to make up stories about these situations. They can be asked whether these "projections," in fact, represent what they, themselves, believe. A third procedure is to ask members directly what their feelings and thoughts are about entering a specified work situation. Some members are likely to be more aware of their reactions than others who can then benefit from considering whether they are in "the same shoes."

The Use of Operant Procedures

The group worker employs operant procedures to increase or decrease the likelihood that a member will act in specified ways. In a concise introduction to a discussion of these procedures Nemeroff and Karoly (1991, p. 122) state:

> Most often associated with the ideas and procedures of B.F. Skinner, the perspective to be elaborated emphasizes freely emitted, overt (observable) actions and the immediate environmental forces that ostensibly "control" these actions. The determinants of behavior are generally thought to consist of (a) signals (or cues) that inform the person (or animal) that a particular response is or is not likely to pay off (in the form of a *reward*; and (b) the pattern of rewards or punishers that are linked to the omission of the response. Skinner's term *operant conditioning* highlights the fact that organisms are active in their interchanges with the world (they *operate* on the environment) and that the frequency or the probability of various operant responses is conditional on the presence of environmental signals (cues) and response contingent events (the prompt delivery of rewards or removal of punishments).

Thus, procedures that make an action more likely to occur are referred to as *reinforcement* while those that make an action less likely to occur are referred to as *punishment*.

Reinforcement occurs through the individual experiencing either a pleasurable *stimulus* (praise, money) or the withdrawal of a punishing one (nagging ceases). Punishment occurs through the individual experiencing a noxious stimulus (criticism) or the withdrawal of a pleasurable one (a fine for an action). Still another category is *extinction* which occurs when a behavior that was previously reinforced no longer is; under this circumstance the behavior diminishes. A group work example occurred when group members agreed not to respond to a member in any way when he made comments that were inappropriate to a discussion in the group that members had chosen to hold.

The group worker or the members can employ one of these procedures to help a member attain a goal. One way this can be done in groups is through the use of a *token economy*. The group worker establishes a token economy by assigning points to members for successfully accomplishing tasks such as doing homework, making specified contributions to group meetings, and so forth. These points can be used to purchase items the agency makes available or may simply gain the member recognition in a group ceremony. This approach is more frequently used with groups whose members have severe psychological or developmental disabilities but any group may find this approach to be novel and interesting.

Group workers also employ reinforcement procedures as a matter of course without even realizing they are doing so when they praise members for accomplishments or reward the entire group with an outing or special refreshments when the members have been working very hard to accomplish group purposes. Criticism in the form of feedback on member actions also occurs "naturally." Workers, however, who use criticism should be aware that there is a great deal of evidence that aversive responses, while momentarily inhibiting an action, can cause the member to become hostile, avoid the group, and see the worker as a negative force. While some criticism may be necessary, on balance workers must seek a solid relationship based on positive interactions to offset the side-effects of punishing responses, although more severe forms of punishment are sometimes required such as asking a member who has become severely disruptive to leave a meeting.

Problem-Solving

One of the most frequently occurring group activities is a problem-solving discussion. Examples are discussions of individual problems such as selecting a training program or overcoming an obstacle such as lack of transportation. Problem-solving discussions may also focus on group problems such as how the group may learn more about a type of job or how the group should handle member absences from the group.

Effective problem-solving takes place in stages. Elsewhere we have identified these stages as follows (Garvin, 1997, pp. 123–124):

1. The problem is specified in detail.
2. The group members determine whether a group problem-solving process should occur.
3. The group members are oriented to problem-solving (the stages of the problem-solving process are taught to those who do not know them).
4. Goals to be attained through problem-solving are specified.
5. Information is sought to help the group members generate possible solutions as well as evaluate such solutions.
6. Alternative solutions are evaluated.

7. One alternative is chosen.
8. Planning the details for carrying out the chosen alternative.

One reason for utilizing the stages of problem-solving approach is that problem-solving often tends to be of very low quality. Members may debate the first idea presented in the group rather than using their energy to discover better solutions than the first one mentioned. They may also select a solution without carefully evaluating each alternative. They may also think they have concluded their work when they have selected a solution and forget that the solution must be implemented and this involves determining who will do what and when.

Group Psychotherapy

While the term "group psychotherapy" is often used to refer to virtually any type of professionally conducted group, except so-called support groups, we think this is too loose a definition. We reserve this term for groups established to help members change deep-seated difficulties in maintaining relationships. This usage is consistent with the definition employed by major group psychotherapy experts (Rutan, 1993; Yalom, 1995). We do not see most vocationally oriented rehabilitation programs as offering this type of group psychotherapy. Nevertheless, some of the techniques used may be applied to other types of groups as a means of helping members adapt better to the work environment when they have problems in relationships.

One of the major techniques is *process commentary*. As Garvin (1997, pp. 164–165) stated:

> Workers introduce this intervention by directing the members' attention to an interaction that has just occurred in the group. This is often referred to as a "here and now" focus. This is a powerful technique because the members cannot easily disguise the behavior they had demonstrated in full view of all the others. This type of reflection in the group ultimately helps members resolve problems outside of the group because of the relationship that is likely to exist between actions and reactions in both places. Members also learn from this experience how to examine interactions in situations of which they are a part, outside of the group. Because of the awareness promoted by a process discussion, the member will experiment with ways of interacting with others that are more likely to meet her or his needs.
>
> Workers may draw attention to processes by questions such as the following:
>
> How did you feel when X said that to you? What did you think Y was saying?
>
> What did X remind you of when s/he said that?
>
> Why did X attack Y?
>
> Why are you not saying anything now?
>
> Why did you laugh when X said that?
>
> Each time I said something tonight, you disagreed with me.
>
> Even though you argue with me, you always sit next to me.

When workers use comments such as these, they should explain to the group why they think such an examination of the process will be useful and the group members should agree to this. Workers should realize that this may produce anxiety and should be prepared to stop using such an approach if it is too upsetting to the group members.

Social Action

It would be a mistake to think of all group services as oriented toward producing changes in the participants. Group members are as likely to experience environmental circumstances that inhibit their attaining vocational goals and they can work in groups to change these. Examples are employment agencies that do not expend enough effort to locate a suitable range of jobs or job training and job sites that discriminate against members because of their gender, ethnicity, sexual orientation, age, or disability. Elsewhere (Garvin, 1997, pp. 177–189) we have provided details on actions such as the following to be used in these circumstances:

1. Providing information to the agency in question.
2. Complaining to people in authority personally or through petition or by issuing an invitation to attend a group session.
3. Collecting and presenting data to the media.
4. Forming coalitions with other groups or organizations seeking the same changes (e.g., the Alliance for the Mentally Ill (AMI), the Welfare Rights Organization, The National Association for the Advancement of Colored People (NAACP), La Raza.

ISSUES IN THE USE OF GROUPS IN EMPLOYMENT SETTINGS

There are many challenges that must be faced by practitioners who seek to utilize the above ideas in employment settings. Offering a group work service is more than following some guidelines. Effective service to groups requires that the practitioners have considerable training in understanding group interventions, stages of group development, and how to assess such group conditions as group structures, processes, norms, climates, and interactions. Furthermore, the practitioner must have a repertoire of group skills and have learned how to apply these through experiential as well as didactic learning. Agencies often must help group workers who lack this expertise to obtain it through continuing education. Agencies must also recognize that offering a group service makes demands on the agency (e.g., appropriate meeting places that are protected from interruptions, resources materials for the groups, consultation for workers on solving group problems). Finally, the integration of employment and mental health services requires that agencies be prepared to experiment with how to adapt traditional group services to the needs of programs that seek to accomplish such integration.

EMPLOYMENT ISSUES THAT ARISE IN OTHER MENTAL HEALTH RELATED GROUPS

The members in any mental health related group are likely to have concerns related to employment; thus the workers should become acquainted with the approaches described in this chapter as they should be utilized in such groups. This requires all group workers to become acquainted with workplace and work training issues. It is with good reason that mental health can be defined as being able to love and to work. Too often, concerns of members are seen as strictly personal issues rather than as interactions between their coping behaviors and the realities of the workplace.

One example of this was a member who described to her group her mourning over the fact that a colleague at work had been diagnosed with cancer. The problem was compounded by the fact that several other coworkers had also become ill with this disease. The member suspected that, since they worked in a laboratory, environmental contamination was a cause. The group worker and the other group members explored options with her such as uniting with other employees to pressure the organization to clean up the contamination. She was convinced that this would lead to her being fired. Other options were then considered such as contacting the union as well as the media.

In another group, a member was an assistant manager of a fast food restaurant. She had allowed an employee she supervised to come late because of illness in his family. Her supervisor wanted her to fire this employee as the efficiency of the restaurant was more important than the needs of an employee. The worker framed this issue as the difference between the attitudes of male supervisors favoring productivity and those of women employees who also considered human needs. The woman member considered the possibility of discussing this issue with other women working in the restaurant with the purpose of getting the business to implement policies related to employees' personal needs.

SUMMARY

This chapter began with a discussion of what group work is, followed by the potential contribution of group work to meeting the employment needs of clients in rehabilitation settings. General principles for working with groups were then presented. The specific purposes that group work can fulfill in such settings were examined. The chapter concluded with information on different group approaches that are applicable to accomplishing these purposes. Finally, attention to employment related issues in other rehabilitation groups was emphasized.

REFERENCES

Bertcher, H. J., & Maple, F. (1985). Elements and issues in group composition. In M. Sundel, P. Glasser, R. Sarri & R. Vinter (Eds.), *Individual change through small groups* (pp. 180–202). New York, NY: Free Press.

Garland, J., Jones, H., & Kolodny, R. (1976). A model of stages of group development in social work groups. In S. Bernstein (Ed.), *Explorations in group work* (pp. 17–71). Boston, MA: Charles Rivers Books.

Garvin, C. (1997). *Contemporary group work* (3rd ed.). Boston, MA: Allyn & Bacon.

Nemeroff, C. J., & Karoly, P. (1991). Operant methods. In F. H. Kanfer (Ed.), *Helping people change: A textbook of methods* (4th ed., pp. 122–160). New York, NY: Pergamon Press.

Rose, S. (1989). *Working with adults in groups: Integrating cognitive, behavioral and small group strategies.* San Francisco, CA: Jossey-Bass.

Rutan, J. (1993). *Psychodynamic group psychotherapy* (2nd ed.). New York, NY: Guilford.

Sarri, R., & Galinsky, M. (1985). A conceptual framework for group development. In M. Sundel, P. Glasser, R. Sarri & R. Vinter (Eds.), *Individual change through small groups* (2nd ed., pp. 70–86). New York, NY: Free Press.

Schwartz, W. (1994). Social work with groups: The search for a method. In T. Berman-Rossi (Ed.), *Social work: The collected writings of William Schwartz.* Itasca, IL: Peacock.

Shulman, L. (1999). *The skills of helping individuals, families, and groups* (4th ed.). Itaska, IL: Peacock.

Sundel, S. S., & Sundel, M. (1980). *Be assertive: A practical guide for human service workers.* Beverly Hills, CA: Sage.

Toseland, R., & Rivas, R. (1998). *Group work practice* (3rd ed.). Boston, MA: Allyn & Bacon.

Yalom, I. D. (1995). *The theory and practice of group psychotherapy* (4th ed.). New York, NY: Basic Books.

CHAPTER 15

The Vocational Development Functions of the Clubhouse

Krista Magaw

INTRODUCTION

This chapter describes how clubhouses assist persons recovering from mental illness to develop readiness in multiple life domains and to enter into employment. Every clubhouse model program adhering to the standards of the International Center for Clubhouse Development (ICCD) provides daily opportunities to develop work readiness by genuinely contributing their efforts to the "work-ordered day" (Beard, Propst, & Malamud, 1982). Activities each day include preparing lunch, answering phones, assisting other clients—called "members"—in performing basic tasks, making outreach calls and visits, and doing computer, house, and yard work. The clubhouse provides a variety of social activities outside of the work-ordered day, including the celebration of holidays, informal gatherings, and recognition of the growth and development of individual participants. Members and staff also perform many case management functions, assisting in the location and maintenance of housing and jobs, and advocating for necessary benefits (Macias, Jackson, Wang, & Schroeder, 1999). Each clubhouse provides Transitional Employment opportunities to promote confidence and work readiness. All these services are provided in a supportive atmosphere of member/staff partnership, where membership is lifelong and unconditional. Indeed, the key to the successful operation of a clubhouse lies in fostering social support among and between members and personnel of the club.

The clubhouse model of psychiatric and vocational rehabilitation has been refined and tested by Fountain House, in New York City, for over 50 years, offering people with mental illnesses unique opportunities for recovery of valued vocational, employment, and social roles. The successful clubhouse is a relevant, flexible, and semipermeable institution that incorporates strongly held cultural values and rehabilitation techniques (Beard et al., 1982). It operates as a milieu that facilitates the transition of people from the clubhouse into the greater society. It is the members of the club who determine their own pace of transition and the direction they wish to go in their rehabilitation.

Krista Magaw • Tecumseh Land Trust, Yellow Springs, Ohio.

Serious mental illnesses rob people of critical developmental opportunities, including the cultivation of successful social and relationship-building skills, vocational and employment skills, and, all too often, the acquisition of a comfortable role or niche in the greater community (Anthony, 1994). The clubhouse provides these developmental opportunities for a surprisingly wide array of members by generating a broad variety of meaningful and necessary activities every day. From sophisticated planning, writing, development, and negotiation tasks to emptying ashtrays, the clubhouse needs and values the contributions of its members. The experience of being needed and appreciated motivates the risk-taking necessary to acquire valued skills and roles, ultimately, in the greater community (Vorspan, 1988).

The staff and members of nearly 400 clubhouses world-wide share responsibility for and ownership of their clubhouses, sharing their challenges and rewards, and filling a unique niche in the field of psychiatric rehabilitation (Anthony, 1994). This "no reject" program has demonstrated its tremendous potential to improve vocational and employment outcomes for persons with mental illness (Drake, McHugo, Becker, Clark, & Anthony, 1996). The recently developed ICCD is strategically committed to overcoming mental health and vocational rehabilitation system barriers to make this model more accessible and to ensure a high standard of quality among clubhouses (Propst, 1992).

CLUBHOUSE HISTORY

Era of Institutionalization (1948–1963)

The clubhouse was born in 1948, during the era of institutionalization when a group of ex-hospital patients in New York City formed a self-help group called "We Are Not Alone." Its members provided each other with the mutual support and resources necessary to re-establish themselves in a rejecting and stigmatizing community. With the support of a generous benefactor, members acquired a brownstone town house with a fountain in its back yard. They hired a radical young social worker, John Beard, to direct their program, and they called it Fountain House (Flannery & Glickman, 1996).

Beard, among the earliest practitioners of psychiatric or psychosocial rehabilitation, had experienced some success in providing employment opportunities to patients of a state hospital near Detroit. Hospital policy in the 1940s required Beard to transport the patients off the state hospital grounds in strait-jackets to their grocery store stocking jobs. Even when only primitive psychiatric medications were available, the value of real, paid work in the community was evident to Beard and to the Fountain House members who hired him.

Beard's belief in real, paid employment quickly translated into the Transitional Employment Program of Fountain House. Unlike partial hospital programs or social clubs, successful clubhouses, based on Fountain House, have always paired accessible opportunities for paid work with meaningful volunteer activity within the clubhouse. Unlike sheltered workshops, which proliferated during this same period, clubhouses have a built-in motivator for community integration. Transitional Employment jobs are in real businesses outside the clubhouse; they are paid at the going community wage; and they are constantly visible to the whole clubhouse community.

The shared history of members and staff in developing the clubhouse model is well documented in books, articles, videos, and the continuing oral history shared in the "clubhouse to clubhouse" colleague training described below. Ester Montanez, an early staff member of Fountain House who remains there today, remembers early members and staff literally inventing the program day by day (Flannery & Glickman, 1996). Ester was initially hired as a house cleaner for the program, but it quickly became apparent that her time was better spent teaching and encouraging members to clean, cook, and make decisions for themselves.

The community (or "house") meeting, a weekly decision-making group of all interested members and staff, evolved early in Beard's nearly 35-year tenure, and continues in clubhouses throughout the world. Issues and decisions, large and small, come to the community meeting. The critical role of members in making decisions for themselves contrasted sharply with the experiences members had in state hospitals (Anderson, 1998). During this era of long-term hospitalizations, many members came to the clubhouse after many years of patient-hood. Many had entered the state hospital in their late teens or early twenties and had very few skills and virtually no work or social experience. Every experience of being wanted and needed, of belonging and being a valued member of the clubhouse, was a powerful antidote to the experience of institutionalization (Beard et al., 1982).

The clubhouse had a similarly powerful effect on staff and community volunteers who became involved in the clubhouse (Anderson, 1998). Most staff hired in the clubhouse had little mental health background or rebelled from their experience with existing institutions. Like Beard, they were dissatisfied with traditional patient/professional roles and found the experimental and intentional nature of the clubhouse community rewarding.

Era of Deinstitutionalization (1963–1993)

As the state of the art of mental health care changed in the 1960s, 1970s, and 1980s, policy-makers and advocates alike pushed for deinstitutionalized care of persons with serious mental illnesses (Torrey, 1997). Fountain House, and a growing number of other clubhouses across the United States, had arguably even more to offer their members during this tumultuous time. The mutual support, opportunities for skills development, and employment connections were obviously needed by even larger numbers of people—quickly and urgently. Hundreds of thousands of persons needed help, discharged to their communities as virtual strangers, often having lost much of their family support and connection over years of hospitalization. Stigma remained a huge problem. The disfigurement of Tardive Dyskinesia drew attention to many ex-patients as they struggled to manage life in the community with few skills and resources.

Clubhouses were not numerous, however, and the model's outsider status in a world dominated by a medical mental health treatment model was a distinct disadvantage as federal and state dollars became available for community programs. Clubhouse staff were not affiliated with or had rebelled against the traditional mental health disciplines of social work, psychology, nursing, and psychiatry, and were thus poorly placed to advocate for the clubhouse model. At the beginning of this era, consumer, family, and advocacy organizations were virtually non-existent. While a philosophical agreement existed that institutional practices of the past had created many evils, the scope and design of community support and the treatment programs needed to take their place was entirely unclear (Anthony, 1994).

Many existing clubhouses grew and some expanded their services to include case management, housing, and a variety of vocational opportunities. After the initial wave of funding for community mental health centers ended, states were stimulated by federal Community Support dollars to develop a variety of non-medical support and outreach programs. A few states, such as North Carolina, saw clubhouses as a good vehicle for community support. In North Carolina, over 30 clubhouses were developed during the early 1980s. A useful network was quickly established among them, supported by the rapidly developing Alliance for the

Mentally Ill and the Mental Health Association. Other states, such as Ohio, however, looked to individual case management as the primary building block of their community support system and devoted nearly all their community resources to the development of a case management system. Yet other states, such as Pennsylvania, looked to residential support programs as the key ingredient in their community support system.

Nationwide clubhouses began to network among themselves and with other psychosocial rehabilitation programs. Clubhouse staff were among the first members of the International Association of Psychosocial Rehabilitation Services (Anthony, 1994). In 1981, Fountain House and its fellow clubhouses began convening biannual International Clubhouse Seminars to disseminate information on the model. Fountain House began training colleagues (both members and staff) from other clubhouses in implementing the model. A set of standards for clubhouse models was developed and disseminated throughout the steadily growing network (Macias, Harding, Alden, Geersten, & Barreira, 1999).

Era of Post- and Trans-Institutionalization (1993 to the Present)

The clubhouse model is more relevant than ever in this era when long-term psychiatric hospitalization is virtually non-existent. Though the treatments potentially available to a person diagnosed with a major mental illness today are significantly different from those available to a person 40 years ago, the fundamental lack of skills, resources, confidence, and support remains astonishingly similar for such persons today (Torrey, 1997). Depending upon a number of factors—access to state of the art health care, adequate insurance coverage, family experience with and attitudes toward mental illness, class, location, personal and family supports, and overall resources—the young person diagnosed with a serious mental illness today may be supported in leading an independent and satisfying life or may end up in prison. Homelessness, drug addiction, and long periods with little or no mental health treatment are all too common (Noble, Honberg, Hall, & Flynn, 1997).

The successful clubhouse community today provides relevant outreach to people who are homeless, substance dependent, and involved with the criminal justice system. The low demand/high expectancy environment in the clubhouse, the supportive, non-status-conscious relationship between members and staff, and the flexibility at matching member strengths with community needs works extremely well in this new era. Engaging the homeless person with mental illness can take months or years, but the clubhouse culture is well suited to this challenge as well. Clubhouses continue to attract staff who are comfortable working outside of traditional institutional boundaries, including many recovering persons, and many members are willing to mentor a person less fortunate (at least at this particular moment) than themselves (Vorspan, 1986).

In addition to homeless persons and persons trans-institutionalized to prisons, jails, or shelters, many persons with mental illnesses today are arguably trans-institutionalized to their own living rooms. Improved access to poverty-level Social Security disability income and Medicaid, coupled with poor or no access to decent private insurance once an individual has been labeled as mentally ill, enforce this kind of permanent holding pattern (Macias & Rodican, 1997). Persons in this situation have few skills and little motivation to take the risk of employment. Many have few friends or social contacts. Stigma and skill deficits have often prevented the acceptance of these persons in churches or social and community organizations. Smoking too many cigarettes, watching too much TV, drinking coffee, staying up late and sleeping all day, loneliness, vulnerability to victimization, multiple health and diet problems, and poverty characterize this lifestyle (Torrey, 1995). The clubhouse that skillfully offers appealing, confidence-building alternatives to this lifestyle can have a huge impact.

Limited access to adequate insurance coverage, timely illness education, support, and treatment significantly worsen the disabling effects of mental illness in the United States and much of the world. Some different results are being seen in countries with universal health-care, such as Ireland, where the best treatment, education and support practices are offered in a timely way with far greater reliability (Torrey, 1997). Despite insurance and treatment access issues, clubhouses in the United States continue to encourage and support their members' employment efforts. Over time, the clubhouse culture's value on work, and the members' hard won skills and confidence, allow many members to escape the trap of disability (Bond, Drake, Mueser, & Becker, 1997).

THE WORK-ORDERED DAY: A PLACE TO BEGIN

At the heart of all Fountain House model clubhouses is the work-ordered day, of approximately eight hours, five days a week. Herein lies the straightforward genius of the clubhouse.

Each work-ordered day provides opportunities for staff to engage every member of the clubhouse in contributing meaningfully to the club. Valued social, vocational, educational, and (in the context of many clubhouses) residential roles are all available to members with any skill level. Each task performed, no matter how big or small, is valued by staff and peers. The urgency of getting each day's work completed provides members with opportunities to risk trying new tasks and activities. Both failures and successes are seen as learning opportunities. While all clubhouses also provide social and recreational activities at evenings and weekends, the work-ordered day is the central vehicle for relationship building, skills teaching, and motivation in the clubhouse (Angers, 1999).

Integration of Psychiatric and Vocational Rehabilitation

The art of the clubhouse lies in the blending of psychiatric and vocational rehabilitation. The clubhouse applies best practices of both—borrowing high acceptance, engagement with staff and peers, direct skills teaching, modeling, and titrated support from the psychiatric rehabilitation field. From vocational rehabilitation, it employs the high cultural value on work roles, the motivation of earning money, and the use of adaptive technologies.

A significant body of research points out the importance of social skills and flexibility to the vocational success of persons with mental illnesses (Anthony, 1984). Mental illness often robs people of the developmental opportunities to learn and practice these skills. The work-ordered day offers innumerable opportunities for social skill development in a supportive, engaging, work-like environment.

Units

Members and staff in each clubhouse develop the work units they need to get their club's unique tasks accomplished (Beard et al., 1982). A small clubhouse may have only one or two units—an administration and education unit, for example. Fountain House currently has 14 units, each with more staff and members than many entire clubhouses. Each clubhouse community must use its own logic to decide which new units are needed and when.

All clubhouses have to perform basic phone-answering, documentation, and mail-opening tasks, so most have some sort of administration or clerical unit. Though most clubhouses do not have a horticulture unit, the relatively small and new Corwin House in Lebanon, Ohio, immediately formed such a unit to care for its historic four and a half acre site. Many members in this semi-rural, tradition-conscious area bring farming and gardening experience to the clubhouse. Corwin House's kitchen unit enjoys using fresh vegetables and herbs raised by the horticulture unit and the neighbors enjoy the flower and perennial gardens surrounding the house.

Each day units begin, and sometimes end, with a meeting to plan the day's work. Staff and members work together to set the agenda and distribute tasks. Members are often paired with other members or staff to learn or perform tasks. Some tasks, such as answering the telephone, occur every day. Others, such as publishing a newsletter, planning events, writing press releases, or orienting new members, occur at different frequencies.

Soon after joining a clubhouse, a member chooses which unit of a clubhouse to join, depending on his or her skills, interests, and goals. Members are generally encouraged to stick with a unit long enough to develop some relationships and confidence there. Unit changes are permitted, and even encouraged. A member with cooking experience might, for instance, join the kitchen unit initially because he/she feels comfortable and useful there. After a few months, he/she might decide to join the education unit and strengthen academic competencies.

Staff and Member Roles

Staff and members work side by side in the units, functioning as coworkers to the greatest extent possible. Staff facilitate the work of each unit but strive to provide as little direction as possible. Instead, they engage members and support them in taking initiative, responsibility, and leadership. The staff role has been described as that of a talent scout. Some members may, in fact, have far better task-specific skills than staff, and are encouraged to use them. A member might be a master chef, a skilled gardener, a teacher, or a computer programmer. Though the member's illness has often prevented recent use of his or her skills in a paid work setting, the member can immediately take pride in contributing valued work to the clubhouse unit.

Members and staff constantly balance the greatest possible level of inclusion of every member—in both decision-making and work—with getting the job done. This balancing act does not come naturally to most staff or members, after a lifetime of messages like "If you want something done right, do it yourself," and "If you can't do the job right, don't do it at all." The risk of failure, even a limited failure, feels devastating to many persons with serious mental illnesses. Often, persons with serious mental illnesses have developed a functional pattern of pulling back from new challenges for fear of failure and the ensuing negative consequences (Wisnick, 1997). Many members have missed out on the developmental benefit of the trial and error of early work experiences, such as summer jobs during their teen years.

Staff make judgment calls all day to maintain this balance. When do they do the work themselves, in favor of expediency? When do they give a member a chance to try something he or she might not be able to complete? How much time does the staff member take to facilitate a good social interaction when lunch is not yet on the stove? The greatest impact of staff may be in modeling this kind of judgment and modeling the patience to exercise it gracefully (Anderson, 1998).

The Community

The clubhouse makes important community decisions as a community (Peckoff, 1992). At least weekly, staff and members meet to address important mutual issues, from setting rules to planning holiday parties. This feature of clubhouse functioning distinguishes it both from traditional staff-directed psychiatric services and from consumer-operated programs such as self-help groups or drop-in centers. Both members and staff—from every part of the clubhouse—contribute to the agenda of the community meeting.

The community works hard to establish and maintain a positive community culture (Anderson, 1998). It evaluates itself and undertakes continuous efforts at improvement. Quality improvement tools from the private sector are a surprisingly good fit to the clubhouse community. Problem-solving techniques, uses of data to detect and correct systems problems, and the pushing of decision-making to the hands-on level are daily features of clubhouse community functioning.

Particularly important to those members with few family or other supportive relation-ships, clubhouses offer social and recreational activities. Chosen by staff and members, all clubhouses plan and carry out holiday celebrations and some weekend and evening activities. Thanksgiving is an especially important holiday for Fountain House and many other club-houses. Summer holiday picnics are a big event for some clubhouses. Social and recreational activities range from photography clubs to hanging out and playing pool.

Most clubhouses publish a weekly or monthly newsletter that publicizes these activities. They can be particularly important for members in need of intense levels of support, for those seeking safe and drug-free social environments, and for members making the transition to community work who need to retain a connection to the clubhouse community.

TRANSITIONAL EMPLOYMENT: THE RIGHT TO WORK

Each clubhouse certified by the International Center for Clubhouse Development must have a Transitional Employment Program (TEP). A TEP guarantees members with little recent or no work history the chance to try out a part-time paid job in a community business. If the member loses the transitional employment (TE) job because he or she cannot, at present, adequately perform it, that member is given a chance at another TE job as soon as one becomes available (Flannery & Glickman, 1996). At least in clubhouses that are parts of well-developed mental health systems, those members who could reasonably be expected to return to work through supported employment or more traditional vocational rehabilitation programs already have done so. A TEP is a real work experience accessible to those who cannot "reasonably" be expected to succeed, based on past performance (Beard et al., 1982).

TE jobs are generally approximately 20 hours each week, and each member gets an opportunity to work six to nine months in the job "slot." This provides the member with a chance to build his or her résumé and evaluate whether he or she is ready to seek a permanent job. It also gives the clubhouse a chance to recycle the TE job slot and give lots of members a chance to try it.

Clubhouse staff look for TEP jobs they believe members will find appealing in commu-nity businesses. Many clubhouse colleagues in training at Fountain House have had the opportunity to visit TEP jobs at the *Wall Street Journal*. The members in these jobs have a chance to return to the real world of work in the heart of the world's business center!

Staff work to find or develop TE positions with clearly defined parameters. Often, TE jobs are carved out of existing jobs in the workplace. For example, a TE job might be created in an office to relieve secretaries of coffee-making and mail-sorting duties. A TE worker might relieve teachers of playground duty during breaks. A restaurant TE might be created to provide additional set up services at peak times of the day. Sometimes a full-time job an employer has had difficulty filling is broken in two (Beard et al., 1982).

Based on the community employer's specifications, two clubhouse staff are trained to perform the duties of the TE job. The clubhouse staff then recommend one of their members to the employer to fill the position. A fairly informal interview is conducted to give the employer a chance to evaluate the recommended member (and vice versa). Generally the recommended member is selected (and the member wants to take the job), though this is not always the case. Once the match is made, the member is trained on the job. Clubhouse staff, who already have a good working relationship with the member, provide training and periodic coaching. If the TE worker is sick, then clubhouse staff will perform the job. If the TE worker cannot successfully learn and perform the job, then clubhouse staff will recommend a new applicant, and, in turn, train him or her. Once the TE worker has completed the entire six to nine month period, clubhouse staff will resume this process, keeping the position filled and performed to the employer's specifications.

The motivation provided by the TEP is tremendous. Opportunities to fill a TE job arise suddenly, and members who fail at TE jobs get many more opportunities to try again. As Ralph Bilby, long the TE director at Fountain House, puts it: "TE is an extremely forgiving system" (Flannery & Glickman, 1996). The peer and staff support for TE is tremendous, and a bit of peer competition is motivating as well. Since staff in the units support the TE placements, the entire unit is aware of and involved in the daily accomplishment of the TE job.

Recent research shows clubhouses to be as effective as other supported employment vehicles at returning persons with mental illness to work (Bond et al., 1997). A TEP seems to contribute to clubhouses' superior results in returning persons to work who did not initially express a desire to do so (Drake et al., 1999). Perhaps the most moving testimony to the motivation of the TEP is the personal account conveyed at Fountain House's weekly TE Dinner. Members hoping to successfully complete a TEP on their second, fourth, or even eleventh try, rise to share their personal story and aspiration to succeed in the world of work (Flannery, 1996).

INDEPENDENT EMPLOYMENT: TITRATING SUPPORT

The clubhouse continues to support members who attain independent employment to the extent they want and need that support. Some working members continue to participate in recreational and even unit activities of the clubhouse on a regular basis. Most diminish their involvement, but play a mentor role for a few fellow members. Some disappear from the clubhouse. All members are welcomed back to the clubhouse anytime they need its support, however. Many members learn from a sequence of failures and successes as they move toward independence and the clubhouse accommodates this process of recovery. Staff and members stand ready to titrate their level of support to meet the individual's needs as they change over time.

Some clubhouses, or their sponsoring agencies, provide formal Supported Employment Programs. Thresholds, in Chicago, for example, provides a full array of support and rehabilitation programs that work in complement to Thresholds' clubhouse. The key expectation, driven by ICCD standards, is that all clubhouses be accessible and supportive to independently employed members (Anthony,1994).

SPECIAL POPULATIONS: MEMBERS WITH MULTIPLE DISABILITIES

The hallmark of the successful clubhouse is its flexibility, both in supporting individuals and in accommodating to service systems changes and expectations over time. Four multiply diagnosed groups present particular challenges to clubhouses in this era of post- and trans-institutionalization: persons with Axis I and Axis II mental illness diagnoses; persons with substance abuse and mental illness diagnoses, people with mental retardation and mental illness, and brain-injured persons with a mental illness diagnosis.

Clubhouses, and most mental health programs, have struggled with the support of persons with Axis II diagnoses, particularly Borderline Personality Disorder (Linehan, 1993). Most are actively working with such members and are seeing them succeed, at least in some areas of their lives. The current thinking of Marsha Linehan and colleagues is quite compatible with clubhouse practice and tradition. The clubhouse provides the emotionally vulnerable person with a validating, yet structured environment, in which he or she can learn and practice the skills necessary to succeed. Staff model these skills and provide cheerleading for members as they practice new skills. Staff, and to the greatest extent possible, members, balance support and respect with humor in a safe, fairly predictable, environment.

Clubhouses have a longer track record of successful work with persons with substance abuse problems and mental illness. In the early 1980s the Club, in New Jersey, pioneered Double Trouble groups, using the Twelve Step approach of Alcoholics Anonymous. Many other clubhouses have established Double Trouble groups, and some have effectively utilized funding targeted for young and/or criminally involved persons with these dual diagnoses. All clubhouses serve some members in this group, parallel to other mental health programs.

From the era of lobotomies to the present, clubhouses have also commonly served persons with mental illness and mental retardation or brain injuries. Often these dually or multiply disabled persons have failed in mental retardation, developmental disability, or traditional medical rehabilitation programs due to their erratic or difficult behaviors. The unique strengths based approach of the clubhouse allows many members with fairly dramatic limitations to find a niche, as long as staff are able to engage them (Macias, Barreira, & Young, 2000).

CLUBHOUSES IN MENTAL HEALTH SYSTEMS

Each certified clubhouse must meet the basic standards set by the ICCD. Each must also adapt to its own community and to its unique mental health system. Depending upon what other mental health and vocational rehabilitation services and supports are available, some clubhouses decide to provide case management, housing, and/or a full array of vocational and psychosocial rehabilitation services. While all clubhouses offer environmental interventions and advocacy on behalf of their members, most strive to support and coach each member to manage his/her own community mental health team.

All clubhouses must work with other agencies in their system or other programs within their auspice agency to coordinate member care. Fountain House, launched far before most state and federal programs of supported or subsidized housing for persons with mental illness, developed an extensive housing operation as large as its other endeavors (Anderson, 1998). Many recently begun clubhouse programs have not needed to enter the housing arena owing to the existence of other adequate housing resources in their mental health and larger communities.

Ideally, funding for the clubhouse supports the blended goals and techniques of the psychiatric rehabilitation and vocational rehabilitation fields. While some clubhouses get funding from their state vocational rehabilitation agencies, most rely on private, state, or local monies directed to providing community support and/or rehabilitation services to persons with mental illnesses. Unfortunately, the outcomes—and particularly timetables for outcomes— sought by different funders are sometimes incompatible. The clubhouse is well suited to provide the long-term, no reject, community support sought by state and local mental health authorities. The cyclical nature of mental illnesses and the long-term skill development needs of many clubhouse members often fit poorly with the federally established vocational rehabilitation payment structure (Noble et al., 1997).

CERTIFICATION AND TRAINING

The International Center for Clubhouse Development recruits and trains an international faculty to train and certify clubhouses. The faculty of staff, members, and board members from certified clubhouses provides a lively network for problem-solving and mutual support and learning. The ICCD, founded in 1994, has quickly improved the quality, consistency, and availability of clubhouses (Macias, Jackson, et al., 1999). Many member and staff colleagues were successfully trained by Fountain House, Independence House, and other training sites over the past four decades. The ICCD, however, has furthered the state of the art dramatically by centrally coordinating training, developing, implementing, monitoring, and marketing certification, and by improving upon the model and marketing it at many levels.

The standard three-week training curriculum for key members and staff of each clubhouse is offered at several ICCD monitored sites throughout the country. Training includes hands-on experience in every aspect of the clubhouse—the work-ordered day, the community meeting, TE, social activities, and member/staff relationships. This intense and experiential form of training bonds participants. Trainees very often form long-term relationships—with the staff and members who train them, and with their fellow trainees. Inclusion of administrators in the third week of training builds in better support for the trainees once they return home.

The ICCD also works with training sites to develop specialized week-long tracks on supervision, TE, and initial clubhouse orientation for potential sites.

ICCD certification is standards-centered and consultative. Recommendations made by the ICCD team are often helpful in clarifying the clubhouses' mission and purpose within the auspice agency, or within the larger local mental health system. The ICCD team has provided even Fountain House with recommendations to keep it true to the clubhouse model! The ICCD faculty and staff provide consultation to state government officials and potential clubhouses as well.

The ICCD's website, its biannual International Seminars, and interim regional conferences undergird a tremendous network of support and information.

START-UP AND MAINTENANCE

Ownership and sponsorship by the local community is very important to the clubhouse, new or old. ICCD staff and faculty are eager to consult with community and interagency groups interested in developing a clubhouse. Obviously, the more central, integrated, and well supported a clubhouse is, the greater its likelihood of impact. New or prospective clubhouse groups often are powerfully affected by visits to existing clubhouses. Often, visitors remark that members of the existing clubs appear better functioning than their own clients (Gunn, 1995). Since most clubhouse members have had severe impairments in the past, this appearance seems attributable to the empowering staff/member partnership in the clubhouse. Use of the strong existing clubhouse network is highly recommended.

Board members from the community can offer the clubhouse a wide array of resources, skills, and connections. From TE prospects, to funding, to real estate, board members can be invaluable.

For maintenance as well, the network and the ICCD are excellent resources. Once staff and members are trained, and the model is established, the principal supervisory task is to support staff as they experience the unique staff/member partnership in the clubhouse. Each staff member must observe his/her personal boundaries and work with their coworkers to meet member needs within the unique set of staff strengths and limitations (Anderson, 1998). Most members come to the clubhouse with some significant interpersonal skill deficits, making the staff role challenging, but potentially very rewarding.

Recruitment of clubhouse staff is important and challenging, particularly because no particular academic discipline exists to train clubhouse staff. The staff/member partnership is as important in the hiring process as it is anywhere else. Most clubhouses evolve a method for in-action evaluation, using the work-ordered day as a means for evaluating potential staff.

Use of students and volunteers in the clubhouse can be of great benefit for recruitment as well good public relations. The skills and value-based fit of staff in clubhouses is extremely important. Recognizing and supporting this fit is perhaps the finest art in clubhouse implementation.

CONCLUSIONS AND IMPLICATIONS FOR PRACTICE

"Membership" conveys a powerful message to persons recovering from mental illness. After many years as a "mental patient," an inmate, a "case," or worse, the four "guaranteed rights" of members (Beard et al., 1982) are highly valued:

- A guaranteed right to a place to come.
- A guaranteed right to meaningful work.
- A guaranteed right to meaningful relationships.
- A guaranteed right to a place to belong.

Membership in the clubhouse serves as a metaphor for membership in the larger world of work and other affiliations. The well-functioning clubhouse provides hope to formerly isolated or unsuccessful individuals. That hope is nurtured, first as the individual engages with staff and members in the clubhouse, then as he or she engages with coworkers, friends, and neighbors in the larger community. The flexibility to support each member's growth, accommodating individual style and pace by providing a variety of opportunities to contribute real assistance to the clubhouse community, is a hallmark of a clubhouse model (Glickman, 1992).

Psychiatric rehabilitation programs of any model can be informed by the 50-year history of consumer empowerment at Fountain House and its successors. This idealistic, strengths-based model suggests answers to some practical questions all contemporary rehabilitation and work programs must address:

1. How can staff be selected and trained to provide the flexible mentorship and support clients need?
2. How can such a complex and diverse community manage itself, and ensure a safe and meaningful role for all its members?
3. How can the momentum toward community integration (and full-time paid employment) be maintained?
4. How can the tendency to get stuck within the boundaries of the supportive program community be transcended?

The ICCD, applying the research and experience of Fountain House and over 400 other clubhouses world-wide, addresses these questions through four unique mechanisms. These mechanisms can inform all practitioners of psychiatric rehabilitation.

First, under the direction of a board of staff and members throughout the world, the ICCD promulgates and revises a set of standards that provide a cohesive value oriented context for all clubhouses. Virtually any question raised in a clubhouse—large or small—can be answered in light of these standards on membership, relationships, space, work-ordered day, employment, functions of the house, and funding, governance and administration. This set of guiding principles provides a practical, research-based model to the field (Macias, Harding et al., 1999).

Second, the experiential three-week "colleague training" offered through the ICCD at several exemplary clubhouses provides effective training for adult staff and members, world-wide, whatever their formal education or experience (Macias, Harding et al., 1999). The ICCD approved curriculum, and ongoing oversight and support of training bases, ensures that all trainees receive consistent and practical training in every aspect of clubhouse operation.

Third, the mentorship among and between members and staff, from one clubhouse to another, starts with training and continues through a variety of mechanisms. The ICCD's biannual International Clubhouse Seminar brings together members and staff world-wide to share experience and research. All clubhouses are invited for input into agenda-setting, and then to present their ideas and findings at the conference. The ICCD also organizes regional conferences to supplement this opportunity. "Clubmail," *The Clubhouse Journal*, and the free exchange of ideas through phone calls, the Internet, and visits, provide continual dialogue on clubhouse cultural and operational issues. Colleague training brings representatives from four clubhouses together within the lively culture of an exemplary training site. That experience alone cements many continuing supportive relationships.

Last, the ICCD certification process models a unique approach to monitoring and improvement of quality. Guided by the clubhouse standards, trained members on the ICCD "faculty" make recommendations to the individual clubhouse based on certification visits at least every three years. Research shows that adherence to clubhouse standards, reflected in ICCD certification, correlates strongly with good work and living outcomes (Macias, Harding et al., 1999).

The values imbedded in clubhouse culture seem to have implications for any program of psychiatric rehabilitation. Whether "consumer operated," professionally staffed, facility based, urban, or rural, the ethos of empowerment—the lived clubhouse experience that every individual can belong and contribute—can inform and challenge every aspect of psychiatric and vocational rehabilitation.

REFERENCES

Anderson, S. B. (1998). *We are not alone: Fountain House and the development of clubhouse culture*. New York, NY: Fountain House.

Angers, M. (1999). Work and meaning conferring context of the clubhouse. *8th International Conference*. ICCD.

Anthony, W. (1984). Predicting the vocational capacity of the chronically mentally ill: Research and policy implications. *American Psychologist, 39*, 537–544.

Anthony, W. (1994). *Psychiatric rehabilitation*. Boston, MA: Center for Psychiatric Rehabilitation, Boston University.

Beard, J. H., Propst. R., & Malamud, T. J. (1982). The Fountain House model of psychiatric rehabilitation. *Psychiatric Rehabilitation Journal, 5*, 47–53.

Bond, G. R., Drake, R. E., Mueser, K. T., & Becker, D. R. (1997). An update on supported employment for people with severe mental illness. *Psychiatric Services, 48*(3), 335–346.

Drake, R. E., McHugo, G. J., Bebout, R. R., Becker, D. R., Harris, M., Bond, G. R., & Qimby, E. (1999). A randomized clinical trial of supported employment for inner-city patients with severe mental disorders. *Archives of General Psychiatry, 56*, 627–633.

Drake, R. E., McHugo, G. J., Becker, D. R., Clark, R. E., & Anthony, W. A. (1996). The New Hampshire study of supported employment for people with severe mental illness. *Journal of Consulting and Clinical Psychology, 64*(2), 391–399.

Flannery, M., & Glickmann, M. (1996). *Fountain House: Portraits of liver reclaimed from mental illness*. Center City, MN: Hazeldon.

Glickman, M. (1992). The Voluntary nature of the clubhouse. *Psychological Rehabilitation Journal, 16*(2), 39–40.

Gunn, T. (1995). *Adventure House* (video). Shelby, NC: Adventure House.

Hallihan, L. (1994). From pedestal to personhood: Staff in the clubhouse. *National Mental Health Services Conference*. Fountain House Online Archives of Conference Proceedings.

Linehan, M. (1993). *Cognitive behavioral treatment of borderline personality disorder*. New York, NY: Guilford.

Macias, C., Barreira, P., & Young, R. (2000). Loss of trust: Correlates of the comorbidity of PTSD and severe mental illness. In H. Harvey & B. G. Pauwels (Eds.), *Post traumatic stress theory, research, and application*. Philadelphia, PA: Bruner.Mazel.

Macias, C., Harding, C., Alden, M., Geertsen, D., & Barreira, P. (1999). The value of program certification for performance contracting: The example of ICCD clubhouse certification. *Administration and Policy in Mental Health, 26*(5).

Macias, C., Jackson, R., Wang, Q., & Schroeder, C. (1999). What is a clubhouse? (Report on the 1996 ICCD Clubhouse Survey). *Community Mental Health Journal, 35*(2), 181–190.

Macias, C., & Rodican, C. (1997). Coping with recurrent loss in mental illness: Unique aspects of clubhouse communities. *Journal of Personal and Interpersonal Loss, 2*, 205–221.

Noble, J. H., Honberg, R. S., Hall, L. L., & Flynn, L. M. (1997). *A legacy of failure: The inability of the federal-state vocational rehabilitation system to serve people with severe mental illness*. Arlington, VA: National Alliance for the Mentally Ill.

Peckoff, J. (1992). Patienthood to personhood. *Psychosocial Rehabilitation Journal, 16*(2), 5–8.

Propst, R. (1992). The standards for clubhouse programs: Why and how they were developed. *Psychosocial Rehabilitation Journal, 16*(2), 25–30.

Torrey, E. F. (1995). *Surviving schizophrenia: A manual for families, consumers, and providers*. New York, NY: Harper.

Torrey, E. F. (1997). *Out of the shadows: Confronting America's mental health crisis*. New York, NY: Wiley.

Vorspan, R. (1986). Attitudes and structure in the clubhouse model. *The Fountain House Annual, 4*.

Vorspan, R. (1988). Activities of daily living: You can't vacuum in a vacuum. *Psychosocial Rehabilitation Journal, 12*(2).

Wisnick, H. (1997). Working, activities, and recovering from serious mental illness. *New Research in Mental Illness*, 1996–1997 Biennium, 13. Columbus: Ohio Department of Mental Health.

CHAPTER 16

Benefit Advisement for Mental Health Consumers Seeking Employment

GARY M. CUSICK

Mental health consumers continue to be among the most difficult population to serve vocationally. Between 1972 and 1988 only 10%–15% of consumers were employed at any level (Anthony, 1994). The Ohio Department of Mental Health's Office of Program Evaluation and Research (Roth, Crane-Ross, Hannon, Cusick, & Doklovic, 1999) surveyed a representative sample of Ohio consumers and found 16 percent were working for pay at any level. The causes of this low percentage working could include stigma, the variability in the course of illness, or poor understanding by the general public (U.S. Health and Human Services Department, 1999).

Although individuals and forms of mental illness vary, diagnosis frequently occurs sometime after graduation from high school. This interrupts a period in the young adult's life that involves gaining education, or experience needed for regular employment. Persons with mental illness coming to vocational rehabilitation programs are therefore older than other clients (Ford, 1995).

The time period between diagnosis, receipt of treatment, and attaining stability is complicated by the high need for support persons with mental illness require. During this time the person applies for federal, state, and county benefits that provide medical care, housing, and food. The person learns the role of sick person (Wright, 1980). They must continue to be ill to receive these essential services and supports, that they cannot obtain through their own efforts.

Paradoxically, the consumer must adopt another role, that of a person able to work, in order to be considered for vocational rehabilitation services. Years of playing the role of a sick person make this new role difficult to master. Beside these two roles, the consumer attempts his/her transition to independence.

Often consumers face assistance agencies that are oriented toward binary eligibility determinations for their services. These agencies understand that if one is unable to work, one

GARY M. CUSICK • Administrator of Planning and Research, Louisville & Jefferson County Health Department, Louisville, Kentucky.

is eligible for social and medical services, but if one is able to work, one is ineligible. The consumer making the transition to work, which may take several months or years, does not fit neatly into this dichotomy. The National Council on Disability (2000) identified this dilemma in their following recommendation to the President:

> Federal income support programs like Supplemental Security Income and Social Security Disability Insurance should provide flexible and work-friendly support options so that people with episodic or unpredictable disabilities are not required to participate in the current "all or nothing" federal disability benefit system, often at the expense of pursuing their employment goals (Chapter 2).

Many consumers are unable to understand the regulations and formulas that the State Medicaid Agency and the Social Security Administration use to determine how benefits and entitlements change when they report work income. Furthermore, as the consumer begins reporting work income, resulting changes in benefits and entitlements create a need for ongoing counseling to understand and anticipate these changes. Managing and disseminating this information to consumers and their families requires someone who has the technical expertise to facilitate the transition of people coping with serious medical illness to employment.

To add to this confusion and anxiety, federal programs have different definitions of what "disabled" means:

> An individual may be eligible for services from one program and ineligible for another, simply because a different definition of disability is applied or because the individual carries a dual diagnosis. As a result, individuals are required to endure a series of application processes (Chapter 2).

Vocational rehabilitation agencies nationwide have seen mental health consumers refuse to participate in vocational rehabilitation programming, or to quit paying jobs because of the effect of work income on their benefits. Consumers are fearful of loss of cash benefits, continuing disability reviews, and healthcare. Increasingly community rehabilitation agencies serving a variety of persons with disabilities are offering a service known as benefit counseling or benefit advisement.

Consumers of mental health services typically consume all their savings and the resources available from family within a short time after developing their disability. At this point they begin looking for other means of support, and usually this means the social welfare system. Unfortunately each consumer may have to learn how to navigate the system without assistance (Dearborn, 1998). After trial and error they eventually find mental health agencies or lawyers that assist them in establishing eligibility for a variety of funds. These funds come from Social Security, the state Medicaid agency, Housing and Urban Development (HUD), and others.

The privation endured for 18–24 months while going through the steps necessary to receive assistance serves to make the consumer reluctant to jeopardize this achievement by attempting work. Mental health case managers will tell consumers not to work, because to do so will cause them to lose their benefits, or to decompensate. The consumer must choose to continue working and risk return to disability, possibly to start the 18–24 month wait for return to assistance, or to quit working and at least remain functional.

When the consumer decides to attempt employment, their rewards from benefit agencies are letters that threaten termination of benefits, a continuing disability review, or an increased spend down amount to keep their Medicaid. The consumer may come to believe that the system is seeking to keep them disabled, or at least in poverty. The Ticket to Work and Work Incentive Improvement Act of 1999 (TTWWIIA) was conceived to repair some of these problems inherent in the work incentives existing before it was signed into law on December 17, 1999.

BENEFIT ADVISORS

Benefit advisors gather information about the consumer's benefit profile and work with the consumer to develop "what if" scenarios so the effect of work income is known or estimable in advance. Continued contact with the consumer is necessary as the person's income or length of employment increases. Consumers need reassurance that their benefits will not be terminated before they can be replaced by income and employer-sponsored medical insurance.

Information on benefits and the impact of work income varies across consumers. Some may only need a detail of a letter explained, while others may need extensive hands-on assistance, including support at the benefit agency offices. ERI of Madison, Wisconsin, provides a range of benefit advisement services depending on the consumer's current need as given below:

1. Information and Referral is limited to brief telephone contact with a beneficiary to answer the most basic questions about benefits, work incentives, and where to get more detailed information.
2. The Benefits Analysis involves an examination of all benefits, entitlements, subsidies and services, and the impact that work will have on:
   - the level of payment, and
   - continued eligibility.
3. Benefits Counseling/Advisement is the process of sharing with the beneficiary the information learned through the analysis. A complete, written summary is presented to the beneficiary in one or more meetings.
4. In Benefits Planning and Follow-Along the beneficiary is provided assistance with accessing work incentive provisions made available through the Social Security Act, HUD, state entitlement programs, etc. When work begins, the beneficiary can plan ahead for changes in benefit status, avoid overpayments and underpayments, and be assured that critical benefits, such as health coverage, are maintained.

Benefit advisors also play a role in advocating for the consumer. Benefit agencies may have line staff that are not well trained in the regulations governing benefit change and termination. In these cases the benefit advisor will have to doggedly advocate for the consumer to get the extended cash benefits and Medicaid or Medicare benefits they are entitled to by regulation. Desk agents may be stubborn. Benefit advisors attempting to remedy an incorrect decision have pointed out regulations in the agency's own handbook without moving the desk personnel from their position on an issue.

Medicaid agency workers often are not aware of the work incentives available to assist a consumer who is transitioning to employment. Some of these incentives have been in effect since the late 1970s, yet caseworkers may be unfamiliar with them. New work incentives coming as a result of TTWWIIA may also take several years to be operative at the state Medicaid agency, unless a change is made in the ongoing training of front-line personnel.

Attorneys have been involved in benefit advisement for some time, particularly Social Security benefits. Attorneys have the advantage of being able to cite legal precedent and to bring legal action against an agency if they believe the consumer's rights have been violated. Availability of legal advice for the non-attorney benefit advisor would be of great value to the rehabilitation agency. Attorneys are often an excellent resource for training benefit advisors in agency regulations and strategies to get consumers their entitlements.

TRAINING AND QUALIFICATIONS OF
BENEFIT ADVISORS

Qualifications for benefit advisors vary across agencies. Typically a human services degree and experience serving persons with mental illness are required as minimum qualifications. Knowledge of benefit regulations is sometimes required, as the learning curve for benefit advisors is steep. Learning the regulations and the contacts needed in the consumer's community may take as long as one year to attain competence. A facility with spreadsheet software is essential so that figures can be easily varied for "what if" scenarios. Minimum qualifications for benefit advisors involve:

1. A bachelor's degree and five years of experience in mental health, vocational rehabilitation, benefits counseling, or a related field, including working with persons with mental illness.
2. Knowledge of community resources, entitlement programs, work incentives, and employment and vocational programs.
3. The ability to communicate effectively about complex and detailed issues, verbally and in writing.
4. The ability to coordinate effectively with a variety of other professionals, clients, and family members.

There has been some discussion about developing a fidelity model of benefit advisement that would provide guidance in hiring and in evaluation of benefit advisors (Virginia Commonwealth University, 2000b). A list of activities benefit advisors might perform include:

1. Assessing the status of the consumer's benefits and entitlements, and the impact that earnings will have on these benefits.
2. Providing education on benefits and entitlements to consumers, families, and mental health service providers.
3. Providing training on benefits monitoring to assist consumers and families in reporting income information to the Social Security Administration.
4. Assisting consumers in developing decision-making skills to access educational and employment services to enhance career development.
5. Advocating on behalf of consumers with the Social Security Administration, the state Medicaid agency, and other providers of subsidies and entitlements.
6. Providing training to staff, clients, and families on various entitlement and subsidy programs.
7. Developing individualized service plans according to client service needs.
8. Linking consumers to community resources.

There have been some efforts to create dedicated software for benefit advisement (Employment Support Institute, 1999). The uniqueness of benefit regulations in every state and community make this a difficult task. Programs that produce easily understood benefit profiles with before and after income and costs detailed would be useful, however. Spreadsheet software can be employed to develop a benefit profile template that may be helpful in organizing the consumer's benefit information, in lieu of a dedicated software package. The trusting, personal relationship necessary for effective benefit advisement that leads to community employment and independence will never be replaced by software.

Crisis situations may be common, particularly when the consumer's medical benefits that provide psychotropic medication are terminated, or when housing subsidies are removed, and the consumer is facing eviction. Perhaps vocational agency benefit advisement work should be split into two tiers: consumers who are unstable due to symptoms or in activities of daily living, and stable consumers who are ready to make the leap to employment.

It is important that the benefit advisor maintain professional boundaries in his/her work with consumers. Having developed a successful rapport with the consumer, there may be some role confusion that may lead the benefit advisor into tasks unrelated to benefits. The work of the benefit advisor should not include that of a case manager. Also, the benefit advisor should not become the representative payee, as this would present a possible conflict of interest or potential infringement of the recipient's rights.

HEALTH CARE ACCESS

A consumer's reluctance to attempt work is based on fear that he/she may lose healthcare benefits, particularly medication. Medication is an essential element in a consumer's recovery from mental illness (Cusick & Carstens, 2000). New, atypical anti-psychotic medications have made community integration a reality for consumers with schizophrenia (Wallis & Willwerth, 1992).

Atypical anti-psychotic medication, and the required labwork that enables consumers to function at a level sufficient to support employment, cost thousands of dollars per year. Without this medication, consumers would most likely be on less effective medication with noxious side-effects, or require frequent hospitalization. Under the pre-TTWWIIA work incentives, consumers will lose their medical benefits through Medicaid or Medicare. Employer-sponsored health care may not cover a pre-existing condition such as schizophrenia or bi-polar disorder, or may not include the consumer's medication in their formulary.

The Balanced Budget Act of 1997 gave states the option of allowing Medicaid beneficiaries to pay for their Medicaid coverage as if they were paying an insurance premium if they were at or below 250% of the federal poverty level. Under the TTWWIIA, states have an option to allow persons from 250% to 450% of the federal poverty level to pay health insurance premiums for their Medicaid/Medicare coverage. This option for states is popularly known as Medicaid Buy-In, and has been adopted by 10 states at the time of this writing. Massachusetts instituted Buy-In in the late 1980s, well in advance of any legislation.

It must be stressed that this provision of TWWIIA is an option, and that states must amend their state plan for Medicaid to bring it about. The paths that states take to Medicaid Buy-In have taken many directions. Minnesota's program came about as a result of work by well-organized disability advocate groups. Iowa employers, facing record low unemployment and an excellent economy, pressed the state to adopt the Buy-In as a way of gaining additional employees.

Funding for the Buy-In will involve careful planning by the state Medicaid agency. The initial start-up cost of Medicaid Buy-In will be returned many times over by consumers entering the workforce, requiring less state and federally funded health care due to the therapeutic nature of work, and paying taxes. States must take this long-term perspective that will add workers to an economy that may stall without them.

The importance of this legislation cannot be overstated. This gives persons with mental illness access to comprehensive medical insurance from which they cannot be turned down because of a pre-existing condition. With guaranteed medical coverage, many persons with mental illness would be willing to work, and would become contributors to the community as active workers.

Medical coverage provided by employers under managed care, even if they cover pre-existing illnesses such as schizophrenia and bi-polar disorder, may not provide coverage sufficient to the consumer's needs. Managed care companies seek low-risk populations, substitute less intensive and less adequate services than those needed, and shift costs to families, public providers, and other care sectors (Mechanic, 1997). In Iowa, however, employers are paying a consumer's Medicaid Buy-In premiums as an employee benefit. This premium is probably less than typical health insurance, and more comprehensive for consumers.

Public opinion on issues such as Medicaid Buy-In and improved work incentives is mixed or worse, generally seeing such programs as an expansion of welfare. Articles in the popular press stress isolated abuses of the SSI/SSDI system, and advocate for limiting the types of mental illness covered by Social Security (Wright, 1995). This may be due to media depictions of persons with mental illness as inherently violent, or to ignorance of mental illness itself (U.S. Health and Human Services Department, 1999).

RIGHTS PROTECTION

Consumers of mental health services are particularly vulnerable to neglect by state and federal agency personnel. When faced with letters perceived as threatening, some may simply not take action, and suffer the consequences. The benefit advisor must develop a personal relationship with each of the consumers on his/her caseload to be truly effective. Consumers will often receive contradictory information from agency personnel, and the benefit advisor must be sufficiently well versed in agency regulations to be able to make a stand with desk personnel.

The marketing of services is important to community mental health provider agencies and to the Social Security and Medicaid offices. Familiarity with the benefit advisor will make timely resolution of differences of opinion regarding regulation interpretation possible. Continued contact with benefit agency personnel will reduce the difficulties experienced at the start of benefit advisement services.

Consumers are frequently distrustful of agency personnel because of past experience. Consumers adopt a stance of tell as little as possible, and lay low. Calling for information typically requires long waits, and may result in information that conflicts with that obtained during previous contacts.

The disincentives inherent in Social Security SSI and SSDI programs extend beyond employment. Beneficiaries are discouraged from saving, parents are discouraged from naming their adult children on SSI as heirs to estates, and consumers are discouraged from marrying, as spousal income can reduce or eliminate some benefits (Martin, Conley, & Noble, 1995). Other disincentives to leave beneficiary roles are found in the arduousness involved in becoming eligible. The evaluation process required for eligibility may be inaccurate, and may actually select against some consumers who are unable to provide necessary information due to their psychopathology (Okpaku, 1985; Okapu, Sibulkin, & Schenzler, 1994).

Eligibility can be simplified through the use of cooperative agreements between the agencies concerned (Kennedy, Tully, Craft, & Ullery, 1990). Mental health agencies carry out evaluations that are equal or superior to the disability evaluations required by benefit agencies. A cooperative agreement between mental health agencies and benefit agencies would prevent unnecessary duplication that may prove detrimental to consumers.

Persons with mental illness are also prey to the winds of fashion. During the Reagan administration, one fourth of all beneficiaries with mental illness were removed from the social security roles following the 1980 presidential election, even though they represent only one ninth of all SSDI beneficiaries (Goldman & Gattozzi, 1988a, 1988b). Class action lawsuits were required to correct this situation (Anderson, 1986).

The experience gained in the Job Incentive Focus Project suggests that Social Security and Medicaid offices are poorly trained to deal with consumers. This is perplexing in that persons with mental illness comprise the largest diagnostic group of disabled beneficiaries of SSI and SSDI (Estroff, Patrick, Zimmer, & Lachicotte, 1997).

SUMMARY

The need for wheelchair ramps in public spaces was once questioned with the logic that persons in wheelchairs were never seen there. If benefit agencies such as Social Security and the state Medicaid agency continue to fail to train their personnel on the regulations regarding work incentives, then consumers will likewise not be seen using work incentives to make the transition to community employment. The TTWWIIA will fail to live up to its name if benefit agencies cannot implement the new regulations. The benefit advisor may provide the best practical training in work incentive regulations that benefit agencies receive.

The importance of a benefit advisor's role in advocating for the consumer will continue throughout the first decade of the new century. Personnel from human services agencies, benefit agencies, consumers, and their families will require extensive education and support to adjust to the new work incentive legislation. Benefit advisors will also play an important role in advocating for work incentives such as Medicaid Buy-In that are optional for states.

Until TTWWIIA is implemented in the consumer's state, the benefit advisor will need to protect the consumer's rights to medical benefits, and provide accurate information for the consumer who is considering community employment. Well-trained benefit advisors can assist consumers in making the transition by limiting the uncertainty and fear the consumer may feel when dealing with benefit agencies. Benefit advisement is the cornerstone of vocational services for the mental health consumer, without which community employment may collapse.

REFERENCES

Anderson, J. R. (1986). Recent developments in assessment of the mentally disabled for Social Security and SSI benefits. *Innovations in clinical practice: A source book*, Vol. 5. Sarasota, FL: Professional Resource Exchange.

Anthony, W. A. (1994). The vocational rehabilitation of people with severe mental illness: Issues and myths. *Innovations and Research, 3*(2), 17–24.

Cusick, G. M., & Carstens, C. (2000). *Myself: The work of recovery.* Unpublished manuscript.

Dearborn, C. (1998). Disability 101. *Sojourner, 24*(2), 24.

Employment Support Institute (1999). WorkWORLD [Computer software]. Richmond, VA: Virginia Commonwealth University, School of Business, Employment Support Institute.

Estroff, S. E., Patrick, D. L., Zimmer, C. R., and Lachicotte, W. S. (1997). Pathways to disability income among persons with severe, persistent psychiatric disorders. *Milbank Quarterly, 74*(4), 495–532.

Ford, L. H. (1995). *Providing employment support for people with long-term mental illness: Choices, resources, and practical strategies.* Baltimore, MD: Paul H. Brookes.

Goldman, H. H., & Gattozzi, A. A. (1988a). Balance of powers: Social Security and the mentally disabled. *Milbank Quarterly, 6*(3), 531–551.

Goldman, H. H., & Gattozzi, A. A. (1988b). Murder in the cathedral revisited: President Reagan and the mentally disabled. *Hospital and Community Psychiatry, 39*(5), 505–509.

Kennedy, C., Tully, R., Craft, L., & Ullery, B. (1990). Expedited Social Security disability determinations: The Ohio experience. *New Directions for Mental Health Services, 45,* 19–27.

Martin, D. A., Conley R. W., & Noble J. H. Jr. (1995). The ADA and Disability Benefits Policy. *Journal of Disability Policy Studies, 6*(2), 1–15.

Mechanic, D. (1997, November/December). Managed mental health care. *Society,* 44–52.

National Council on Disability (2000). *From privileges to rights: People labeled with psychiatric disabilities speak for themselves.* [On-line], Washington, DC: Author. Available: http://www.ncd.gov/newsroom/publications/privileges.html

Okpaku, S. O. (1985). A profile of clients referred for psychiatric evaluations for Social Security Disability Income and Supplemental Security Income: Implications for psychiatry. *American Journal of Psychiatry, 142*(9), 1037–1043.

Okapu, S. O., Sibulkin, A. E., & Schenzler, C. (1994). Disability determinations for adults with mental disorders: Social Security Administration vs. independent judgements. *American Journal of Public Health, 84*(11), 1791,1795.

Presidential Task Force on Employment of Adults with Disabilities (1999). *Recharting the course: If not now, when?* Washington, DC: Author.

Roth, D., Crane-Ross, D., Hannon, M., Cusick, G. M., & Doklovic, S. (1999). A longitudinal study of mental health services and consumer outcomes in a changing system Unpublished raw data. Columbus: Ohio Department of Mental Health Office of Program Evaluation and Research.

U.S. Health and Human Services Department (1999). *Mental health: A report of the Surgeon General.* Washington, DC: U.S. Health and Human Services Department, Public Health Service.

Vash, C. L. (1981).*The psychology of disability.* Springer Series on Rehabilitation, (Vol. 1), New York, NY: Springer.

Virginia Commonwealth University Rehabilitation Research and Training Center (2000a, Spring/Summer). *SPI Connections,* 6.

Virginia Commonwealth University Rehabilitation Research and Training Center, (2000b). Topical conference on the Ticket to Work and Work Incentive Improvement Act, February 28–29.

Wallis, J. & Willwerth, J. (1992). Awakenings: Schizophrenia. A new drug brings patients back to life, *Time,* July 6, 52–57.

Wright, C. M. (1995, November). The supplemental security income program: The welfare state's black hole, *USA Today Magazine,* 14–16.

Wright, G. N. (1980) *Total Rehabilitation,* Boston, MA: Little Brown.

CHAPTER 17

Workplace Socialization of People with Disabilities

Implications for Job Development and Placement[1]

D AVID P. M OXLEY, J OHN R. F INCH, AND
S TUART F ORMAN

INTRODUCTION

The Americans with Disabilities Act and recent changes to the Rehabilitation Act strengthen the focus on helping people with disabilities to secure competitive employment in the community and makes the effective execution of placement and development services even more important than in the past (Fabian, Luecking, & Tilson, 1995). But the development of employment opportunities for people with disabilities is a complex process and requires rehabilitation and mental health personnel to meet both the needs of employers and the needs of workers who are disabled (Fabian & Waugh, 2001). Researchers who inquire into this important area of rehabilitation suggest that success is a function of the belief systems of professionals who engage in job development and placement activities (Fabian & Waugh, 2001). They must achieve proficiency in three areas of performance: addressing and resolving employer concerns, identifying and resolving employment barriers, and marketing placement services (Fabian & Waugh, 2001). It is critical, according to these researchers, to ensure that professionals involved in the provision of employment services believe that they have or can master these essential skills and can achieve positive placement outcomes. Such a concern with the self-efficacy of placement professionals is relevant today as it has been in the past given the continued low levels of workplace participation that still persist among people with disabilities (Bowe, 1988; U.S. Department of Labor, 1997).

An emphasis on marketing of employment services raises a fundamental question involving what it is that rehabilitation and mental health personnel that offer these services

---

[1]This chapter is an expanded verison of "Social work strategies and tactics in the workplace." Published in the *Journal of Social Work in Disability and Rehabilitation, 1*(3), 2002.

D AVID P. M OXLEY • Wayne State University School of Social Work, Detroit, Michigan.   J OHN R. F INCH • Rehabilitation Consultant, Columbus, Ohio.   S TUART F ORMAN • Wayne State University, Detroit, Michigan.

actually market. Job placement and development represents a bundle of discrete tasks and activities of relatively broad scope. These tasks and activities focus on fostering the readiness of job seekers for employment, identifying the availability of employment within the community and within specific markets, fostering the readiness of employers to work with people with disabilities, and preparing the workplace to include the employee who is disabled. Ultimately, once a person has secured a job he/she often requires assistance to transition into the workplace.

Ideally, the aim of these services is to help people to secure employment in competitive work situations in which the person with a disability becomes included as a regular and permanent member of the workforce. As the paradigm of rehabilitation increasingly incorporates ideas pertaining to the normalization of work, and the inclusion of people in mainstream work settings, those rehabilitation and mental health personnel who address the employment needs of people with disabilities must think about how the development of work opportunities contributes to the aims of inclusion. Accommodations, the provision of supports, and the use of technologies that increase the probability of successful work performance suggest that the work environment can be engineered to become inclusive.

Given the current emphasis within many fields of disability to help people to participate in inclusive employment settings, the authors suggest that job development and placement activities should be executed within a normative framework of organizational membership. That is, within such a framework, the principal aim of the development of employment opportunities for people with disabilities is to help them become inclusive members of work settings and that the achievement of this objective is the principal product these personnel are marketing to job seekers and potential employers.

Rehabilitation and mental health personnel who are involved in facilitating the employment of people with disabilities likely adopt a person-in-environment perspective and this, in turn, can make them sensitive to the importance of facilitating a match between the person with a disability and the work environment in which the person must function. And, rehabilitation and mental health professionals who are sensitive to the person's movement into a new employment role will focus on the facilitation of a successful transition. However, what is the nature of this transition? Rehabilitation and mental health personnel who are involved in the development of inclusive employment opportunities for people with disabilities can frame this transition as the facilitation of the socialization of the person into a specific work setting and organizational culture. The facilitation of organizational socialization, therefore, is an important aim of rehabilitation practice that seeks to produce viable employment outcomes for people with disabilities.

AN OVERVIEW OF ORGANIZATIONAL SOCIALIZATION

A normative framework of organizational membership suggests that newcomers need to learn to be effective members of a work community. However, the effectiveness of this learning is a function of the extent to which the workplace invests in the process of socializing newcomers as organizational members who acquire the behaviors, skills, knowledge, and competencies to perform their work roles effectively. Within contemporary organizational theory this process of learning to be an effective worker within a specific worksite is referred to as organizational socialization. The aim of this chapter is to place employment development and support into the context of organizational socialization and to identify the contribution rehabilitation and mental health professionals can make to workplace socialization of people with disabilities.

Schein (1978, 1988) introduced the concept of organizational socialization into the literature and emphasized that effective socialization of workers enabled them to gain an understanding of a particular organization's culture and how to function effectively within this culture. He pointed out in this early work that many organizations neglected to socialize newcomers systematically and effectively. Although, as Anakwe and Greenhaus (1999) point out, thinking about organizational socialization has been quite narrow and often confined to a change in attitudes or an adaptation to work norms on the part of the person who is entering the organization as a new member. Wanous (1992) suggests that organizational socialization involves an internalized commitment to the aims and success of the employing organization. Few investigators have taken such a comprehensive view of organizational socialization that Schein (1978) originally proposed.

Effective socialization of a newcomer requires the new employee to learn about the nuances of how to function within a given setting (Chao, O'Leary, Wolf, Klein, & Gardner, 1994). Newcomers enter a complex situation and they are likely uncertain about how to behave and how to function within this new social setting. They must learn much both informally and formally to become effective workers and contributors. Workplace socialization involves complex social learning and requires newcomers to adapt to performance requirements, new task structures and routines, work group norms, new roles, and a new culture. Ultimately workplace socialization requires workers to be personally flexible and adaptive, if not ingenious, about how to function in a new territory that relatively inexperienced workers can find threatening and anxiety-provoking (Anakwe & Greenhaus, 1999).

Of course, some people enter new work settings with considerable social capital about how to perform effectively in most any organizational context. They have garnered numerous work-related competencies through a number of different employment experiences and the receipt of mentoring and supervision has helped them to learn about themselves, how to read an organizational culture, and how to move quickly to establish themselves in a specific work group. Other newcomers may have benefited from informal vocational and work guidance within their families, and their parents may have served as role models not only within the world of work but within specific careers. Facilitating successful organizational socialization of these individuals is an internalized self-efficacy about work performance and success and specific expectations about their success in their new jobs. These individuals come to employment not only with vocational maturity but also with career sophistication and skills in career self-management.

Unfortunately, for a variety of reasons, people with disabilities may simply lack social capital and job-related assets. People with disabilities are under-represented in the workforce and, therefore, likely lack long-term exposure to a variety of work roles and, perhaps more importantly, to a variety of work settings. From a career perspective, this may lower their vocational maturity since they do not have the direct experience with the world of work that is so essential to adult maturity (Super, 1977, 1994).

Unlike many of their non-disabled peers, individuals with disabilities may have never had the advantage that previous work-oriented mentoring and supervision offers individuals in work settings. Recent research on the career insight and development of youth with disabilities suggests that although they have aspirations similar to non-disabled youth they simply lack the career sophistication their non-disabled peers possess (Ochs & Roessler, 2001). Thus, many people with disabilities may lack what Herr (1993) refers to as personal flexibility within a work setting, namely those skills, abilities, and insights into how someone functions productively and effectively within a specific job context.

A program of organizational socialization may be most important for those newcomers who are new to the world of work or who are in transition from other roles in which their involvement in the world of work was somewhat abbreviated. Secondary students making a transition to full-time employment, post-secondary students making a transition to their first professional job, people who have spent considerable time out of the job market, and people with disabilities may be very appropriate candidates for an intensive program of organizational socialization. Those individuals who are more experienced in the world of work, who have clear vocational identities seasoned by multiple job experiences, and workers who are in the middle or late stages of their careers may require different socialization experiences (Van Eck Peluchette & Jeanquart, 2000).

Organizational socialization can be differential in its focus and effort. It can deploy different learning experiences based on an appraisal of career maturity, vocational identity, and readiness for employment, factors that may be fundamental to job development and placement personnel in forging good matches between job seekers with disabilities and their potential employers.

FIVE STRATEGIES OF WORKPLACE SOCIALIZATION

There are five strategies of workplace socialization that are relevant to framing the development of employment options and job placement assistance for people with disabilities. Anakwe and Greenhaus (1999) identify these strategies to conceptualize fully workplace socialization. The authors make use of these strategies to expand the understanding of mental health and rehabilitation personnel about how to approach the development of employment options as a natural process of socialization within inclusive work settings. Although the authors focus on people with disabilities, they assume that any workplace socialization program itself can be inclusive in its delivery and differential in its design by focusing on the development of work-related assets that are relevant to people at different levels of career maturity and career involvement. The five strategies of workplace socialization are helping new workers to:

1. master the tasks of their jobs and gain an understanding of performance expectations;
2. understand work group functioning;
3. gain knowledge of the organizational culture and come to accept how the organization functions to achieve success;
4. learn about the personal consequences of work and how to manage them; and
5. achieve role clarity.

Mastery of Tasks and Expectations

This strategy likely is at the core of successful organizational socialization and perhaps is one of the most challenging rehabilitation and mental health personnel can face in focusing on the development of employment options for people with disabilities. Although older models of workplace socialization suggest that it is incumbent upon the worker to enter the work setting already prepared in the substantive tasks that a specific job calls for, many organizations increasingly search for workers who have the potential and motivation to master specific tasks and to mature into a particular work role. Employers increasingly place emphasis on workplace learning and many corporations and businesses make significant investments in workplace learning opportunities that facilitate their employees' acquisition of relevant academic and job-related skills.

During the decades of the 1980s and 1990s, many organizations shifted the design and flow of work and the basic parameters of the technology of work within their organizations. These changes, undertaken with the aim of improving quality and productivity, led to substantive changes in the design of jobs so that many workers were expected to participate in structured learning activities and to achieve educational outcomes. Training in these decades became more salient and was linked to the core business mission of the organization.

An effective program of organizational socialization, therefore, helps workers to integrate into the socio-technical framework of learning that exists within the workplace and to take advantage of those formal and informal learning opportunities that the corporation, professional associations, and labor groups increasingly offer within the worksite. These training opportunities not only address the acquisition of task-related skills but also likely emphasize the acquisition of expectations pertaining to quality management and quality improvement.

This first strategy of organizational socialization has several implications for mental health and rehabilitation professionals who are engaged in the development of employment opportunities. In assessing the appropriateness of a job within a particular setting, rehabilitation and mental health personnel may need to assess the practices of the work setting relevant to socializing the new employee with a disability into the task structure and performance expectations a specific job demands of its incumbent. Such an assessment can focus on the time the work setting commits to this socialization process, opportunities for individualized instruction and coaching delivered on the job, and how and when a new employee is evaluated in the acquisition of a desired level of performance. A sound and supportive process of task socialization that is open to all new employees may be important to a job seeker with a disability who is anxious about performance on a new job and in a new setting with challenging expectations. It is exactly these performance expectations that the rehabilitation and mental health personnel must assess and understand within the context of whether and to what extent the employing organization offers substantive supports to help new workers or workers in transition to master these expectations.

Alternatively, marketing job seekers with disabilities to potential employers can FOCUS on the employer's commitment to organizational socialization of new employees. The employer does not have to be promised a worker who is ready to engage in high-level task performance immediately upon entry into the workplace. Marketing to the employer can emphasize the readiness of the worker to learn essential tasks within the framework of the socialization structure of the workplace. Rehabilitation and mental health personnel can show employers how individualized learning processes, technological accommodations, and job redesign or engineering can be used as tactics to facilitate organizational socialization within the area of task performance and the achievement of task-related performance expectations. The marketing process can extend the applicability of these tactics beyond the immediate aim of employing a new job seeker. Those rehabilitation and mental health personnel who are committed to the development of inclusive workplaces can illuminate how these tactics fit into the learning system of the organization. They can show potential employers how such supports are relevant to other employees who are in transition in their own health or functioning, or who are returning to the workplace after a long hiatus.

This strategy of organizational socialization should help newcomers to achieve self-confidence in relation to task performance and to experience a subjective sense of efficacy on the job. Indeed, it is this sense of job-specific self-efficacy that rehabilitation and mental health personnel must help people with disabilities to gain since it is an important predictor of subsequent success in a work setting. Job-specific or career self-efficacy may be one of the most important assets a person with a disability may acquire from a work experience.

Functioning Effectively within a Work Group

This strategy of workplace socialization amplifies the amount of informal learning new-comers must undertake in an organization. Shifts in workplace design and the organization of work have placed considerable responsibility for the execution of work on teams. Team-based work is a reality in many sectors of the economy including industry and manufacturing, health and human services, the military, service industries, leisure and tourism, and education.

As organizations increase the diversity of their membership, teams themselves become more diverse, and this change requires members at the group level to learn to work together effectively using differences among themselves as strengths. As these groups learn to function effectively they develop their own norms, practices, perspectives, and subcultures within the larger matrix of organizational culture. Current research on knowledge management within complex organizations illuminates the manner in which team-based work units formulate their own indigenous knowledge bases involving specific insights into how to engage in productive activity and deliver products that earn them favorable endorsement within the larger organiza-tion. Often, for a variety of reasons, these teams do not share their indigenous knowledge with other teams. Within teams, members are socialized into such knowledge through on-the-job teaching (oversight, coaching, and instruction), rewards for the proper execution of tasks and work, and informal sanctions for unwanted deviation from standards and norms.

Programs of organizational socialization may view this form of team-based learning as "learning by the ropes." Typically, newcomers are immersed immediately into a team or work group and they must learn first hand about how job-related tasks are performed within a specific context in which the norms of the group and the expectations or demands of the larger organization intersect. New workers may learn to rotate among tasks and learn about the norms that govern productivity and performance. Perhaps, more importantly, new workers learn about the importance of social skills and interaction in terms of how employees get along on the job, how coworkers interact, how the team relates to supervisors and superiors, and how others in the work group and in the general workplace come to value them as fellow workers (Anakwe & Greenhaus, 1999). Effective programs of workplace socialization facili-tate this form of social learning so that teams gain competencies in how to incorporate new members into their work routines and perhaps, subsequently, how to use for their own benefit the diversity that members bring to teamwork.

A measure of the effectiveness of organizational socialization involves the extent to which the new employee can achieve integration into the work group and earn the trust and respect of other group members. Rehabilitation and mental health personnel who develop job opportunities likely will need to understand how particular employers socialize new employ-ees into work groups and how they ensure that particular teams function in respectful and inclusive ways.

Perhaps one of the most significant challenges rehabilitation and mental health person-nel face is to facilitate the inclusion of their job seekers into the social system of the workplace. They may need to help employers identify specific ways of making what Gates, Akabas, and Oran-Sabia (1998) refer to as "relationship accommodations" within the workgroup. It is these accommodations that enable people to manage stress, establish tolerable levels of social involvement, adjust to social interaction, and receive the support they find useful to their job performance. Some new employees with disabilities may be overwhelmed by the amount of interpersonal interaction that occurs on the job, the complexities of informal interactions, and the nuances involved in the informal manner in which people communicate about task com-pletion. Many new workers may need support to decipher these communications and gain insight into their cultural meaning.

In meeting this challenge successfully, rehabilitation and mental health personnel may find that the diversity policies of those organizations that seek to recruit people from many different backgrounds and with different demographic qualities or attributes can facilitate the inclusion of people with disabilities in the work setting. Rehabilitation and mental health personnel have much to offer employers. They can assess the needs of employers in the areas of diversity, assess the disability content of their learning systems, and offer specific resources to support the inclusion of content about disabilities into the educational curriculum of the organization.

Alternatively, in helping specific job seekers to become new organizational members, rehabilitation and mental health personnel may demonstrate to employers how the group-oriented and interpersonal assets of their job candidates contribute to the effectiveness of the work-group structures of the organization. Social skills, collaborative work skills, awareness of and respect for social norms, and sensitivity to others may be important assets for particular employers who may express a strong interest in job seekers who possess these qualities.

Understanding and Acceptance of the Organizational Culture

Schein (1997) outlines the dynamics of organizational culture and how members come to ignore this culture even though it influences and directs their behavior in the workplace and on the job. More and more organizations, however, are seeking to illuminate their organizational cultures and shape them through the leadership activities of key individuals. For these organizations, the culture is the matrix in which organizational beliefs and values influence how work is performed and success is measured (Schein, 1997). Anakwe and Greenhaus (1999) highlight the importance of employees learning about organizational culture as an aspect of their socialization into the workplace.

According to Schein (1988), explicit learning about the organizational culture enables new employees to understand the situation they are in and it offers them a schema for understanding and interpreting mundane or everyday events in the workplace. Such learning may be at an explicit level as more senior and experienced members of the organization describe to newcomers the culture and how it functions. Eventually, however, individuals achieve a tacit incorporation of the culture and it is from this tacit incorporation that a new self-identity as a bona fide member of the organization emerges (Schein, 1988). Newcomers learn about essential social norms and under successful conditions of organizational socialization they come to internalize them to guide and/or direct their behavior on the job.

New employees may find that the organizational culture is one of the most difficult aspects of organizational life to decipher. By definition it is one of the most amorphous features of an organization and Schein (1997) himself notes how difficult it is for newcomers to gain an understanding of the culture in which they are immersed.

Effective programs of workplace socialization not only make the organization's culture explicit but also foster its acceptance by newcomers. An aim of workplace socialization is to help new members to acquire the knowledge of the organizational culture that is so important for effective functioning. It helps newcomers to begin the process of internalization from which a new self-identity can emerge (Schein, 1988).

Rehabilitation and mental health personnel in employment services will be interested in how the employer socializes the new worker into the organizational culture, which is probably a process of many different kinds of interactions workers experience during the early part of their tenure within the organization. The employer's commitment to this strategy of organizational socialization signifies a commitment to helping a new worker to become a member of the organization and not merely an employee. Membership communicates something more than employment. It suggests that the person makes a strong commitment to the social system in which one participates and seeks to make this system effective in the achievement of its aims. Alternatively, membership means that workers are helped to join groups and to achieve acceptance as members of teams.

Some readers may find the idea of acceptance to be unrealistic or unreasonable. However, reflection on this aspect of effective workplace socialization suggests that workers who do not personally legitimize their work setting and internalize its practices may experience considerable conflict. This conflict can result in the worker experiencing tension on the job, considerable stress, the absence of job satisfaction, and ultimately ill health. The achievement of congruence between the individual and the culture may be a critical aspect of any successful or effective social group or system (Bolman & Deal, 1997).

Rehabilitation and mental health personnel can undertake specific tactics to facilitate the socialization of job seekers with disabilities into the organization's culture such as the provision of follow-along counseling and guidance sessions that increase the new employees' understanding of the organizational culture and its norms. This counseling can help employees with disabilities to learn how to function within the culture and how they can contribute to organizational success. Rehabilitation and mental health personnel also can offer troubleshooting conferences to new employees who may experience tension in the workplace as a result of conflict that is a product of the gap between their beliefs and values and those operating within the culture of the employing organization. Rehabilitation and mental health personnel can ensure new employees and their employers that they will offer continuous oversight of the work situation during the early period of socialization. And they can ensure both parties that they will be available to facilitate the transition of the person out of the organization if the integration of the new employee into the organizational culture is not successful.

But rehabilitation and mental health personnel can prevent this contingency from occurring if they achieve an understanding of the organization's culture and the values and beliefs of employers and are able to help the job seeker to appraise this culture through anticipatory guidance. Rehabilitation and mental health personnel can offer specific assessment services to both job seekers and potential employers that help both parties to make better decisions about whether to stay the course of employment. Job seekers can gain awareness of what constitutes an organizational culture and clarify the attributes of the organizational culture they value or find acceptable. Rehabilitation and mental health personnel can communicate to employers that they take seriously their efforts to create a culture that is right for their organization. They can communicate to employers that they respect these efforts through the referral of candidates who not only know something about the basic cultural practices of the organization but also are willing to invest in the success of the organization and its enterprise.

Learning about the Personal Consequences of Work and How to Manage Them

Entry into and execution of work roles in specific work settings can set in motion many consequences for the incumbents of these roles. Effective programs of organizational socialization incorporate opportunities that enable newcomers to gain an understanding of the consequences their work can and does create for them on and off the job. Perhaps one of the most important outcomes of an effective organizational socialization program is that it results in a diminution of uncertainty that movement into new roles and settings often create for people.

Some individuals thrive on this uncertainty and enjoy deciphering it and finding out how work settings actually operate. Others may experience considerable anxiety in the face of this uncertainty, while still others may experience serious depression if they feel that their mastery of the work is thwarted.

An effective socialization program can facilitate the awareness of how one functions in the workplace and help new employees to gain a broader understanding of the world of work, how one fits into this world, and the conditions under which one performs in an effective manner. This form of personal learning facilitates the expansion of the self-identity Schein (1988) highlights as an important outcome of the process of internalizing the organizational culture. It is the kind of learning that broadens vocational identity. This kind of learning can foster career maturity (Anderson & Brown, 1997; Ochs & Roessler, 2001), particularly for people with disabilities who may require an array of exploratory opportunities to extend their understanding of the world of work and to increase their familiarity with how work demands influence their functioning and adaptation (Fisher & Harnisch, 1992). Rehabilitation and mental health personnel should keep in mind that many people with disabilities come to work settings with little background in the world of work but with high expectations for their performance and success (Herr, 1993).

Rehabilitation and mental health personnel involved in employment services are strategically placed to assess continuously the personal consequences employment creates for new employees with disabilities and the extent to which personal learning unfolds as part of the process of workplace socialization. It is likely that they continue to interact with the people they serve long after placement, and a commitment to the provision of follow-along services enables rehabilitation and mental health personnel to monitor personal adjustment and adaptation to what their clients will likely experience as new, if not novel, organizational settings. Indeed, these personnel have considerable expertise to contribute here; expertise employers may want to tap in helping other employees address the personal consequences of employment making rehabilitation and mental health personnel good candidates to offer employee assistance services for workers who experience a range of work challenges and difficulties.

It is likely that some people with disabilities who have limited exposure to the world of work and/or who have struggled to obtain responsive rehabilitation services may formulate negative expectancies about their success in the workplace and about the support they will receive from employers. People with such backgrounds may possess considerable anxiety about their work performance and develop personal doubts that only serve to undermine their confidence in the workplace.

Thus, personal learning is most likely an important area of workplace socialization for people with disabilities. This form of learning offers new employers opportunities to reflect on their work, to identify areas of uncertainty, to address their anxiety about performance, and to help them resolve on-the-job tensions. As Anakwe and Greenhaus (1999) emphasize, personal learning is an avenue through which an effective program of workplace socialization enables new workers to learn about themselves and how they function in the workplace.

The supportive reflection, evaluation, and action that personal learning can stimulate may figure in the work lives of people with disabilities in important ways. It can help people with disabilities to strengthen their career self-concepts. It can equip them with a new understanding of the workplace and their role in it and, as a consequence, help them to formulate positive expectancies or beliefs about their performance and effectiveness in the workplace (Abery, 1994; Anderson & Brown, 1997; Betz & Voyten, 1997). Reflection that enables new workers with disabilities to think about their situations and to identify and evaluate strategies that will enable them achieve job-related success can further increase self-efficacy. Reflection on what people learn about the personal consequences of work can help new workers with disabilities to process their experience in the workplace. These workers can gain insight into how a workplace operates, and, as a result, help them to achieve higher levels of career maturity and insight (Super, 1994). Reflection that leads to purposeful actions new workers take to foster the management of the personal consequences they experience on the job may increase the subjective sense of self-efficacy even more.

Rehabilitation and mental health personnel can reach out to employers by offering them services that will facilitate the coping effectiveness of new workers and, as a result, strengthen workplace socialization. For employers, rehabilitation and mental health personnel can amplify their relevance through the preparation of good employees who are learning about self-management on the job. And, to job seekers, rehabilitation and mental health personnel can offer counseling and guidance that helps them to explore their personal experiences in the workplace the insight from which can contribute to the realization of tangible career development, career maturity, and vocational identity outcomes.

Fostering Role Clarity

This fifth strategy of an effective program of workplace socialization identifies the importance of helping people to achieve role clarity within the workplace. The achievement of role clarity enables newcomers to achieve a specific focus on their responsibilities and the nature of their contribution to the workplace. Role clarity means that new workers achieve a clear sense of what is expected of them, the level of performance they must achieve, and how to link their work role to the organizational role set within the teams in which they operate. The opposite of role clarity, that is, role ambiguity, may serve as a significant source of distress for workers. Role ambiguity introduces uncertainty into the work setting and can make highly skilled and motivated workers appear inefficient and ineffective. The replacement of role ambiguity with role clarity enables new workers to adjust to the work setting and to function within a work group effectively.

Rehabilitation and mental health personnel have numerous methodologies they can use to facilitate the achievement of role clarity including the assessment and evaluation of specific jobs, carving out jobs, and task analysis of how a specific job is to be undertaken to achieve favorable ratings by others in the worker's role set. These methodologies can assist new workers with disabilities to clarify their roles and to understand the expectations they must meet in particular work teams. Role clarity and task mastery may go hand in hand since specific roles encompass groups of tasks that new workers must learn to execute effectively in particular work settings. Helping new workers to clarify their understanding of their roles and to understand the tasks and expectations their roles encompass may further strengthen self-efficacy and result in higher levels of performance. Role clarity likely contributes to technical proficiency in a particular job.

Rehabilitation and mental health personnel who offer employment services can facilitate the achievement of role clarity. They can help potential employers to understand how job assessment, evaluation, and design activities contribute to the organizational socialization of new employees. Rehabilitation and mental health personnel can help new employees to achieve an understanding of how a job is to be executed at a given level of performance or at a desired level of quality.

The achievement of role clarity may vary by the kind of job a person undertakes. So, it is important to clarify for workers with disabilities the nature of the work, its contributions to workplace performance, and its ultimate purpose.

CONCLUSION

An important theme of this chapter is that by facilitating the participation of new workers with disabilities in an effective program of workplace socialization these workers can begin to accumulate career and vocational assets they may otherwise be unable to acquire. Mastering the essential tasks of a job, learning to function within a work group, acquiring knowledge of organizational culture and learning to participate in this culture, expanding personal awareness of self as a worker, and achieving role clarity are tangible assets that workers can acquire through formal and informal participation in workplace socialization experiences an organization offers its newcomers.

Rehabilitation and mental health personnel can make important contributions to the enhancement and effectiveness of the socialization of employees and, as a result, facilitate the augmentation of important career assets among people with disabilities. One of the most important outcomes of an effective program of workplace socialization is the augmentation of workers' job-specific self-efficacy. Such an outcome can increase the self-confidence of workers and contribute to their expectancies for success on the job and in the organizations that employ them.

Rehabilitation and mental health personnel in disability and rehabilitation can extend their understanding of how people function in social systems to employment settings since the strategies of workplace socialization this chapter presents is an extension of the profession's use of a person-in-environment paradigm. By facilitating the process of socialization into work roles rehabilitation and mental health personnel can help organizations increase their competencies in the employment of people with disabilities. The five strategies of workplace socialization suggest that rehabilitation and mental health personnel can be proactive in the vocational development and employment of people with disabilities and in the development of inclusive work settings, an important aim of rehabilitation and mental health practice given the low rates of workforce participation people with disabilities continue to experience.

REFERENCES

Abery, B. H. (1994). A conceptual framework for enhancing self-determination. In M. F. Hayden & B. H. Albery (Eds.), *Challenges for a service system in transition: Ensuring quality community experiences for persons with developmental disabilities* (pp. 345–380). Baltimore, MD: Brookes.

Anakwe, U. P., & Greenhaus, J. H. (1999). Effective socialization of employees: Socialization content perspective. *Journal of Managerial Issues, 11*(3), 315.

Anderson, S., & Brown, C. (1997). Self-efficacy as a determinant of career maturity in urban and rural high school seniors. *Journal of Career Assessment, 5*, 305–315.

Betz, N. E., & Voyten, K. K. (1997). Efficacy and outcome expectations influence career exploration and decidedness. *Career Development Quarterly, 46*, 179–189.

Bolman, L. G., & Deal, T. E. (1997). *Reframing organizations: Artistry, choice, and leadership* (2nd ed.). San Francisco, CA: Jossey-Bass.

Bowe, F. (1988). Recruiting workers with disabilities. *Employment Relations Today, 15*, 107–111.

Chao, G. T., O'Leary, A. M., Wolf, S., Klein, H. J., & Gardner, P. D. (1994). Organizational socialization: Its content and consequences. *Journal of Applied Psychology, 79*(5), 730–743.

Fabian, E., Luecking, R., & Tilson, G. (1995). Rehabilitation and employers' perceptions of employment: Implications for job development. *Journal of Rehabilitation, 61*(1), 42–57.

Fabian, E. S., & Waugh, C. (2001). A job development efficiency scale for rehabilitation professionals. *Journal of Rehabilitation, 67*(2), 42.

Fisher, A., & Harnisch, D. (1992). Career expectations and aspirations of youth with and without disabilities. In D. Harnisch, T. Wermuth & F. Rusch (Eds.), *Selected readings in transition* (pp. 31–64). Champaign, IL: Transition Research Institute.

Gates, L. B., Akabas, S. H., & Oran-Sabia, V. (1998). Relationship accommodations involving the workgroup: Improving work prognosis for persons with mental health conditions. *Psychiatric Rehabilitation Journal, 21*, 264–273.

Herr, E. L. (1993). Contexts of and influences on the need for personal flexibility for the 21st century, Part II. *Canadian Journal of Counselling, 27*, 219–235.

Ochs, L. A., & Roessler, R. T. (2001). Students with disabilities: How ready are they for the 21st century? *Rehabilitation Counseling Bulletin, 44*(3), 170.

Schein, E. H. (1978). *Career dynamics: Matching individual and organizational needs.* Reading, MA: Addison-Wesley.

Schein, E. H. (1988, Fall). Organizational socialization and the profession of management. *Sloan Management Review*, 53–64.

Schein, E. H. (1997). *Organizational culture and leadership* (2nd ed.). San Francisco, CA: Jossey-Bass.

Super, D. E. (1977). Vocational maturity in mid-career. *Vocational Guidance Quarterly, 25*, 294–302.

Super, D. E. (1994). A life-span, life-space perspective on convergence. In M. L. Savickas & R. W. Lent (Eds.), *Convergence in career development theories* (pp. 63–71). Palo Alto, CA: Consulting Psychologists Press.

U.S. Department of Labor (1997). *Handbook of labor statistics.* Washington, DC: U.S. Government Printing Office.

Van Eck Peluchette, J., & Jeanquart, S. (2000). Professionals' use of different mentor sources at various career stages: Implications for career success. *Journal of Social Psychology, 140*(5), 549.

Wanous, J. P. (1992). *Organizational entry: Recruitment, selection, and socialization of newcomers.* Reading, MA: Addison-Wesley.

SECTION IV

SUSTAINING EMPLOYMENT AND DEVELOPING SELF-EMPLOYMENT OPTIONS

The seven chapters that comprise this section are authored by professionals who come from a variety of disciplines and represent different theoretical perspectives. In addition, some of the authors come from a rehabilitation background while others represent the mental health professions. All the chapters have one common attribute: they focus on the work setting and how to address issues in the immediate workplace so that people can retain their jobs and sustain employment.

In Chapter 18, Tyrell, Burns, and Zipple discuss organizing supports in the workplace to sustain employment. Although they focus on using supports to sustain the employment of people coping with disabilities, the strategies they offer are relevant to any worker who faces serious challenges to their functioning effectively on the job. Erlandson offers in Chapter 19 a set of exciting guidelines for making employment accessible to people with serious disabilities through the application of assistive technologies and universal design principles. Erlandson illustrates quite dramatically the effects of various technologies on work performance and he shows through the use of specific examples how the quality of work as well as productivity can be enhanced through technological innovations.

Chapter 20, authored by Raider and his colleagues, focuses on how clinical interventions can be targeted on employment-related mental health concerns to achieve practical outcomes for workers and supervisors. These authors identify stressors that can occur within and outside of the workplace and they show how interventions can be tailored to facilitate the resolution of these issues so that they do not become chronic and disruptive. What is important about this chapter is that the authors show how mental health professionals address job-related issues through the clinical process and illuminate specific methods they use to resolve these issues, and the outcomes they seek to achieve.

In Chapter 21, Sullivan links case management practice to the achievement of employment outcomes. Both mental health and rehabilitation professionals often undertake important case management roles in relation to the formulation and implementation of a comprehensive package of services. Recognizing some of the limitations of case management, Sullivan offers guidelines on how to optimize the case management process and the important contributions this form of practice can make to the facilitation of employment.

Favorini addresses substance abuse problems in the workplace in Chapter 22 and offers a comprehensive overview of the issue and its dynamics in the context of the world of work. The author makes practical recommendations relevant to identification, assessment, entry into treatment, and coordination of care. She also illustrates key interfaces between substance abuse treatment and employee assistance programs and other mental health services.

Addressing acute mental health concerns, in Chapter 23 Hoffman and his colleagues discuss how to sustain employment during short-term mental health episodes that may constitute substantial crises within the workplace. The authors of this chapter discuss short-term interventions, crisis intervention, consultation within the workplace, and critical incident debriefing as important methods of intervention designed to resolve work-related problems or problems that emerge within the workplace.

Finally, in Chapter 24 Allen and Granger focus on how people with disabilities can develop consumer-run businesses. This chapter is particularly important in the field of rehabilitation and mental health practice since consumers themselves may initiate their own employment options and create free-standing businesses, consumer-run cooperatives, and home-based enterprises. The authors offer a set of best practices that are relevant to business start-ups and describe the actual process consumers can undertake to develop their own businesses.

Thus, the authors of the chapters that comprise this section address strategies for sustaining employment options under a variety of circumstances. Taken collectively the chapters examine practical ways to help people to move into employment situations, to sustain employment under challenging circumstances, and resolve issues that can threaten the stability of employment.

CHAPTER 18

Organizing Supports in the Workplace to Sustain Employment

WAYNE TYRELL, MATTHEW BURNS, AND
ANTHONY ZIPPLE

The costs of mental illness are exceedingly high. The direct costs of mental health services in the United States in 1996 totaled $69.0 billion. This figure represents 7.3% of the total health spending. An additional $17.7 billion was spent on Alzheimer's disease and $12.6 billion on substance abuse treatment and rehabilitation nationwide (U.S. Department of Health and Human Services, 1999).

Diagnosis of mental disorders is made on the basis of a multidimensional assessment that takes into account observable signs and symptoms of illness, the course and duration of illness, response to treatment, and degree of functional impairment. One problem has been that there is no clearly measurable threshold for functional impairments (U.S. Department of Health and Human Services, 1999).

HISTORY

Traditional psychiatric diagnoses have also failed to provide meaningful data as to an individual's work potential (Rubin & Roessler, 1995). Throughout most of the past 200 years in both Europe and America, the basic medical belief about serious mental illness was that it was incurable and usually prevented people from achieving occupational success. Rubin and Roessler (1995) describe a prevailing negative societal treatment of persons with mental illness who were usually tightly secured in either (1) the home of their family, (2) an alms-house, (3) the local jail, or (4) a mental hospital. The degree of family wealth often dictated in which location the individual with a mental illness resided. The living conditions found in mental hospitals in the 18th century would make some of the worst present-day jails and prisons look like country clubs in comparison. An early champion of persons with mental illness was Dorothea Dix. She was reported to have visited hundreds of jails and mental institutions advocating human treatment for those inmates with psychiatric disabilities. In 1854,

WAYNE TYRELL • Boston University Department of Rehabilitation Sciences, Boston, Massachusetts.
MATTHEW BURNS AND ANTHONY ZIPPLE • Vinfen Corporation, Boston, Massachusetts.

Dorothea Dix's advocacy activity almost produced federal government financial support. Unfortunately, President Franklin Pierce vetoed the legislation. Treatment modalities consisted of isolating individuals with mental illness in large, rural, warehouse-type buildings and restraining those who were unable to vocationally contribute or having those patients who were able to work assist in maintaining their daily life necessities (food, clothing, heat, etc.). The role of work was not a focus in institutional treatment and patients were unable to participate in decision-making on their own behalf when work activities were involved.

Even in more recent years the emphasis for persons with mental illness has not been on meaningful activity or employment. Until the broad implementation of the Community Mental Health Centers Act in the late 1970s, most individuals with severe and persistent mental illness were segregated for protracted periods of time. Individuals incarcerated within institution settings were considered a liability to themselves and others and therefore relegated to servitude and mistreated within these facilities (Rubin & Roessler, 1995). Well into the 20th century it was common to enlist patients at these facilities to work in the surrounding fields of these institutions to grow produce and tend livestock to become totally self-sustaining hospitals. While this was often promoted as "therapeutic," little was learned that translated into community employment. With the introduction of psychotropic drugs in the 1950s, improved legal protections, the introduction of Supplemental Security Income (SSI), and increased funding of community-based alternatives to hospitalization the focus of treatment shifted. Only in the past thirty years has attention been given to improving the functional abilities of persons with mental illness in integrated community settings instead of segregating them (Anthony, Cohen, & Farces, 1990). Early outpatient community mental health interventions tended to consist of a variety of theoretical approaches spanning the range from Freudian, Neo-Freudian, Adlerian, Gestalt, to Stimulus-Response paradigms. Most of these clinical interventions focused on symptom reduction, not the vocational abilities or strengths of clients. Interventions aimed at changing attitudes toward work also have little impact on competitive employment outcomes. Although counseling may motivate people to seek employment, if the counseling is not accompanied by direct assistance in helping people find jobs, then increased motivation to work does not translate into higher employment rates (Blankertz & Robinson, 1996; Growick, 1976). There was also a growing recognition that the population of persons with psychiatric disabilities is quite diverse and includes sub-populations, such as young adults (e.g., Bachrach, 1982), persons who are homeless (e.g., Farr, 1984), senior citizens (e.g., Gaitz, 1984), people with both severe physical disability and severe psychiatric disability (e.g., Pelletier, Rogers, & Thurer, 1985), persons who are also developmentally disabled (e.g., Eaton & Menalasciro, 1982; Reiss, 1987), and persons with severe substance abuse problems (e.g., Bachrach, 1990; Foy, 1984; Talbot, 1986). This heterogeneous population of individuals possessed the same hopes and desires to make their lives meaningful and productive as many others in our society who pursued meaningful work-related activities. The early 1970s saw the development of social policy positions such as the principle of "normalization" (Wolfensberger, 1972) which became a driving force to evaluate services, accomplishments, and outcomes for people with disabilities based on the same values used to evaluate services, accomplishments and outcomes for people without disabilities.

According to Pumpian, Fisher, Cento, and Smalley (1997), the formal establishment of supported employment policies and programs affirmed the use of new, effective approaches to broaden opportunities for people with disabilities in the workforce and within the workplace. A growing recognition by mental health advocates and individuals with psychiatric disabilities and policy-makers that employment is one of the primary mechanisms for participation in our society began to find its way into legislative language. For example, there was recognition of the need to change an ongoing problem of unacceptably high unemployment rates for people with disabilities. The current unemployment rate for people with severe disabilities of over 70% has remained unchanged for a decade (Fesko & Temelini, 1997; Louis Harris & Associates, 1998), while improvements in employment outcomes, in many ways impressive over the last 10–15 years, have not significantly increased for the majority of citizens with serious disabilities (Fesko & Temelini, 1997; Louis Harris & Associates, 1998). Some speculate that the unemployment rate for persons with psychiatric disabilities is closer to 90% (Marrone, 1993).

LEGISLATION

A key legislative response to this chronic unemployment problem occurred in the early 1980s. The concept of supported employment was first introduced and defined in the Developmental Disabilities Act of 1984. At the time, supported employment was:

> Paid employment which (1) is for persons with developmental disabilities for whom competitive employment at or above the minimum wage is unlikely and who because of their disabilities, need ongoing support to perform in a work setting; (2) is conducted in a variety of settings, particularly worksites in which persons without disabilities are employed; and (3) is supported by any activity needed to sustain paid work by persons with disabilities, including supervision, training, and transportation (p. 2665).

In July 1990, President Bush signed into law the Americans with Disabilities Act (ADA). It was hailed as the most significant piece of civil rights legislation ever written and addresses the needs of all Americans with disabilities. The ADA has put in place legal pathways to address employment discrimination for persons with disabilities and many cases are actually under review. However, almost a decade later the promise of reducing the unacceptably high rates of unemployed persons with physical and psychiatric disabilities has gone unfulfilled.

Many advocates quickly hailed the formal development of supported employment programs, services, and funding sources as a historic development in integrated employment access and placement which provided an alternative to adult daycare programs (Mank, 1994; Rucker & Bower, 1993; Wehman & Kregel, 1989).

Fabian and Widened (1989) point out that although federal authorization and funding of supported employment for severely psychiatrically disabled persons were clarified by the 1986 Rehabilitation Act Amendments, it is only recently that program descriptions and models have emerged in the psychiatric rehabilitation literature. Anthony and Blanch (1987) identified technology adaptation issues in the delivery of supported employment services to psychiatrically disabled persons, and Isbisten and Donaldson (1987) reviewed program development issues. Danley and Mellon (1987) discussed staff training and staff competencies for supported employment for this population and, in a thoughtful review at the time, Bond (1987) compared supported employment to transitional employment in the delivery of vocational services to individuals with long-term mental illness.

MODELS OF EMPLOYMENT SUPPORT

Supported employment has grown rapidly. In 1984 there were fewer than 10,000 people involved. By 1995, more than 140,000 people were in supported employment programs (Wehman, Revell, & Kregel, 1996). Economic benefits and integration for those in supported employment far exceed the outcome of those with similar disabilities in traditional activity centers and sheltered workshops (Coker, Osgood, & Clouse, 1995). Recent supported employment data (Wehman et al., 1996) indicate that 79% of people in supported employment are in individual jobs rather than group placements. Their mean hourly wage is $4.53 (with average monthly earnings of $464.10) (Monk, Cioffi, & Yovanoff, 1997).

In spite of the large quantity of reserves put into supported community employment over the last decade in the United States much remains undone (McGaughey, Kiernan, McNally, Gilmore, & Keith, 1994; Monk, 1994). Many programs and models considered "exemplary" have achieved paltry results in terms of jobs, hours worked, and wages (Bond & McDonel, 1991; Monk, 1994; Vandergoat, 1987). Seventy percent of the approximately one million individuals served by day and employment services nationally spend their days in facility-based programs, and not in the community (Gilmore, Schaloch, Kiernan, & Butterworth, 1997). Often programs funded to help people with disabilities get community jobs have low placement rates, and even individuals who obtain employment through the efforts of these service providers are often under-employed (Kiernan, Gilmore, & Butterworth, 1997; Mank, 1994).

In the early 1990s vocational rehabilitation services were designated a priority for persons with psychiatric disabilities (National Institute of Mental Health, 1991; National Institute on Disability Rehabilitation and Research, 1992). Although programs often focused on vocational preparation and finding employment, many experts have noted that persons with psychiatric disabilities have at least as much difficulty maintaining jobs as finding jobs (Anthony & Blanch, 1987; Black, 1988; Bond & McDonel, 1991; Cook, 1992; General Accounting Office, 1993; MacDonald-Wilson, Revell, Nguyen, & Peterson, 1991). Even with ongoing support a central theme of supported employment, many persons with psychiatric disabilities experience unsatisfactory job termination (Cook, 1992; Fabian & Wiedefeld, 1989; MacDonald-Wilson et al., 1991). A common view held among rehabilitation professionals is that people with severe disabilities benefit most from programs that offer a range of protected employment options, such as mobile work crews, affirmative industries, agency-run businesses, set-aside jobs, transitional employment (i.e., temporary jobs in the community paying minimum wage and supervised by the rehabilitation staff), and volunteer jobs (Campbell, 1988; Dincin, 1995; Levin, Chandler, & Barry, 1998; Marrone, 1993; Prieve & DePoint, 1987). By having many options, the theory has been that consumers can find the level of work that best suits their capabilities (Black, 1988). Under this formulation, people with the most severe disabilities are placed in the less demanding work settings, on the assumption that they will eventually gain the skills and confidence to work competitively. For years professionals relied on these intermediate program options to build and become the necessary support system leading toward competitive employment for consumers. If the goal is increasing the number of consumers getting and maintaining competitive employment, then these intermediate program options and supports were lacking from a public policy and treatment perspective. For instance, the evidence against an agency investing heavily in sheltered workshops is extensive (Bond, 1998). Observers have noted that if an agency operates a sheltered workshop, then it has significant incentives to employ its best workers (Black, 1988; Salkind, 1971). Many early surveys would confirm that clients at rehabilitation facilities with sheltered workshops have dismal prospects for competitive employment (Greenleigh Associates, 1975). As a matter of fact, the supported employment movement was a reaction to the limitations of sheltered workshops (Wehman & Moon, 1988). National surveys of supported employment have documented impressive competitive employment rates for people with severe disabilities who, prior to the advent of this innovation, might have been placed in sheltered employment (Wehman, Revell, & Kregel, 1997).

Many of the same people who were part of the tumultuous civil rights struggles of the 1960s found themselves, through personal predilection, directing and designing human services in the 1970s and 1980s. Not surprisingly, they took with them strong ethics of social justice and individual self-determination and applied them to working with disabled people who seemed to be mired in stultifying "sheltered" settings. Vocational rehabilitation programs and practices, once seen as progressive and protective of people with disabilities, became, to a large degree, recast as regressive and in many cases, repressive. Thousands of people with a wide range of different disabilities and often-questionable diagnoses were working at low or no pay in facility-based work that often went on for decades with no change. Notions of a continuum of services that led from isolated underpaid piecework to eventual mainstream employment proved, in reality, to be fiction (Wiek & Strully, 1991). Most "sheltered" workers remained in that category for life. A vast majority of sheltered workshops did not employ job developers at all and when job placement professionals were employed they often found their work frustrated by facility production managers who coveted their most productive disabled employees and blocked their "promotion" to outside jobs.

It was against this backdrop that the responsibility was shifted from the consumer, who had been expected to acquire and demonstrate proficiencies before moving into employment, to the rehabilitation professional. The principles of supported employment now rest on the proven assumption that almost all disabled people who strive to work in regular community-based jobs can do so given adequate resources and technology.

Supported employment is a promising approach to vocational rehabilitation that prescribes ongoing supports (Federal Register, 1992). The question of what supports are most effective remains. Supports such as continued vocational services (Danley, Rogers, MacDonald-Wilson, & Anthony, 1994; McFarlane, Stastny, Deakins, & Dushay, 1995) and continued support from a job counselor were strong predictors of extended employment over time (Rosenberg, 1993). The promising practice of using natural supports in the work environment continues to bring consumers closer to working in regular places of business with non-disabled workers as it reinforces community integration into adult roles, which is a fundamental goal of rehabilitation (Wolfensberger & Tullman, 1982).

FACILITATIVE EMPLOYMENT SUPPORT

In its purest form the job of the supported employment professional is to put into place whatever supports are necessary to make the work experience a success for both the worker and the employer. Supported employment is a unique vocational rehabilitation service option because it seeks to establish and maintain consistent services and work supports over the longevity of a person's employment tenure (Brooke, Revell, & Green, 1999). Since each employee and every employment site is unique, every set of supports is made up of a singular mixture of conditions that require ongoing resourcefulness, flexibility, and creativity. Unlike earlier sheltered and facility-based approaches to employing people with psychiatric disabilities, integrated, community-based work requires an understanding of the matrix in which the consumer of mental health services carries on his life. A move into a new job, often after a long hiatus, can have meaning in all realms of the employee's day-to-day existence. Habits and attitudes of family and friends and service providers can be uplifting and encouraging and can provide crucial support through the transition to work and as the job matures. Room mates, spouses, parents, and house staff can encourage the new worker to take the risk of changing his/her life and move in the direction of self-sufficiency. They can help with the new and sometimes unfamiliar demands of a job-oriented life such as scheduling, laundry, and transportation. Most of all they can provide a feeling of stability and a reassurance that the material and non-material benefits and comforts of a life out of work will not be lost, and indeed can be improved with the move to the new job.

For these reasons it is important to assess the attitudes and resources in place within the prospective worker's current support system as part of the employment support planning process and to understand what the impact of the new job will be. Fears, apprehensions, and negative fantasies can often give way to support through careful discussion and exploration with all the different people who will likely feel the impact of the change.

Relatives may be concerned about a change in benefit levels brought about by paid work as well as a possible reduction in of other kinds of support the new worker usually provides at home. Underlying these concerns there is often the fear that the ill family member will suffer a setback as a result of his/her move out into the world of work. The supported employment professional must communicate that changes in substantial areas such as benefits and taxes are understood and manageable and that the worker will continue to be followed and supported in his/her job over time. Many people with disabilities in the United States depend on monthly income and associated medical insurance from the SSI and Social Security Disability Income (SSDI) programs. Both programs are administered through the Social Security Administration and both provide targeted incentives designed to encourage program recipients to return to work. Features such as trial work periods and extended medical benefit eligibility can ease the transition and provide substantial reassurance to both the new worker and his/her family. It is important for the employment professional to develop a thorough understanding of the applicable rules. In his demeanor and in the accuracy and consistency of his communication the professional models the attitude that change and risk are healthy and life affirming.

Residential arrangements such as group homes and supported apartments will also figure in the total system of support and here too the impact can be empowering or discouraging. Residential staff who are used to a daily schedule of shopping, household chores, and other routine activities of daily living that take place during "normal business hours" may find the new work schedule disruptive. Staff's customary hours of work may need to be changed. New schedules designed around consumers' jobs may represent a jarring change. New duties focused on facilitating transportation or early morning routines may seem to be out of the realm of their usual work. In describing an active supported employment program in Baltimore, Isbister and Donaldson (1987) reported, "Therapists from community mental health centers have argued or refused to change patient appointment times in order to accommodate work schedules. Housing providers have failed to support rehabilitation plans to wake passive clients for work."

Often the supported employment professional can enlist program directors, housing managers, and clinical coordinators in an effort to educate line staff about the benefits of helping consumers to become integrated into the employment mainstream. Often, an open discussion about the underlying values of empowerment, inclusion, and choice brings to light strivings on the part of program staff to be part of consumers moving ahead. The employment professional must be aware that program staff may cling to familiar routines even when they feel frustrating. The positive message the employment professional has to convey is that the move into the new job with its attendant need for flexibility and new opportunity for enthusiasm has the potential to be as empowering for service providers as it does for the newly employed consumer. The aim is to create the opportunity for a natural set of supports to evolve in the consumer's off-work hours that complement his work activities.

NATURAL SUPPORT IN THE WORKPLACE

Because people are social animals, most worksites are very social settings. Typically, employees interact with their supervisors and coworkers about job-related matters such as job tasks that need to be done and the best way to accomplish these tasks throughout the work day (Chadsey-Rusch & Gonzalez, 1988). Almost every job is made up of a network of supports in which people interact, and provide direct and indirect aid as they go about their jobs. Workers may complete each others' work, give reminders or "cover" for a mistake, change their jobs to accommodate the needs of a coworker, provide transportation, help with apartment or house hunting, give medical and dieting advice, arrange dates, and provide literally countless other forms of support to one another (Hagner & Dileo, 1993). The typical workplace is based on a division of labor with individual workers specializing in providing various supports to coworkers that contribute to getting the job done. Some supports are formal, such as the folks in the mailroom distributing the mail or the bagger at the supermarket helping the cashier to keep the line moving. Other supports are social and emotional, sometimes contributing directly to production and sometimes maintaining a "livable work culture." In a survey of research on job satisfaction among workers in supported employment, Moseley (1988) found that "Among the most frequent reasons cited for placement failure was the inability of workers with disabilities to adjust to the social aspects of the employment situation." So although integration in terms of physical presence is one stated goal of supported employment it is vital that the supported employment professional focus on the texture of participation and the richness of opportunity to become an equal participant in the workplace (Rusch, Chadsey-Rusch, & Johnson, 1991).

Assessing the working culture is often difficult for the job coach. Many if not most informal customs and social links are hard to observe over a short time. Often they are intentionally hidden from the initial observer. It is a safe bet that the more an employee is identified as different or special at the outset, the higher will be the initial barrier to full inclusion in the workplace culture. Note that the new employee as a member of an often-stigmatized group such as the mentally ill may raise the barrier to social inclusion further. This reality presents a paradox. Supported employment is based on the provision of a set of on-the-job supports that may in themselves militate against full inclusion. The job coach must be aware of the inescapable stigmatization that comes with each provision of "special services" such as on-one-job training provided by the job coach or worksite accommodations that isolates or underlines the uniqueness of the mentally ill worker. The job coach needs to balance his priorities and think in terms of transferring supports to the natural support system on the job whenever possible. Since few if any workers in a typical business function fully independently, the idea of training to independence may actually be destructive. The eventual transition is, instead, in the direction of independence from special outside supports and toward full and equal competitive employment. Often employers insist that their own training regimens will be workable for the worker with a disability. They have trained many employees in the past, they know their business, and they feel they can handle it best. Under these circumstances the job coach has the opportunity to act as a consultant to the employer. The job coach needs to remember that the best service a job coach can sometimes provide is to not get in the way of an already existing support system.

From the first contact with the employer the supported employment service sets the tone for how the potential employee will be seen. Brochures and marketing materials that emphasize the competence and reliability of the service may be less effective than materials that talk about specific successful workers who are doing a job well. Most employers are concerned about whether or not a worker will be able to produce the work that is needed and whether or not the worker will "fit in." When targeted accommodations are required, such as modified work schedules or employee specific training for supervisors, it is important to present them as what they are, namely adjustments of routine business activity to ensure the smooth flow of work and the quality of the work environment. Caring and consideration are generally not qualities that need to be modeled for employers or coworkers. Human service providers are not unique in their wish to aid and extend themselves to other people. A consultative approach that respects and tacitly acknowledges the competence and expertise of the business tends to lower resistance to suggested adjustments and ease the way into the natural support system already in place. Of course this does not mean that the job coach adopts a passive role while facilitating natural supports any more than he does while carrying on other facets of work training. In fact, helping with integration into the culture at work may become a primary focus of the coach's efforts.

Providing support with the goal of accomplishing integration requires that the job coach continually assesses the effects of his consultations and interventions in the workplace while providing education, support, reality testing, and social skills building to the employee.

In a study of 30 individuals in supported employment the most frequently identified accommodation was orientation and training of supervisors to provide necessary assistance (Fabian, Waterworth, & Ripke, 1993). Support provided to the "system" at the workplace is usually preferable to individually targeted on-site training by a job coach. Whenever possible the job coach meets with the supported worker off the job site. When the job coach does provide training to the employee on site he dresses in a way that is normal to the culture and he defers to local experts as sources of information and guidance about "the way things are done around here." In doing so he is setting the stage for the usual ongoing informal coworker to coworker communication that everybody at work relies on to get through the day and get the job done.

The nature of psychiatric disabilities dictates that some social skills will not align as easily to the workplace culture as they may for the average non-disabled employee. Even the most scrupulous attempts to enable the normal integrative mechanisms of the job culture to include the new worker may need to be augmented with off-site socialization coaching. Isbister and Donaldson (1987) cite nine psychosocial areas in which the job coach may be expected to provide training: "1) reality testing; 2) self/other concept; 3) regulation and control of drives; 4) interpersonal relationships; 5) defense mechanisms; 6) thought processes; 7) mastery competence; 8) autonomous functioning; and 9) synthetic integrated functioning." These kinds of interpersonal and internal psychological issues can often be effectively addressed in a variety of forums individually with the employee at the supported employment service, in a coffee shop near work, or in employment support groups. Nate Azrin pioneered the use of job clubs where current and aspiring employees come together and talk about their experiences on the job, in interviews, and in social situations at work (Azrin, 1979). The job coach can facilitate, and problem-solving, story-telling, mutual affirmation, and encouragement can take place and new behaviors and responses can be tried out. Routine weekly or biweekly get togethers that allow group members to keep "up to date" about each other's progress and experiences at work often prove valuable and popular. The context of the group helps convey to the supported employee that problems can be tackled and worked out together with peers and that increasing competencies and comfort levels can be achieved through talk and cooperation. This may be both the message and an important goal of integration into the mainstream of work life.

In short, it is clear that vocational success depends on a combination of the skills that we bring to the workplace and the support that we receive in the workplace. While professionals can provide supports, these supports are expensive and less effective than reliance on natural networks of support within the workplace. Developing effective peer supports, employer supports, and family supports should be a central focus of one's professional efforts. It is the logical next step in a 30-year history of empowering consumers and supporting community integration.

SUMMARY

The preceding review of current research and contemporary program models suggests four key lessons regarding the role of natural supports in the workplace. First, while unemployment is extraordinarily high among U.S. citizens with disabilities and other related special needs, there is ample evidence that supported employment services can be effective in helping individuals with disabilities to get and keep quality jobs. In spite of these conditions, this high level of unemployment persists.

Second, there is mounting evidence that supported, real jobs that are fully integrated in workplaces are more effective in promoting long-term improved vocational outcomes than job training programs or jobs in preparatory settings. While better vocational outcomes for people with disabilities are strongly associated with integration in the workplace, they are not necessarily associated with increased levels of professional support. This suggests that the role of natural supports in the workplace may be even more important than direct professional assistance. While this conclusion seems valid, the field has not adjusted to the reality and as much as 70% of vocational service for people with disabilities is still facility-based.

Third, better outcomes are associated with successful transitions from social service supports to natural supports. As noted earlier, providing more professional supports does not necessarily result in improved outcomes. However, better outcome is strongly associated with more extensive natural support networks. Effective programs are characterized by their ability to intervene in a strategic manner to help consumers to get into integrated work settings and transition quickly from dependence on professionals to dependence on natural supports.

Finally, learning to integrate individuals with disabilities into the workforce has significant and generalized advantages for employers. The kinds of interventions that integrate and support disabled employees in the workplace are no different from the kinds of structures that are associated with more satisfied, effective, and efficient employees in general. By learning better strategies for building natural supports for people with disabilities, employers also learn strategies for building better peer support networks for all employees in their organization.

These conclusions suggest strategies for improving our ability to build natural supports for people with disabilities. We need better strategies for convincing private employers to hire people with disabilities and other special needs using a place–train approach rather than a train–place approach. Interventions by practitioners should be focused on assisting employers to build better networks of support, including the training of coworkers as peer supports. Again, more professional support is not necessarily associated with better outcomes. Instead, intervening strategically with employers to build more supportive workplaces may yield better results.

Real jobs in integrated settings consistently yield better vocational outcomes than jobs associated with training or preparatory environments. Therefore, there are significant advantages to placing consumers as quickly as possible into integrated job settings. Successful job placement also needs to acknowledge the preferences of the disabled worker. Practitioners need to focus on assessing the job preferences and choices of people with disabilities and work towards getting them jobs that are consistent with these preferences. Historically, we have tended to focus on matching people's limitations with jobs. In the future, we need to focus on matching people's preferences and career aspirations with job–place characteristics.

Vocational practitioners need to become much more adept at building natural support networks for disabled workers. As noted earlier, this means working with employers and coworkers to enhance these natural networks of support. In addition, it means recognizing the importance of natural supports in individuals' social and residential lives as well. Just as practitioners need to become more strategic in working with employers to build natural supports for disabled workers, practitioners also need to become more strategic in working with family members, friends, and community contacts as key job supports for people with disabilities.

Practitioners need to become more knowledgeable about the relationships between the interventions that they propose for disabled workers and generic high-quality interventions for all employees. The kinds of interventions associated with better outcomes for people with disabilities are also frequently associated with better outcomes for all employees. In many respects, working on natural supports means developing strategic human resource-based interventions.

The field needs to shift its research and training focus from professional supports and facility-based interventions to natural supports and jobs in integrated settings. Training and research need to occur in partnership with consumers and employers focused on consumer preferences and matched with employer needs. They should also consider the workplace itself more as the intervention site and intervene more strategically but less intensively.

We need to increase our efforts to develop interventions that will be effective in serving individuals with the most challenging disabilities. This includes people with autism, significant behavioral problems, and serious and persistent mental illness. Applying the principles discussed in this chapter can be effective with these populations, but pose particular challenges. As practitioners we need to rise to the occasion.

The challenge for us is to move aggressively in these directions now. During much of the 1990s, the United States experienced the longest continuing period of economic expansion and employment opportunity of the last 40 years. We need to take advantage of this opportunity before the inevitable downturn in the economy occurs. Every individual with a disability that can be moved into integrated work settings and supported by natural networks today becomes a person who is less likely to experience the adverse consequences when unemployment rates rise. Increased employment has obvious advantages in terms of the disabled person's ability to contribute to society through work and employment taxes. More fundamentally, it has the advantage of increasing the dignity of people with special needs as they work side by side with non-disabled individuals providing and benefiting from the natural and normal supports in the mainstream workplace.

The future supported employment prospects for individuals with severe mental health issues remains unclear. Public policy and federal legislation are in place to bring about significant changes in the way the United States, in both its private and public sector employment arenas, responds to persons with psychiatric disabilities who want competitive employment. However, spending for mental health care has declined as a percentage of overall health spending over the past decade. Furthermore, public payers have increased their share of total mental health spending. Some of the decline in resources for mental health relative to total health care may be due to reductions in inappropriate and wasteful hospitalizations and other improvements in efficiency (U.S. Department of Health and Human Services, 1999). It is paramount that we as a society realize that individuals with mental illness have the ability to be productive and gainfully employed in spite of their illness. It is said that attitudes are the most difficult barriers to overcome. Unfortunately this may be all too true with respect to providing all persons with psychiatric disabilities their right to become and remain productive working citizens.

REFERENCES

Anthony, W. A., & Blanch, A. (1987). Supported employment for persons who are psychiatrically disabled: An historical and conceptual perspective. *Psychosocial Rehabilitation Journal, 11*(2), 5–23.

Anthony, W., & Farkas, M. (1990). *Psychiatric rehabilitation.* Boston MA: Center for Psychiatric Rehabilitation.

Bachrach, L. (1982). Program planning for young adult chronic patients. In B. Pepper & H. Ryglewicz (Eds.), *The young adult chronic patient* (New Directions for Mental Health Services, No. 14, p. 254). San Francisco CA: Jossey-Bass.

Bachrach, L. (1990). The context of care for the chronic mental patient with substance abuse problems. *Psychiatric Quarterly.*

Black, B. (1988). *Work and mental illness: Transitions to employment.* Baltimore MD: Johns Hopkins University Press.

Blankertz, L., & Robinson, S. (1996). Adding a vocational focus to mental health rehabilitation. *Psychiatric Services, 47*, 1216–1222.

Bond, G. (1987). Supported work as a modification of the transitional employment model for clients with psychiatric disabilities. *Psychosocial Rehabilitation Journal, 11*(2), 55–73.

Bond, G., & McDonel, E. (1991). Vocational rehabilitation outcomes for persons with psychiatric disabilities: An update. *Journal of Vocational Rehabilitation, 1*(3), 9–20.

Brooke, V., Revell, G., & Green, J. H. (1998). Long-term supports using an employee-directed approach to supported employment. *Journal of Rehabilitation, 64*(2), 38–45.

Butterworth, J., Kiernan, W., Schalock, R., & Hagner, D. (1996). Natural supports in the workplace: Defining an agenda for research and practice. *Journal of the Association for Persons with Severe Handicaps, 21*, 103–113.

Campbell, J. (1988). Rehabilitation facilities and community-based employment services. In P. Wehman & M. S. Moon (Eds.), *Vocational rehabilitation and supported employment* (pp. 193–202). Baltimore MD: Paul Brookes.

Coker, C., Osgood, K., & Clouse, K. (1995). *A comparison of job satisfaction and economic benefits of four different employment models for persons with disabilities.* Menominic, WI: University of Wisconsin–Stout RRTC.

Cook, J. (1992). Job ending among youth and adults with severe mental illness. *Journal of Mental Health Administration, 19*, 158–169.

Danley, K., & Mellon, V. (1987). Training and personnel issues for supported employment programs which serve persons who are severely mentally ill. *Psychosocial Rehabilitation Journal, 11*(2), 87–102.

Danley, K., Rogers, E., MacDonald-Wilson, K., & Anthony, W. (1994). Supported employment for adults with psychiatric disability: Results of an innovative demonstration project. *Rehabilitation Psychology, 39*, 269–276.

Dincin, J. (1995). A pragmatic approach to psychiatric rehabilitation: Lessons from Chicago's thresholds program. *New Directions for Mental Health Services, 68*, whole issue.

Eaton, L. F., & Menolascion, F. J. (1982). Psychiatric disorders in the mentally retarded: Types, problems, challenges. *American Journal of Psychiatry, 139*, 1297–1303.

Fabian, E., & Widened, M. (1989). Supported employment for severely psychiatrically disabled persons— A Descriptive Study. *Psychosocial Rehabilitation Journal, 13*(2), 53–60.

Farr, R. K. (1984). The Los Angeles Skid Row Mental Health Project. *Psychosocial Rehabilitation, 8*(2), 64–76.

Federal Register (1992). *Vocational Rehabilitation Act amendments of 1992* (29 United States Code 706) (18). Washington, DC: U.S. Government Printing Office.

Fesko, S., & Temelini, D. (1997). What consumers and staff tell us about effective job search strategies. In W. E. Kiernan & R. L. Schalock (Eds.), *Integrated employment: Current status and future directions* (pp. 67–81). Washington, DC: AAMR.

Foy, D. W. (1984). Chronic alcoholism: Broad-spectrum clinical programming. In M. Mirabi (Ed.), *The chronically mentally ill: Research and services* (pp. 273–280). Jamaica, NY: Spectrum.

Gaitz, L. M. (1984). Chronic mental illness in aged patients. In M. Mirabi (Ed.), *The chronically mentally ill: Research and services* (pp. 273–280). Jamaica, NY: Spectrum.

General Accounting Office (GAO) (1993). *Vocational rehabilitation: Evidence for federal program effectiveness is mixed* (PEMD-93-19). Washington, DC: Author.

Gilmore, D. S., Schalock, R., Kiernan, W. E., & Butterworth, J. (1997). National comparisons and critical findings in integrated employment. In W. E. Kiernan & R. L. Schalock (Eds.), *Integrated Employment: Current Status and Future Directions* (pp. 49–66). Washington, DC: AAMR.

Greenleigh Associates (1975). *The role of sheltered workshops in the rehabilitation of the severely disabled.* New York, NY: Department of Health, Education and Welfare.

Growick, B. S. (1976). Effects of a work-adjustment program on emotionally handicapped individuals. *Journal of Applied Rehabilitation Counseling, 7*, 119–123.

Isbister, F., & Donaldson, G. (1987). Supported employment for individuals who are mentally ill: Program development. *Psychosocial Rehabilitation Journal, 11*(2), 45–54.

Kiernan, W., Butterworth, J., Schalock, R., & Hagner, D. (1993). *Enhancing the use of natural supports for people with severe disabilities.* Boston MA: The Children's Hospital, The Training and Research Institute for People with Disabilities.

Kiernan, W. E., Gilmore, D. S., & Butterworth, J. (1997). Provider perspectives and challenges in integrated employment. In W. E. Kiernan & R. L. Schalock (Eds.), *Integrated Employment: Current Status and Future Directions* (pp. 97–100). Washington, DC: AAMR.

Levin, S., Chandler, D., & Barry, P. (1998). The menu approach to employment services, Pt I, Philosophy manuscript. Submitted for publication.

Louis Harris & Associates (1998). National Organization on Disability/Harris survey on employment of people with disabilities. New York, NY: Author.

MacDonald-Wilson, K., Revell, W., Nguyen, N., & Peterson, M. (1991). Supported employment outcomes for people with psychiatric disability: A comparative analysis. *Journal of Vocational Rehabilitation, 1*(3), 30–44.

Mank, D. (1994). The underachievement of supported employment: A call for reinvestment. *Journal of Disability Policy Studies, 5*(2), 2–24.

Mank, D., Cioffi, A., & Yovanoff, P. (1997). Analysis of the typicalness of supported employment jobs, natural supports, and wage and integration outcomes. *Mental Retardation, 35*(3), 185–197.

Marrone, J. (1993). Creating positive outcomes for people with severe mental illness. *Psychosocial Rehabilitation Journal, 17*(2), 43–62.

McGaughey, M., Kiernan, B., McNally, L., Gilmore, D., & Keith, G. (1994). *Beyond the workshop: National perspectives on integrated employment.* Boston, MA: ICI.

National Institute of Mental health (1991). *Caring for people with severe mental disorders: A national plan of research to improve services* (DHHS Publication No. ADM 91-1762). Washington, DC: U.S. Government Printing Office.

National Institute on Disability and Rehabilitation Research (NIDRR) (1992). *Consensus Validation Conference: Strategies to secure and maintain employment for persons with long-term mental illness.* Washington, DC: Department of Education.

Pelletier, J. R., Rogers, E. S., & Thurer, S. (1985). The mental health needs of individuals with severe physical disability: A consumer advocate perspective. *Rehabilitation Literature, 46*, 186–193.

Prieve, K., & DePoint, B. (1987). *Making it work: Supported employment for persons with severe and persistent mental illness.* Minneapolis, MN: Rise.

Pumpian, I., Fisher, D., Certo, N., & Smalley, K. (1997) Changing jobs: An essential part of career development. *Mental Retardation, 35*(1), 39–48.

Reiss, S. (1987). Symposium overview: Mental health and mental retardation. *Mental Retardation, 25*, 323–324.

Rosenberg, M. (1993). *Society and adolescents self image.* Princeton, NJ: Princeton University Press.

Rubin, S., & Roessler, R. (1995). *Foundations of the vocational rehabilitation process* (4th ed.). Austin, TX: Pro-Ed.

Rucker, R., & Bower, D. M. (1993). From shelter to integrated employment: Current public practice and future directions. In *Consensus Validation Conference: Supported employment for people with severe disabilities* (Resource papers). Washington, DC: NIDRR.

Salkind, I. (1971). Economic problems in the workplace. In H. R. Lamb & Associates (Eds.), *Rehabilitation in community mental health* (PP71–91). San Francisco, CA: Jossey-Bass.

Talbot, J. (1986). *Chronically mentally ill young adults (18–40) with substance abuse problems: A review of relevant literature and creation of a research agenda.* Report submitted to Alcohol, Drug Abuse, and Mental Health Administration, Washington, DC.

U.S. Department of Health and Human Services (1999). *Mental health: A report of the Surgeon General.* Rockville, MD: U.S. Department of Health and Human Services, Substance Abuse and Mental Health Services Administration, Center for Mental Health Services, National Institutes of Health, National Institute of Mental Health.

Vandergoot, D. (1987). Review of the placement research literature: Implications for research and practice. *Rehabilitation Counseling Bulletin, 30*(4), 243–272.

Wehman, P., & Kregel, J. (1989). Supported employment: Promises deferred for persons with severe disabilities. *Journal of the Association for Persons with Severe Disabilities, 14*(4), 293–303.

Wehman, P., & Moon, M. (Eds.) (1988). *Vocational rehabilitation and supported employment*. Baltimore, MD: Paul Brookes.

Wehman, P., Revell, W., & Kregel, J. (1996). *Supported employment from 1986–1993: A national program that works*. Richmond, VA: Virginia Commonwealth University, Rehabilitation, Research, and Training Center.

Wehman, P., Revell, G., & Kregel, J. (1997). Supported employment: A decade of rapid growth and impact. In P. Wehman, J. Kregel & M. West (Eds.), *Supported employment research: Expanding competitive employment opportunities for persons with significant disabilities* (pp. 1–18). Richmond, VA: Virginia Commonwealth University, Rehabilitation, Research, and Training Centre.

Wolfensberger, W. (1972). *The principle of normalization in human services*. Toronto, Canada: Human Policy.

Wolfensberger, W., & Tullman, S. (1982). A brief outline of the principle of normalization. *Rehabilitation Psychology, 27*, 131–145.

CHAPTER 19

Accessible Design and Employment of People with Disabilities

ROBERT ERLANDSON

Factors such as worker demographics, evolving legislation, global business practices, and technology are combining to create an environment that promotes greater accessibility in the workplace and jobs for individuals with disabilities. While increased accessibility is necessary, it is not sufficient to guarantee job creation, retention, and advancement opportunities for individuals with cognitive disabilities. Essential to the employment of anyone is their job performance and productivity. Hence it is important to establish the connection between the aforementioned factors, accessible design principles, improved job performance, and job creation for individuals with cognitive disabilities.

PRODUCTIVITY: JOB RETENTION AND PERFORMANCE IMPROVEMENT

The ability to do the essential functions of a job, unaided or with reasonable accommodations, is a key issue with respect to the competitive employment of individuals with disabilities. The importance of production for individuals with disabilities is often underestimated because it is not an isolated factor with respect to securing and retaining a job. Production, with regard to securing employment for people with disabilities, is associated with psychological and social factors. Studies by Greenspan and Shoultz (1981) and Hanley-Maxwell, Rusch, Chadsey-Rusch, and Renzaglia (1986) found that persons with disabilities most often lost their jobs for social reasons. The Hanley-Maxwell et al. study (1986) examined factors reported to contribute to job termination of adults with disabilities. There were 51 subjects and 103 reasons for termination given. Statistical analyses showed that the distribution of reasons was not random. The single most frequent cause for job termination was production, closely followed by character. These results focus attention on the multifaceted nature of the sustained employment of individuals with disabilities. The Hanley-Maxwell et al. study showed that a mix of social awareness, character, and/or production accounted for more than 80% of the terminations. Thus, while social and/or character reasons were given, they were typically coupled with

ROBERT ERLANDSON • Wayne State University College of Engineering, Detroit, Michigan.

production. In this way production came to be the single most frequent cause for job termination.

Many studies on the lack of job success among people with disabilities have focused on individual-centered problems, including social skills and behavioral excesses. Lagomarcino and Rusch (1988) analyzed applied research on adults with mental retardation in competitive employment situations and found the studies dealt exclusively with changing the behavior of the person with mental retardation. This unidimensional approach results in a restricted view of the factors impeding successful employment performance as well as the identification of subsequent solutions (Lagomarcino, 1990).

A mid-1980s project called VECTOR (Vocational Education, Community Transition, Occupational Relations) sought to increase the employability of severely to mildly mentally handicapped students (aged 18–21) in transition from school to work in the greater Minneapolis, Minnesota, area (Lindskoog, 1987). VECTOR's objectives were to develop a long-range planning mechanism, incorporate a vocational counseling program, and develop universal work skills such as social/interpersonal skills, independent living skills, and occupational skills. VECTOR also sought to enhance the attitudinal development of handicapped students and develop support services to ensure the successful transition from school to work (Lindskoog, 1987). These objectives reflect a traditional approach.

Project VECTOR found the development of new community-based employment sites problematic. They relied heavily on service occupations and experienced partial success in the printing industry, health care, and packaging occupations. In many other potential areas, however, the production requirements were highlighted as a major factor making inroads for job openings very difficult. The traditional approaches, with a focus on universal work skills, were not sufficient for job placement and retention.

Lagomarcino reports on an analysis of data from 318 job terminations of persons with disabilities from 70 agencies implementing supported employment across Illinois between 1985 and 1988. This study reported that the majority of persons with severe or profound mental retardation lost their jobs for production-related reasons. These production-related reasons included a slow work rate, and the need for continual prompting.

Lagomarcino (1990) discusses possible solutions for production difficulties, including job redesign and rehabilitation engineering services. These techniques have evolved from the earlier work of Gold (1968, 1972, 1973), who pioneered the use of assistive technologies and skills training methods for individuals with cognitive impairments. This focus implies an assembly line or mass production type of process. It presumes a fixed product or process into which the individual must be fitted or placed. Gold (1968) and others (Sowers & Powwers, 1991) argue that with the right kind of training, individuals with cognitive disabilities can in fact be trained to perform a variety of relatively complex tasks. The individual might need an adaptation, such as a special jig or color-coding of parts, to facilitate their performance, but this adaptation was solely for the disabled individual.

While there are still an abundance of assembly jobs, the mass production model is no longer adequate (Womack, Jones, & Roos, 1990). Lean production models are expanding under the influences of QS and International Organization for Standardization (ISO) certification, Occupational Safety and Health Administration (OSHA) standards, and relentless competition (Tidd, 1991; Womack et al., 1990). Lean production involves cross-training, job rotation, and other strategies that challenge employment opportunities for individuals with cognitive disabilities (Womack et al., 1990). OSHA ergonomic standards also encourage cross-training and job rotation as a way to reduce ergonomic risks (Occupational Safety and Health Administration, 1999). Hence issues of productivity and employment must be addressed in the context of mixed production models, some still oriented toward mass production, but a growing number moving toward lean production.

Vocational rehabilitation and job placement specialists typically tend to address production issues with social/human supports, which are areas of strength in their educational programs. They tend to use the terms *social supports* and *natural supports* interchangeably. Social supports include people networks, personnel support groups, job coaches, job trainers, supportive coworkers, supervisors, and mentors (Hagner, Rogan, & Murphy, 1992). Natural supports include coworker support, peer support, and other forms of informal support (Hagner et al., 1992). A slightly broader conceptualization of natural support, called *natural workplace support*, is suggested by Fabian, Edelman, and Leedy (1993). Natural workplace supports focus on training efforts for persons with disabilities within the functional context of the work environment.

Use of the terms *natural supports* and *natural workplace supports* to include only social/human supports is limiting and needs to be expanded to include *process supports*, which are built into a workplace and the product/process. Noel (1990) discusses the importance of linking workers with disabilities to available supports in the work environment. For example, he suggests changing the focus from what the individual needs to what the environment can provide. This perspective emphasizes how to use what is available in the work environment, rather than emphasizing how to help the individual fit into the work environment. This approach comes closer to an engineering approach based on accessible design principles, which emphasizes changing the job to better accommodate people (Grandjean, 1991; OSHA, 1999).

The utilization of accessible design principles allows the creation of system supports which include the traditional social/human supports as well as inherent process supports that can be designed into processes and jobs. This is precisely what the *kaizen* (continuous improvement) techniques are designed to accomplish. Jobs and work processes designed using *kaizen* techniques allow the worker to enter into a dialogue with the processes themselves. This dialogue facilitates fast, on-the-job learning, essential for cross-training and job rotation. The dialogue helps to reduce errors and maintain high-quality products and services.

ACCESSIBLE DESIGN

Accessible design means designing processes, products, and services so that as many people, with as broad a spectrum of abilities as possible, can access and use the processes, products, or services. This section discusses the principles of accessible design, which are listed below, as well as the effectiveness of their application.

1. Design to reduce the physical demands of the task.
2. Design to reduce the cognitive demands of the task.
3. Design to reduce the inherent variability of the task.
4. Design to reduce the errors associated with the performance of the task.
5. Design to reduce the non-value-added activities of the task.

Accessibility has the following dimensions: social, economic, and human factors. Societal values are made explicit by a nation's laws. The Americans with Disabilities Act of 1990 (ADA) made explicit the societal value that one cannot discriminate against individuals with disabilities with respect to employment (Access Board, 1999; National Institute on Disability and Rehabilitation Research, 1992). It also requires that buildings, facilities, and jobs must be made accessible. The Telecommunications Act of 1996, Section 255, makes explicit the social value that telecommunication devices and services must be made accessible to individuals with disabilities (Federal Communications Commission, November 19, 1999). These laws are important because they provide a legal matrix which supports all other efforts.

In addition to the legal matrix, the advance of QS and ISO quality assurance processes and certification requirements are accelerating the application of *kaizen* techniques and quality tools (Hoyle, 1997; Imai, 1986, 1997; Ishiwata, 1991; Randal, 1995). OSHA's new work-related musculoskeletal disorders (MSDs) standards reduce the ergonomic stress of jobs and renders them more accessible (OSHA, 1999). The *kaizen*/quality techniques and ergonomic standards are closely related in that they all embody accessible design principles targeted at the human factors dimension. The human factors dimension is the focus of this discussion.

BASIC CONCEPTS

Human Factors

Human factors deal with the physical and cognitive demands of a job as they relate to the physical and cognitive abilities of the worker. One central accessible design principle is to design for physical accessibility. The lifting and handling requirements of a job have implications for who can perform the job. There are very specific strategies available to analyze the physical demands of jobs. OSHA has a great deal of material available to help businesses conduct ergonomic assessments (OSHA, 1999).

Another accessible design principle is to design for cognitive accessibility. Reading, performing mathematical operations, or the memorization of long sequences of actions or codes place constraints on who can perform a job. An analysis of the cognitive demands of jobs is more difficult than an analysis of physical activity. Workers who cannot read, who are color blind, or who cannot remember code or action sequences may develop complex strategies to hide this from an employer. Typically cognitive issues are noticed indirectly by increased errors, a decrease in productivity, and other symptomatic indicators.

Variation

Another fundamental principle of accessible design is to reduce the inherent variability of a job. Every job, task, and process naturally has a certain amount of variability or variance. Deming (1982) termed this variability as *common cause*. Everyday occurrences, such as traffic volume and the timing of traffic signals, contribute to the time variability associated with one's drive to work. An accident or severe storm, however, are exceptional events, not common to the process. Deming termed these events *special cause*. In terms of jobs and the work environment one needs to plan for the occurrence of special cause events, but we typically have no control over such events. On the other hand, we do have the ability to reduce common cause events and the problems associated with such variability.

Consider the task of balancing a broom on the open palm of your hand, broom bristles up. The laws of physics introduce a great deal of variability. An accomplished balancer has the expertise and skills necessary to balance the broom; however, most of us would scurry around trying, with no avail, to keep the broom balanced. We do not possess the skills necessary to overcome the variation inherent to the process to successfully perform this job.

If we redefine the process, hold the broom in two hands, and introduce some technology, such as bracing the broom handle against a desk top, many more people can successfully perform the task. The redefined process and use of *enabling technology*, which is technology that enables improved performance, makes the task more accessible by reducing the variation inherent to the process. This illustrates a typical strategy for reducing the variability associated with job processes: redefine the processes and incorporate enabling technology.

Quality—Error Reduction

Error reduction is a fundamental principle of accessible design. Human errors and machine malfunctions are two examples of how mistakes and errors contribute to product defects and process inefficiencies. Error-proofing has always been central to high-risk operations. Two examples of such error-proofing strategies are (1) the completion of pre-flight checklists by commercial pilots, and (2) the safety checks and balances used by nuclear power plant controllers (Rasmussen, 1986; Woods & Roth, 1988). The idea is to design systems and processes that facilitate "doing the right thing."

The pressures of lean production and higher quality standards imposed by the QS and ISO certification requirements are accelerating the introduction of error-proofing strategies into assembly, manufacturing, office, and service jobs (Imai, 1997; Japan Human Relations Association, 1992). High-quality products and services are fundamental to lean production. Ideally one strives for zero defects in products or services

Design for assembly (DFA) (Boothroyd & Dewhurst, 1991) and similar concepts (Crow, 1989) are related to error-proofing in that they reduce or eliminate the probability of an incorrect assembly (Shimbun, 1988). The changing demographics of the workforce, cross-training, and job rotation require that work process and jobs provide more feedback and support to the workers to not only reduce error, but also speed up on-the-job learning.

QS and ISO certification requires the implementation of quality improvement strategies; error-proofing is a core element of such strategies. Relatively inexpensive electronics and smart sensors with embedded microcomputers can be integrated into assembly, packaging, sorting, and counting tasks to provide feedback to the workers. Color coding, icons, and other visual controls can be used as error-reducing tools in office and service jobs (Shimbun, 1988).

Error-proofing is a core strategy for achieving the objectives associated with lean production and quality control programs. For workers without disabilities the error-proofing strategies fight boredom, fatigue, and other distractions. For individuals with disabilities, the error-proofing strategies provide an essential dialogue between the job and person, enabling the person to actually perform the job.

Waste—Non-Value-Added Activity

Another fundamental issue is waste, with waste meaning non-value-added activity, and the design principle being reduce or eliminate waste. Work can be viewed as a series of processes or steps. Work steps can add value to the product. For example, in manufacturing, a piece of steel is milled into a shape. In an assembly task, parts are joined together. In the service sector, information is added to a document, French fries are added to the customer's plate, or purchased merchandise is placed into a bag for the customer. Other steps do not add value to the product. Such non-value-added steps include parts waiting for transport to the next manufacturing or assembly step, lifting heavy parts from the floor to a table top, a restaurant dinner order sitting on the counter getting cold waiting for a server to take it to the customer, or inspection of a part after an assembly operation. Hence the process resources, which are people and/or equipment, either add value or do not add value.

For manufacturing or assembly jobs non-value activity has been classified according to seven categories: overproduction, inventory, repair/rejects, motion, processing, waiting, and transport (Imai, 1997). Similar non-value-added categories can be associated with service sector jobs. The reduction of non-value-added activity complements and in some cases overlaps the other accessible design principles. For example, by reducing errors, and reducing the physical demands of a job (lifting, transporting) one also reduces the non-value-added components of the job.

Interventions

The five principles of accessible design are intended to: reduce the physical and cognitive demands of jobs, reduce the inherent variability of jobs, reduce job-related errors, and reduce waste or non-value-added activities. The following intervention strategies address the factors targeted by the accessible design principles. The application of these strategies can create a win–win scenario with respect to improved business operations and improved job performance and job creation for individuals with disabilities.

Process Analysis and Redesign

Kaizen terminology includes the term "making it visible." Problems, issues, and relationships cannot be dealt with if they cannot be made visible. That is, the topics under consideration must be clearly stated, represented, or articulated. This idea can be illustrated by the blindfolded men "viewing" an elephant metaphor. Each man feels a different part and offers a different description.

Even seemingly simple work processes can be quite complex when analyzed in detail. Added to this, productivity and job performance issues are typically ill-defined and vague. This complexity and vagueness, along with potential personality conflicts among participating individuals, make it extremely difficult to arrive at a consensus as to the problems and issues, much less an approach to solving the problems.

There are a variety of process analysis tools and techniques available (Peach & Ritter, 1996). A description of these tools and techniques is beyond the scope of this discussion, but knowledge of these tools and techniques is important if vocational rehabilitation, job placement professionals are to effectively communicate with industry managers and supervisors.

Poka-Yoke

Poka-yoke, a Japanese term for error-proofing, accepts that human beings are forgetful and tend to make mistakes. Shimbum, a Japanese proponent of *poka-yoke*, states that "too often we blame people for making mistakes. Especially in the workplace, this attitude not only discourages workers and lowers morale, but it does not solve the problem. Poka-yoke is a technique for avoiding simple human error at work" (Shimbun, 1988).

The concept of *poka-yoke* has existed in many forms for a long time. The Japanese manufacturing engineer Shigeo Shingo developed the idea into a tool for achieving zero defects and eventually eliminating the need for quality control inspections (Shingo, 1986). Shingo coined the term *poka-yoke*, generally translated as "mistake-proofing" or "fail-safing" (Shingo, 1986).

Poka-yoke is a fundamental accessible design strategy. An example of a *poka-yoke* principle at work is the 3.5 in. memory diskette for computers. It only goes into the disk drive one way. Its dimensions prohibit insertion sideways, a sliding key mechanism prevents insertion upside down or backwards. These physical attributes prevent the error of wrong diskette insertions.

Another example of a *poka-yoke* approach is the use of a fixed height fixture to hold the paper rolls for coins. When counting dimes it is easier, faster, and less error-prone to use pattern recognition. For example, using the height of the roll of dimes as an indicator of the correct count. Again this technique relies on the physical uniformity of dimes. In both the computer diskette and coin-rolling examples there is a dialogue between the worker and the process. The process provides feedback as to the correctness of the actions. The disk/drive design prohibits an error. The dime-rolling case allows errors if the worker cannot recognize the pattern; the standard height.

The two types of feedback or dialogue are important. In one case the process does not allow an error. In the other the process warns of an error, but the worker must be able to perceive and recognize the warning. These represent *prohibitive error controls* and *warning error controls*. The type of error control used depends on the application, the risk or cost associated with making an error, and the cost of implementing the error-proofing technique.

It is important to make a distinction between a *poka-yoke* intervention and an accommodation. Currently, most interventions are accommodations. Accommodations represent a very narrow approach to productivity enhancement and are targeted at the worker with a disability. There is really no substantial business advantage for individual worker accommodations. That is why state or federal job placement and support agencies typically subsidize the cost of such interventions. On the other hand, a *poka-yoke* intervention is designed to improve overall process productivity and quality. There is a direct and potentially substantial business benefit.

An intervention for a worker with a disability may or may not be a *poka-yoke* intervention. If the intervention reduces error and improves the performance for everyone doing the task, then it is a *poka-yoke* intervention. If the intervention were to slow down or hinder a worker who does not have a disability, then it is an accommodation. For example, a specialized fixture designed to hold open the clamps on a pants hanger used in clothing stores so that an individual with the use of only one hand can perform the task of placing pants on a hanger is an accommodation. Workers with the use of two hands would be hindered by this device.

There are a number of books targeted at industry that discuss *poka-yoke* principles and provide a wealth of examples (Shimbun, 1988; Shingo, 1986). The Enabling Technologies Laboratory (ETL) web site has examples of *poka-yoke* applications as well as links to other sites dealing with *poka-yoke*, and error-proofing techniques (Erlandson, Bradow, & Sant, 1999).

Sensory Controls (Visual, Auditory, Tactile, Olfactory)

Visual and auditory controls are found everywhere: from traffic control lights and signs, to train crossing gates and bells, back-up warning buzzers on fork lifts and buses, police warning lights and sirens, exit and entrance signs, to the food preparation charts used in fast food restaurants. Visual controls include lights, color coding, icons, and words. Auditory controls include buzzers, bells, and tones. Tactile controls include the vibration alarms on pagers, rippled shoulders on roads to vibrate the car, and raised or depressed points on push buttons. Natural gas has an additive with a distinctive smell so as to warn people of gas leaks. Any sense has the potential to serve as a control or communication mechanism.

Use of icons and color coding reduces the cognitive processing load of reading words. Many offices at General Motors Technical Center in Warren, Michigan, use a centralized office supply system. The storage cabinets in these locations use icons to represent the contents of the drawers. An Occupational Therapist seeing this system inquired as to why they used icons instead of words. The answer was that with words the drawers were left in a mess after a short period of time. People would open drawers, rifle through and leave the contents in a mess. With icons there was no such mess. Apparently, with a written description of the drawer's contents, a trial-and-error retrieval strategy was preferred. Icons, on the other hand, produced a different retrieval strategy. This example illustrates the power of visual or sensory controls to organize the workplace and reduce errors for all workers regardless of their intelligence or levels of education.

Workplace Organization

Workplace organization starts with cleaning up, keeping it clean, getting things organized, and keeping them organized (Imai, 1997). The *kaizen* strategy for workplace organization is termed the *5S's* (Imai, 1997). Table 19-1 summarizes the 5S's. Following this strategy makes common sense, but the discipline to actually do it, and standardize it into the regular work routine, is much more difficult.

Workplace organization also means storing working materials and positioning tools in ways that minimize ergonomic risks and arranging the flow of materials and people so as to avoid the non-value-added activities of unnecessary transport, walking, or storage. It may mean the use of *kits*. Kitting is an effective way to group all the materials required for a job in one location ready for use.

One principle for workplace organization is to create an organization that is "self-managing." Consider a parking lot in a busy shopping mall. The parking lot has clearly marked parking places and people conform to the standardized practice of parking within the marked parking spaces. On winter days when the parking lot is covered with snow, before it is plowed away, cars tend to be parked much more chaotically. People try to align themselves, but usually end up in curving lines of cars and inefficient use of parking lot space. The visual controls organize the parking lot and create, to a high degree, a self-managing system.

Visual controls such as shadow diagrams on peg boards for tools are effective ways to create a "self-managing" workplace. Any worker can quickly see if the tool they want is

Table 19-1. The 5S's. Taken from Imai (1997, chapter 5)

1. Sort	Separate out all that is unnecessary and eliminate it
2. Straighten	Put essential things in order so that they can be easily accessed
3. Scrub	Clean everything—tools and workplaces—removing stains, spots, and debris and eradicating sources of dirt
4. Systematize	Make cleaning and checking routine
5. Standardize	Standardize the previous four steps to make the process one that never ends and can be improved upon

available. At the end of the work period the supervisor in charge of tools can quickly see if any tools are missing and take appropriate action.

Another example of a self-managing system can be found in many offices at the General Motors Technical Center in Warren, Michigan. They use a "pull system" for inventory control. Office supplies are stored in a central location and when workers need such supplies, they go to the storage cabinet and take what they need. There are markers in the office supplies that indicate an order point. For example, in the stack of paper pads there is a marker about three-fourths of the way down the full stack. Who ever hits this marker, removes it and places it in a basket on the front of the storage cabinet. On a regular schedule, someone is charged to retrieve these markers and place an order for the required items. No person has to sort or count office supplies to figure out what to order. The process informs workers when an action needs to be taken.

Workplace organization can address all the factors targeted by the accessible design principles. Workplace organization can include all the interventions mentioned thus far. Lastly, workplace organization leads to the creation of structured, consistent, predictable work environments which form the basis for standardized work procedures.

Standardized Work

Standardized work is another basic *kaizen* strategy (Imai, 1997). Standardized work or standard operating procedures stabilize a job. In process terms, standardized work reduces a job's inherent variability. Standardized work is not an isolated technique, but rather coordinated with workplace organization, visual, and *poka-yoke* controls. From a business perspective standardized work is an effective tool in quality assurance and a cost-effective way to do the job.

Table 19-2 lists some of the key features of standardized work.

Standardized work procedures, such as the OSHA ergonomic standards and QS and ISO requirements, have a spin-off effect with respect to the employment and job performance of individuals with disabilities. Standards reduce inherent process variability by creating a structured, safe, consistent environment. Such an environment is important for the successful employment of individuals with cognitive disabilities.

APPLICATIONS

There is a large body of literature documenting the success of product and process designs following the application of *kaizen, poka-yoke,* and other related principles (Boothroyd &

Table 19-2. Key Features of Standardized Work (Imai, 1997)

1. Represent the best, easiest, and safest way to do a job
2. Offer the best way to preserve know-how and expertise
3. Provide a way to measure performance
4. Show the relationship between cause and effect
5. Provide a basis for both maintenance and improvement
6. Provide objectives and indicate training goals
7. Provide a basis for training
8. Create a basis for audit or diagnosis
9. Provide a means for preventing recurrence of errors and minimize variability

Dewhurst, 1991; Crow, 1989; Dingwelki, 1988; Eppinger, Whitney, Smith, & Gebala, 1990; Gardner, 1989; Hammer, 1990; Imai, 1997; Ishiwata, 1991; Poli, Graves, & Groppetti, 1986; Shimbun, 1988; Tidd, 1991; Wiest & Kregel, 1977; Womack et al., 1990). These have focused on workers without disabilities in competitive work environments. However, it was not at all clear how individuals with cognitive impairments would perform with a redesigned job process. The following applications demonstrate that the use of accessible design principles can yield the same improvements in job quality and performance when the workers are people with disabilities as when the workers are people without disabilities. Also, the applications consistently found that when workers with disabilities performed competently on the job, they demonstrated pride in their work and exhibited fewer behavioral problems. This linking of productivity with social behavior should not be surprising based on the linkages presented in the Productivity section.

Design for Assembly (DFA)

In *Product Design for Assembly*, Boothroyd and Dewhurst (1991) present a systematic procedure for analyzing the design of a device with respect to specific features of the assembly process. The intent, among other things, is to reduce the number of parts, avoid screws in favor of snap-on fasteners, avoid ergonomically awkward assemblies, and provide guides, notches, and other aids for insertion of parts or alignment of parts. If followed, these principles can dramatically reduce assembly time. For example, a dot matrix printer redesign went from 185 parts to 32 and the assembly time went from over 30 min to slightly over 3 min (Dingwelki, 1988).

Pilot studies conducted by the ETL, Wayne State University, found similar results where the workers were individuals with cognitive impairments (Erlandson & Phelps, 1995). The studies included 12 workers ranging in age from 15 to 44 years old, with IQ scores ranging from 10 to 57. After a very short training period the workers were asked to perform two pneumatic piston assemblies. While these devices were functionally equivalent and could be interchanged in the final product, they were strikingly different. The old design had seven parts, two of which were small screws. The new design, based on DFA principles, had four parts, no screws, and used snap-on fasteners.

This application showed a dramatic improvement in worker performance with the new design over the old design. With the old design there were 47 unsuccessful assembly attempts and 42 assemblies at about 10 times the normative rate—an unacceptable performance for employment. With the new design, every worker could perform the assembly. There were 72 assemblies in the above normative range, but the associated assembly times averaged about 30% above the normative rate—a significant improvement over the old design. There were 13 assemblies within 15% of the normative rate and 4 assemblies actually were faster than the normative rate. Professionals involved in the pilot study were surprised at the dramatic improvements in performance. They also believed that the majority of the workers could be trained to perform this assembly task with the new design within the normative + 15% time range.

Industry is embracing the use of such design approaches because it is good business practice. By reducing the ergonomic demands of the assembly process and by reducing the cognitive complexity of product assembly, the product is less expensive and of higher quality. Also, the assembly process is made easier and less error-prone for all workers. As with the *kaizen* techniques they have the added benefit of making the assembly process more accessible to individuals with a wider range of physical and cognitive abilities.

The utilization of DFA techniques creates new job opportunities for individuals with disabilities. Assembly jobs which were once not feasible are now becoming increasingly accessible. Job placement specialists, vocational rehabilitation specialists, and those in related professions must become aware of these opportunities.

Process Redesign: Commercial Bakery

The Josephine Brighton Skills Center, Wyandotte, Michigan, provides vocational services to over 200 individuals, 16–25 years old, who have a broad range of physical and cognitive disabilities. The center runs a commercial bakery which produces a variety of cookies and baked goods for the community. After training in *kaizen* and process improvement techniques, staff at the facility decided to re-engineer the bakery's operations. The central goal was to increase worker independence as measured by fewer interventions by bakery staff (Powell, Hardin, & Erlandson, 1998).

The redesigned operations primarily incorporated visual controls, workplace organization, and standardized work procedures. These are overlapping strategies. Visual controls were designed to provide process cues that would direct the employees step-by-step through a process, allow all materials and tools to be identified and located easily, and indicate a place, by icons or shadow diagrams, for everything. For example, all recipe sheets dealing with oatmeal cookies have a green sticker. After baking, the cookies are packaged. Packaging kits were created, identified by color coding, which contained all the materials required for packaging, such as bags, an ink stamp and ink pad for marking "oatmeal cookies" on the bag, and ties.

Materials required for specific tasks such as packing, measuring ingredients, and rolling dough were collected and placed at associated worksites. The worksites were designed to provide a controlled flow of people and materials. Employees entered the bakery, turned left to hang up coats, then proceeded straight ahead to the job board, where the day's job assignments were posted. The job assignments included the employee's name and multiple representations of his/her jobs, a written statement, an icon, and color code. Employees then moved to their respective worksites where essentially all the required materials were located.

This timing and flow of people, the associated visual controls, and workplace organization created a standardized work procedure for the bakery which created a structured, consistent, predictable sequence of activities and actions.

The process redesign had a dramatic impact. As part of the baseline and assessment process, staff had video taped the bakery operations before and after modifications. Since their goal was increased worker independence, they counted the number of staff interventions during three 5-min segments: start-up, halfway through the work period, and clean-up. The number of staff interventions during start-up went from 89 (before) to 3 (after); similar reductions were recorded for the mid-point and clean-up. Staff interventions were reduced because workers could now "read" and follow their recipe cards, workers were more independent in locating and re-shelving tools and materials, and they could independently set up and perform complex operations such as weighing ingredients (Powell et al., 1998).

Productivity increased dramatically. Cookie production rose from about 300 dozen cookies per week with the old process to over 700 dozen cookies per week with the new process (Powell et al., 1998). Such an increase in productivity, without it being a specific objective, is a typical finding.

The staff also noted behavioral changes. The workers demonstrated more pride in their work and exhibited fewer discipline problems. Based on worker comments to staff there was a significant rise in worker self-esteem (Powell et al., 1998).

The *kaizen* techniques used in the bakery reduced the inherent variability of the jobs, rendered the jobs less physically and cognitively demanding, and reduced employee errors and mistakes. The employees were more independent and competent, which led to fewer discipline issues and a dramatic increase in productivity. These are precisely the same effects seen with the application of *kaizen* techniques where the workers are people without disabilities.

Talking Scale: Weighing Task

Services To Enhance Potentials (STEP), a non-profit organization serving approximately 1,000 developmentally disabled adults in Wayne County, Michigan, operated a community employment site at C. Itho. C. Itho is a supplier of building and construction materials located in Detroit, Michigan. The STEP workers were to package 1- and 5-lb boxes of nails. The nails were emptied from a large rotating drum into 1- or 5-lb boxes in approximate weights. STEP workers took the grossly overfilled boxes, placed them onto a large mechanical scale, then added or removed nails to bring the box weight to within specified tolerances. The task required that the worker be able to read and understand the scale dial.

D.J., a 43-year-old woman functioning in the moderate range of mental retardation, was cognitively unable to perform the weighing function on the packaging line. She could not discern from the values on the scale dial whether she should add or remove nails to achieve the desired weight. Many training aids were attempted. For example, the job coach tried color coding, purposeful under- or overfilling, and a digital readout. None of these aids proved successful. The only intervention that worked was verbal prompting provided by a job coach for every weighing attempt. The job coach was essentially doing the job. This intervention was not financially and behaviorally viable for the long term. D.J. did not like having someone always looking over her shoulder, telling her what to do with the product in front of her. She recognized that none of the other workers was getting the same kind of personal attention. She also recognized that her difficulties with the scaling function slowed down the productivity of the line she was working on and felt bad for her coworkers who wanted to produce more (Erlandson & Sant, 1998).

The talking scale configuration consists of a digital scale, a microprocessor-based controller, and a Cheaptalk voice output device (Erlandson & Sant, 1998). The supervisor enters the acceptable low and high weights into the process controller along with a specified prompt time. The prompt time is a period of time for which the controller detects no change in values from the digital scale. If this occurs it is assumed that the worker's attention has wandered. The controller then activates the voice output device to play a message to get the worker's attention back to the task at hand. As material was presented for weighing, the system would prompt her as to whether she should add nails to or remove nails from the box until the specified tolerance was reached.

The talking scale proved to be an effective accommodation for D.J. Her cognitive ability was such that the voice prompting allowed her to perform the task in a timely fashion. She progressed from being unable to perform this task independently to working independently at production rates comparable to her coworkers using mechanical scales. Training with the talking scale system was minimal. Staff demonstrated the system's operations on two boxes and then monitored her work very closely for about half a day. After that she received no more staff attention than her coworkers.

There were many positive results from this successful intervention, one being that D.J.'s self-esteem improved. D.J.'s supervisor reported that "she started to arrive at work smiling every day with a higher level of motivation to work and a more positive attitude" (Erlandson & Sant, 1998). She liked being able to work independently and seemed much more comfortable socializing with her "high producing" coworkers. D.J.'s accuracy proved to be better on average than her coworkers on the mechanical scales due to the digital scale's tare function (accounts for weight of the box) and her ability to respond appropriately and in a timely manner to the cues provided by the system. D.J.'s supervisor also appreciated D.J.'s growing confidence. D.J. no longer exhibited the occasional behaviors from frustration seen prior to using the talking scale. Most significantly, the supervisor really liked being able to depend on D.J. to keep up with her coworkers on the packaging line while maintaining above-average accuracy with little intervention.

The digital scale system is an error-proofing system in that the weight of the empty nail box could be discounted when the scale was configured and hence the weight displayed was the actual weight of the nails. Workers, including D.J., using the digital scale system had zero weight errors. D.J. required the voice prompting to perform at a required level. The voice prompt could be turned off if not required by another worker.

Counting

Visions Unlimited, Farmington Hills, Michigan, is a post-secondary educational program that serves 18–26-year-old young adults with developmental and physical disabilities. Visions Unlimited provides vocational skills training, both on site and at local area businesses. One agreement with a local supermarket was to recycle returnable cans. Workers used can crushers, adapted for single switch use, to crush the cans. The recycling center required 240 crushed cans per container when submitted. Staff at Visions Unlimited tried a variety of techniques to help workers with this counting task. The technique in place prior to intervention replaced counting with pattern recognition. The cans were first crushed then the crushed cans placed into a box or bin. Workers then took the crushed cans and placed them into the 12 holes in plastic muffin containers. It took 20 filled containers to count out the required 240 crushed cans. The stacked-up empty and then filled muffin containers took considerable workbench space. Staff had to check the filled muffin containers to make sure they were all filled and then they had to dump the 240 crushed cans into another container for delivery. Lastly, staff returned the empty muffin containers to a student worksite for the next round of counting.

This procedure prohibited workers from being able to work independently for long periods of time. It required considerable space to store the crushed cans, the empty muffin containers, the filled muffin containers, the empty can collection containers, and the filled can collection containers. The procedure was staff time and energy intensive in non-value-added ways. With the redesigned system a worker places the crushed cans, one at a time onto a small conveyor belt (Erlandson & Sant, 1998). A through-the-beam sensor at the end of the conveyor counts the cans as they fall into the recycling box. When the proper count is reached, the conveyor belt stops, and a voice message indicates the end of the job. Staff can now remove the filled container and restart the counting process.

Staff can configure the Poka-Yoke Controller for the specified number of counts. They can also specify a prompt time for loss of attention messages. If no cans pass through the infrared beam with a moving conveyor belt within the allotted "prompt time," then the controller will activate a prompting device, which, in this case, is a light or voice prompt.

This application required a *poka-yoke* intervention which used a control function—stop the conveyor belt to ensure a proper count. Counting 240 cans is an error-prone job. The *poka-yoke* intervention would ensure error-free operation for any worker. As a result of the *poka-yoke* intervention, the workers were able to work more independently (Erlandson & Sant, 1998). Several of the workers have commented that they really like being able to work independently. Additionally, there were several workers who could not perform this task with the muffin container or other pattern recognition techniques but can perform the counting tasks with this configuration.

The material handling and storage requirements of the new configuration are significantly less than previous methods. Also, staff no longer need to recount the final filled container since the count is accurate. These are significant impacts in terms of staff time and energy and work area space required for the job. This configuration has also been used for a variety of other counting tasks at Visions Unlimited, such as counting and packaging Christmas ornaments, bows, and other products made by students.

This application reiterates the worker-related findings of the previous applications, but also highlights staff-related benefits that have occurred with this and the other applications. With the new process staff did not have to engage in a lot of non-value-added activity. Staff did not have to transport and maintain the empty muffin containers or large inventory of crushed cans. Staff did not have to closely monitor and inspect the work in progress or the finished product. With the new process, staff had the time to engage in more value-added activities. These value-added activities depend on the work environment. In a training environment it can mean more individual staff time with workers needing focused attention. In a competitive work environment it may mean that a job coach is not required or that a supervisor can attend to other duties. Such staff-related benefits are an important consequence and have been consistently observed with all the ETL applications (Erlandson, Kierstein, & McElhone, 1998b; Erlandson, Noblet, & Phelps, 1998a; Erlandson & Phelps, 1993, 1995; Erlandson & Sant, 1998; Powell et al., 1998).

Assembly Operation: Fuel Filter Clamp

The job in this study consisted of placing adhesive back pads onto fuel filter clamps with very little margin for error (Erlandson et al., 1998a). The workers ranged in age from 15 to 22 years and in IQ from 45 to 86. A visual inspection was the only checking used to determine if the rubber pad was properly placed. If the pad was not properly placed, it had to be removed and reapplied. This was a time-consuming task that severely limited daily production rates.

The original fixture, provided by the company subcontracting the work, allowed the metal clamp to be placed onto the supporting structure in several orientations. Improper placement of the clamp increased the likelihood of improper placement of the rubber pad. Also, the metal clamps as supplied by the manufacturer exhibited considerable variation. Hence, even with the clamp placed in the proper orientation, movement of the clamp hindered accurate placement of the sticky-backed pad. The original fixture design made it difficult for everyone to perform this assembly without errors.

From a *kaizen* point of view, the fixture promoted errors rather than hindered them. The fixture introduced considerable variation into the assembly process. While this inherent variation made it difficult for all workers to perform the assembly task, it made it virtually impossible for the workers who have cognitive impairments. The high degree of variability and error promotion features made any kind of standardized work procedure impossible. Under these conditions the workplace organization was of little consequence. The workers tried to avoid this task. They were not pleased with their own work. They tried very hard to perform the task, but the job process itself was too much to overcome.

The fixture was redesigned to accommodate the variability of supplied blank clamps and yet still allow for accurate placement of the pad. The addition of two pad placement guide rails and physical constraints made it impossible to improperly place the metal clamp onto the fixture and concurrently made it possible to precisely place the rubber pad onto the clamp. Data comparing production rates and error rates for individuals with cognitive impairments between use of the old fixture and the new showed that the production rate increased by about 80% and the error rate dropped from above 50% to about 1%. These are dramatic results. More significantly, a large number of individuals who could not perform the assembly task with the old fixture were able to competently perform the task with the new fixture (Erlandson et al., 1998a).

In addition to increased productivity, the supervising staff reported that the workers demonstrated improved morale and motivation to work using the redesigned fixture. The positive impact on workers' self-esteem, feelings of self-worth, and attitude toward work are significant. The participating workers earned more money because they were more productive. They were at their jobs before the starting time, which was rare before the fixture's redesign. The workers started a "1,000" club for workers hitting over 1,000 assemblies in a standard 2-hour work period. At the end of the day workers would "high five" each other because of the high productivity rates (Erlandson et al., 1998a).

The participating individuals were proud of their work. They established their own production goals (Erlandson et al., 1998a). These behaviors followed from their production success. They knew what they did with the old fixture and they knew how much better they were with the new fixture. The workers started to organize their work areas. They personalized use of the fixtures. A number of individuals laid the fixture on its side, others used it upright. Each person had a preferred fixture placement. Workers positioned the blank metal clamps and rubber pads for fast access to get higher production rates.

CONCLUSIONS

Five principles for accessible design were presented. The design should aim to keep both the physical and cognitive demands of the job as low as possible. The design should keep the inherent variability of the job low and incorporate *poka-yoke* interventions to reduce or eliminate job-related errors. Lastly, the design should aggressively seek to minimize non-value-added activities.

The existing legal matrix, which includes the ADA, Section 255 of the Telecommunications Act 1996, and OSHA ergonomic standards, encourage and mandate accessibility and the use of accessible design principles. The QS and ISO quality standards require the use of *kaizen* techniques, which embody accessible design principles. Thus, we have a social and business environment that demands the application of accessible design techniques.

What is not generally recognized is that application of *kaizen* techniques not only produces beneficial business effects but concurrently creates jobs for and improves the job performance of individuals with disabilities. Vocational rehabilitation and job placement specialists need to be aware of this win–win scenario and educate themselves and their respective business contacts to the potential advantages for all concerned.

There is considerable evidence of the benefits of applying *kaizen* techniques in jobs where the workers are people without disabilities. The applications presented in this chapter demonstrate that the use of accessible design principles improves the job performance of workers with disabilities, but, more importantly, jobs were created for individuals with disabilities. The redesigned processes dramatically changed the essential functions of the job so that people who could not perform the job prior to redesign could perform the job at productivity levels acceptable for their employment situations.

A major objective of all the scenarios presented was increased worker independence. In all cases, this objective was achieved. Moreover, in every case there was a dramatic increase in worker productivity. Also, in every application there were significant improvements in the social behavior of the workers with cognitive disabilities. Disruptive behavior decreased, workers were more focused and demonstrated a pride in their work, and, in many cases, the workers set their own higher-than-required production rates. These worker-related changes allowed for significant, positive changes in staff activities. The accessible design changes to the jobs complemented existing human and social supports. The use of accessible design techniques created process supports that complement natural supports and demonstrated a direct impact on productivity.

As mentioned in the Lagomarcino study, slow work rates and the need for continual prompting were two major reasons why persons with mental retardation lost their jobs. The counting and weighing applications illustrate how prompting and pacing can be incorporated with *poka-yoke* and quality control techniques. Also recall from these examples that, as workers with cognitive disabilities improved their job performance, there were positive changes in behavior.

The combined, synergistic impact of process supports as offered by accessible design techniques and traditional social/human supports is the important outcome. This combined approach represents a philosophical shift in worksite accommodations and a movement away from customized worksite modifications targeted at one individual to modifications of the environment, the process, or product that can create job opportunities for a greater number of individuals with disabilities. Furthermore, this approach represents a win–win scenario in that the methods and techniques were designed to improve business performance and the quality of the products and services being offered. This combined approach is not only feasible, but is supported by today's legal and business environments.

ACKNOWLEDGEMENTS.   The work presented was supported by grants from the National Science Foundation (BSE-9707720 and DUE-9972403), and contracts from the Region IV Assistive Technology Consortium. I would also like to acknowledge the editorial support provided by Ms. Kristine Bradow.

REFERENCES

Access Board (1999). *Americans with Disabilities Act accessibility requirements*. Washington, DC: Author.

Boothroyd, G., & Dewhurst, P. (1991). *Product Design for Assembly* (3rd ed.). Wakefield, RI: Boothroyd Dewhurst.

Crow, K. A. (1989). *Design for manufacturability: It's role in world class manufacturing*. Palos Verdes Estates, CA: Defense Resource Management Associates.

Deming, W. E. (1982). *Out of crisis* (15th ed.). Cambridge, MA: Massachusetts Institute of Technology.

Dingwelki, D. (1988). Design for manufacturability, Paper presented at the Second International Conference on Design for Manufacturability: Building in quality. Orlando, FL.

Eppinger, E., Whitney, D. E., Smith, R. P., & Gebala, D. (1990). *Organizing the tasks in complex design projects*. Cambridge, MA: Massachusetts institute of Technology.

Erlandson, R. F., Bradow, K., & Sant, D. (1999, January 11). *Enabling Technologies Laboratory web site: Resources.* Available: ecc.eng.wayne.edu/etl.

Erlandson, R. F., Kierstein, I., & McElhone, D. (1998b, March 5–7). *Assembly techniques to sheltered workshops and community worksites: Working smarter not harder.* Paper presented at the Council on Exceptional Children Annual State Conference, Grand Rapids, MI.

Erlandson, R. F., Noblet, M. J., & Phelps, J. A. (1998a). Impact of Poka-Yoke device on job performance of individuals with cognitive impairments. *IEEE Transactions on Rehabilitation Engineering, 6*(3), 269–276.

Erlandson, R. F., & Phelps, J. A. (1993). *Mechatronic systems As vocational enablers for persons with severe multiple handicapps.* Paper presented at the Proceedings of the RESNA '93 Annual Conference, Las Vegas.

Erlandson, R. F., & Phelps, J. A., (1995, June 11–16). *Simplification of essential functions using design for assembly techniques.* Paper presented at the RESNA '95 annual conference, Vancouver, BC.

Erlandson, R. F., & Sant, D. (1998). Poka-Yoke process controller designed for individuals with cognitive impairments. *Assistive Technology, 10,* 102–112.

Fabian, E. S., Edelman, A., & Leedy, M. (1993). Linking workers with severe disabilities to social supports in the workplace: Strategies for addressing barriers. *Journal of Rehabilitation, July/August/September* 29–34.

Federal Communications Commission (1999, November 19). Access to telecommunications service, telecommunications equipment and customer premises equipment by persons with disabilities. *Federal Register, 64*(223), 63235–63258.

Gardner, R. (1989). Sapphire introduces design for assembly software for the Mac. *MacWeek, December 12.*

Gold, M. (1968). Preworkshop skills for the trainable: A sequential technique. *Education and Training of the Mentally Retarded, 3,* 31–37.

Gold, M. (1972). Stimulus factors in skill training of the retarded on a complex assembly task: Acquisition, transfer, and retention. *American Journal of Mental Deficiency, 76,* 517–526.

Gold, M. (Ed.) (1973). *Research on the vocational habilitation of the retarded: The present, the future* (Vol. 6). New York, NY: Academic Press.

Grandjean, E. (1991). *Fitting the task to the man* (4th ed.). New York, NY: Taylor & Francis.

Greenspan, S., & Shoultz, B. (1981). Why mentally retarded adults lose their jobs: Social competence as a factor in work adjustment. *Applied Research in Mental Retardation, 2*(10), 23–38.

Hagner, D., Rogan, P., & Murphy, S. (1992). Facilitating natural supports in the workplace: Strategies for support consultants. *Journal of Rehabilitation, January/February/March,* 29–34.

Hammer, M. (1990). Reengineering Work: Don't automate, obliterate. *Harvard Business Review, July/August,* 104–112.

Hanley-Maxwell, C., Rusch, F. R., Chadsey-Rusch, J., & Renzaglia, A. (1986). Reported factors contributing to job termination of individuals with severe disabilities. *JASH, 11*(1), 45–52.

Hoyle, D. (1997). *QS 9000 quality systems handbook.* Newton, MA: Butterworth–Heinemann.

Imai, M. (1986). *Kaizen* (1st ed.). New York, NY: McGraw-Hill.

Imai, M. (1997). *Gemba Kaizen* (1st ed.). New York, NY: McGraw-Hill.

Ishiwata, J. (1991). *I.E. for the shop floor 1: Productivity through process analysis.* Cambridge, MA: Productivity Press.

Japan Human Relations Association (Ed.) (1992). *Kaizen Teian 2* (1st English ed.). Portland, OH: Productivity Press.

Lagomarcino, T. R. (1990). Job separation issues in supported employment. In F. R. Rusch (Ed.), *Supported employment models, methods, and issues* (pp. 301–316). Sycamore, IL: Sycamore.

Lagomarcino, T. R., & Rusch, F. R. (1988). Competitive employment: Overview and analysis of research focus. In V. B. VanHasselt, S. Strain & M. Hersen (Eds.), *Handbook of developmental and physical disabilities* (pp. 150–158). New York, NY: Pergamon Press.

Lindskoog, W. (1987). *VECTOR a new direction: Excellence in education* (Final report) (ERIC Document Reproduction Service No. ED 293 234). Minneapolis, MN: Hennepin Technical Centers.

National Institute on Disability and Rehabilitation Research (1992). *ADA; Q&A—The Americans with Disabilities Act: Questions and answers.* Washington, DC: U.S. Department of Justice Civil Rights Division, U.S. Equal Employment Opportunity Commission.

Noel, R. T. (1990). Employing the disabled: A how and why approach. *Training and Development Journal, 44*(8), 26–32.

Occupational Safety and Health Administration (1999). Ergonomics program: Proposed rule. *Federal Register, 64*(225), 65768–66078.

Peach, R. W., & Ritter, D. S. (1996). *The memory jogger 9000.* Methuen, MA: GOAL/QPC.

Poli, C., Graves, R., & Groppetti, R. (1986, August 21). Rating products for ease of assembly. *Machine Design.*

Powell, K., Hardin, S., & Erlandson, R. F. (1998, October 23). *Stop the juggling act: Structure for success.* Paper presented at the Closing the Gap, St Paul, MN.

Randal, R. C. (1995). *Randall's practical guide to ISO 9000: Implementation, registration, and beyond.* Reading, MA: Addison-Wesley.

Rasmussen, J. (1986). *Information processing and human–machine interaction: An approach to cognitive engineering* (Vol. 12). New York, NY: North–Holland.

Ringwelski, D. (1998, November 13–15). Paper presented at the the Second International Conference on Design for Manufacturability: Building in Quality. Orlando, FL.

Shimbun, N. K. (Ed.) (1988). *Poka-yoke: Improving product quality by preventing defects.* Cambridge, MA: Productivity Press.

Shingo, S. (1986). *Zero quality control: Source inspection and the Poka-Yoke system.* Portland, OR: Productivity Press.

Sowers, J., & Powwers, L. (1991). *Vocational preparation and employment of students with physical and multiple disabilities.* Baltimore, MA: Paul H. Brookes.

Tidd, J. (1991). *Flexible manufacturing technologies and international competitiveness.* London, UK: Pinter.

Wiest, M. D., & Kregel, J. (1977). *A management guide to PERT/CPM* (2nd ed.). Englewood Cliffs, NJ: Prentice-Hall.

Womack, J. P., Jones, D. T., & Roos, D. (1990). *The machine that changed the world.* New York, NY: Harper-Collins.

Woods, D. D., & Roth, E. M. (1988). Cognitive systems engineering. In M. Helander (Ed.), *Handbook of human–computer interaction* (pp. 3–43). New York, NY: North–Holland.

CHAPTER 20

Clinical Interventions into Employment-Related Mental Health Concerns

MELVYN RAIDER, ALISON FAVORINI, AND MARGARET BRUNHOFER

INTRODUCTION

Based on the National Co-Morbidity Survey, fully 30% of the U.S. population are diagnosable with a mental health or substance abuse disorder in any given year (Kessler et al., 1994). Many of these individuals are in the workforce. For example, about 60% of those with a diagnosis of depression work full time or part time (Rouse, 1998). Estimated costs to the workplace of untreated mental health conditions are about $150 billion a year (Rouse, 1998). Furthermore, according to the National Alliance for the Mentally Ill (NAMI), the number one reason for hospital admissions in the United States is a psychiatric condition. In addition, there are millions of individuals with alcohol, drug abuse, or mental health conditions associated with job-related stress due to downsizing, job reconfiguration, plant closings, and other changes.

This chapter addresses interventions for people with stress-related mental health problems generated in large part by work-related factors, and secondarily with pre-existing mental health conditions exacerbated by, and possibly disruptive of, the workplace.[1] Owing to the increasing difficulty in accessing long-term or more intensive treatment, our focus is primarily on briefer treatments. The chapter aims to:

1. describe the types and sources of workplace stress;
2. discuss the bi-directional causal influences of workplace stresses on mental health and well-being, and of mental health status on the workplace; and
3. describe the primary clinical interventions used for work-related mental health problems, focusing on short-term and brief approaches.

[1]Substance abuse is dealt with in Chapters 26 and 27.

MELVYN RAIDER AND MARGARET BRUNHOFER • Wayne State University School of Social Work, Detroit, Michigan. ALISON FAVORINI • Huntington Woods, Michigan.

The primary clinical interventions discussed are time-limited psychotherapy, crisis intervention, and brief ego supportive therapy, each with an illustrative case vignette. A cross-cutting and particularly useful set of strategies to improve stress-coping—skill development techniques—can be employed within each of these modalities and will also be discussed.

EMPLOYMENT-RELATED MENTAL HEALTH PROBLEMS

Factors in Job Stress

Because so much of our time is spent at work and we define ourselves in terms of our careers, job stresses and pressures can affect the mental health and well-being of any employee, not just those with pre-existing mental health problems. According to Kahn and Aidinoff (1999, p. 12), "the workplace is a frequent source of physical and psychological stressors that trigger emotional disorders, and … is frequently where emotional disorders produce symptoms and reduced function." Following Ross and Altmaier (1994), we define *occupational stress* as "the interaction of work conditions with characteristics of the worker such that the demands of work exceed the ability of the worker to cope with them" (p. 12).

While much of the occupational research literature has focused on job satisfaction and commitment, investigators have also examined the impact of job stress and workplace characteristics on mental and physical health (Caplan & Jones, 1975; Ivancevich, 1986; Karasek, Gardell, & Lindell, 1987; LaRocco, House, & French, 1980; Margolis, Kroes, & Quinn, 1974). This research stems from the perspective of the *person-in-environment* model or, more narrowly, person–role fit.

JOB AND ROLE CHARACTERISTICS. Many aspects of jobs have been studied for their possible role as stressors for individuals. These include work overload or underload, role ambiguity, role conflict, work pace, task repetitiveness or variety, social interaction required, degree of responsibility, and the control workers have over their work—autonomy (Ross & Altmaier, 1994). These job characteristics interact with individual traits to produce a variety of stress-strain reactions on the job. French (1973) conceptualized this as *person–role fit*, defined as the fit of the individual's skills to job demands and the degree to which the individual's needs are fulfilled by the job environment. Either form of misfit can cause job dissatisfaction and mental health strain (French, 1973). Under the adverse organizational conditions described later, poor person–role fit can become widespread.

Research has confirmed that work overload, role ambiguity or conflict, task repetitiveness, and lack of control over the job do, in fact, increase stress and decrease job satisfaction (Karasek et al., 1987). In a study of air traffic controllers, Tattersal and Farmer (1995) reported that workload and organization climate strongly predicted job stress, and higher workload adversely affected mental health. Lack of control over job conditions and performance has been identified as one of the key factors in stress-related physical and mental health disorders (Margolis et al., 1974; Karasek, 1979; House, McMichael, Wells, Kaplan, & Landerman, 1979).

PERSONAL CHARACTERISTICS. Personal traits have received less attention than job and organizational factors as antecedents or moderators of job stress. Both *demographic factors*—age, gender, education, job status, job tenure—and *personality traits*—type A behavior, locus/sense of control, self-esteem—have been studied (Jackson & Schuler, 1985; Ross & Altmaier, 1994). Emotional problems have not often been examined in the organizational literature except as dependent variables; their status as complicating factors in stress and job difficulties will be discussed later in the chapter. Job stress is less often reported by older, longer tenured, better educated, and higher level employees, and job satisfaction is higher (Billings & Moos, 1982; Jackson & Schuler, 1985). These demographic factors thus may be moderating variables that diminish job-related stress or enhance coping skills. Women are more likely to experience work–family role conflict than are men (Wortman, Biernat, & Lang, 1991) and have more spillover of job stress into family life (Ross & Altmaier, 1994). Type A personality is associated with emotional distress (House et al., 1979) and low self-esteem with role ambiguity (Jackson & Schuler, 1985). For personality traits, two-way causality may well be operating.

ORGANIZATIONAL CONTEXT FACTORS. These factors may be ongoing characteristics of the organization—organizational climate and management style—or due to events within the organization.

Organizational Climate. Climate factors generating job stress include high production pressures or competitiveness, poor communication (leading to role ambiguity and uncertainty), adversarial labor-management relations, widespread discrimination and harassment, and significant interpersonal conflict at the workplace. Also important are how career transitions, training, and career development are dealt with in the organization (Lowman, 1993).

Organizational Events. These events include downsizing, mergers and acquisitions, workplace violence, serious accidents, significant technology changes, and mandatory overtime. Mergers and acquisitions, for example, result in new reporting arrangements, organizational goal changes, layoffs, and job insecurity, and can generate role ambiguities and job conflict (Kent, 1999). Organizational events can cause long-term or short-term change in other job-related factors influencing stress (e.g., organizational climate and job conditions). Accidents and workplace violence often cause post-traumatic stress disorder (PTSD).

Supervisory Style. Research suggests that supervisors who create structure for their employees, but are also considerate of them, have less stressed and more satisfied employees. Clear communication of expectations and regular performance feedback cut down on role ambiguity and fear of termination, and may diminish job conflict (Jackson & Schuler, 1985; Ross & Altmaier, 1994). Higher stress due to a maladaptive supervisory style could result in chronically high cortisol[2] levels in employees, further contributing to difficulties handling stress (Ember, 1998).

SOCIETAL TRENDS CONTRIBUTING TO JOB STRESS. The global economy has precipitated downsizing and mergers, in turn creating more individual stressors such as job loss or insecurity. Our society is now experiencing more income inequality than at any time in the past 50 years and more than other industrialized nations (Mishel, Bernstein, & Schmitt, 1997). As a result, many couples both work of necessity and not by choice, in turn escalating childcare and work–family issues. Other job-related stress factors are inadequate health benefits and the frightening workplace and community violence that scars so many communities. Such factors compound stress already felt by employees.

---

[2]Increased cortisol is a byproduct of stress and is produced by the adrenal glands. It is a known factor in depression.

Lowman (1993) describes a case which illustrates the impact of many job stressors noted here and also suggests a different line of treatment. Paul was a manager referred for depression after moving from private to public-sector work. Paul's department oversaw an industry that was in decline, and he had to lay off several people. The agency gave managers very little autonomy and yet expected departments to show a positive balance sheet.[3] Paul's loss of control over work conditions led to a sense of helplessness and situational depression. Antidepressants were not effective for Paul, but a solution-focused intervention geared to the job situation proved beneficial.

Prior Mental Health Problems: Interactions with Job Stress and Performance

Other individuals are more vulnerable to stress by nature or show behavior patterns that can produce work dysfunction. Adult children of alcoholics (ACOAs) are often perfectionistic and have a strong desire to control their environment, due to having lived in a chaotic family of origin (Woititz, 1983). Frequently they make very dedicated employees, but these traits can result in conflict with other employees who resent their efforts to control others' behavior. Individuals with Type A behavior patterns are usually overly committed to work and impatient with others, putting the employee at risk for burnout. While not formal diagnoses, these traits generate stress that annoy or antagonize others and can even trigger the development of mental illness in predisposed individuals.

Employees with mental health diagnoses are more vulnerable to stress and may show behavior patterns that create stress, as well. For example, depression is associated with increased cortisol levels and an exaggerated stress response (Ember, 1998). Employees with depression need to pace themselves, not overwork, and develop social supports (Billings & Moos, 1984). Individuals with any of the mental health diagnoses discussed here often need to develop "stress hardiness" (Maddi & Kobasa, 1991) and can benefit from the therapeutic approaches described here, as well as from medication. Those with obsessive compulsive personality disorder (OCPD)[4] or traits may be overly rigid about how tasks should be done, may have trouble with teamwork, or take too long to complete projects. Bipolar individuals may show erratic behavior that puzzles coworkers. When hypomanic, the employee may be productive and optimistic but can also become irritable, grandiose, or obsessive. When depressed, bipolar and unipolar employees may miss work, have trouble concentrating, and be far less productive. Many of these individuals are productive and dedicated employees when not in acute episodes.

Employees with anxiety disorders may be burdened with occasional panic attacks at work or suffer from performance anxiety. Those with borderline personality often have trouble functioning independently and may become overly attached to a coworker or supervisor and later lash out at them. Resentment of authority can be a feature in many types of mental illness. Individuals with personality disorders, for example, narcissism, are often insensitive to or unaware of how their behavior affects others, causing job conflict or avoidance by others (Lowman, 1993). Impulse control problems often occur in hypomanic or manic workers, with antisocial personality, in head trauma victims, and in alcoholics not in recovery.

---

[3]Any resemblance between this scenario and the mental health system is purely coincidental....
[4]OCPD is less severe than OCD, which manifests repetitive compulsive actions and is brain-based.

CLINICAL INTERVENTIONS

Time-Limited Therapies

Time-limited psychotherapy is rapidly becoming the treatment method of choice in employment-related mental health problems. Although family therapists and social workers have been using short-term or brief models of treatment since the 1970s, they have gained widespread adherents since the proliferation of managed care in the late 1980s and 1990s. For many years, family therapists utilized strategic and solution-oriented therapies (Haley, 1976) because they believed such approaches were more effective than more lengthy treatments. Similarly, social workers utilized task-centered casework and related approaches (Reid & Epstein, 1972) for the same reasons. In contrast, many practitioners on panels of managed care organizations use brief therapy models because managed care organizations limit the number of sessions subscribers are entitled to have. Today, time-limited therapy consists of many psychotherapeutic approaches which have in common the use of relatively few therapy sessions, usually less than 20 (Fanger, 1995).

COMPONENTS OF BRIEF THERAPY.   Assessment is a key component of all therapeutic models and typically includes appraisal of both person and environmental variables. In brief therapy, this process focuses on the presenting concern, its duration, and coping methods used by the client to manage the resulting distress. The practitioner engages in limited exploration of past experiences and attempts to gain an understanding of the client's strengths and resources. Behavior and psychiatric rating scales (e.g., SCL-90-R, the Clinical Global Impressions Scale, Montgomery–Asberg Depression Rating Scale, and the Beck Depression Inventory—II[5]) may be used to gain information in a rapid manner. The practitioner should include analysis of the work situation and history as part of the assessment to pinpoint client behavior or cognition needing modification, and to identify stressful work conditions (Kahn & Aidinoff, 1999). It is also desirable to gauge the attitudes of supervisors and coworkers to the employee's mental illness, if feasible,[6] and assist the employee with explaining the condition and obtaining job accommodations.

Time-limited therapies generally have a number of defining characteristics. They are symptom focused, goal directed, problem-solving, focus on person–environment fit, have a delimited definition of the target of therapy, utilize active intervention, and often have measurable outcomes. Some brief therapies also utilize homework assignments between sessions, seek to alter cognitions, and help clients develop coping skills and strategies.

The most important therapeutic task of time-limited therapies is helping clients to identify specifically what they hope to accomplish in treatment. This is designed not only to help motivate the client to actively pursue change but also to serve as a framework to keep therapy focused. A written or oral treatment plan clearly specifying the goal(s) of treatment is often utilized.

Time-limited therapies seek to help clients resolve specific symptoms or problems which are obstacles to normal functioning in the client's social environment. Even though the solution to a problem may eventually lead to client growth or personality change, the intent is more modest. The intent is to help clients manage or resolve a problem which is causing

[5]See Derogatis (1977) re the SCL-90-R. The CGI is now available for bipolar illness (Spearing, Post, Leverich, Brandt, & Nolan, 1997). See Muller, Szegedi, Wetzel, and Benkert (2000) on the MADRS and contact the Psychological Corp. at 1-800-211-9378 about the BDI-II.

[6]A therapist or EAP counselor must have client consent to talk with a supervisor; client can also assess these attitudes.

uncomfortable symptoms and stresses. Unlike long-term therapies which focus on resolution of intrapsychic conflicts, time-limited therapies "often use a developmental model of change wherein the task of therapy is seen as helping clients overcome a particular developmental snag and then resume their lives" (Fanger, 1995, p. 325).

The client's definition of the problem and the client's priorities in resolving the problem are generally accepted in time-limited therapy models. Clients are active participants in establishing a plan of treatment and agree to take an active role in working toward managing or solving the problem. Time-limited therapies are often regarded as respectful therapies since they view the client as an expert with regard to knowing they are motivated to change.

For time-limited therapies derived from a cognitive–behavioral framework, goals are established that have measurable outcomes. Clients may be asked how they would know they are ready to terminate treatment. Generally, the problem to be changed must be defined in a solvable form. "It should be something that can be objectively agreed upon, e.g., counted, observed, or measured, so that one can assess if it has actually been influenced" (Stanton, 1981). Measurable goals help to keep therapy on task by avoiding goals which are too ambitious, vague, or unachievable.

By definition, time-limited therapies limit the length of the treatment period. Therefore, goals of change must be attainable in that time frame. Time-limited therapies generally operate from either a systemic perspective or a psychodynamic perspective. For those therapies operating from a systemic perspective, a small change influences the family or social system which in turn affects the client and produces larger change. Eventually small changes may produce larger systemic changes. Psychodynamic therapy utilizes client strengths and available resources to bolster adaptive capacity.

In some time-limited therapies, clients are encouraged to carry out an activity or accomplish a task between therapy sessions. These are labeled "homework assignments." Homework assignments are agreed upon by both client and therapist, and there is a verbal contract in which the client commits to task accomplishment. The use of homework assignments potentially increases the likelihood of achieving treatment goals in a time-efficient manner. They also help the client to develop skills to solve the problem while the therapist is available to serve as coach and teacher.

The therapist's role in many time-limited therapies is that of one who is knowledgeable about the change process. Therapists help to develop coping skills and strategies, as well as to educate and coach their clients. They also serve as facilitators helping to structure the solving of problems. In order to accomplish client problem-solving, therapists often reframe and seek to alter dysfunctional cognitions. Clients are encouraged to avoid focusing on negative emotions and to take action to do something about the problem. In brief ego supportive therapies, insight into intrapsychic processes may emerge, but insight is not a major focus of therapy. In some time-limited therapies, therapists rely on a cognitive–behavioral approach in which change occurs as a result of new behaviors or reframing of beliefs rather than as a result of insight or awareness of one's defenses or personality structures.

CASE VIGNETTE—TIME-LIMITED THERAPY. Bob held the position of Assistant to the Vice President of Marketing of a large telecommunications company. He was in his late fifties and his wife had recently retired from her job as a teacher of high school science. His wife Miriam was a golf enthusiast and, after retiring with a generous pension from the school district, she hoped to relocate to a golf club retirement community in Scottsville, Arizona. Miriam was encouraging Bob to retire also so that they could sell their home in the Northeast and move to Arizona. Bob had occupied his position for 30 years and was totally committed to his work. He couldn't imagine himself not going to the office each day and was not confident that the Vice President could manage without him, signs of a possible Type A personality. He contacted his Employee Assistance Program (EAP) representative after he developed sleep problems, aphasia and, most recently, panic attacks. The representative referred Bob to a local outpatient mental health clinic. His managed care provider limited his psychotherapy to eight sessions.

Bob's therapist asked him to complete a brief questionnaire called the EAPI (*Employee Assistance Program Inventory*; Anton & Reed, 1994) and was able to hypothesize that many of his symptoms were related to anxiety stemming from his perceived loss of identity if he were to retire. Bob was caught in a bind. He wanted to please his wife as well as meet his own needs for status, purpose, and self-actualization.

The therapist asked Bob to imagine that he awoke the next morning and his problem had been resolved. She asked him to describe the details of what this would be like. Bob responded by indicating that his wife would not continue to pressure him to retire and he would be able to continue in his current position for several more years. The therapist asked Bob what it would take for his wife to stop pressuring him to retire. The answer to that question became the problem-solving framework Bob developed over the next few sessions to seek a compromise solution that would enable Miriam to meet her needs. It would also enable Bob to rekindle his interest in writing fiction, an interest he abandoned some time ago. Bob could work more slowly toward retirement while developing an identity and sense of self-worth that was not exclusively related to his career. Within several months, Bob's symptoms were significantly reduced.

Crisis Intervention

In response to the stresses and challenges created by work and employment, a brief therapy most likely to be of benefit to the employee is Crisis Intervention. Workplace events most likely to precipitate a crisis are situational and are often uncommon and extraordinary events that an employee has no way of forecasting or controlling (Gillilard & James, 1993). Examples include an industrial or work-related accident; corporate buyout or loss of employment; transfer, change of shift, hours of work, or duties and responsibilities; work-related critical illness or injury; and violence in the workplace such as murder, kidnapping, random shooting, assault, and rape. These events are shocking, sudden, intense, and catastrophic.

Other precipitant events are developmental, characterized by the employee moving through stages of the life cycle. Examples include promotion, changes in the direction of a career, and retirement. Some events precipitating a crisis may be work-related or family-related psychological and emotional anxieties and conflicts. Examples include job stress and burnout, sexual harassment, competition among work groups, supervisor relationships, and job demands versus family responsibilities. It is important to keep in mind that individuals in the workplace perceive these events through their own perceptual system. What may be viewed as a crisis by one person may not be perceived the same way by another employee. Individuals possess different coping skills and environmental resources. Therefore, the perception of a crisis is unique to each individual.

Kathleen Ell describes a crisis as "a severe emotional upset, frequently accompanied by feelings of confusion, anxiety, depression, anger and disorganization in usual relationships and social functioning" (Ell, 1995, p. 661). Slaiken (1990) points out that the crisis state is evidenced by increased psychological vulnerability, reduced defensiveness, and a severe breakdown in coping and problem-solving ability. Potential dysfunctional responses of an individual in crisis are: (1) emotional detachment, coldness, and aloofness, (2) emotional explosiveness and unpredictability, (3) helplessness, (4) unwillingness to communicate, (5) unwillingness to ask for or accept help, (6) inability to examine alternatives to old ways of coping, (7) inability to make decisions or solve problems, (8) inability to alter roles, responsibilities, or expectations during crises, (9) scapegoating and blaming, (10) substance abuse, and (11) denial and withdrawal (Steele & Raider, 1991). Crises usually are six to eight weeks in duration.

Crisis intervention strategies and techniques "are distinguished from other forms of psychologically focused brief treatments in the extent to which the intervention focuses on breakdown of individual or family coping in the presence of a distinguishable precipitant event" (Ell, 1995, p. 662). Practice principles are derived from a range of theoretical frameworks, including psychodynamic, cognitive–behavioral, problem-solving, and systemic theoretical frameworks.

PHASES OF CRISIS INTERVENTION.   There are essentially eight phases or components of crisis intervention. Although it may appear that the practitioner should proceed through each phase sequentially, in practice this is not possible. The practitioner will move in and out of different phases, depending upon circumstances, but upon completion of the process will have touched upon each phase or component. Some sessions may focus more on specific phases than others.

The first phase focuses on structuring the interviews to clarify ground rules, roles, responsibilities, and expectations. The therapist seeks to establish their credibility while working toward minimizing further breakdown of adaptive capacities. Other tasks of this phase are to define the parameters of the crisis intervention and the type of interaction expected between practitioner and client. The most important task of the first phase is to help the employee commit to working on the crisis to manage the situation or solve the problem.

The second phase is concerned with understanding how the client perceives the crisis and the nature of the problem. In doing so, it is important to identify ways in which the client may be distorting perceived causes of the crisis, as well as threats the crisis is precipitating. It must be kept in mind that the client's perceptions may not reflect objective observations of the presenting problem. Perceptions, however, do reflect the client's own sense of what is real. It is this perception of the problem that initiates a client's responses to a crisis situation. The primary therapeutic task is to reframe the problem or change the client's cognitions of the problem.

In phase three the practitioner compares the client's perception of the crisis with a more objective description. The practitioner's understanding of the nature of the crisis and its causes, coupled with his or her sense of the client's perception of it, will help the intervention to become more focused and result in clearer, more realistic expectations of what can be accomplished.

Phase four focuses on gaining an understanding of the client's family system, and social and community environment. This phase enables the therapist to further identify those factors that will either become potential barriers to resolution or enhance the likelihood of a healthy resolution of the crisis. Phases two, three, and four become the basis for the initial assessment.

Phase five is concerned with assessing the potential for suicide or homicide or other destructive or assaultive behavior. In any crisis, hopelessness and decompensation may create the potential for behavior which puts the client or others at risk, and therefore must always be addressed. When the potential for homicide or suicide exists, providing whatever safeguards are possible becomes the first order of business.

The focus of phase six is to normalize emotional responses to the crisis, thereby minimizing anxiety related to loss of control. It is critical to those in crisis to understand that their reactions are not unlike reactions others have had in similar situations. Clients need to accept their emotional reactions as normal reactions to fear, vulnerability, and a sense of powerlessness and hopelessness. Next, it is important to provide an explanation of the crisis situation that suggests the crisis can be stabilized, resolved, or managed. This is essentially cognitive reframing or restructuring of the crisis situation.

Phase seven involves engaging the client in the problem-solving process. First the client must be helped to understand that developing problem-solving skills offers the mechanism with which he/she may manage or resolve the crisis. Next, clients need to be helped to develop problem-solving skills, which is primarily an educative task. When an individual is in crisis, effective solutions are often not obvious. Clients must be assisted in identifying what might appear to the practitioner to be very obvious solutions. Clients need to be taught how to go about using problem-solving skills when their usual methods of coping are ineffective.

The final phase of crisis intervention involves rehearsing the chosen solution and setting a timetable for implementation. Rehearsing the chosen solution is a behavioral intervention which builds confidence and empowers the client to understand the specific steps necessary to carry out the solution.

CASE VIGNETTE—CRISIS INTERVENTION. John contacted the company's EAP representative due to his heightened anxiety and inability to focus on his work. He was highly distressed after learning that his former wife, the custodial parent of his only child, had left the state and abandoned their 13-year-old son. He was overwhelmed with concerns for his son, and also with a resurgence of painful memories about his own experience with childhood abandonment. He was particularly concerned about how these reactions interfered with his concentration on work assignments. Recently he had received a reprimand from his supervisor for marginal performance on an important assignment. He feared his current preoccupation with this personal crisis would interfere with his performance on another major assignment.

During the initial meeting the practitioner clarified John's expectation about crisis services and focused on understanding John's fears and concerns for his son while assessing his psychosocial functioning. Active listening, empathy, and interest in the client were interventions used to develop the therapeutic alliance. John was encouraged to describe his perception of the crisis and its impact on his son. With pressured, rapid speech, he discussed his anger and outrage with his former wife and his own experience of abandonment. The practitioner provided this opportunity for John to ventilate his feelings and describe his concerns. Then, in response to the practitioner's questions, John described his son's reactions to his mother's abandonment and his own observations of his son's behavior.

During this session the practitioner assessed John's coping capacities by clarifying his functioning at work, his reality testing and problem-solving skills, eating and sleeping patterns, potential for suicide, and his social support network. The practitioner acknowledged the anguish that John demonstrated as he discussed his own and his son's abandonment and normalized the range of feelings John experienced. John was engaged in the problem-solving process and helped to identify ways to assist his son in coping with his mother's absence. His role as a concerned and supportive parent was underscored. The practitioner described normative emotional and behavioral reactions to his son's loss in an effort to educate and assist John in helping his son. Differences between his own experience with maternal abandonment and his son's current situation were stressed. John appeared relieved and seemed less distressed.

As a result of the crisis intervention, he was able to manage this difficult, unexpected life event and quickly returned to his former level of job performance.

Skill Development Training

Skill development training is proactive and can be used with any of the three therapeutic approaches discussed here. It is designed to equip employees with stress-coping skills to (1) change the stressful situation, (2) reappraise stressors and resources, or (3) change arousal under stress (Folkman & Lazarus, 1991; Lowman, 1993). Strategies addressing these three phases of the stress response process are useful in ameliorating job conflict or other problems dealing with supervisors and coworkers. Often the employee is not fully aware of what situations trigger the stressful reactions or does not know how to identify emotional strain until it is overwhelming. Therefore, a first step is *identifying stress–strain patterns* using a stress diary, which helps break the pattern into small steps to identify triggers and points of intervention. Relaxation training can also help people become aware of when they are tense.

CHANGING THE STRESSFUL SITUATION.   Several studies have found that action to change the situation, based on problem-solving strategies, is more effective than avoiding or denying the stress (Billings & Moos, 1984; Koeske, Kirk & Koeske, 1993; Latack, 1986; Shined & Morch, 1983).

Approaches which can be directed to preventing or ameliorating stressful situations are assertiveness training, social skills training, and problem-solving skills training. A major focus in all three of these approaches is improving communication skills. In *assertiveness training*, clients learn that they have a right to say "no," and they role-play specific techniques of doing so such as the "broken record" and "fogging." They learn the differences between passive, aggressive, and assertive communication, and that others are not necessarily entitled to a reason why they cannot or wish not to do what is asked. These techniques can be especially useful in harassment situations.

Social skills training is valuable for those with limited workplace communication skills—anxious or shy clients and those with social skills deficits or poor social supports. Typical skills learned include initiating and maintaining conversations, making and refusing requests, giving and receiving criticism or compliments, and interpreting non-verbal behavior. Instructional methods include modeling behavior, role-playing, "homework" assignments, and feedback (Lowman, 1993).

Problem-solving skills training employs cognitive–behavioral strategies and breaks the process down into discrete steps. The focus is on generating a solution that meets everyone's needs and not on winning. The training is especially useful for supervisors, impulsive individuals, and work environments involving extensive teamwork. Participants are encouraged to analyze problems, brainstorm action options, and consider consequences of actions before acting.

CHANGING APPRAISAL OF STRESSORS.   A second set of strategies focuses on changing appraisal of stressors and coping resources by using cognitive–behavioral techniques, thus transforming a perceived threat into a challenge. One technique is to ask the client to imagine the worst possible consequence of a stressful event and then assist them in developing a more effective and reality-based approach to the problem. In *cognitive restructuring*, individuals are encouraged to change irrational beliefs and replace dysfunctional cognitions (beliefs, thoughts) with functional ones. This process may involve taking responsibility for their own feelings and recognizing that they cannot control the actions of others. *Stress innoculation training*, developed by Meichenbaum, combines these cognitive techniques with coping skills training and behavioral rehearsal. Positive self-talk is used to counteract negative beliefs (Lowman, 1993).

CHANGING EMOTIONAL AROUSAL.   Emotional arousal can be reduced by the approaches described above, but several techniques *directly* target emotional arousal both during stressful situations and preventively (cf. Folkman & Lazarus, 1991). Deep breathing, muscle relaxation, meditation, guided imagery, biofeedback training, and exercise are all methods for increasing stress tolerance by reducing emotional reactions (Lowman, 1993). The techniques should be practiced regularly for best effect.

Anger management training is productive for individuals prone to angry outbursts. Individuals are assisted in identifying triggers for their anger and paying attention to early warning signs of mounting anger. This training is very useful for workplace violence prevention and reduction of job conflict. Skill development, cognitive restructuring, relaxation training, and desensitization to triggers are used jointly to facilitate more successful ways of dealing with stress without angry outbursts (Puig, 1995). Similar strategies can be used to assist people in managing other emotions such as panic or depressive reactions to situations.

While skill development may be used more frequently in time-limited approaches and crisis intervention, it can be used as an adjunct to ego supportive therapy.

CASE VIGNETTE—SKILL DEVELOPMENT TRAINING.   George was a 51-year-old male employed as a mechanic in an automotive plant. He had experienced a traumatic brain injury after a fall at work. As a result of the injury, George was prone to angry outbursts. At times he would throw his tools, or yell and curse at coworkers. He was fearful that he would be terminated and requested help from his EAP representative. Following an assessment of his work difficulties, the practitioner and George focused on anger management techniques. He was offered encouragement that he could develop skills to manage his anger and decrease the outbursts. Work with George focused on identifying triggers to his loss of control. Through examination of his work performance and prior angry outbursts, he identified his difficulty with assignments that required immediate attention and inspection by his supervisor. George was instructed in "time-out" techniques. He learned to retire to his work cubicle for 10–20 minutes and focus on calming himself. He was instructed to take short walks around the plant to decrease his tension and agitation. George used these methods successfully and reported fewer episodes of loss of control.

Brief Ego Supportive Therapy

Brief ego supportive therapy is derived from more traditional, intensive psychodynamic therapy. In order to understand brief ego supportive therapy, it is necessary to summarize the important attributes of intensive psychodynamic psychotherapy. Intensive therapy focuses on understanding the client's current life difficulties in terms of past experience with significant others. Basic propositions of this perspective assert that individuals develop internalized images of significant figures during early development and experience the world based on these. Essentially, one relives the past in present interpersonal interactions. Long-term psychodynamic therapy considers the influence of the unconscious mind and the multiple meanings of behavior.

The therapeutic alliance is considered a critical factor in the progress of therapy. The practitioner and client explore the adaptive and non-adaptive ego functions reflected in the client's interpersonal functioning and seek to modify non-adaptive modes of functioning over the course of therapy. A central feature of the therapy is to expand the client's awareness of unconscious conflicts that interfere with interpersonal functioning and to interpret defensive strategies used to ward off uncomfortable emotions evoked by these conflicts. The transference relationship—the client's experience of the therapist as significant figures from early childhood—is a defining feature of this therapeutic approach. Over the course of therapy the transference relationship is explored, interpreted, and worked through (Wachtel & Messer, 1997).

In contrast, a brief ego supportive therapy has more modest goals than long-term, intensive therapy. It seeks to assist clients to master life stresses and work toward the development of more adaptive coping methods. The practitioner, while maintaining a focus on the here and now, can further the client's awareness of key conflicts that contribute to the client's maladaptive responses to current work problems. While the primary goal may be the reduction or resolution of symptoms, the purposes the symptoms serve may be considered and better understood by the client. In contrast to long-term therapeutic approaches, this briefer approach furthers a positive transference or relationship with the client and stresses the realistic aspects of the helping relationship (Goldstein, 1995). Although transference issues are not explored, a collaborative partnership is formed with the client, and the practitioner maintains an active focus in order to sustain this partnership.

The workplace presents many stressors and requires one to manage a range of interpersonal dynamics, some hierarchical and others of a peer nature. Conflict in the workplace with supervisors, coworkers, and/or supervisees can trigger and replicate unresolved, painful issues related to early experience with significant figures. Confrontations with authority and peer rivalries can parallel family experiences and result in serious interpersonal distress in the workplace. Woodburn and Simpson (1998) suggest that workers bring their own unique needs to the workplace with expectations that the needs will be fulfilled by other employees. These expectations may be unrealistic and contribute to the difficulties that employees experience at the workplace.

THE ASSESSMENT PROCESS.   When clients enter therapy with chief complaints regarding workplace issues, the assessment should obtain relevant information about the client (person) and the work situation (environment). The client's strengths and resources, both psychological and environmental, should be clarified. Details about the current work difficulty and history should be gathered. The number of employers, absences or work leaves, firings, and problematic relations with coworkers should be clarified and explored. This information can be quickly gained through questions posed in both written intake materials and focused questions in the initial meeting. This data allow the practitioner to determine whether the work problem is the primary concern or secondary to other psychological difficulties (Lowman, 1993).

Brief ego supportive therapy uses a here-and-now approach with the focus on current concerns. Comparatively little historical material is elicited or explored. The practitioner attempts to help stabilize the client by reducing anxiety and other presenting symptoms and by supporting the client's sense of mastery and competence. The client's ego functions—for example, reality testing, judgment, and emotional regulation—are assessed and techniques are used to restore and enhance these. Encouragement and reassurance, exploration and ventilation of emotion, and suggestion and advice-giving are employed. Education and information-giving are other useful interventions that further the client's sense of competence and understanding of their situation. Partializing problems (breaking down into concrete steps) and the use of time limits help mobilize client strengths (Wood & Hollis, 2000).

Since practitioners often work within the constraints of managed care, they may identify core conflicts and transference themes but not address these due to the time constraints. The case that follows provides an example of brief ego supportive therapy.

CASE VIGNETTE—BRIEF EGO SUPPORTIVE THERAPY. Fred was a 44-year-old salesman referred by his internist after he placed Fred on short-term disability leave. The physician determined that Fred's physical symptoms, headache, chest pain, cold sweats, and stomach aches, were related to the severe work stress Fred reported. Fred also related difficulties with concentration, periods of intense anger, agitation, mood swings, and recent suicidal ideation. He was concerned that he had displayed considerable anger at home, frightening his wife and sons.

During the early phase of therapy, Fred related details about his prior discharge from his job. He viewed his discharge as unjust and based on his failure to reach sales quotas during a period when he was recovering from major surgery. After rehiring by his employer, he indicated that he became increasingly angry over the embarrassment and humiliation he suffered following the discharge. The firing threatened his status as the family bread winner and position in his family of origin as the successful one. Fred shared his feelings and beliefs that he was not valued sufficiently by his employer nor given the attention he deserved for his history of outstanding sales performance. This treatment contrasted with his experience in a family as the only male child who was nurtured and indulged by doting parents and grandparents. He expected that allowances would be made for his lateness with monthly reports and weekly sales statistics. He became outraged that his failure to complete required reports and meet deadlines served as the grounds for his initial dismissal, since these patterns were tolerated when his sales quotas were achieved. Prior to his disability leave, Fred had been given a written reprimand that continued lateness with paperwork would result in another, and final, dismissal from his sales position.

As the therapy progressed, Fred detailed his fantasies of retaliation against the perceived unfair treatment by his employer. He talked of blowing up the business, having a shouting match with his boss, and disrupting the workplace by destroying physical property. All of these thoughts frightened him since he had no history of aggressive behavior. He was able to ventilate these intense feeling and express his rage during the therapy sessions. Over time, his rage lessened and his somatic symptoms abated.

Fred came to expect that others would gratify his needs for attention and special treatment as his family had. When these needs were unmet in the workplace, Fred responded with frustration and anger at his boss and coworkers. The therapy focused on his presenting symptoms and worked toward their resolution. Family themes and experiences were explored. The therapist suggested that these experiences contributed to the intense rage that Fred experienced when the workplace did not provide the same level of acknowledgment and gratification. Fred gained some awareness of these dynamics during the therapy.

Fred was seen for 23 sessions over a five-month period. Because of the intensity of his presenting symptoms, he was seen twice a week during the first two months of therapy. The therapy ended when he took a position with a new employer and had no psychosomatic complaints.

CONCLUSION

Work has many real and symbolic meanings unique to the individual. Work experiences offer opportunities to achieve, excel, gain acknowledgment and ego gratification, as well as financial rewards. One's social status, societal power, and authority are closely related to one's work endeavors. Work problems, therefore, threaten these benefits and often result in significant psychological distress for the individual. This chapter addressed brief interventions for people with stress-related mental health conditions. It also described skill development training which cuts across and complements many brief therapies. Utilizing these effective and efficient techniques, practitioners can have a positive impact on individual and work unit morale and productivity, and advance the quality of work life.

REFERENCES

Anton, W. D., & Reed, J. R. (1994). *EAPI—Employee Assistance Program Inventory. Professional manual.* Odessa, FL: Psychological Assessment Resources.

Billings, A. G., & Moos, R. H. (1982). Work stress and the stress-buffering roles of work and family resources. *Journal of Occupational Behaviour, 3*, 215–232.

Billings, A. G., & Moos, R. H. (1984). Coping, stress and social resources among adults with unipolar depression. *Journal of Personality and Social Psychology, 46*, 877–891.

Caplan, R. D., & Jones, K. W. (1975). Effects of work load, role ambiguity, and Type A personality on anxiety, depression and heart rate. *Journal of Applied Psychology, 60*(6), 713–719.

Derogatis, L. R. (1977). *SCL-90: Administration, scoring & procedures manual for the revised version.* Baltimore, MD: Clinical Psychometric Research.

Ell, J. (1995). Crisis intervention: Research needs. In R. Edwards & J. Hopps (Eds.), *Encyclopedia of Social Work* (pp. 245–267). Washington, DC: NASW Press.

Ember, L. (1998). Surviving stress. *Chemical and Engineering News, 76*(21), 12–24.

Fanger, M. (1995). Brief therapies. In R. Edwards & J. Hopps (Eds.), *Encyclopedia of Social Work* (pp. 323–344). Washington, DC: NASW Press.

Folkman, S., & Lazarus, R. S. (1991). Coping and emotion. In A. Monat & R. S. Lazarus (Eds.), *Stress and coping: An anthology* (3rd ed., pp. 207–227). New York, NY: Columbia University Press.

French, J. R. P. (1973). Person–role fit. *Occupational Mental Health, 3*, 15–20.

Gillilard, B. E., & James, R. K. (1993). *Crisis intervention strategies.* Pacific Grove, CA: Brooks/Cole.

Goldstein, E. (1995). *Ego psychology and social work practice.* New York, NY: Free Press.

Haley, J. (1976). *Problem solving therapy.* New York, NY: Harper Colophon Books.

House, J. S., McMichael, A. J., Wells, J. A., Kaplan, B. H., & Landerman, L. R. (1979). Occupational stress and health among factory workers. *Journal of Health and Social Behavior, 20*, 139–160.

Ivancevich, J. M. (1986). Life events and hassles as predictors of health, symptoms, job performance, and absenteeism. *Journal of Occupational Behavior, 7*, 39–51.

Jackson, S. E., & Schuler, R. S. (1985). A meta-analysis and conceptual critique of research on role ambiguity and role conflict in work settings. *Organizational Behavior and Human Decision Processes, 36*, 16–78.

Kahn, J. P., & Aidinoff, S. (1999). Occupational psychiatry and the employee assistance program. *EAPA Exchange, 29*(1), 11–13.

Karasek, R. A. (1979). Job demands, job decision latitude, and mental strain: Implications for job redesign. *Administrative Science Quarterly, 2*(1), 285–309.

Karasek, R. A., Gardell, B., & Lindell, J. (1987). Work and non-work correlates of illness and behavior in male and female Swedish white collar workers. *Journal of Occupational Behaviour, 8*, 187–207.

Kent, W. (1999). Employee response during organizational change. *EAPA Exchange, 29*(3), 89.

Kessler, R. C., McGonagle, K. A., Zhao, S., Nelson, C. B., Hughes, M., Eshleman, S., Whittanen, H. U., & Deneller, K. S. (1994). Lifetime and 12-month prevalence of DSM-III-R psychiatric disorders in the U.S. (Report on National Co-Morbidity Survey). *Archives of General Psychiatry, 51*, 8–19.

Koeske, G. F., Kirk, S. A., & Koeske, R. D. (1993). Coping with job stress: Which strategies work best? *Journal of Occupational and Organizational Psychology, 66*, 319–335.

LaRocco, J. M., House, J. S., & French, J. R. P. (1980). Social support, occupational stress, and health. *Journal of Health and Social Behavior, 21*, 202–218.

Latack, J. C. (1986). Coping with job stress: Measures and future direction for scale development. *Journal of Applied Psychology, 71*, 377–385.

Lowman, R. L. (1993). *Counseling and psychotherapy of work dysfunctions*. Washington, DC: A.P.A. Press.

Maddi, S. R., & Kobasa, S. C. (1991). The development of hardiness. In A. Monat & R. S. Lazarus (Eds.), *Stress and coping: An anthology* (3rd ed., pp. 245–257). New York, NY: Columbia University Press.

Margolis, B. L., Kroes, W. H., & Quinn, R. P. (1974). Job stress: An unlisted occupational hazard. *Journal of Occupational Medicine, 16*(10), 659–661.

Mishel, L., Bernstein, J., & Schmitt, J. (1997). *The state of working America, 1996–97*. Economic Policy Institute. Armonk, NY: M.E. Sharpe.

Muller, M. J., Szegedi, A., Wetzel, H., & Benkert, O. (2000). Moderate and severe depression. Gradations for the Montgomery–Asberg Depression Rating Scale. *Journal of Affective Disorders, 60*(2), 137–140.

Puig, A. (1995). *Dealing with the anger dyscontrol worker in the workplace: Implications for EAP's* (Presentation at the 1995 Employee Assistance Professionals Association conference). Seattle, WA.

Reid, W. J., & Epstein, L. (1972). *Task centered casework*. New York, NY: Columbia University Press.

Ross, R. R., & Altmaier, E. M. (1994). *Intervention in occupational stress*. Thousand Oaks, CA: Sage.

Rouse, B. A. (Ed.) (1998). *Substance abuse and mental health statistics sourcebook*. Rockville, MD: U.S. Department of Health & Human Services, Substance Abuse and Mental Health Services Administration.

Shined, M., & Morch, H. (1983). A tripartite model of coping with burnout. In B. A. Farber (Ed.), *Stress and burnout in the human service professional*. New York, NY: Pergamon Press.

Slaiken, K. (1990). *Crisis intervention: A handbook for practice and research* (2nd ed.). Boston, MA: Allyn & Bacon.

Spearing, M. K., Post, R. M., Leverich, G. S., Brandt, D., & Nolen, W. (1997). Modification of the Clinical Global Impressions (CGI) Scale for use in bipolar illness: the CGI-BP. *Psychiatric Research, 73*(3), 159–171.

Stanton, D. M. (1981). Strategic approaches to family therapy. In A. Gurman and D. Kriskern, *Handbook of family therapy*. New York, NY: Brunner/Mazel.

Steele, W., & Raider, M. (1991). *Working with families in crisis*. New York, NY: Guilford.

Tattersall, A. J., & Farmer, E. W. (1995). The regulation of work demands and strain. In S. L. Sauter & L. R. Murphy (Eds.), *Organizational risk factors for job stress* (pp. 139–156). Washington, DC: A.P.A. Press.

Wachtel, L., & Messer, S. B. (Eds.) (1997). *Theories of psychotherapy: Origins and evolution*. Washington, DC: A.P.A. Press.

Woititz, J. G. (1983). *Adult children of alcoholics*. Deerfield Beach, FL: Health Communications.

Wood, M., & Hollis, F. (2000). *Casework: A psychosocial therapy*. Boston, MA: McGraw-Hill.

Woodburn, L. T., & Simpson, S. (1998, May/June). Coping with the stages of job stress. *EAP Digest*, 22–25.

Wortman, C., Biernat, M., & Lang, E. (1991). Coping with role overload. In M. Frankenhaeuser, U. Lundberg & M. Chesney (Eds.), *Women, work and health*. New York, NY: Plenum Press.

CHAPTER 21

Mental Health Case Management and Employment Outcomes

Patrick Sullivan

INTRODUCTION

For consumers, families, professionals, and policymakers, the inadequacies of the mental health service system are regularly illustrated in bold relief. Indeed, many on the front line of helping see only those most in need and struggling to survive day to day. While this alone can be frustrating this feeling of powerlessness is elevated when the heroic efforts of all are stymied by a populace who seemingly holds an "out of sight, out of mind" philosophy of care.

At such moments it is good to step back and reflect on the progress that has been made in mental health treatment. In fact, when one scans the past two decades there have been considerable gains made in the quality and range of care available to those challenged by serious and persistent mental illness. While there is little reason to remain satisfied with the status quo, there is, however, cause for optimism. It appears that we are on the verge of an exciting frontier in the evolution of mental health services as new medications, new treatment modalities, and most important, a new vision of human possibilities takes root.

Beginning in the late 1970s the system of services for those facing serious mental illnesses was transformed. Simply stated, the locus of care shifted from the hospital to the community, and concomitantly, a new generation of innovative programs emerged to support consumers. While it is true that the community mental health center movement began more that a decade earlier, it became painfully obvious that the cleavage between the necessary technology and philosophy of care, and the demands of those most in need, was having a deleterious impact on consumers and families. It was the tireless work of these same consumers and families, along with the support of concerned professionals, that paved the way for some significant changes in the mental health system. In the heady days that followed, new or re-energized treatment modalities, such as psychosocial rehabilitation, community support programs, and day treatment, began to flourish. And from the beginning, case management has been a keystone service in the panoply of mental health programming.

Case management became such a popular concept that a wide range of practice models emerged—a trend that continues today with the rise of managed behavioral health care. What

Patrick Sullivan • Indiana University School of Social Work, Indianapolis, Indiana.

differentiated case management from other typical "treatment" services was the clear and *direct* focus on the problems of living and community functioning of consumers. Furthermore, in a unique twist absent since the early days of social casework, much of the work actually occurred in the community and in the homes of clients. Accordingly, as considered here, case management can be defined as a creative and collaborative process requiring skill in assessment, counseling, teaching, modeling, and advocacy that aims to enhance the social functioning of consumers (Sullivan, Wolk, & Hartmann, 1992).

Case management became an integral part of the spectrum of mental health services at the time when more consumers exited State psychiatric services and as efforts to avoid hospitalization intensified. The popularity of case management is an outgrowth of the natural conceptual fit of this service and the needs of consumers. When consumers resided in inpatient settings the range of professional services as well as the basic needs of life were covered. For some consumers and families the situation changed dramatically when discharge occurred. Suddenly, it was necessary to arrange these same services and resources—a process that could be taxing emotionally and economically. Case management, it was envisioned, could smooth this process in a proactive and rational manner, and as a result, increase the odds for successful community adjustment.

Yet, with time simple community adjustment was no longer an acceptable goal, and in some respects the focus of case management evolved in commensurate fashion (Moxley, 1997; Mueser, Bond, Drake, & Resnick, 1998). Critics of the direction of mental health policy decried the substandard living conditions and quality of life experienced by the most seriously ill. Arguably at the opposite end of the spectrum, consumers gained their voice and began advocating for rights and opportunities, and in some cases developed support groups and alternative programs. Regardless of the place where one stands, most would agree that true community integration requires participation in the common activities of daily life. In simple terms, consumers, like all people, desire a home, friends, and meaningful activities.

Some models of case management, notably the strengths model, purported to address the goals that consumers deemed important. It followed that the key life domains of work, shelter, and leisure would figure prominently in the plans of action mutually developed by clients and case managers working from strengths principles (Rapp, 1998; Rapp & Chamberlain, 1985). While the goals, functions, and activities of case management vary by model, for the most part all direct practice case managers devote attention to the community functioning of consumers. Therefore, it is reasonable to ask if case management, broadly defined, has positively affected this aspect of consumers' lives.

Before turning directly to the key question under consideration in this chapter, namely the impact and role of case management services in advancing the vocational aspirations of consumers, one additional trend must be examined. It is important to delineate the changing contextual backdrop for case management and mental health services for those facing serious and persistent mental illnesses. Case management does not occur in a vacuum. Certainly, public opinion, policy considerations, and delivery system organization all impact the way case managers perform.

In the early days of case management the sentiments embodied by this service modality were not universally embraced. Everything from in-home intervention to the advisability of encouraging consumer desires to work and live independently was questioned. At times these conflicts reflected real disagreements in treatment philosophy. In other cases these debates exposed divergent expectations for consumers. For embedded in the values and functions of case management was a prevailing belief that persons facing serious mental illnesses could improve and, as a result, could assume adult roles in the community.

Over the past two decades the public mental health system, particularly community mental health, has devoted more attention to those facing severe disorders. Simultaneously, case management, once a maverick service offering, has proliferated. The growth of case management, as noted above, is consistent with the increased pressures, necessity, and desire to serve those most in need in community settings. However, the depopulation of state psychiatric hospitals, and the development of community-based programming has occurred at different rates across the nation. How case management services are configured at a given locale is likely the result of the demand, culture of the host organization, and selective exposure to various models of care.

Nonetheless, if there has been one universal goal of case management in mental health it has been to prevent unnecessary hospitalization. Yet, it was quickly realized that while preventing hospitalization serves as a good starting point, as an overall mission for services it is insufficient. If case management services are to make a true difference, more, it seemed, should be accomplished. If jobs, friends, and housing are needed, case management programs are often viewed as the means to accomplish these outcomes. At times, too much is expected of case management (Mueser et al., 1998). Case management is but one service that functions within a larger context, and these contextual factors have always served to bolster or hamper the ability of case managers to be successful. Rarely are the optimum conditions for success present.

As model programs and pilot projects are launched they often operate within a set of conditions that are at variance with the day-to-day world of mental health practice. To illustrate, for broker models to be successful, a lush array of easily accessible resources must be available to address consumer needs and goals. Intensive models of case management, which demand a greater time commitment, require case loads to be relatively small and manageable. Furthermore, the skills needed by case managers, particularly when they provide face-to-face service, are often drastically underestimated. In comprehensive models of case management these professionals ideally posses excellent clinical and advocacy skills, must have a firm grasp on resource creation and acquisition, and display a level of creativity and resilience that is rare indeed. Now that case management has emerged as a common entry-level mental health job, it is increasingly rare to find professionals who have true zeal for the work as well as the range of talents described above.

While there is danger in overestimating the impact of case management and other community-based mental health services the fact remains that the overall mission has become more expansive and the gold standard for success has been rightfully elevated. Consider the mere fact that the vocational activity of consumers is not only an area of focus but *is* an accepted barometer of program performance. In the 1950s to be diagnosed with schizophrenia was to face the possibility of lengthy institutionalization, and if one worked at all they did so in the service of the hospital. Over time, as was true with other stigmatized groups, sheltered workshops and other types of alternative employment settings were developed. Later, in the first rush to expand specialized community mental health programs new employment models emerged including work teams and work enclaves—and here consumers could be afforded the opportunity to participate in sponsored programs that generally fell into the work categories of food, filth, or folding. Even in the presence of specialized work programs professionals often discourage consumers from working, fearing that the stress of employment will exacerbate symptoms and result in relapse (Bond, 1998; Torrey et al., 1998). Today, while vestiges of the traditional thinking remain, new expectations and programs set forth a course that emphasizes that people facing serious mental illness are not simply patients, clients, or consumers—they are citizens. Most citizens choose to participate in the world of work; thus, it stands to reason that effective community-based programs should strive to help individuals reach this goal as well.

WORK AND RECOVERY: THE ROLE OF CASE MANAGEMENT

During the last decade the concept of recovery has joined the vernacular of mental health services. This development is the result of longitudinal research as well as the reports of current and former consumers of mental health services which points to the ability of many to live "a satisfying, hopeful, and contributing life even with the limitations caused by illness" (Anthony, 1992, p.15). The rise of the term recovery in mental health services reflects more than a mere change in lexicon, it signals "a revolution in mental health services" (Corrigan, Giffort, Rashid, Leary, & Okeke, 1999, p. 232).

With the concept of recovery now in place, the challenge confronting all stakeholders is to discover those activities, attitudes, and behaviors, initiated by self or others, that are essential to success (Sullivan, 1994). Which leads to the role of work in recovery. Work can be viewed as an example of recovery. When consumers are active in the workforce it can be surmised that the process of recovery is underway—that the person is, in fact, surmounting the potential devastation that comes with serious mental illness. On the other hand, work can be seen as an activity that *contributes* to recovery. This would suggest that the ability to participate in some form of meaningful vocational activity (including education) stimulates the process of recovery. In the former model one looks to behavioral manifestations of recovery. In the latter recovery may be more an intrapersonal process that is reflected in a host of attitudes and behaviors.

However configured, it seems certain, based on consumer narratives, that work is central to this phenomenon we now term recovery. To work bolsters self-esteem, helps one feel like a citizen, and of course, has instrumental value as well. This chapter will examine the role of case management in improving the vocational experience of mental health consumers. In this journey the direct and indirect impact of case management services will be explored as well as the organizational context that supports and/or hinders the efforts of case managers.

Any review of personal narratives and formal explorations of consumer desires indicates that many consumers wish to work (Bailey, 1998; Drake, 1998; Jackson, 1992; Sullivan, 1994; Waters, 1992). Equally important, empirical work indicates that the career goals and work expectations of consumers tend to be realistic, and that when career goals and actual opportunities are congruent job tenure is enhanced (Becker, Bebout, & Drake, 1998). So it seems fair to suggest that the emphasis on vocational performance embedded in many case management models is appropriate.

CASE MANAGEMENT AND VOCATIONAL PERFORMANCE: A REVIEW OF THE RESEARCH

For a service modality that has been so widely embraced there is a relative dearth of research assessing the effectiveness of case management. Issues of treatment fidelity and organizational context become key factors when examining the role and impact of case management in the vocational life of consumers. Mueser et al. (1998) have compiled an extensive review of case management services and have identified three ideal types of case management models: standard, which encompasses traditional broker and clinical models; rehabilitation, including the strengths model; and comprehensive, notably represented by Assertive Community Treatment (ACT) teams. There are natural areas of overlap between these models conceptually, and certainly commonalities present in the real world of practice.

The majority of the research reviewed by these authors suggests that case management programs have little direct impact on vocational activity and other areas of social functioning. The research does suggest that case management tends to reduce the use of psychiatric hospitals and that case managers seem to help buffer the stress experienced by consumers. Furthermore, there is some evidence that there is a modest association between case management involvement and symptom reduction. Obviously, while case management is often designed to have a clear and dramatic impact on social functioning, each of the items noted above is an important ingredient to the process of recovery and hence the ability to engage in work activity.

While the bulk of the research on the relationship between case management and the vocational life of consumers has been disappointing, isolated studies have suggested that such services are indeed beneficial in this life domain. As noted earlier, the strengths model explicitly targets vocational improvement as a key outcome area to assess effectiveness. In a study that examined the results of several of early demonstration projects implementing the strengths model, Rapp and Wintersteen (1989) report that nearly 19% of all goals established by case managers in 12 demonstrations fell in the vocational/education arena and that over 87% of these goals were accomplished. It is important to note that these goals include necessary steps to gain employment and other objectives that were designed to impact a larger overarching vocational goal. In a more recent analysis, Stanard (1999) reports that the strengths model was more effective than the generalist (or standard) model in the area of educational and vocational outcomes. In this study vocational activity was also broadly conceived to include such items as volunteer work and homemaking.

Select studies have also indicated a relationship between improved vocational activity and involvement with ACT teams (Mueser et al., 1998). However, Bond (1992) has suggested that these results are, in part, positively influenced by the presence of active vocational programs that operate in consort with ACT teams. It is interesting to note that the difference between the strengths model of case management and ACT is largely structural. Where ACT is a team model with members representing a wide array of disciplines, the strengths model is a pure case management model with the functions provided by a lone professional. However, in terms of the overall treatment philosophy and values there is a great deal of congruence between the two approaches.

While there may be a lack of evidence that case management, as a discrete intervention, has a significant impact on overall social functioning, this does not indicate that services are unimportant to the process or recovery and/or that they do not augment other vocational programs. In fact, research on the process of recovery in general, and vocational services more specifically, provide some important suggestions on the potential role of case managers and specialized teams.

THE CENTRALITY OF THE CONSUMER–CASE MANAGER RELATIONSHIP IN VOCATIONAL INITIATIVES

A primary consideration in any exploration of the impact of case management is the nature of the relationship between these professionals and consumers—and here case managers appear to excel. McGrew, Wilson, and Bond (1996) have explored consumers' views on the most helpful aspects of ACT programs. Using an open-ended interviewing method these authors found that the areas consumers deemed most useful were the relationship with a case manager and the personal attributes of these same professionals. McGrew and associates express some surprise at these results given the team approach that is central to ACT. These results are similar to those found by Sullivan (1994) in an exploratory study examining the process of recovery. Using an open-ended interviewing method as well, consumers in this study also stress the importance of their relationship with case mangers. In this study consumers tended to highlight the areas of support and encouragement that case mangers offer, and a sense that case managers treated them with respect and dignity. Here consumers spoke of case managers who never give up on them or treat them like a friend. These same case managers are seen as always available, and willing to do simple tasks, such as helping arrange an apartment or work out a daily routine. In reality it appears that the seemingly simple things that case mangers do to help consumers in their day-to-day life matter greatly. This becomes even more important when one considers that these types of activities have largely fallen on the shoulders of exhausted family members and are only rarely performed by other professionals.

These results are hardly startling, although they do indicate that any model of case management that ignores the importance of the relationship and/or the potential therapeutic or clinical aspects of the role is likely wanting. The centrality of the case manager/consumer relationship is a bedrock principle in the strengths model, and obviously a key facet of clinical models of case management (Harris & Bergman, 1987; Roach, 1993). In the strengths model it is recognized that the close nature of the work, and the stated belief that consumer choice prevails, requires the development of a healthy professional relationship. In the classic clinical model, the centrality of the relationship is defined in a manner similar to that of a psychotherapist. Here the case manager may exert more control initially, and by actively modeling and teaching the consumer problem-solving skills, demonstrates a proactive and orderly approach to life issues.

Consumer narratives are reminding us anew that what Goering and Stylianos (1988) coin the therapeutic alliance is a key ingredient to rehabilitation work and the process of recovery. Intriguingly, these reports also hint at the possibility that the model one employs is far less important than the ability of case managers to connect with a consumer at the personal and human levels. In this regard it not surprising that research indicates that good case management is associated with overall satisfaction with community mental health services (McGrew et al., 1996; Mueser et al., 1998). However, the quality of the consumer/professional relationship may be best considered as necessary but insufficient when the goal is improved outcomes. McGrew et al. (1996) concur noting that, "although a warm, caring relationship may be important for clients to feel satisfied with services, the elements most instrumental to preventing hospitalizations may be the mundane attention to details of everyday living that are the hallmark of the ACT approach" (p. 20).

Several observations can be made at this point. First, for many consumers case management is a critical ingredient to the process of recovery—an assertion that is supported by first-person accounts. Second, the development of a positive relationship is associated with overall satisfaction with services, and maybe important in "mediating a favorable response to community care" (Mueser et al., 1998, p. 66). Finally, case management operates within a context of services that may help or hinder consumer goal attainment in a diverse array of life domains including vocational activity.

Bond (1998) notes that a wide range of programs, including case management, do not appear to have any impact on consumer outcomes beyond those for which they are specifically designed, and this is especially true in the area of employment. Thus, case management and other forms of helping may ready a person for employment, but direct assistance is needed if employment gains are to be made. Ideally, it follows, intensive case management services, including ACT, are offered in the context of a formal vocational program. This is particularly important when other conditions for success, such as manageable caseloads and professional autonomy, are absent.

In the following sections concrete examples will be offered to detail how case managers can help consumers attain their vocational goals. Embedded in this discussion will be a review of model vocational programs, the research on these models, and an articulation of the various roles for case managers within these models. It is hoped that the activities and principles set forth are useful to case managers who work from team or individual practice models, and in a diverse array of organizational settings.

PRACTICING CASE MANAGEMENT TO IMPROVE VOCATIONAL SUCCESS

One of the best predictors of consumer vocational success is a past work history, followed by other indicators of positive pre-morbid functioning (Regenold, Sherman, & Fenzel, 1999). In such instances the consumer may have a clearer notion of the types of jobs they prefer and the requirements of the world of work. Others, particularly those who have faced illness since early adulthood, may not have an appreciable work history. In many cases the first task of the case manager is to kindle or rekindle an interest in work and assist the consumer as he/she focuses on the kind of work that interests him/her.

Assessment

Most helping processes in mental health begin with a period of diagnosis and assessment, and case management practice is no different. Yet, in intensive case management this assessment is squarely focused on the community functioning of clients and is closely coupled with an early exploration of the consumer goals (De Jong & Miller, 1995). This establishes the focus of case management at the onset, and also signals that there is an expectation that the consumer can recover and assume accepted adult roles. Hence, if the overall goal is to improve client outcomes in the activities of daily life, the assessment process should ascertain consumer interests and activities (past and present) in a wide range of life domains. To immediately and directly link the assessment to an action plan, the case managers and consumer should define some potential goals in these same life domains and also identify the resources that are needed to accomplish these goals. It is also preferable to complete this assessment in a natural setting, such as the consumer home or an agreed upon community location. This setting often puts the consumer at ease and also is a reminder that the work between a consumer and the case manager is conducted in the community (Rapp, 1998).

Several strengths-based assessment tools are designed to capture the information essential to an intensive case manager and the consumer as they proceed in their work together (Cowger, 1997; McQuaide & Ehrenreich, 1997; Rapp, 1998). In all cases the completion of the strengths assessment is seen as a mutual activity, one where consumers should feel valued and heard. In the strengths model the assessment is not an activity that precedes helping; it is instead seen as a key element of helping. Involving consumers from the beginning affirms their competencies and indicates that they can take charge of the recovery process. The mere fact that there is a discussion about strengths, abilities, and life goals is a relatively new experience for many consumers, particularly those with long treatment histories. This alone can be empowering for consumers whose previous interaction with professionals has usually centered on their problems and deficits. It is here that case managers should begin to actively investigate the previous work history of consumers and aspirations they have in this area. As was noted previously, many consumers are interested in beginning or returning to work and see this as a way to improve the quality of their life (Arns & Linney, 1993; Vorspan, 1992).

Using well-tested assessment tools is certainly helpful, but the process and style employed in this initial phase is also an important consideration. Rapp (1998) has offered some useful guidelines for completing assessments that have utility in the vocational rehabilitation world as well. Given the challenges presented by serious mental illness it may be difficult for many consumers to maintain their concentration during the assessment phase. The use of a conversational style and an expectation that the initial assessment will be completed over several settings is certainly helpful. In all cases, the assessment should reflect the consumer voice, and where possible, interests and desires should be recorded in a diverse array of life domains such as work, leisure time, health, and daily living. During the data-gathering period every opportunity to highlight and underscore personal accomplishments should be exercised as the consumer has spent ample time discussing their struggles and disappointments. The product should also be highly individualized, to the degree that all professionals who have contact with the client should be able to immediately recognize the consumer when reviewing the document.

Goal Setting and Case Planning

The next step for the case manager and the consumer is to define concrete and specific vocational goals and detail the steps needed to complete them. Goal setting is a key aspect of good case management practice. Goals provide direction for future work and serve as a gauge to monitor client progress and program success. How goals are written has clinical significance as well. Serious mental illness impacts one's ability to process information, and life tasks that others take for granted overwhelm many consumers. On close inspection it became clear that the behaviors and skills needed to ride a bus or cook a meal are complex. Imagine, or better yet remember, how daunting the process of finding a job is when you have little or no experience doing so.

There are a few quality standards for establishing well-formed goals that are useful to case managers working to advance the vocational aspirations of consumers (De Jong & Miller, 1995; Rapp, 1998). It is vitally important that the goals selected are those that the client has identified as important. Other professionals and interested parties will be quick to offer their suggestion on areas that demand attention. Oftentimes, such suggestions are designed to service the illness and focus on obvious client deficits. This pull toward deficits is so pervasive in many clinical settings that attention is ultimately diverted from the very activities, such as work, that can contribute to recovery. To be successful case management practice should be consumer-driven (Moxley & Daeschlein, 1997; Moxley & Freddolino, 1997). Recall that research has indicated that consumers tend to have realistic vocational goals. Yet, even when these goals seem to be unrealistic, they can be broken down into a series of smaller achievable steps. In written form all goals should be concrete, specific, and measurable. The later standard allows both the consumer and the case manager to assess progress that has been made and to use this data to guide future planning. Professionals often get discouraged when consumers do not seem to improve. Using a clear goal-setting method allows the consumer and professional to reflect on progress that has been made and to discern any patterns in the fits and starts of recovery.

If possible, it is desirable to establish an initial goal that the consumer is likely to achieve with little or minimal difficulty. An early success can help boost the self-confidence of consumers and provide encouragement to take the next step in recovery. Recent work underscores the importance of self-efficacy in the vocational activity of consumers (Regenold et al., 1999). Self-efficacy involves the perception that one has the capacity to accomplish significant tasks in spite of present obstacles. It is also is reflected in a proactive and organized approach to life, and a pervasive belief that one will succeed. This spirit is reflected in the success narratives of current and former consumers of mental health services. Case managers can actively model efficacious behavior and use goal setting to demonstrate how one breaks a complex task into a series of achievable steps. Other skills may be useful when consumers begin to ponder employment including role-playing and self-instruction (Regenold et al., 1999). Therefore, in the vocational realm, early goals may include things as simple as reading the want ads or completing a résumé. As basic as these goals may appear, the self-initiative of many consumers is stymied through the forces of illness, medication, and inactivity making any active task an important first step toward recovery.

CASE MANAGEMENT IN CONTEXT: COMPLEMENTARY VOCATIONAL PROGRAMMING

In spite of such potentially modest beginnings, the intent is to quickly move toward an employment outcome for consumers and to avoid a lengthy prevocational stage. The presence or absence of an active complementary vocational program influences how this phase proceeds. If the case manager and consumer operate independently, the task of securing employment may be arduous. In this scenario the consumer and case manager must locate possible jobs or volunteer activities, arrange transportation, and other fundamental but time-consuming details. Even if successful, experience indicates that consumers are likely to need ongoing support and encouragement—often at the job site. Needless to say this is a difficult task when helping a single individual, but it becomes nearly impossible when caseloads climb to 30 and above.

Early vocational programs in community mental health centers customarily featured a range of prevocational programs focusing on skill building. Over time it was not uncommon for a center to create a range of work crews—janitorial work or grounds crew programs became mental health favorites—while others adopted a wider and more imaginative range of in-house program opportunities. In the early days of the community support program movement efforts to establish beneficial linkages with traditional vocational rehabilitation (VR) services proved instructive. It quickly became clear that the challenge presented by serious mental illness did not match the prevailing model operating in standard VR programs (Bond, Drake, Mueser, & Becker, 1997).

Then a series of innovative programs arrived on the scene, which challenged a host of sacred assumptions in VR. The first volley in this significant change was supported employment (Anthony & Blanch, 1987). This model set forth the proposition that all consumers, regardless of their disability, could engage in productive and meaningful work if provided the necessary supports. Furthermore, it was suggested that failures arose when there was an improper job selection and failure to provide necessary supports, not due to the disability. Finally, it was argued that support was a function, not a setting. Thus, isolated, and segregated vocational programs were not a necessity (Anthony & Blanch, 1987). The stage was set for what has become the chose, get, and keep model of VR.

While there is variation among models, common components of supported employment include client choice, a goal of competitive employment, minimal prevocational programming, and individualized placement. Most importantly, these programs appear to effective in the quest to help consumers obtain and retain jobs (Bond et al., 1997; Drake, 1998). Recent reviews of the individual placement and support (IPS) model continue to show promise and point to areas where case management services can augment vocational program initiatives (Bond, 1998).

A key difference in the new models of VR is a move to a place then train model of employment as opposed to the classic train then place paradigm. This principle can be defended empirically as research indicates that there is little support for a lengthy prevocational service phase including skill training (Bond, 1998). At the heart of the IPS model is a rapid job search and placement philosophy, with an immediate goal of competitive employment. In ACT and other team models of care a vocational specialist may be one of the multidisciplinary members. If a vocational specialist is not present, then case managers can be invaluable by helping consumers identify a job preference and provide the instrumental and emotional support necessary at the onset.

It is here that the assessment process becomes so important. One key feature of the strengths model of case management is the notion that assessment is continuous (Rapp, 1998). This is vital to the long-term success of a vocational effort for an assessment should not only help guide the consumer and case manager in the selection of a job, but also provide clues for how to keep it. The strengths model has long been predicated on exploiting the potentialities of the person and the environment (Cowger, 1997; Sullivan, 1997). Likewise, Bond (1998) observes that a key ingredient in the success of the IPS model is the quality of the person/environment fit at the workplace. Is there a need for accommodations? What characteristics of an individual should be considered when finding a good job match? These kinds of questions are important in ensuring the long-term vocational success of consumers.

The ongoing assessment of the person/environment fit is a cogent issue in the development of IPS programs as research suggests that job retention is still an area of needed improvement (Bond, 1997). What appears to be important to increasing job tenure is time-unlimited support, in particular outreach to the consumer. Job coaches and job sharing have been staples in supported and transitional employment models for many years. In the case of job coaches it is obvious that financial constraints limit the time that can be spent on this direct intervention. In some vocational programs professional staff are expected to fill in for workers who are temporarily incapacitated to both fulfill obligations to employers and ensure that the job remains available to the client. These types of job supports can be formally incorporated into a vocational program but for the majority of mental health programs in the country these arrangements are rare. In transitional employment programs, which are by definition time limited, consumers often share job sites (Bilby, 1992).

Regardless of the manner in which it is provided, ongoing support and contact is a valuable adjunct to vocational programming (McHugo, Drake, & Becker, 1998). It is here that the outreach services, a traditional feature of case management, can be particularly useful. An active case manager has regular contact with the consumer in those environments where consumers live, work, and recreate. Here, more than in formal service settings, case managers can see those areas where consumers excel and where they struggle. The case manager can help consumers incorporate new skills and insights into their daily life. These same case managers should recognize and respond to those idiosyncratic indicators that things are not going well for consumers. What can be done? Perhaps medications need adjusting, or the consumer is temporarily overwhelmed and some activities should be cut back or temporarily curtailed. While there will be variation in the specific needs of individual clients, case managers should be poised to react quickly. The ability to work side-by-side with consumers through turbulent times deflects unnecessary setbacks and increases consumer confidence in their ability to recover.

Case managers should be active in the community and, with permission, have regular contact with employers. Conversations and negotiations between all parties can result in modifications to the work environment, an arranged vacation, or any number of potential interventions that can help the consumer maintain a job. The case manager can also translate the expectations of the job to the consumer, and work on those skill areas that need shoring up. As a member of the multi-disciplinary team, case managers can provide insights and observations on the life of the consumer outside the walls of the agency and keep others informed of the goals and progress being made. The ebbs and flows of the work between the consumer and case manager may reflect the ongoing job of managing an illness and/or the personal adjustment that arises when there are greater demands to perform in newly acquired roles. With this knowledge, other professionals should be prepared to gear their interventions in a manner that supports the goals of the consumer.

CONCLUSION

We return to the key question addressed in this chapter: Is there a role for case management in the vocational habilitation and rehabilitation of consumers? The answer is yes—but with the caveat that case management is no panacea. Case managers cannot de-fragment a system nor provide each and every service that a consumer needs. It appears that there are several important considerations that must be addressed if case management services are to positively impact consumer outcomes in the area of employment.

First, as the research indicates the magic of case management still pivots on the power of the relationship. Case managers who can forge positive and supportive relationships with consumers, who are honest, reliable, and compassionate are successful. For many consumers to enter or re-enter the world of work requires them to fight their anxieties and fears, as well as the strong forces of stigma and social rejection. Case managers who are there at every step can be enormously helpful.

Second, case management services appear to be most beneficial when offered within the context of, or in conjunction with, specialized vocational services. The existence of a vocational program underscores employment as a valued consumer outcome. Furthermore, the current realities of practice preclude case managers from engaging in the full range of development and recruitment activities that create viable opportunities for consumers. However, case management services can fruitfully augment vocational services, particularly through outreach and support activities.

Finally, in the era of managed care and increased demands for services future research must not only determine if and how case management is effective, but also who is likely to benefit from this service and who is not. Case management must not become the 21st-century version of individual therapy where all consumers get it regardless if they need it or want it.

Without a doubt vocational opportunity is a pathway to recovery. It is incumbent on mental health programs to develop a wide range of employment services for consumers and demonstrate confidence that consumers can succeed. Advocates must implore policymakers and, more importantly, the general public, to open the door to consumers. Those affected by mental illness, like all people, desperately desire to make a contribution to society and this desire should not be thwarted.

It is clear from the narratives of consumers that case managers are important to them. They help by being fully human. They help by treating consumers as people with talents and abilities, and with respect. They make a difference by helping consumers tackle the day-to-day challenges of life. Perhaps most important, they matter by believing that consumers can recover.

REFERENCES

Anthony, W. A. (1992). Recovery from mental illness: The guiding vision of the mental health system in the 1990's. *Psychosocial Rehabilitation Journal, 16*(4), 11–23.

Anthony, W. A., & Blanch, A. (1987). Supported employment for persons who are psychiatrically disabled: An historical and conceptual perspective. *Psychosocial Rehabilitation Journal, 11*(2), 5–23.

Arns, P., & Linney, J. (1993). Work, self, and life satisfaction for persons with severe and persistent mental disorders. *Psychosocial Rehabilitation Journal, 16*(4), 63–79.

Bailey, J. (1998). I'm just an ordinary person. *Psychiatric Rehabilitation Journal, 22*(1), 8–10.

Becker, D., Bebout, R., & Drake, R. (1998). Job preferences of people with severe mental illness: A replication. *Psychiatric Rehabilitation Journal, 22*(1), 46–50.

Bilby, R. (1992). A response to criticisms of transitional employment. *Psychosocial Rehabilitation Journal, 16*(2), 69–82.

Bond, G. (1992). Vocational rehabilitation. In R. P. Liberman (Ed.), *Handbook of psychiatric rehabilitation* (pp. 244–275). New York, NY: Macmillan.

Bond, G. (1998). Principles of the individual placement and support model: Empirical support. *Psychiatric Rehabilitation Journal, 22*(1), 11–23.

Bond, G., Drake, R., Mueser, K., & Becker, D. (1997). An update on supported employment for people with severe mental illness. *Psychiatric Services, 48*(3), 335–346.

Corrigan, P., Giffort, D., Rashid, F., Leary, M., & Okeke, I. (1999). Recovery as a psychological construct. *Community Mental Health Journal, 35*(3), 231–239.

Cowger, C. (1997). Assessing client strengths: Assessment for client empowerment. In D. Saleebey (Ed.), *The strengths perspective in social work practice* (2nd ed., pp. 59–73). New York, NY: Longman.

De Jong, P., & Miller, P. (1995). How to interview for client strengths. *Social Work, 40*(6), 729–736.

Drake, R. (1998). Whither supported employment? *Psychiatric Rehabilitation Journal, 22*(1), 1.

Goering, P., & Stylianos, S. (1988). Exploring the helping relationship between the schizophrenic client and the rehabilitation therapist. *American Journal of Orthopsychiatry, 58*(2), 271–280.

Harris, M., & Bergman, M. (1987). Case management with the chronically mentally ill: A clinical perspective. *American Journal of Orthopsychiatry, 57*, 296–302.

Jackson, R. (1992). How work works. *Psychosocial Rehabilitation Journal, 16*(2), 63–67.

McGrew, J., Wilson, R., & Bond, G. (1996). Client perspectives on helpful ingredients of assertive community treatment. *Psychiatric Rehabilitation Journal, 19*(3), 13–21.

McHugo, G., Drake, R., & Becker, D. (1998). The durability of supported employment effects. *Psychiatric Rehabilitation Journal, 22*(1), 55–61.

McQuaide, S., & Ehrenreich, J. H. (1997). Assessing client strengths. *Families in Society, 78*(2), 201–212.

Moxley, D. (Ed.) (1997). *Case management by design.* Chicago, IL: Nelson-Hall.

Moxley, D., & Daeschlein, M. (1997). Properties of consumer-driven forms of case management. In D. Moxley (Ed.), *Case management by design* (pp. 111–133). Chicago, IL: Nelson-Hall.

Moxley, D., & Freddolino, P. (1997). A model of consumer-driven case management in psychiatric rehabilitation. In D. Moxley (Ed.), *Case management by design* (pp. 134–144). Chicago, IL: Nelson-Hall.

Mueser, K., Bond, G., Drake, R., & Resnick, S. (1998). Models of community care for severe mental illness: A review of research on case management. *Schizophrenia Bulletin, 24*(1), 37–74.

Rapp, C. A. (1998). *The strengths model.* New York, NY: Oxford University Press.

Rapp, C. A., & Chamberlain, R. (1985). Case management services to the chronically mentally ill. *Social Work, 30*(5), 417–422.

Rapp, C. A., & Wintersteen, R. (1989). The strengths model of case management: Results from twelve demonstrations. *Psychosocial Rehabilitation Journal, 13*(1), 23–32.

Regenold, M., Sherman, M., & Fenzel, M. (1999). Getting back to work: Self-efficacy as a predictor of employment outcome. *Psychiatric Rehabilitation Journal, 22*(4), 361–367.

Roach, J. (1993). Clinical case management with severely mentally ill adults. In M Haris & H. Bergman (Eds.), *Case management for mentally ill patients.* Langhorne, PA: Harwood Academic.

Stanard, R. (1999). The effect of training in a strengths model of case management on client outcomes in a community mental health center. *Community Mental Health Journal, 35*(2), 169–179.

Sullivan, W. P. (1994). A long and winding road: The process of recovery from severe mental illness. *Innovations and Research, 3*(3), 19–27.

Sullivan, W. P. (1997). On strengths, niches, and recovery from serious mental illness. In D. Saleebey (Ed.), *The strengths perspective in social work practice* (2nd ed., pp. 183–197). New York, NY: Longman.

Sullivan, W. P., Wolk, J., & Hartmann, D. (1992). Case management in alcohol and drug treatment: Improving client outcomes. *Families in Society, 73*(4), 195–203.

Torrey, E. F., Bebout, R., Kline, J., Becker, D., Alverson, M., & Drake, R. (1998). Practice guidelines for clinicians working in programs providing integrated vocational and clinical services for persons with severe mental illness. *Psychiatric Rehabilitation Journal, 21*(4), 388–393.

Vorspan, R. (1992). Why work works. *Psychosocial Rehabilitation Journal, 16*(2), 49–54.

Waters, B. (1992). The work unit: The heart of the clubhouse. *Psychosocial Rehabilitation Journal, 16*(2), 41–48. October 12, 1999.

CHAPTER 22

Addressing Substance Abuse Problems in the Workplace

ALISON FAVORINI

BACKGROUND AND INTRODUCTION

The purposes of this chapter are to acquaint the reader with the societal and workplace consequences of substance abuse and to discuss identification of employee substance abuse, intervention techniques, treatment options, issues in serving dual diagnosis clients, and workplace issues encountered throughout this process from identification to reintegration or termination.

Prevalence and Costs of Substance Abuse

One in four Americans has a substance abuse problem during his or her lifetime, with alcohol abuse being the most common. Between 12 and 18 million Americans need treatment for alcohol abuse or dependence (Brandeis University, 1993; Substance Abuse and Mental Health Services Administration (SAMHSA, 1999a). Alcohol use and abuse among adults has been stable in the past decade (SAMHSA, 1999a), but the annual cost to U.S. society in lost productivity, healthcare, crime, accidents, and workplace violence exceeds $165 billion a year (Rouse, 1998). Among illicit drugs, marijuana and cocaine are the most popular, but use of designer drugs and heroin is rising, especially among young adults. Due partly to purer, more powerful drugs, emergency room episodes involving drugs have risen over the past decade (Rouse, 1998). The estimated annual cost to U.S. society of drug abuse, excluding alcohol, is $110.4 billion (Rouse, 1998). Only 10% of alcoholics and 9% of drug addicts receive treatment in any given year (Grant, 1997).

For its victims, the costs of substance abuse in human suffering are incalculable.

Workplace Prevalence, Costs, and Consequences

An estimated 70% of illicit drug users are employed, and the proportion for alcoholics and heavy drinkers is probably higher (SAMHSA, 1998b). Nearly 8% of full-time employees

---

ALISON FAVORINI • Huntington Woods, Michigan.

report current illicit drug use (past month), and the number of self-reported heavy drinkers is similar (SAMHSA, 1998b).[1] Much higher rates are found among employed young adults, age 18–25 (SAMHSA, 1999b).

Annual costs of substance abuse to the U.S. workplace have been estimated at between $100 billion and $200 billion (Rouse, 1998; Harwood et al., 1998). About half of employed illicit drug users and a third of employed heavy drinkers and alcoholics work in small businesses (less than 25 employees), which are least likely to have employee assistance programs (EAPs) and adequate treatment benefits (SAMHSA, 1998a, 1998b). Substance abuse is highest in male-dominated occupations such as construction, manufacturing, and trucking and in fields with less employee supervision such as outside sales (National Institute on Alcohol Abuse and Alcoholism (NIAAA), 1999).

Workplace consequences of substance abuse include higher absenteeism (two to three times that of other workers), arriving late, more accidents (two to four times), higher job turnover (SAMHSA, 1998a), more conflict on the job, lower productivity, and higher healthcare costs (Holder & Hallan, 1986; Mangione et al., 1999). In addition, these problems affect employee morale and take significant management time to resolve. Such consequences have been a major factor in the development and spread of EAPs and drug testing in the workplace.

SUBSTANCE ABUSE IN THE WORKPLACE

Often the workplace is the last arena in the employee's life to show significant impairment. Signs of a potential substance abuse or addiction problem include:

1. Frequent Monday or unexplained absences and arriving late.
2. Taking long lunch hours or breaks.
3. Accidents on the job and undue risk-taking.
4. Deterioration in quality or timeliness of work.
5. High medical costs (a late-stage sign).
6. High family medical costs (stress-related).
7. Conflict or fights on the job and emotional volatility.
8. Poor judgment in job-related decisions.
9. Disappearance/theft of equipment or materials.
10. Evidence of significant financial problems.
11. Association with known "users" at the workplace.

The last three items are associated particularly with drug abuse. A *pattern* of such events indicates a substance abuse problem, since family stress or medical problems can account for some of them.

Intervention at the Workplace

The supervisor should carefully document any performance and other work-related problems of the employee. Confrontation or discussion with the employee should be based on job performance and not on suspected substance abuse, which is harder to prove. The

---

[1] Alcoholics and heavy drinkers typically underestimate their consumption, so the true percentage is probably higher.

substance abuse may occur only outside work, but research shows that it does affect job performance (Mangione et al., 1999). The supervisor can recommend a visit to the EAP counselor for confidential guidance concerning personal or work-related problems that interfere with work performance. The EAP counselor can then identify the substance abuse. Substance abuse at work is explicitly identified, citing company policy and invoking disciplinary procedures. When the employee's job is at stake, this should be clearly indicated, emphasizing behavior changes necessary to keep the job. Potential job loss may motivate the employee to seek help when other efforts have failed.

Organizational Factors in Workplace Substance Abuse

Based on research, a number of worksite factors have been linked to employee substance abuse (NIAAA, 1999): workplace culture, low worker morale and alienation, availability of drugs and alcohol; degree of supervision, and the nature of company drug and alcohol use policies.

WORKPLACE CULTURE AND EMPLOYEE MORALE. A permissive attitude concerning drinking or even drug use is associated with more use during or after work. Drinking is often an integral part of social events that foster worker bonding (Sonnenstuhl, 1996), particularly in predominantly male firms (Hoffman, Larison, & Sanderson, 1997), but it can become an expectation rather than an option. In a dysfunctional workplace culture employees typically are not valued as individuals, decision-making is "top down," and unrealistic expectations prevail (Schaef & Fassel, 1988). In such a firm, employees lack job autonomy and morale suffers, often resulting in alienation, stress-related problems, and addiction. Repetitive, boring, or stressful work and isolation from others can also contribute to substance abuse.

ALCOHOL AND DRUG AVAILABILITY. In many companies it is relatively easy to bring alcohol and even drugs to the worksite. Drug dealing is common in some workplaces, particularly in large manufacturing firms with repetitive work and low job control.

WORKER SUPERVISION. Limited supervision is associated with higher levels of substance use (Ames, Grube, & Moore, 1997), and such situations are sought out by many alcoholics and addicts. Examples include jobs such as sales, where employees spend all day out in the field.

ORGANIZATIONAL SUBSTANCE USE POLICIES. Formal employer policies, particularly concerning illicit drugs, are far more common now than 20–30 years ago. A clearly written and consistently enforced substance abuse policy can be a significant deterrent to worksite use, especially when coupled with drug testing.

SUBSTANCE ABUSE AND ADDICTION
TREATMENT

A Brief History

The term "alcoholism" originated in the mid-19th century shortly before the first inebriate homes were established (White, 1999). By the end of the 19th century, several large treatment institutes had been built, but many closed with the advent of Prohibition. A half-century passed before a national network of professional treatment institutions was formed again (White, 1999). The primary reason for this delay was that health insurance did not cover addiction treatment until about 30–35 years ago, due to the prevailing belief that addiction was a moral failing and not a disease.

In 1966, the American Medical Association recognized alcoholism as a disease, and in the early 1970s the NIAAA and the National Institute on Drug Abuse (NIDA) were created. As a result of NIAAA and state alcoholism agency efforts, in less than 10 years 33 states had mandated that group health plans offer alcoholism treatment coverage as an option. Similar laws concerning drug abuse treatment were passed by 18 states (McNeece & DiNitto, 1994). Addiction treatment had "arrived."

Treatment Trends and Models

Until the past decade, the gold standard for chemical dependency treatment was 28-day inpatient rehabilitation provided in hospitals or residential programs. These "Minnesota Model" programs were/are abstinence-oriented and based on Alcoholics Anonymous (AA) principles. They flourished because many health insurers covered only inpatient care and not outpatient care (McNeece & DiNitto, 1994). Content included education about chemical dependency, group and individual counseling, in-house self-help groups, and outpatient aftercare. These four components remain the cornerstone of treatment today.

In the mid-1980s, business and the insurance industry became concerned about annual, double-digit healthcare cost increases and the concept of "managed healthcare" was born. A few years later, the insurance industry focused on behavioral healthcare and made radical changes in what would be funded, bolstered by research suggesting that outpatient, day care, and shorter inpatient treatment were as effective as four-week inpatient care (Edwards & Guthrie, 1966; Longabaugh et al., 1983; and others). In the 1990s, inpatient care shrank from four to two weeks to a few days in "detox" (detoxification), dictated by medical necessity. A typical step-down treatment plan today might include outpatient detox, followed by an intensive outpatient program (IOP), outpatient group therapy and AA or Narcotics Anonymous (NA). The vast majority of addiction treatment episodes are now provided in outpatient settings. This presents a challenge since today's clients enter treatment with more poly-drug use, mental health problems, and life skills deficits.

Although treatment is now more individualized, the briefer and less intense treatment that insurance covers is inadequate for more severely ill addicts and alcoholics (Filstead & Parella, 1990).

THE TREATMENT PROCESS AND
LEVELS OF CARE

In the great majority of settings, the treatment process has sobriety as its primary goal— the *abstinence model*. Most programs treat alcoholics along with drug abusers; programs for a single drug are unusual, except for methadone maintenance. After referral, the following phases or components of treatment typically occur: assessment, breaking through denial, treatment planning and level of care decisions, implementing the planned treatment stages, provision of adjunctive services, and aftercare and relapse prevention.

Assessment

The goals of assessment are to gain an understanding of the client's pattern of use and its consequences, to arrive at a diagnosis, and to assess medical and other complications affecting level of care. The assessment should be biopsychosocial in nature and may use an open-ended, agency-developed measure or employ structured instruments such as the *Addiction Severity Index*, which assesses drinking, drug use, and life functioning (McLellan, Luborsky, Woody, O'Brien, & Kron, 1980). Either might be supplemented by more detailed drug and alcohol questions from an instrument such as the *Substance Abuse Disorder Diagnosis Schedule* (SUDDS) (Harrison & Hoffman, 1989).

Ideally the assessment should cover the following topics (McNeece & DiNitto, 1994):

1. educational history and school adjustment
2. employment history, with attention to job changes and influence of substance use
3. medical history and examination
4. drinking and drug history, including past treatment, current use, withdrawal symptoms, and efforts at sobriety
5. legal history (automobile DWI offenses, disorderly conduct, family and other violence)
6. mental health and psychiatric history
7. family of origin background, including substance abuse and
8. current family and social relationships, including co-dependence, family violence.

Clients are viewed within the context of systems in which they participate (family, work, friends) to gauge positive supports and negative forces. Assessment takes place over two or three sessions to allow for a more relaxed pace and to build a therapeutic alliance.

Breaking through Denial

Ending the client's denial of substance abuse and addiction is crucial to the success of treatment and prevention of relapse. The power of addiction is equaled only by the strength of the client's denial. Getting the client to admit powerlessness over drugs and alcohol is a vital, but challenging task since being in control is often a key element in the addict's personality. This issue is typically not resolved until the client is in group therapy and is confronted by group members about his or her denial. Motivational interviewing is a technique that can be used as an alternative to a more confrontational approach (Miller, W. R., 1995). In this approach the counselor does not discount the client's views and the client is asked for his or her perspective on substance use, allowing assessment of the client's attitudes toward treatment. The client may be reluctant to enter treatment because s/he will miss work. Here, the encouragement of the EAP counselor can be helpful.

Treatment Planning

The assessment information, details about insurance coverage, and client preferences are the building blocks for the treatment plan. A medical detoxification will be needed if the client has ever experienced DTs (delirium tremens) or seizures during withdrawal or has other significant medical or psychiatric problems. After detox, inpatient or residential care is preferred if a patient has severe addiction or the home and social environment are very detrimental to maintaining sobriety. If the patient participates in treatment planning and agrees to the plan, there is less likelihood of dropout before treatment is completed. The treatment plan should be reviewed periodically and updated. The client's employer may ask for details of the client's treatment plan and progress, but must be told that federal confidentiality regulations prohibit sharing this information. The EAP counselor can say that the client is getting treatment but can give no details.

Level of Care Determination

Level of care decisions are a key component of the treatment planning process and are often based on the American Society of Addiction Medicine (ASAM) criteria. "Level of care" refers to both the setting and intensity of services provided, especially medical care.

The levels of care[2] in descending order of intensity and cost include:

- Acute detoxification (hospital-based)
- Intensive inpatient (hospital-based)
- Sub-acute detoxification (residential setting)
- Residential inpatient (in a free-standing residential program)
- Ambulatory detoxification
- Extended care
- Partial or day hospital
- Intensive outpatient (IO)
- Halfway houses
- Traditional outpatient
- Methadone maintenance or tapering
- Self-help groups (AA, NA, etc.)

DETOXIFICATION.   At one time nearly all detoxification was hospital-based. Owing to costs and insurance restrictions, there are now three levels of care used for detox. Hospital-based detoxification is used for patients in acute withdrawal (DTs or seizures), with other serious medical problems, or with unstable vital signs. Acute detox now lasts only two to three days, except for heroin addicts. For patients with fewer problems, sub-acute detox in a residential setting can be utilized.

Patients in either setting may require medication to ease withdrawal trauma. These typically include benzodiazepines for alcohol, Catapres for opiates, and amantadine or bromocriptine for cocaine withdrawal. The most life-threatening withdrawals occur with alcohol and barbiturates. Heroin withdrawal is very unpleasant and usually requires medication, while cocaine withdrawal less often does.

Ambulatory detox can be used when withdrawal symptoms are not severe, no serious medical problems exist, and the patient is motivated to cooperate. Research shows that detox alone without additional care usually is not effective (Gerstein & Harwood, 1990). In addition, many alcoholics and addicts are not good risks for compliance with ambulatory detox, but such considerations are often ignored under current managed care criteria for "medical necessity."

---

[2]The terminology used here is less technical than ASAM's, but the types are similar to theirs.

INPATIENT OR RESIDENTIAL CARE VS. OUTPATIENT TREATMENT. The next five levels of care—intensive inpatient, residential, extended care, partial or day hospital, and IO—are the choices for the second phase of treatment after the patient has been detoxed. *Intensive inpatient* and *residential* care are used when the patient is unable to maintain abstinence outside a controlled environment and is seriously impaired in social, family, or vocational functioning. Most managed care firms now require that the patient fail in lower levels of care before receiving inpatient or residential care. Exceptions may be made if the patient met criteria for acute detoxification. Hospital-based care is generally used if the patient has significant medical or psychiatric problems.

Extended care refers to a therapeutic community (TC) program or other long-term residential programs usually supported by public funding. Ninety-day TC programs are sometimes covered by insurance. Extended care is not less intensive than inpatient or residential care, but involves less medical management. Additional phases of TC care include halfway house and outpatient care.

In any of these three settings, clients participate in group and individual therapy, "didactics" (substance abuse education), self-help meetings, and often family sessions. Residential and extended care will also include recreational and occupational therapy and vocational services. When clients do not meet the medical necessity criteria for inpatient or residential care, day hospital or IOP are options. *Day hospital* meets five days and 25–40 hr per week. It is helpful for clients with poor life skills and social supports, but is a less common model for substance abuse than for mental health clients. *Intensive outpatient* (IO) usually takes place in a clinic setting three days and 9–12 h per week. This treatment, which did not exist 10 years ago, is the most common form of substance abuse treatment today. It includes individual and group therapy, didactics, and family groups, and is held during the day or at night, convenient for, and often preferred by, working clients. IO is less disruptive to the patient's life and permits dealing with real-life issues as they occur, but does not remove the client from negative influences in his social environment. Today, most outpatient settings include periodic drug testing in order to satisfy accountability requirements of the justice system and managed care.

LESS INTENSIVE LEVELS OF CARE. These include halfway houses, traditional outpatient, methadone treatment, and self-help groups. *Halfway houses* are residences for recovering individuals who have completed more intensive care but are not yet ready to live independently. They are a good choice for clients with poor social supports, a problematical job history, or limited life skills. Research is mixed on the effectiveness of halfway house treatment (McNeece & DiNitto, 1994, pp. 124–125), but a well-run program builds life skills and fosters vocational advances.

Traditional outpatient typically involves weekly group and sometimes individual therapy. As a first stage of treatment it is used for clients with less serious substance abuse. More often, weekly outpatient care is provided after a client has completed a more intensive level of care. Major themes in outpatient care include relapse prevention, forming healthier relationships, regular AA and NA attendance, avoiding "stinking thinking," and grief and loss issues. The therapy is typically more confrontational than that used in mental health. Outpatient therapy as a stand-alone treatment for substance abuse is less effective than more intensive levels of care, except for the least severe clients (Simpson, 1984).

Methadone tapering or maintenance is used for heroin addicts when drug-free treatment has failed. Methadone is an addictive opiate but does not produce the high that heroin does. Its purpose is to prevent physical withdrawal symptoms, which lead to further heroin use.

Psychological craving and lifestyle issues must be addressed in outpatient therapy. Methadone is offered through specialized clinics because most treatment programs oppose using addictive drugs as treatment. However, when other treatments fail, it is an effective deterrent to relapse and reduces criminal behavior.

Self-help group attendance, considered to be a sine qua non by most addiction professionals, is usually included in the treatment plan. A standard saying in the field is "90 and 90," which means that the patient should attend 90 meetings in 90 days after completing treatment. Alcoholics typically attend AA, while drug abusers are encouraged to attend NA or Cocaine Anonymous. These groups espouse the 12 steps and 12 traditions as principles to live by to remain sober. Twelve-step groups, and indeed most support groups, rely on the support, candor, and encouragement of peers to confront the person who is not "working the program" and support those who are. If someone relapses, however, they are welcomed into the fold again. Other self-help groups, which eschew the spiritual bent of AA, include Rational Recovery and Secular Organizations for Sobriety (SOS).[3]

Progression through Treatment

Two threats to implementation of the treatment plan are client dropout and managed care restrictions.

DEALING WITH DROPOUT.   Clients who drop out before completing treatment are far more likely to relapse than treatment completers (Daley & Zuckoff, 1999). Women are especially at risk due to family responsibilities. Dropout prevention has therefore been a key concern in the field. Many studies show that longer time in treatment is a strong predictor of remaining sober (De Leon, 1985; Washton, 1993). To increase continuity of care and prevent dropout, clients should participate in a single system of care for all substance abuse services they receive.

Additional tools used to decrease dropout by meeting clients' needs include motivational interviewing (confrontation before a bond is formed may lead to early dropout), on-site child-care, and having minority or multi-lingual counselors available. Since most substance abuse clients who drop out leave in the first month of treatment (Daley & Zuckoff, 1999), it is important to engage clients early on. Zuckoff and Daley (1999) recommend discussing attendance with the client and resolving obstacles to regular attendance at the outset. Attendance can be built directly into the client–counselor contract. Dramatic dropout reduction occurred in a program addressing attendance and dropout openly using cognitive–behavioral and problem-solving strategies (Goldapple & Montgomery, 1993).

DEALING WITH MANAGED CARE.   When the client's insurance will pay only for brief intervention, it is essential that treatment be problem-oriented and goal-focused (Schreter, 1997). A strengths-oriented perspective, while unusual in addiction treatment, may help to empower the client for earlier change. Joint goal-setting and monitoring of goal attainment engages the client more in the treatment process. Cognitive–behavioral counseling can be used effectively as a short-term strategy with substance abuse (Project MATCH, 1997). The impact of brief treatment is bolstered by client participation in 12-step groups and those dealing with related problems, such as codependency or domestic violence.

---

[3]Rational Recovery is based on Albert Ellis's rational emotive therapy principles and permits controlled drinking.

Provision of Adjunctive Services

Adjunctive services include pharmacotherapy, nutritional supplements, exercise, vocational services, acupuncture, and meditation. These are increasingly used to improve treatment outcome.

PHARMACOTHERAPY. Pharmacological adjuncts are used to manage withdrawal, control or prevent craving, to antagonize or block the abused drug's effects, and to manage depression and anxiety. We will discuss these agents briefly according to the drugs for which they are used.

Alcoholism. To manage withdrawal, benzodiazepines are typically employed (Rone, Miller, & Frances, 1995). Anticonvulsants are used for withdrawal seizures, and thiamine for neurological symptoms. Most alcoholics do not receive additional medications after detox, but there are options available when craving is overpowering. *Antabuse* (disulfiram), used mainly with severe alcoholism, inhibits drinking by making the client very sick if he drinks. If the client stops taking it, he cannot drink for 4–7 days, making impulsive decisions to drink less likely (Fuller, 1995). Antabuse is contraindicated with cardiovascular disease, has significant long-term side-effects, and interacts with many medications (Fuller, 1995; Miller, N. S., 1995). Clients must be motivated enough or required to take it every day. Clients on Antabuse report significantly fewer drinking days than placebo control groups (Fuller et al., 1986).

ReVia (naltrexone) reduces craving for alcohol, decreases drinking frequency, and shortens periods of relapse. It may act by blocking the effects of TIQ[4], an addictive agent formed by the interaction of acetaldehyde and dopamine (Miller, N. S., 1995). A promising new medication used successfully in Europe is *acamprosate*, which does not make users sick if they drink (Alcohol Dependence..., 1997). In controlled research, 272 detoxified alcoholics in outpatient counseling were assigned to either acamprosate or placebo and followed for one year (Sass, Soyka, Mann, & Zieglgansberger, 1996). Acamprosate patients more often remained in treatment a year after intake (58% vs. 40%), and nearly half did not relapse (45% vs. 25% in placebo group).

Antidepressants and mood stabilizers have been used to reduce craving in alcoholics, but are effective primarily with unipolar and bipolar patients. Typically, alcoholics showing post-withdrawal depression are not given antidepressants unless suicidal or they have a known history of depressive illness. Withdrawal-related depression normally remits in two to four weeks (Rone et al., 1995).

Opiate Addiction. For detoxification, *Catapres* (clonidine), an opiate antagonist, is given to stabilize vital signs and reduce withdrawal discomfort (Inaba, Cohen, & Holstein, 1997). Clonidine and naltrexone (*Trexan*) are used together for rapid opiate detox in 3–4 days (Center for Substance Abuse Treatment (CSAT), 1997).

Craving is powerful in recovering heroin addicts, who also become addicted to the lifestyle. Methadone maintenance or tapering can be utilized to control heroin craving, and research has shown its effectiveness in reducing both heroin use and crime (Treatment..., 1995). Drawbacks include the need for daily dosing, methadone dependence, and possible liver damage. A long-acting form of methadone called LAAM[5] permits dosing every three

---

[4]Tetrahydroisoquinolines. Acetaldehyde is a byproduct of alcohol metabolism.
[5]Levo-alpha-acetylmethadol.

days and eliminates the need for take-home methadone, which is often sold on the street. It is also preferred over regular methadone by many clients (Gordon, 1997).

An alternative to methadone is *Trexan* (naltrexone), a narcotic antagonist used to block opiate action. Unfortunately research on Trexan's effectiveness with heroin has not been encouraging, since clients on Trexan show lower treatment retention than those on methadone (27% vs. 87% in one study) (CSAT, 1997). Since this medication has been effective with alcoholics, additional research with heroin addicts may be needed.

Cocaine Addiction. For cocaine dependence, bromocriptine reduces craving and improves treatment retention, but amantadine may be more effective (Blum, Trachtenberg, & Kozlowski, 1989). Anticonvulsants are used to treat cocaine-induced seizures (Johnson & Vocci, 1993), and beta-blockers for cardiac symptoms. Antipsychotics can be used to treat withdrawal hallucinations. Antidepressants have efficacy for treating the extended dysphoric phase during abstinence and also reduce craving. Calcium channel blockers assist with cocaine-induced heart problems and block some of cocaine's effects (Johnson & Vocci, 1993).

Nutritional Supplements, Meditation, and Exercise. Amino acid precursors may be given to replenish neurotransmitters depleted by cocaine and alcoholism, improving mood, and reducing craving.[6] A nutritional supplement, Tropamine, is reported to increase synthesis of depleted neurotransmitters and combat depression and stress (Blum et al., 1989). The compound includes several amino acids, B-vitamins, folic acid, and minerals which help with synthesis of depleted neurotransmitters. Blum's team and independent researchers report higher treatment retention and less relapse among Tropamine-treated cocaine addicts than among controls.

Meditation and yoga have a calming effect, while active exercise increases endorphins and fights depression. Both are ways of taking care of one's health, and can highlight that substance abuse is inconsistent with that objective.

Acupuncture. Acupuncture has been increasingly used as an adjunct to reduce craving in both alcoholics and drug addicts and has even been tried as a withdrawal agent. In one study, 100 heroin addicts in outpatient detoxification were randomly assigned to receive acupuncture or "sham" acupuncture in which needles were placed on the ear, but not on the preferred locations (CSAT, 1997). The acupuncture group attended twice as many days of outpatient detox as the controls and remained in treatment longer but most did not have clean urines throughout the study. Based on these and other results, acupuncture may have some potential as an adjunct to treatment.

Vocational Services. Having a job is one of the best predictors of avoiding relapse after addiction treatment (Mattson et al., 1995; Walker, Donovan, Kirlahan, & O'Leary, 1983). Job retention is a powerful motivator used by EAPs to get employees to enter and complete treatment. Residential programs and TCs often include job readiness training and sometimes other vocational services, although a recent study noted that a sample of substance abuse clients said their greatest unmet needs were vocational and educational and were not adequately addressed in their treatment programs (Deren & Randell, 1990).

---

[6]The neurotransmitters are dopamine, norepinephrine, serotonin, enkephalins, and GABA, and their precursors include tyrosine, phenylalanine, tryptophan, lecithin, and glutamine (Inaba et al., 1997).

If the client's work history has not already been explored during the assessment, it should be during outpatient treatment or in a halfway house. Substance abusers tend to change jobs more, have "checkered" employment records, and are often loners or mavericks who do not like working for others and might prefer self-employment. On the other hand, many alcoholics and even drug addicts have been productive and loyal employees prior to the worst stage of their addiction.

To provide vocational assistance, the counselor needs to explore the pluses and problems of prior jobs, client skills and strengths in the job market, and types of work preferred. Counselors can assist the client in seeing that addiction was a major cause of job performance problems, help the client regain confidence, and assist with developing realistic vocational goals and identifying needed training and education. This preliminary vocational exploration lays the groundwork for additional vocational services later received in the community.

Substance abusers in recovery are recognized as disabled by the federal Rehabilitation Services Administration, which funds state vocational rehabilitation systems. When a client is referred to a vocational rehabilitation agency, they should ideally receive a diagnostic work evaluation, job readiness and work adjustment training, or other training and education, and job placement services. Supported employment may sometimes be indicated. However, thorough diagnostic work skills assessments appear to be more unusual than in the past due to cost, and there is an emphasis on getting the client placed in *any* job since payment for services is often made only if the client is placed for at least 90 days.

High functioning clients in recovery can be referred directly to mainstream job placement agencies, to additional skilled training, or return to their pre-treatment job. These clients are usually not difficult to place but should not be short-changed by placing them in entry-level jobs.

The CSAT has included several vocational service options in its *Fifty Strategies for Substance Abuse Treatment* (CSAT, 1997). In the Job Seekers' Workshop (JSW), clients receive guidance in preparing résumés and job applications, job interviewing (videotaped role-plays), following up on job leads, and dealing with difficult issues such as a criminal record. Three studies of recovering opiate abusers, in which clients were randomly assigned to JSW or no job services, used raters "blind" to client status to rate their performance in interviews and job applications. The three JSW groups were rated significantly higher and were significantly more likely to obtain employment than were control groups (50% vs. 14%, 54% vs. 30%, and 86% vs. 54%) (CSAT, 1997, pp. 91–92).

Use of *employment specialists in drug abuse programs* has been studied by NIDA. Thirty-nine treatment programs were assigned to receive either (1) a full-time employment specialist (FTES), (2) an employment specialist shared with two other programs (PTES), or (3) no employment specialist (CSAT, 1997, p. 93). Programs with employment specialists were significantly more likely to retain clients in treatment for at least four months[7] than were the control programs (59% of FTES, 47% of PTES, and 43% of control clients). Nearly two thirds (62%) of the FTES group became drug free or reduced use, compared with 45–47% of clients in the other two conditions. However, the three groups did not differ in percent employed after services or in length of time on the job, probably due to the limited vocational counseling background of the staff.

Recovering chemical dependency (CD)[8] clients receiving *supported work services* (on-the-job support) were 50% more likely to find jobs than control clients and more often

[7]Programs appear to be mostly public funded and probably included some longer-term TCs.
[8]The term "chemical dependency" is used interchangeably with substance abuse in reference to treatment.

worked full time (CSAT, 1997). Supported work may be necessary and most effective for clients with limited work histories and weak social support systems.

The potential value of vocational services in CD treatment programs is suggested by these research findings. To expand the number of programs offering these services, CSAT may need to provide financial incentives by tying treatment dollars to long-term client outcomes.

Aftercare and Relapse Prevention

AFTERCARE.   During aftercare the client and counselor work to consolidate and extend the gains made in treatment. This phase typically includes attending a recovery group and several 12-step meetings each week. The outpatient group focuses on maintaining sobriety—relapse prevention; resisting triggers; coping with stress, anger, and other feelings; establishing new friendships based on sobriety; and establishing new patterns of family interactions. Avoiding "stinking thinking"—black-and-white thinking, projecting blame, not taking responsibility, and believing one can "use" moderately—is a major theme. Groups are effective because members give each other support, confront rationalizations and distorted thinking, and offer a haven where the recovering person's behavior and needs are understood. Many clients, especially those with early onset of addiction, will show delayed social and emotional development, which must be addressed in individual and group therapy. Some clients need individual therapy also to address sensitive issues such as childhood physical or sexual abuse, mental illness, or divorce.

Self-help groups such as AA, NA, Rational Recovery, and SOS have many of the same benefits but provide an extra sense of empowerment because they are not professionally led. Clients can try many different groups and are encouraged to find a sponsor to assist in their recovery. Some AA groups are held at the worksite, which is convenient and strongly reinforces sobriety. Several studies of AA have found that it decreases relapse rates and is an important aftercare component (Pettinati, Sugerman, DiDonato, & Maurer, 1982; Cross, Morgan, Mooney, Martin, & Rafter, 1990).

Several studies have established the value of aftercare in optimizing client outcomes. In two General Dynamics studies, clients regularly attending aftercare had significantly fewer work absences than non-participants, and none of the aftercare group was terminated from his/her job, compared with 50% of the no-aftercare group (Yandrick, 1992). Aftercare attendance was the best predictor of long-term outcome. In a study of alcoholics in Veteran's Administration Treatment Programs (Walker et al., 1983), clients completing aftercare were far more likely to abstain during the follow-up period than were those who dropped out of aftercare (70% vs. 23%). Other important predictors of abstinence were employment and residential stability. In another study, EAP referrals for substance abuse were randomly assigned to frequent aftercare contacts with EAP counselors or to the usual more limited follow-up. The aftercare group had 15% fewer CD hospitalizations and 24% lower treatment costs (Foote & Erfurt, 1991). Note that each of these studies was work-related.

RELAPSE PREVENTION.   Relapse prevention is the primary focus during the aftercare phase. Successful sobriety requires changes in thought patterns, behavior, and lifestyle. The difficulty of this task is dramatized by the fact that 90% of alcoholics relapse at least once in the four years following treatment (NIAAA, 1989). Three quarters of crack addicts have been reported to relapse in the first month (Wallace, 1992). Many of the various pharmacological adjuncts reviewed earlier can be used to prevent relapse or reduce severity, particularly for heroin and cocaine addiction. The major theories of relapse prevention focus on the individual's responses to high-risk situations.

Alan Marlatt, the first to systematically investigate relapse, contends that how a recovering client handles a *lapse* affects whether *relapse* occurs. Relapse results from an interaction of high-risk environmental situations, skills to cope with them, perceived personal control (self-efficacy), and anticipated positive consequences of substance use (Marlatt & Gordon, 1980). High-risk situations include those producing frustration and anger, social pressure, and personal temptation. Coping with such situations requires modification of lifestyle, learning to identify internal and external cues to "use," and acquiring self-control strategies. Cognitive behavioral and skill-building strategies are typically used to achieve these goals.

Predictors of relapse include individual and environmental factors and the interaction between them. *Personal characteristics* associated with relapse include psychiatric illness (McLellan, Luborsky, Woody, O'Brien, & Druley, 1983; Yates, Booth, Reed, Brown, & Masterson, 1993), severity of substance dependence (NIAAA, 1989), early age of onset, motivation to stay sober, denial, and evasion (Gorski, 1987), self-efficacy (Rychtarik, Prue, Rapp, & King, 1992), painful emotional states, coping skills (Mackay & Marlatt, 1991), positive expectations of using, and impulse control (Gorski, 1987). Motivation for sobriety, self-efficacy, coping skills, and impulse control are protective factors. Low self-efficacy was found to be a significant predictor of earlier relapse in a study of male alcoholics (Rychtarik et al., 1992). Gorski has identified additional individual traits or behaviors predictive of relapse: avoidance and defensive behavior, inadequate recovery program, isolating behavior, loss of constructive planning, wishful thinking, loss of daily structure, self-pity, low self-confidence, discontinuing AA and treatment, trying "controlled" drinking or use, and guilt and shame.

Environmental and social predictors of relapse include changes in life circumstances (e.g., divorce, job loss) (Tucker, Vuchinich, & Gladsjo, 1991), social pressure, interpersonal conflict (Gorski, 1987), weak social supports (Moos & Finney, 1983), and triggers to use (Tucker et al., 1991). These situations are stress-producing, although it is the individual's perception of them that is crucial. Dealing with triggers is a special challenge for recovering cocaine and crack addicts. An additional environmental risk factor, seen especially in heroin addicts, is a high-risk lifestyle exposing the person to many triggers (Gorski, 1987). Social pressure may take the form of drinking or drug-using coworkers urging the recovering employee to imbibe. A protective factor is developing alternative activities besides drinking or "using" (Gorski, 1987).

Several models of relapse have been proposed and two are discussed here:

1. *Stress-coping models* such as those of Marlatt and Gordon and of Annis. Marlatt places more emphasis on developing coping behaviors through cognitive–behavioral techniques (modeling, behavior rehearsal and cognitive reframing), while Annis highlights expectancy effects about "using" and coping skills for high-risk situations (Annis & Davis, 1988).

2. *Psychosocial intervention.* Catalano and Hawkins (1985) have developed a model of relapse prevention and a 9-month program called Projects Skills, which aims to develop social supports, involvement in productive roles, recreation and leisure pursuits, skills to cope with stress and deal with high-risk situations, and prevent slips from becoming relapses. This program involves pairing the recovering person with a non-using volunteer to introduce him/her to new activities and friends. Clients also meet with their counselor at least weekly.

Regardless of model, relapse prevention programs used in treatment facilities tend to emphasize the following components or objectives:

- Avoidance of triggers through lifestyle change
- Regular attendance at aftercare and 12-step meetings
- Avoiding "stinking thinking" (denial, blaming others, black-and-white thinking, etc.)
- Forming a network of non-using friends
- Personal life goal-setting and productive involvement (school, work, etc.)
- Development of skills to handle emotions, stress, and temptation
- Developing other interests besides "using" (recreation, hobbies)
- Recognizing that pain and disappointment are part of life and need not be viewed as catastrophes
- Building self-esteem, self-efficacy, and a sense of purpose in life.

Cognitive–behavioral strategies can be used to attain some of these goals, while others can be forged through the group process in which members confront denial and dishonesty and support effort, success, and self-worth. It is important to recognize that many addicts and alcoholics have been raised in abusive or otherwise dysfunctional families who themselves had limited coping skills and destructive lifestyles. The recovering person may therefore be learning some coping strategies for the first time. As C. C. Nuckols says, "habilitation," not rehabilitation, may be needed (Nuckols, 1989).

DUAL DIAGNOSIS AND TREATMENT

Prevalence

Co-occurrence of substance abuse and mental health disorders has been noted and researched for at least 30 years. At the same time that these researchers were establishing that co-occurrence was prevalent (1970s, early 1980s), the substance abuse treatment community continued to treat addiction without dealing with co-occurring mental disorders. Two large-scale studies—the Epidemiological Catchment Area (ECA) study (Regier et al., 1990) and the National Comorbidity Study (Kessler et al., 1994)—gave evidence too compelling to ignore. Thus, in the late 1980s and 1990s, treatment facilities began efforts to establish dual diagnosis programs. In this discussion we use the term "dual diagnosis" loosely since many patients have three or more diagnoses.

The National Comorbidity Study, using a structured diagnostic instrument, assessed a national sample of nearly 9,000 individuals and found that nearly half (48%) had had a mental or substance abuse disorder during their lifetimes, and 14% had had both types (Kessler et al., 1994). About 30% of the sample had these diagnoses in the past year.

The ECA study interviewed over 20,000 adults in five cities using the Diagnostic Interview Schedule (Regier et al., 1990). They found high lifetime rates of mental disorders among substance abusers affecting:

- 37% of alcoholics and alcohol abusers;
- 65% of alcoholics in treatment (NIAAA, 1993);
- 53% of drug abusers;
- 76% of cocaine abusers; and
- 50% of marijuana abusers.

Drug abusers are 4.5 times as likely as the general population to have a mental disorder (Regier et al., 1990). A separate study of over 500 opiate abusers found that 70% had a *current* psychiatric disorder (Rounsaville, Weissman, Kleber, & Wilber, 1982).

Conversely, lifetime prevalence of substance abuse/dependence among those with mental disorders was as follows (Regier et al., 1990):

- 29% of those with any mental disorder;
- 47% of schizophrenics;
- 84% of those with antisocial personality disorder;
- 61% of bipolar clients;
- 32% of those with any affective disorder; and
- 24% of those with any anxiety disorder.

These data dispel the myth that substance abuse and mental health treatment programs do not have to deal with both types of disorders. Mental health clients with untreated substance abuse are *eight* times as likely to be medication non-compliant (Dixon & De Veau, 1999).

Furthermore, the presence of a psychiatric diagnosis in substance abuse clients is associated with earlier dropout (De Leon, 1974) and poorer prognosis for recovery (McLellan et al., 1983; NIAAA, 1993). For example, alcoholics with major depression relapse much earlier on average than non-depressed clients, but those discharged on antidepressants are less likely to relapse (Greenfield, 1998). Other studies have also found that treating the mental disorders of substance abuse clients improves treatment outcomes (e.g., Nunes & Quitkin, 1997).

Assessment

The high rates of mental health problems among substance abuse clients necessitate screening for mental disorders at intake (Dixon & De Veau, 1999) and for substance abuse disorders in psychiatric patients (Mueser, Drake, & Miles, 1997). When clients enter substance abuse treatment, it is quite difficult to distinguish between drug-induced symptoms and genuine mental illness. Stimulant, PCP, or LSD users may be psychotic at intake, and cocaine users are often euphoric and grandiose, mimicking mania. Depression is common in alcoholics and heroin addicts, and in cocaine addicts after withdrawal. If these symptoms continue beyond two weeks, psychotropic medication may be indicated. If the patient is in an IOP, it is important to look for suicidal intent and provide medication and/or inpatient care. Differential diagnosis can be aided by requesting prior treatment records and asking family members for details of the mental health history.

Since two thirds of substance abusers in treatment report being physically, sexually, or emotionally abused in childhood (SAMHSA, 2000), it is important to be alert for signs of post-traumatic stress disorder (PTSD) and to ask about abuse when clinically feasible. For example, cocaine addicts and patients with borderline personality disorder are especially likely to have a history of sexual abuse. Many substance abusers appear to be self-medicating for prior traumas or mental illness (Khantzian, 1985; SAMHSA, 2000).

Drug and alcohol abuse is common among bipolar patients in a manic phase and contributes to their stopping medications. Since over half (61%) of these patients have a history of substance abuse, it is important to assess for current use. Depressed bipolar or unipolar patients are less likely to drink to excess or take drugs because their energy level is usually low. Those in a mixed state or with an agitated unipolar depression would be more at risk for use. Anyone on antidepressant medication should not be drinking alcohol. Treatment personnel should never assume that patients already know about these risks; frequently they do not.

Dual Diagnosis and the Treatment System

It is apparent that many dual diagnosis patients present with complicated and multiple problems and that treatment must take these into account. Historically, and even today, treatment of dual diagnosis (comorbidity) has taken place in two separate systems (Shulman, 1995) and typically involves sequential or parallel episodes in each type of facility rather than a single episode in an integrated setting. Research suggests that separate programs are less effective (Mueser et al., 1997). There is a definite shortage of true dual diagnosis programs in which both substance abuse and mental illness are treated with equal skill and attention (Shulman, 1995). Cross-training of staff is essential if dual diagnosis treatment is to become more than a marketing device.

The shortage of true dual diagnosis programs is also due to historical and philosophical factors. Mental health treatment providers have adhered to a medical model and hired degreed staff, while CD treatment facilities more often have used recovering staff and espoused a drug-free ethos. Medical programs are hierarchical and formal, while the atmosphere in CD programs is more egalitarian. Now mental health programs are paying more attention to consumers and families as partners (but seldom as staff), while CD programs are hiring more credentialed and degreed staff than before.

As managed care and other forces have strongly encouraged more collaboration and integration, formerly separate units are now merging into "behavioral health" programs. As trust builds and ideologies and training become more similar, the barriers to joint programs have begun to come down. This is none too soon for dual diagnosis patients, who have suffered greatly by being ping-ponged between two systems and sometimes rejected by both.

TREATMENT ISSUES AND OPTIONS.   A major issue in treating substance abusers with mental health diagnoses is individualization of treatment geared to the interplay among the various disorders (Dixon & De Veau, 1999; Shulman, 1995). Each dual or multi-diagnosis client should have a case manager who can pull together an individualized array of services for the client (Mueser et al., 1997). Such patients more often need inpatient treatment, have a longer course of treatment than addiction-only clients, and are often adjusting to new medications. An important component of treatment for dual diagnosis clients is assertive outreach to ensure treatment attendance (Mueser et al., 1997). Some clients may need an ACT[9] team to come to their homes to assist with activities of daily living.

Substance abuse programs have traditionally been rather confrontive with clients and some make little allowance for being late, absences, and inconsistent behavior. Staff need to be less confrontational, more supportive, and more flexible when treating dual diagnosis patients (Shulman, 1995). The mantra that sobriety is the only key to recovery may not ring true for these clients. Zuckoff and Daley (1999) report good results using motivational interviewing techniques for dual diagnosis clients. In contrast to regular CD treatment, these clients will need *individual therapy* and may not be ready to be in a group at first. Issues such as child abuse, ACOA[10] issues, codependence, and relationships must be dealt with, as with other CD clients.

Medication options for dual diagnosis clients may be restricted, as compared with CD-only or mental health-only clients. For example, benzodiazepines (Xanax, Valium, Librium, etc.) should be avoided. Buspar (buspirone) can be used for anxiety, if effective, or

---

[9]Assertive community treatment, a mental health system service.
[10]Adult children of alcoholics.

Klonipin (less addictive than most benzodiazepines). Clients with an addiction history may need a larger dose of many medications than other mental health clients.

Family Issues. With dual diagnosis clients, the need to involve the family in treatment is probably greater than with CD-only clients. Many addicts and mental health patients live with their parents well into adulthood, and parents may be monitoring medications, bringing the client to appointments, and assisting with needs and skills of daily living. Enmeshment and over-protectiveness in such a situation is not uncommon and must be dealt with constructively so that the client will have supports but be allowed to grow as an independent person. Enabling behavior of family, with respect to drinking and drug use, must be addressed also. If the family environment is too stressful and family members are uncooperative with treatment, then it may be necessary for the client to move to a group home or apartment after treatment. Families can get advice and support from support groups such as those of the National Alliance for the Mentally Ill (NAMI).

Other Treatment Options. Dual diagnosis clients are more likely than other clients to attend a day hospital program after residential or inpatient treatment and may participate in club-house activities. In addition to 12-step groups, they should attend a mental health support group such as those of Recovery, Inc., the Depressive and Manic Depressive Association (DMDA), or Schizophrenics Anonymous. These groups are peer-led and can be very effective in supporting members and urging them to comply with their treatment. The counselor should steer the client toward 12-step or other CD self-help groups whose members will not tell the client to stop taking their psychotropic medications.[11]

REINTEGRATION INTO THE WORKPLACE

For clients returning to work after treatment, it is important for the EAP and supervisor to assist the client in reintegrating into the workplace. Although substance abuse has some stigma, discrimination in the workplace is more likely to result from a client's mental illness. Education of the supervisor may be required but is possible only with client consent due to confidentiality policies and laws. Accommodations will be needed for the client to attend aftercare appointments, and a flexible schedule or rest periods may be necessary at times. At times, the client may need to work at home rather than at the worksite. The workplace may present temptations to use, especially if drinking or drugging is widespread. The client will need assistance in resisting peer pressure to use. Some worksites have 12-step and other support groups which can be important in preventing relapse.

Both the EAP and the worker's supervisor should monitor the returning employee—the former for maintaining sobriety and the latter for job performance. This monitoring should be done discretely and with confidentiality in mind. Union EAP representatives, when present, will often provide much of the follow-up, or recovering colleagues may offer support. These individuals also model acceptance of the recovering employee and can counteract stigma. The supervisor must understand that it will take awhile for reintegration to occur, and the recovering worker may not be able to sustain the pace or stresses tolerated in the past. Particularly for dual diagnosis clients, assignment to a less demanding and stressful job may

---

[11]AA has a policy stating it does not oppose use of psychotropic medications, but not all members know this.

be needed. The employee must put his/her recovery first, above peer, supervisor, family, or internal pressures to perform. Support groups or continued outpatient treatment can be invaluable in maintaining this focus.

REFERENCES

Alcohol dependence: A new treatment (1997). *The Harvard Mental Health Letter*, March, 6.

Ames, G. M., Grube, J. W., & Moore, R. S. (1997). The relationship of drinking and hangovers to workplace problems: An empirical study. *Journal of Studies on Alcohol, 58*(1), 37–47.

Annis, H. M., & Davis, C. S. (1988). Self-efficacy and the prevention of alcoholic relapse: Initial findings from a treatment trial. In T. B. Baker & D. S. Cannon (Eds.), *Assessment and treatment of addictive disorders.* New York, NY: Praeger.

Blum, K., Trachtenberg, M. C., & Kozlowski, G. P. (1989, January/February). Cocaine therapy: The "reward cascade" link. *Professional Counselor*, 27–30, 52.

Brandeis University, Institute for Health Policy (1993). *Substance abuse. the nation's number one health problem: Key indicators for policy.* Princeton, NJ: Robert Wood Johnson Foundation.

Catalano, R. F., & Hawkins, J. D. (1985). Project skills: Preliminary results from a theoretically based aftercare experiment. In R. S. Ashery (Ed.), *Progress in the development of cost effective treatment for drug abuse,* Rockville, MD: NIDA.

Center for Substance Abuse Treatment (CSAT) (1997). *Fifty strategies for substance abuse treatment* (DHHS Publication No. (SMA) 96-8029). Rockville, MD: SAMHSA.

Cross, G. M., Morgan, C. W., Mooney, A. J., Martin, C. A., & Rafter, J. A. (1990). Alcoholism treatment: A ten-year follow-up study. *Alcoholism: Clinical and Experimental Research, 14*(2), 169.

Daley, D. C., & Zuckoff, A. (1999). *Improving treatment compliance: Counseling and systems strategies for substance abuse and dual disorders.* Center City, MN: Hazelden.

De Leon, G. (1974). Phoenix House: Psychopathological signs among male and female drug-free residents. *Addictive Diseases, 1*(2), 135–151.

De Leon, G. (1985). The therapeutic community: Status and evolution. *International Journal of the Addictions, 20*(6,7), 823–844.

Deren, S., & Randell, J. (1990). The vocational rehabilitation of substance abusers. *Journal of Applied Rehabilitation Counseling, 21*(2), 4–6.

Dixon, L. B., & De Veau, J. M. (1999 April/May). Dual diagnosis: The double challenge. *NAMI Advocate*, 5–6.

Edwards & Guthrie, S. (1966). A comparison of inpatient and outpatient treatment of alcohol dependency. *Lancet, 1,* 555–559.

Filstead, W. J., & Parella, D. P. (1990). *Inpatient vs. outpatient treatment for alcoholism: Examining the debate.* Park Ridge, IL: Parkside Medical Services Corp.

Foote, A., & Erfurt, J. C. (1991). Effects of EAP follow-up on prevention of relapse among substance abuse clients. *Journal of Studies on Alcohol, 52*, 241–248.

Fuller, R. K. (1995). Antidipsotropic medications. In R. K. Hester & W. R. Miller, *Handbook of alcoholism treatment approaches: Effective alternatives* (2nd ed., Chapter 7) Boston, MA: Allyn & Bacon.

Fuller, R. K., Branchey, L., Brightwell, D. R., Derman, R. M., Emrick, C. D., Iber, F. L., James, K. E., Lacoursiere, R. B., Lee, K. K., Lowenstam, L., Maany, I., Neiderheiser, D., Nocks, J. J., & Shaw, S. (1986). Disulfiram treatment of alcoholism: A Veterans Administration cooperative study. *Journal of Nervous and Mental Disease, 256*, 1449–1455.

Gerstein, D. R., & Harwood, H. J. (Eds.) (1990). *Treating drug problems*, Vol. 1. Washington, DC: National Academy Press.

Goldapple, G. C., & Montgomery, D. (1993). Evaluating a behaviorally based intervention in therapeutic community treatment for drug dependency. *Research on social work practice, 3*, 21–39.

Gordon, C. O. (1997, Fall). Publication offers diverse strategies to treat substance abuse. *SAMHSA News*, 3–5.

Gorski, T. T. (1987). The developmental model of recovery: The Relapse/Recovery Grid. Homewood, IL: CENAPS.

Grant, B. F. (1997). The influence of comorbid major depression and substance use disorders on alcohol and drug treatment: Results of a national survey. In L. S. Onken, J. D. Blaine, S. Genser, & A. M. Horton (Eds.), *Treatment of drug-dependent individuals with comorbid mental disorders* (NIDA Research Monograph 172). Rockville, MD: NIDA.

Greenfield, S. F., Weiss, A. D., Muenz, L. R., Vagge, L. M., Kelly, J. F., Bello, L. R., & Michael, J. (1998). The effect of depression on return to drinking: A prospective study. *Archives of General Psychiatry, 55*(3), 259–265.

Harrison, P. A., & Hoffman, N. G. (1989). *SUDDS, Substance Use Disorder Diagnosis Schedule manual.* St. Paul, MN: Ramsey Clinic.

Harwood, H., Fountain, D., Livermore, G. et al. (1998). *The economic costs of alcohol and drug abuse in the United States.* Rockville, MD: National Institute on Drug Abuse, National Institute on Alcohol Abuse and Alcoholism.

Hoffman, J. P., Larison, C., & Sanderson, A. (1997). *An analysis of worker drug use and workplace policies and programs.* Rockville, MD: Substance Abuse and Mental Health Services Administration.

Holder, H. D., & Hallan, J. B. (1986). Impact of alcoholism treatment on total health care costs: A six-year study. *Advances in Alcohol and Substance Abuse, 6*(1), 1–15.

Inaba, D. S., Cohen, W. E., & Holstein, M. E. (1997). *Uppers, downers, and all arounders* (3rd ed.) Ashland, OR: CNS Publicatons.

Johnson, D. N., & Vocci, F. J. (1993). Medications development at the National Institute on Drug Abuse: Focus on cocaine. In F. M. Tims & C. G. Leukefeld (Eds.), *Cocaine treatment: Research and clinical perspectives* (NIDA Research Monograph 135). Rockville, MD: NIDA.

Kessler, R. C., McGonagle, K. A., Zhao, S., Nelson, C. B., Hughes, M., Eshelman, S., Wittchen, H. U., & Dendler, K. S. (1994). Lifetime and 12-month prevalence of DSM-III-R psychiatric disorders in the United States. *Archives of General Psychiatry, 51*, 8–19.

Khantzian, E. (1985). The self-medication hypothesis of addictive disorders: Focus on heroin and cocaine dependence. *American Journal of Psychiatry, 142*(11), 1259–1264.

Longabaugh, R., McCrady, B., Fink, E., Stout, R., McAuley, T., Doyle, C., & McNeil, D. (1983).Cost-effectiveness of alcoholism treatment in partial vs. inpatient settings: Six-month outcomes. *Journal of Studies on Alcohol, 44*, 1049–1077.

Mackay, P. W., & Marlatt, G. A. (1991). Maintaining sobriety: Stopping is starting. *International Journal of the Addictions, 25*(9A, 10A), 1257–1276.

Mangione, T. W., Howland, J., Amick, B., Cote, J., Lee, M., Bell, N., & Levine, S. (1999). Employee drinking practices and work performance. *Journal of Studies on Alcohol, 60*(2), 261–270.

Marlatt, G. A., & Gordon, J. R. (1980). Determinants of relapse: Implications of the maintenance in behavior change. In P. O. Davidson & S. M. Davidson (Eds.), *Behavioral medicine: Changing health lifestyles.* New York, NY: Brunner-Mazel.

Mattson, M. E., Allen J. P., Caldwell, F., Fertig, J. B., Litten, R. Z., Lowman, C., Marshall, L. A., & Nickless, C. (1995). Recognition and therapy of alcohol use and addiction: Research findings. In Norman S. Miller & Mark S. Gold, *Pharmacological therapies for drug and alcohol addictions* (Chapter 24). New York, NY: Marcel Dekker.

McLellan, A. T., Luborsky, L., Woody, G. E., O'Brien, C. P., & Kron, R. (1980). An improved diagnostic evaluation instrument for substance abuse patients: The Addiction Severity Index. *Journal of Nervous and Mental Disease, 168*, 26–33.

McLellan, A. T., Luborsky, L., Woody, G. E., O'Brien, C. P., & Druley, K. A. (1983). Predicting response to alcohol and drug abuse treatments: Role of psychiatric severity. *Archives of General Psychiatry, 40*, 620–625.

McNeece, C. A., & DiNitto, D. M. (1994). *Chemical dependency: A systems approach.* Englewood Cliffs, NJ: Prentice-Hall.

Miller, N. S. (1995). Pharmacotherapy in alcoholism. In Norman S. Miller, *Treatment of the addictions: Applications of outcome research for clinical management* (Chapter 8). New York, NY: Haworth.

Miller, W. R. (1995). Increasing motivation for change. In R. K. Hester & W. R. Miller (Eds.), *Handbook of alcoholism treatment approaches: Effective alternatives* (2nd ed., Chapter 5) Boston, MA: Allyn & Bacon.

Moos, R. H., & Finney, J. W. (1983). Expanding the scope of alcoholism treatment and evaluation. *American Psychologist, 38*, 1036–1044.

Mueser, K. T., Drake, R. E., & Miles, K. M. (1997). The course and treatment of substance use disorders in persons with severe mental illness. In L. S. Onken, J. D. Blaine, S. Genser, & A. M. Horton, *Treatment of drug-dependent individuals with comorbid mental disorders* (NIDA Research Monograph 172). Rockville, MD: NIDA.

National Institute on Alcohol Abuse and Alcoholism (NIAAA) (1989). Relapse and craving. *Alcohol Alert,* October.

National Institute on Alcohol Abuse and Alcoholism (1993). Psychiatric comorbidity with alcohol use disorders. In *Eighth Special Report to the U.S. Congress on Alcohol and Health* (Chapter 2). Rockville, MD: Author.

National Institute on Alcohol Abuse and Alcoholism (1999). Alcohol and the workplace. *Alcohol Alert, 44*, 1–4.

Nuckols, C. C. (1989, January/February). Negotiating the minefield: Recovery and the 'new' cocaine addict. *Professional Counselor*, 39–40.

Nunes, E. V., & Quitkin, F. M. (1997). Treatment of depression in drug-dependent patients: Effects on mood and drug use. In L. S. Onken, J. D. Blaine, S. Genser, & A. M. Horton (Eds.), *Treatment of drug-dependent individuals with comorbid mental disorders* (NIDA Research Monograph 172). Rockville, MD: NIDA.

Pettinati, H. M., Sugerman, A. A., DiDonato, N., & Maurer, H. S. (1982). The natural history of alcoholism over four years after treatment. *Journal of Studies on Alcohol, 43*(3), 201–215.

Project MATCH Research Group (1997). Matching alcoholism treatments to client heterogeneity: Project MATCH post-treatment drinking outcomes. *Journal of Studies on Alcohol, 58*(1), 7–29.

Regier, D. A., Farmer, M. E., Rae, D. S., Locke, B. Z., Keith, S. J., Judd, L. L., & Goodwin, F. K. (1990). Comorbidity of mental disorders with alcohol and other drug abuse. *JAMA, 264*(19), 2511–2518.

Rone, L. A., Miller, S. I., & Frances, R. J. (1995). Psychotropic medications. In R. K. Hester & W. R. Miller (Eds.), *Handbook of alcoholism treatment approaches: Effective alternatives* (2nd ed., Chapter 16) Boston, MA: Allyn & Bacon.

Rounsaville, B. J., Weissman, M. M., Kleber H., & Wilber, C. (1982). Heterogeneity of psychiatric diagnosis in treated opiate addicts. *Archives of General Psychiatry, 39*, 161–166.

Rouse, B. A. (Ed.) (1998). *Substance abuse and mental health statistics source book*. Rockville, MD: SAMHSA, Department of Health and Human Services.

Rychtarik, R. G., Prue, D. M., Rapp, S. R., & King, A. C. (1992). Self-efficacy, aftercare and relapse in a treatment program for alcoholics. *Journal of Studies on Alcohol, 53*, 435–440.

Sass, H., Soyka, M., Mann, K., & Zieglgansberger, W. (1996). Relapse prevention by acamprosate: Results from a placebo-controlled study on alcohol dependence. *Archives of General Psychiatry, 53*, 673–680.

Schaef, A. W., & Fassel, D. (1988). *The Addictive Organization*. San Francisco, CA: Harper & Row.

Schreter, R. K. (1997, May). Essential skills for managed behavioral health care. *Psychiatric Services, 48*(5), 653–658.

Shulman, G. D. (1995). Reorienting CD treatment for dual diagnosis. *Behavioral Health Management*, September/October, 200–204.

Simpson, D. D. (1984). National treatment system evaluation based on the Drug Abuse Reporting Program (DARP) following research. In F. M. Tims & J. P. Ludford (Eds.), *Drug abuse treatment evaluation: Strategies, progress and prospects* (NIDA Research Monograph No. 51). Rockville, MD: NIDA.

Sonnenstuhl, W. J. (1996). *Working sober: The transformation of an occupational drinking culture*. Ithaca, NY: Cornell University Press.

Substance Abuse and Mental Health Services Administration (SAMHSA) (1998a). Rates of illicit drug use higher among workers in smaller businesses. *SAMHSA News*, Winter, 4–6.

Substance Abuse and Mental Health Services Administration (1998b). Worker drug use and workplace policies and programs: Results from the 1994 and 1997 NHSDA. Available http://www.samhsa.gov.

Substance Abuse and Mental Health Services Administration (1999a). *Highlights of the 1998 national household survey on drug abuse*. Available http://www.samhsa.gov/OAS/NHSDA.

Substance Abuse and Mental Health Services Administration (1999b). *National household survey of drug abuse: Population estimates, 1998*. Rockville, MD: Author.

Substance Abuse and Mental Health Services Administration (2000). Two-thirds in substance abuse treatment report physical, sexual, or emotional abuse during childhood. *SAMHSA News* Release, February 15. Available http://www.samhsa.gov.

Treatment of drug abuse and addiction, Part I. (1995). *The Harvard Mental Health Letter, 12*(2), 1–4.

Tucker, J. A., Vuchinich, R. E., & Gladsjo, J. A. (1991). Environmental influences on relapse in substance use disorders. *International Journal of the Addictions, 25*(7A,8A), 1017–1050.

Walker, R. D., Donovan, D. M., Kirlahan, D. R., & O'Leary, M. R. (1983). Length of stay, neuropsychological performance and aftercare: Influences on alcohol treatment outcome. *Journal of Consulting and Clinical Psychology, 51*, 900–911.

Wallace, B. C. (1992). Treating crack cocaine dependence: The critical role of relapse prevention. *Journal of Psychoactive Drugs, 24*(2), 213–222.

Washton, A. M. (1993). Outpatient treatment of cocaine and crack addiction: A clinical perspective. In F. M. Tims & C. G. Leukefeld (Eds.), *Cocaine treatment: Research and clinical perspectives* (NIDA Research Monograph 135). Rockville, MD: NIDA.

White, W. L. (1999). A lost world of addiction treatment. *The Counselor, 17*(2), 8–11.

Yandrick, R. M. (1992). Taking inventory: Process and outcome studies. *EAPA Exchange, 22*(7), 22–29.

Yates, W. R., Booth, B. M., Reed, D. A., Brown, K., & Masterson, B. J. (1993). Descriptive and predictive validity of a high-risk alcoholism relapse model. *Journal of Studies on Alcohol, 54*, 645–651.

Zuckoff, A., & Daley, D. (1999). Dropout prevention and dual diagnosis clients. *The Counselor, 17*(2), 23–27.

CHAPTER 23

Sustaining Employment during Acute Mental Health Episodes

LOREN HOFFMAN, ROGER W. MANELA, AND
SANDRA SCHIFF

INTRODUCTION

Traditional norms about work and career are being redefined, and job-related stress is on the rise, sometimes creating mental health crises for workers and compromising their ability to function at full capacity on the job (Ciulla, 2000). Mental health problems can slowly erode worker effectiveness and undermine productivity. They also can erupt in violent headline-grabbing crises, which force a wide range of employees to seek referrals to mental health services for help dealing with what happened. Sometimes, employees must successfully complete therapy before they can return to their jobs. Devastating personal tragedies also can compromise employees' ability to function effectively on the job, and employees may need mental health counseling to help them cope with events such as the death of a loved one, divorce, or severe physical injury.

Mental health and mental illness in the workplace have long been of interest to employers, employees, mental health service providers, and researchers in occupational health and medicine. (Brodsky, 1976; Ferry, 1990; House, 1980; Kornhauser, 1965; McLean, 1970; Rogg & D'Alonzo, 1965; Warr, 1987). Once primarily of academic interest, mental health issues in the workplace are now at the forefront of occupational health and safety concerns in major corporations, insurance companies, and labor unions. In many countries, legislation about worker compensation includes coverage for mental illness and job-related stress (Brodsky, 1976; Kessler & Frank, 1997; Warr, 1987). A continuing challenge for employers is to ensure that employees with acute emotional and mental health problems can access appropriate treatment.

In the last 20 years, Employee Assistance Programs (EAPs), which initially were developed to meet the internal needs large corporations had for addressing the alcohol-related problems of their employees, have evolved to the point where many of them now offer contractual services to both large and small employers in corporations, public service organizations, and

LOREN HOFFMAN AND SANDRA SCHIFF • Wayne State University School of Social Work, Detroit, Michigan.
ROGER W. MANELA • Detroit Public Schools, Detroit, Michigan.

government agencies, and the services they provide have expanded from focusing primarily on alcohol and drug-related problems to embrace a whole spectrum of employee emotional and behavioral health issues.

EAPs are funded, in part, because there is convincing data supporting their ability to help employees recover from stress-related mental health problems in a cost-effective manner. But, EAPs also reach beyond bottom-line concerns and respond to employees on a personal and humane level with skillful and timely interventions.

Recent advances in behavioral health have revolutionized the treatment of mental illness and increased the recognition that mental health problems should be a reason to seek treatment, not a source of shame (Adams, 1999; Satcher, 1999). The fear of stigma and negative labeling, however, still keeps some workers from seeking the mental health services they need. To counter misunderstandings and negative stereotypes about mental health problems and their treatment, practitioners of occupational medicine have devoted considerable time and effort to documenting the effectiveness and benefits of providing mental health care and prevention services to employees (Ettner, Frank & Kessler, 1997; McLean, 1970; Rogg & D'Alonzo, 1965). This has convinced a growing number of employers and their employees that access to mental health services makes sense. But, despite increased access, despite improved treatment modalities, and despite more enlightened attitudes about mental health problems and their treatment, the impact of mental health problems on the workplace remains significant enough to support continued development of more effective intervention strategies.

THE EXTENT OF THE PROBLEM

Nearly two million disabling injuries occur at work annually, and 70,000 of them result in permanent impairment. Every year, there are over 11,000 work-related fatalities. Mental and emotional problems, especially those related to stress, are major contributors to these statistics. Stress-related disorders are among the fastest growing disease categories (deCarteret, 1994). It has been estimated that over 14% of the 400,000 workers who receive annual workers' compensation benefits have stress-related disorders. The direct cost of such disorders is approximately $20,000 for each worker (Ferry, 1990). And, stress-related medical claims cost the U.S. economy approximately $150 billion per year in absenteeism, lost productivity, retraining, and health care.

The 1999 Mental Health Report of the U.S. Surgeon General highlights that one in six adults obtains some kind of mental health service in a given year, and approximately 10% of these people receive mental health services from a mental health specialist or general medical provider (Satcher, 1999). In 1996, the direct treatment of mental disorders, substance abuse, and Alzheimer's disease cost the United States $99 billion, and the direct costs of mental disorders alone totaled $69 billion. Depression costs the United States over $47 billion a year in treatment costs and lost or reduced productivity. This translates into costs of $180 per employee and about $3,000 for each depressed worker (Tracey, 1995). In addition, the emotional problems of troubled employees cost companies large sums of money through tardiness, absenteeism, lost productivity, errors, accidents, and compensation claims. And, this problem is not limited to just the United States. Mental disorders account for 4 out of 10 of the leading causes of disability in established market economies worldwide.

Work-related mental health episodes can be both personally disastrous for workers and costly for employers (Ettner et al., 1997). Even when an employee's mental health concerns are not job-related, business and industry have come to recognize that mental health treatment significantly reduces employee mental and emotional health problems, and the cost effectiveness of intervention is a compelling reason for companies to refer their employees for treatment (Tracey, 1995).

INTERVENTION CHALLENGES POSED BY DIFFERENT ASPECTS OF DEPRESSION AND ANXIETY

Stressful events can produce acute mental health episodes, which are particularly damaging to productivity in the workplace. Depression, anxiety, panic disorder, adjustment disorder, acute stress disorder, crisis-related stress, sometimes known as critical incident or traumatic incident stress, and post-traumatic stress disorder, along with stress related to the risk of injury at work or to witnessing the injury or death of a coworker, all can produce acute emotional and mental health problems among employees.

More than 19 million adult Americans over age 18 experience some form of depressive illness (American Psychiatric Association, 1994). Depression, in its various manifestations, accounts for more days of disability, absenteeism, and lost productivity than all chronic physical complaints, such as heart disease, hypertension, diabetes, and low back pain (Conti & Burton, 1995; Greenberg, Kessler, Nells, Finkelstein, & Berndt, 1996). The cost of depression is so great that many employers encourage employees to voluntarily participate in the annual National Depression Screening Day (NDSD) (Jacobs, 1999).

Depression can range from a slight change in normal mood, which may disrupt a work routine, to a complete loss of the ability to function in the workplace. Three of the most frequently encountered diagnoses of depression in the workplace are adjustment disorder with depressed mood, dysthymic disorder, and major depression. While employers may have a difficult time differentiating the various forms of depression, when job performance deteriorates and absenteeism increases, supervisors should refer the employee to an EAP.

Adjustment Disorder

Adjustment disorder with depressed mood refers to emotional or behavioral symptoms of depression in response to an identifiable social stressor or combination of stressors. A significant number of people who experience changes in their personal, social, or work environments have difficulty adjusting, and if they are not helped, adjustment disorder may develop into "full blown" clinical depression (Levy, 1996).

> *A case of adjustment disorder:* William, age 24, was recruited to work for a large firm located in a major urban metropolitan area. After two months on the job his supervisor suggested he contact the company EAP. William seemed to be a different person from when he was hired. In meetings, he was not able to express himself and kept falling asleep. He appeared to be sad all the time and was withdrawn. William was in danger of being fired, when the EAP referred him to a mental health counselor for an evaluation.
>
> William grew up in a rural community where he had been active in high school sports and church activities. His family was very religious, and church affiliation was important to him. After completing an MBA at a regional campus of a state university, he worked for a small company near his family home. In taking the job with his current employer,

William relocated some distance from his family and community. William started work at his new job before he had completely adjusted to his new environment. He had not yet found a church, and although he had met a woman in whom he was interested, he stated that he was afraid to develop a close relationship. On weekends he drove home, about 500 miles each way. He told the counselor that he felt inferior to his colleagues, confused, upset, and unable to express himself at work.

William's situational change required him to make a difficult and stressful adjustment. The mental health counselor guided William through his adjustment crisis by helping him understand his feelings about the major changes he was going through. William and the counselor identified the goal for counseling as restoring a level of functioning that reflected the strengths William had demonstrated in the past. Intervention focused on helping William develop insight into his problem, so he could understand that the problems he was facing were based on his difficulty adjusting to the differences between the values and life style of his family of origin and those of a large city and a corporate culture. As long as William felt that his personal values, beliefs, and ethics were being threatened, he would have a hard time adjusting to his new life. Helping this young man develop strategies for coping with and adjusting to his new environment and helping him understand how the stress of the changes he was going through was affecting him, was an important part of the counseling process.

For many people, the multiple personal, legal, and social stressors associated with divorce pose serious adjustment problems, and there is a clear relationship between marital distress and work loss, particularly among men. Even when an employee is not getting divorced, obtaining family or marital therapy to ameliorate or prevent marital problems can result in both psychosocial benefits for the employee and economic benefits for the employer (Forthofer, Markman, Cox, Stanley, & Kessler, 1996).

> *A case of adjustment disorder during divorce*: Richard, 32, a physician two years out of a residency in trauma medicine, was working 12-hour night shifts on the ER staff at a large hospital. The unit's senior physician received a number of patient complaints about Richard's insensitivity, verbal abusiveness, and hostility. Although Richard had a two year record of competent patient care, an investigation of these complaints turned up information that was disturbing enough for the hospital chief of staff to suspend Richard for an indefinite period, making his return to the ER contingent upon his seeking assessment of his problem and the recommendations of the EAP which served the hospital. Richard, shocked by the severity of the sanction he had received from his supervisors, indicated to the EAP counselor that he was going through a painful divorce and was embroiled in a custody fight over visitation rights to see his two children. He also admitted that he had been drinking heavily at times, often before coming to begin his 12-hour evening shift.

The EAP counselor realized that alcohol was probably affecting Richard's behavior and emotional state on the job. Without a prior history of severe emotional problems or alcohol abuse, the prognosis was good that Richard would respond to short-term counseling, if he recognized the seriousness of his developing drinking problem and stopped turning to alcohol to cope with other problems in his life. Therefore, Richard's counselor made it a condition of his treatment and return to work that Richard attend Alcoholics Anonymous (AA) meetings and work with AA to assist other physicians who had drinking problems. Richard also joined a divorce adjustment group, which helped him put the end of his marriage in perspective and sped his return to effective performance in his professional role on the job.

The death of a family member or a loved one is another highly stressful event which can be emotionally devastating. Bereavement is often so incapacitating that the bereaved person has trouble functioning on the job long after the death of a loved one. EAP counselors often need to look beyond the workplace when searching for the sources of an employee's emotional distress. For example, a fifth of all pregnancies end in miscarriage, and for many men and women the premature death of a child they had been expecting can lead to depression and anxiety severe enough to affect their performance on the job (Lee & Slade, 1996).

The death of a coworker also can affect workers, even those who do not work directly with the person who died (Breslau et al., 1998; Murphy, 1997; Zisook, Chentsova-Dutton, & Shuchter, 1998).

> *Bereavement issues at a worksite*: The human resources department of a large accounting firm sought the help of a mental health counselor following multiple unrelated deaths, which affected both professional and clerical employees over a two-month period in one of their branch offices. Sadness pervaded the emotional climate at the workplace. Employees were missing work, and when at work, they were finding it difficult to get the job done following the accumulation of losses from the accidental death of an associate's spouse, the sudden fatal heart attack of a young associate, and the murder of a secretary's grandchild, who was killed on the way to school in another city. The national EAP firm serving this firm contracted with a local affiliate counselor to complete a worksite assessment and develop a strategy of response. The intervention consisted of group sessions at the worksite to address issues related to the dynamics of coping with grief and loss. Material was distributed to help those who attended better understand the reduced emotional, cognitive, and physical functioning which can follow tragic losses. Each session included responses to the individual questions and concerns of attendees. At these sessions educational material was shared about bereavement and stress symptoms associated with trauma and loss. The EAP counselor was available to make individual appointments for counseling at the worksite as well as away from the worksite, depending on a staff member's preference.

Witnessing or being in close proximity to the violent death of another also can produce extreme stress reactions. When a class of graduate students at an urban university witnessed the murder of their professor by a disgruntled doctoral student, some experienced depression for some time afterward. Some students experienced acute stress disorder and had trouble returning to their student and occupational roles. When the university offered counseling to students and staff in the wake of this event, those who sought help included both witnesses to the murder and students who had been in proximity to the murder but did not see it or its aftermath. Many of these students had nightmares and intrusive thoughts of death, which interfered with their ability to concentrate and sleep, to the point where they were considering not returning to school.

Dysthymic Disorder

Dysthymic disorder, or dysthymia, describes a cluster of depressive symptoms which persist over two years or more. These symptoms include poor appetite, insomnia, low energy or fatigue, low self-esteem, poor concentration, and feelings of hopelessness. Dysthymic depression begins slowly and can increase over time, especially when one is under stress. It results in a loss of interest in most activities of daily life and can be a warning sign about more severe mental health problems. In the psychiatric literature, dysthymia is sometimes referred to as endogenous depression, or depression caused more by the internal and biologically based nature of the individual than by external stressors. However, external environmental and social stressors contribute to the severity of this condition.

> *A case of dysthymic depression*: Mary, age 38, worked for 10 years with county government and had been promoted a number of times. During the past two years she became disinterested in her marriage, and focused more and more on developing her career.

She recently was served with divorce papers and discovered that her husband had a long-standing affair. Over the course of the past two years, fellow employees noticed that Mary appeared depressed most of the workday, had trouble concentrating, making decisions, and completing tasks. She was frequently exhausted. Mary reported that she no longer got pleasure from her job. While there were short periods when Mary's functioning improved, they never lasted more than a couple of weeks. When referred to the mental health counselor, Mary said she felt guilty and responsible for her marriage failing. As her feelings of worthlessness grew, she withdrew from family and from friends at work. Although Mary's salary was substantial, the thought of working to support herself after a divorce overwhelmed her.

Mary was experiencing dysthymia, a deeper level of depression than adjustment disorder. The most effective treatment strategy for such long-standing depression combines appropriately prescribed medication with counseling. Most psychiatrists focus on treating the biological symptoms of depression through the use of a combination of medication and counseling. Many also work in conjunction with social workers and other mental health counselors, often working in the same clinic, who supplement the psychiatrist's services with additional counseling. The mental health counselor can coordinate contact with the psychiatrist, and, if symptoms persist or if the employee is concerned about side-effects from the medication, the counselor can make sure the psychiatrist meets with the employee and addresses issues or concerns the employee may have.

Major Depressive Disorder

The symptoms of a major depressive disorder are even more severe than those of dysthymia and may include recurring thoughts of suicide and even a plan for committing suicide.

A case of major depressive disorder: Mr Leon, a 52-year-old engineer, had seen a counselor seven years earlier, when he was going through a divorce. Recently, he again sought help from the company EAP counselor, who referred him for a psychiatric evaluation, after he reported having recurring thoughts about suicide. Mr Leon's career with his employer was successful until he had a closed head injury from an automobile accident. He believed he had been demoted at work because of cognitive impairments caused by the accident. Since his divorce, Mr Leon felt that he was a failure, and he could derive no pleasure from life. Although he had been in a relationship with a woman for the past three years, he reported that he had no sex drive. Also, he no longer enjoyed watching sports, something that had given him pleasure in the past. When first seen by the counselor, Mr Leon did not care about losing his job, and he said he did not care if he lost his life. He blamed himself for making mistakes in life that he could not correct. After three months of outpatient treatment Mr Leon agreed to see the consulting psychiatrist for an evaluation of his depression. The psychiatrist prescribed Prozac, and Mr Leon reported that after he began using this medication, he felt a significant improvement in his mood, and he was functioning more effectively at work and in his personal life.

The employee in this case initially would not follow the counselor's recommendation and obtain psychiatric evaluation. However, the mental health counselor pursued the need for consultation with a psychiatrist, and the counselor and Mr Leon entered into a contract in which Mr Leon agreed not to commit suicide and to call a local crisis line if he was feeling suicidal and unable to reach the therapist. After a period of time in therapy, Mr Leon came to trust the counselor enough to follow through with the recommended psychiatric evaluation and the prescribed medication. This dramatically improved his mood and the quality of his life. Eventually, individual counseling was reduced to an as-needed basis, with medication reviews continued by the psychiatrist.

MANIC-DEPRESSIVE OR BIPOLAR DISORDER. A major depressive disorder may involve extreme swings in mood from euphoric (manic) states to deep depression, with increased risk of suicide. With this condition, it is important that a psychiatric evaluation is completed to assess suicidal risk and the possible need for hospitalization. In the wake of a crisis, when an employee has disclosed to a counselor serious thoughts and/or plans for suicide, the appropriate response is to make a direct referral to a psychiatric hospital or to the emergency room of a general hospital.

> *A case of manic depression*: Joe, age 29, recently trained for a position with a casino. After completing a degree in elementary education he taught for a couple of years, while working evenings as an insurance salesman. Joe decided that he did not enjoy working in education, quit teaching, and worked at a variety of jobs. The casino world excited him, and initially, he loved his work in the casino business. Feeling excited and upbeat, he imagined that he would quickly be promoted. In conversations with friends and family he exaggerated his position and the amount of money he was earning. He seemed to enjoy the 24-hour routine of the casino, and he sought out work at night. Often, even when he was off work, Joe would not sleep at night. After working at his new and exciting job for several months, he became ambivalent about his work, and he eventually became depressed and started drinking heavily. After he expressed thoughts of suicide to another employee, Joe said he was willing to see an EAP counselor and complete an initial assessment. The counselor suspected major depression, possibly bipolar (manic) depression, and made a referral to a mental health clinic for evaluation.

DEPRESSION AND THE RISK OF SUICIDE. EAP counselors need to be on the alert for indications of suicidal ideas and intentions when a worker's clinical depression is severe enough to affect his or her functioning in the workplace, since such severe depression can lead to thoughts and even attempts at suicide. If the counselor suspects a problem with a potential suicide, then he or she should intervene immediately and coordinate both medical and non-medical treatment to help the employee obtain both psychiatric care from a physician/psychiatrist and supportive counseling.

A reliable screening tool counselors can use to help them identify major depression is the Hamilton Depression Rating Scale (HDRS) (Jacobs, 1999). The HDRS is an efficient tool for identifying dimensions of depression, including depressed mood, feelings of guilt, ideas of suicide, low involvement in work and interests, agitation, psychic anxiety, somatic anxiety, and loss of libido.

After screening for depression and engaging the employee in the treatment process, the mental health counselor has the important task of educating the employee about the nature of depression and strategies for treating it. This psycho-educational component of treatment involves providing the employee with factual information about depression and educating him or her about the nature of depression. In this "cognitive" treatment strategy it is important to establish a framework for positive outcomes from short-term treatment by helping the employee understand what he or she is going through. It is also important to help the employee learn to recognize when the depression is getting worse, and learn how to take steps to deal with the depression before it becomes extreme.

Anxiety Disorders

With anxiety disorders, an individual experiences excessive worry, has difficulty concentrating, is easily fatigued, and has difficulty sleeping (American Psychiatric Association, 1994). The economic consequences of anxiety-related problems can be as great as those of depression, since anxiety can completely compromise an individual's ability to function on the job. Anxiety disorders are affected by workplace and other life stressors, but they are one of the most misunderstood and untreated mental health conditions (DuPont et al., 1996).

> *A case of anxiety disorder*: Karen, age 39, who had been working as a third grade teacher for 15 years, was referred to an outpatient mental health clinic by a medical social worker, after she came into the emergency room of a local hospital with chest pains. Heart problems were ruled out. In spite of her devotion to her students, Karen felt that her work was not valued by her principal. During the summer, Karen started to worry about returning to her classroom and developed chest pains and stomach aches. Her physician could find no physical cause for these problems. Karen did not know if she wanted to stay in teaching. As the summer progressed she had trouble getting to sleep. Karen felt on edge all the time and was tearful during her sessions with the counselor. During the course of the initial counseling sessions, Karen mentioned her concern about her husband's health following his heart surgery. She also worried about her parents' health. Karen tried to be helpful to her parents, although her father was very critical of her and others.

Through insight-oriented therapy Karen learned to recognize and develop strategies for coping with the personal and social pressures that created anxiety for her. She responded to the short-term counseling she received and was able to return to work at the beginning of the school year.

ACUTE STRESS AND POST-TRAUMATIC STRESS

Research on emotional stress in the aftermath of disasters laid the foundation for the behavioral health strategies that have been adopted for helping employees exposed to a wide range of catastrophic events. When dealing with disasters, like airplane or train accidents, or when faced with traumatic incidents of accidental or violent death in the workplace, both victims and rescuers may need mental health support (Frederick, 1981).

People who are exposed to disasters often have intense fears and feelings of helplessness and horror. Sometimes, these reactions are immediate and devastating. At other times they are delayed and may occur weeks or even months later (American Psychiatric Association, 1994). A person may re-experience a traumatic event with recurring thoughts, images, dreams, illusions, and flashback episodes. Other common symptoms include difficulty sleeping, poor concentration, hypervigilance, a sense of impending disaster, looking over one's shoulder, and waiting for a reoccurrence of the trauma. This kind of disturbance can cause significant impairment in a person's ability to function socially and at work. Social impairment can inhibit a person from seeking help or even talking with friends or family about the experience.

> *Stress after a traumatic event*: Ben, age 26, a postal carrier for three years, was referred by the post office EAP to an outpatient mental health clinic following a robbery. Ben was covering his daily mail delivery route and delivering monthly social security checks when a man approached him as he got out of his delivery vehicle, put a gun to his head and said that he would kill him if Ben did not turn over all the checks he was to deliver that day.
>   Ben was seen by the mental health counselor within two days of the incident. He was physically shaken by what had happened and was afraid to return to work, especially in the neighborhood where he had been robbed. Ben feared that the gunman may have believed that he had recognized him and that the gunman would try to kill him to prevent identification. Ben was also afraid that the gunman was high on drugs at the time of the robbery

and could have pulled the trigger without any hesitation. When seen by the counselor, Ben was exhausted. He had not slept the previous two nights and kept replaying the incident over and over again in his head. When he did drift off to sleep, Ben would be aroused by disturbing dreams. He was worried that the gunman knew where he lived and would come after him. He was constantly looking around and was afraid he was being stalked. His stomach was in knots and he could not eat. Immediate intervention was necessary to help limit Ben's symptoms from growing to the point of disabling him from ever returning to work.

The significant difference between acute stress disorder and post-traumatic stress disorder (PTSD) is essentially the duration of symptoms. If symptoms last for longer than one month, the diagnosis is PTSD. It is important to refer an employee who expresses concerns about acute stress symptoms for help immediately, since obtaining treatment for acute stress disorder is the best defense against the exacerbation of symptoms and the development of PTSD.

HIGH STRESS OCCUPATIONS.   Employees in high stress jobs, such as emergency medical technicians or emergency room staff, face stressful events on a daily basis. When job stress accumulates, a single incident can push the employee over the emotional edge. If the employee does not receive help, then he or she may lose confidence and find it difficult or impossible to function effectively in their work role. The triggering event could be a real or perceived threat to the employee's safety. It might be sexual harassment on the job, or it could be a significant emotional blow to an individual who is already coping with high levels of stress.

> *Coping with the accumulation of stress on the job*: Robert, a 42-year-old emergency medical service worker, with 23 years experience, including combat time in the military medical corps, was proud of his ability to respond cooly in any emergency. But, things became too much for him when he and his partner answered a call to help an elderly woman having chest pains at a private residence. As Robert and his partner began to examine the patient, the son of the woman suddenly appeared with a shotgun. He was delusional and believed the paramedics were there to harm his mother. He ordered them to lay on the floor face down. When police and other emergency medical service staff arrived at the scene they were held at bay, while the gun was held to Robert's head. After an hour of negotiating with police, the woman's son put down the shotgun, and he was transported by police to a state forensic psychiatric facility.
>
> After this hostage incident, Robert was not able to report to duty and was unable to sleep or eat. He described himself as a "physical and emotional wreck." He spent a lot of time during the day drinking, both at bars and at home, describing his use of alcohol as an attempt to get to sleep. Robert became increasingly irritable and would get angry at coworkers and supervisors who encouraged him to return to work. He said they did not understand or appreciate what he had been through. When Robert did try to work, he could barely do so, and refused to enter private residences.

INTERVENTION APPROACHES WITH EMPLOYEES FACING JOB-RELATED STRESS

In many circumstances, work related trauma can lead an employee to seek help with his or her emotional reactions. When traumatic events happen to an employee while he or she is working alone, the likelihood that the employee will experience a stress-related disorder increases. When an employee making a delivery or a bank deposit is robbed at gunpoint, he or she is at high risk for a stress-related disorder. Postal workers who have been robbed or attacked when they are alone are more susceptible to stress-related disorders than when they are accompanied by a colleague. When a bank is robbed with only one teller singled out as the hold-up victim, that teller is likely to experience a stress-related disability. Truck drivers who have been robbed while making solo deliveries often see themselves as uniquely singled out and especially vulnerable. It seems that, when a person is isolated in a threatening situation, feelings of helplessness escalate and stress reactions intensify.

An employee who has experienced or witnessed an event significantly beyond the normal range of his or her experience, such as the accidental death of a coworker or a violent event at work which may have been life threatening to the employee, is at much greater risk of acute traumatic stress than employees who were not witness to or involved in such events.

Workplace events that contribute to acute stress disorder include industrial accidents, especially when an employee is killed on the job, and the tragedy is witnessed by coworkers. In occupational settings where workers have a high risk of accident, counselors are alert to respond to acute stress disorder in the wake of accidents and severe injury. Railroad EAP programs have protocols for responding to locomotive engineers who are involved in a suicide on the tracks or a tragic accident at a railroad crossing. It is not uncommon for employees affected by such trauma to be afraid to return to work and to have difficulty with day-to-day job-related and personal activities.

If acute stress disorder and anxiety disorders are not treated early, then they can lead to PTSD and significant—perhaps permanent—disability (Mitchell & Everly, 1997). In the wake of threatening, violent, or catastrophic experiences, employees should be informed by the EAP about mental health resources and referred to counseling which can help them deal with what they have been through. If they are not referred by an EAP counselor soon after the traumatic event, then employees may be referred by their primary care physician who they see about acute physical, but stress-related, symptoms such as chest pain, shortness of breath, feelings of panic, and fear of going crazy in the aftermath of a workplace trauma.

After completing a comprehensive assessment of the employee's occupational functioning, an important function for the mental health counselor is, with the employee's consent, to help the employee communicate with the employer's human resources department and supervisory personnel. The EAP or mental health counselor should advocate for the employee at work to limit pressure for job performance or attendance until the employee has regained the ability to function effectively on the job.

Another task for the counselor helping an employee cope with acute emotional distress is the coordination of a return to work or a "fitness for duty" evaluation. Such evaluations may be requested or even required by an employer. If the employee agrees to participate in such an evaluation, it could be completed by a mental health counselor, but some employers may want a report in writing from a psychiatrist or primary care physician as well. If this is the case, the counselor can facilitate the process, arrange for the evaluation, and possibly consult with the psychiatrist or physician about the employee's emotional capacity to function on the job.

CISD—AN EFFECTIVE INTERVENTION FOR STRESS-RELATED DISORDERS

After going through a traumatic event, employees need help working through their feelings and regaining equilibrium. Critical Incident Stress Debriefing (CISD) is a structured intervention designed to educate individuals affected by trauma about the nature of stress and support them through the critical post-trauma period of adjustment. The CISD intervention model was developed from crisis intervention theory and then evaluated and revised by Jeffrey

T. Mitchell especially to assist emergency medical service workers, police, fire fighters, and their families (Mitchell & Everly, 1997). The CISD model has been further adapted as a response strategy to trauma for many different employee groups and for the community at large. This intervention technique is also referred to as Traumatic Incident Stress Management (TISM).

The term "debriefing" in CISD comes from the military, where psychological debriefings were first developed. During World War II, psychiatric casualties were the highest incidence of combat disability, and the military pioneered many developments in psychiatric care and behavioral health in their efforts to help military personnel cope with combat and to help veterans recover from the long-term effects of PTSD.

Public safety personnel are at particularly high risk of stress reactions when children are killed, especially if the employee has children the same age at home. The death of a child is a particularly distressing tragedy for anyone, but public safety workers, who face this tragedy on a recurring basis, are confronted over and over with the realization that their own loved ones are also at risk. Also, when a firefighter or law officer dies in the line of duty, it is impossible for coworkers to avoid a sense of loss heightened by the realization of their own risk and mortality.

Help for people who have faced extremely traumatic events should be provided soon after the event. When such help is provided within three weeks of the event, the cost for treatment of a severely traumatized person is about $5,000. If help is delayed beyond three or four weeks, a severely traumatized person or his employer might be faced with health care bills of up to $200,000 (Mitchell & Everly, 1997; Mitchell, 1988a).

The CISD takes place in a highly structured psychological and educational support group. The process is conducted by a specially trained mental health professional who is supported by peer counselors who have also been trained in the CISD process. A debriefing usually takes place within 72 hours of the incident and addresses the immediate response of employees to the trauma.

The CISD process focuses on helping each employee, through a non-critical peer review process, manage any acute stress symptoms and psychologically innoculate the employee against long-term disability as a result of PTSD. Before a debriefing, the mental health counselor reviews all the facts surrounding the incident. The information-gathering process usually includes visiting the scene of the incident, since visual familiarity with the setting is helpful in later discussions with employees. This increases the counselor's credibility and reduces the feeling that the counselor is an outsider, unfamiliar with the job and what people experience on the job. In preparing for the debriefing, the counselor selects a setting at which to conduct the debriefing which is located away from the everyday work scene. Employee CISD groups may vary in size from 8 to 18 and should be made up of individuals who share a common profile or theme. For example, the group may be made up of those who were at work at the time of the incident, or those who were direct witnesses, or those who were not at work, etc. During the introduction to the debriefing, confidentiality is stressed, and it is emphasized that the process is not a critique of what happened or should have happened.

Some employees who have participated in a critical incident stress debriefing will also require additional follow-up and individual counseling. The astute counselor learns to identify which individuals might benefit from follow-up contact and counseling after the debriefing.

A case of CISD debriefing: Gary, an emergency medical service specialist, was summoned to the scene of a brutal execution-style killing of three adults and two infant children. As he checked a baby, who was totally covered in blood and resting in the arms of a woman dead from a gunshot wound, Gary was startled when the child opened her eyes and was apparently unharmed. During the CISD debriefing session, it was apparent that Gary was particularly shaken by this episode. He talked about feelings resurfacing from a similar incident several years ago when he rescued a baby who had miraculously survived an airline disaster. Gary asked for a referral to a mental health professional, and during counseling he said he was not able to eat and had constant indigestion. He also was exhausted from recurring nightmares that disrupted his sleep. Gary talked about the airline disaster as much as he talked about the recent experience at the homicide scene. He was upset that there had been no debriefings after the airline disaster. Gary was preoccupied with thoughts of his own three children ages 5, 3, and 10 months, and he was growing increasingly angry with his wife. He also was angry with his oldest child when she would not take care of her dolls.

Gary required individual counseling that went beyond the CISD debriefing to help him address unresolved issues related to the airline disaster. Counseling also helped Gary examine his behavior toward his wife and children. Family counseling with his wife helped the members of Gary's family better understand and deal with what he was going through.

Mental health counselors interested in developing CISD skills need to obtain formal training and invest the time and effort necessary to learn to use the process. If they plan to work with employees routinely exposed to traumatic stress, counselors need to get to know them and the lives they lead. Periodically riding on calls with emergency response teams helps the counselor become familiar with their work and culture (Mitchell, 1988b). If a counselor is to provide CISD services for emergency personnel, police, or firefighters it is imperative that he or she understand that the CISD intervention is a response to the reaction of normal people in the face of abnormal events. It is not a service for a person with a diagnosed mental health problem.

INTERVENTION FROM A STRENGTHS PERSPECTIVE

Counselors seeking to help employees resolve emotional and mental health problems that can undermine effectiveness on the job may achieve concrete results in a relatively short time. The key is to help employees see their problems in the context of their success on the job before the current problems surfaced. By orienting employees toward their strengths, counselors can help them focus on getting back to being strong, competent, and effective.

When the foundation for intervention is rooted in the belief that employees have the resources and strengths necessary to resolve current problems, the counselor is able to focus on treatment strategies that do not always need to address the cause of an employee's problem to resolve it. In this approach counselors ask questions about how people have successfully coped with different kinds of problems in the past. This positive emphasis helps employees recognize that they already have been able to meet challenges and triumph in the face of adversity, and it strengthens their belief that they will successfully meet the challenges of their current problems. A strength-focused perspective also orients counselors toward active engagement with their clients and the implementation of robust interventions that help employees develop and extend coping strategies that have proven to be effective for them in the past (Moxley, 1997).

Addressing Concerns about Confidentiality and Stigma

Employees in need of mental health services are often concerned about the confidentiality of what transpires between them and their mental health counselor. Many are especially concerned about whether or not the counselor will contact a supervisor or physician in the health department at work. These concerns should be addressed early, especially if an employee fears that seeking help for emotional and mental health problems may have a negative impact on the ability to keep his/her job, to advance within the workplace, or on the attitudes and actions of supervisors or coworkers.

It is important for a mental health counselor to be able to reassure employees that no information will be shared with anyone at the worksite, unless the employee gives written consent for information to be shared with a specific party. In order to give such assurances, the mental health counselor needs to understand the legal and company policy issues related to EAP referrals. The company may expect some sort of feedback or even a written fitness for duty evaluation, and the counselor should get clarification about such expectations, explain them to the employee, and obtain employee consent for such feedback before proceeding with treatment.

From the time an employee decides to seek help for his or her emotional or mental health problems, the employee is likely to have concerns about how others will react when they find out that he or she has sought mental health counseling. It is usually best for an employee to raise these concerns early in the counseling process so that they can be resolved and do not stand in the way of effective treatment.

Employees also may fear that, when they return to work after a mental health episode, the response of coworkers, people in the community, and even family members will reflect negative preconceptions about mental illness. Sometimes employee concerns about social stigma are coupled with their own fears that their mental health problems are incurable. Mental health counselors must encourage employees to voice these concerns whenever they surface, so the counselor can address them and not allow them to derail the treatment process. If an employee has been away from work for some time, at the end of treatment it may be necessary for the mental health counselor to work with the family and with the EAP to help smooth the employee's reintegration into the routines of work, life with family, and participation in the community.

Fear, Confusion, and Misunderstanding

Employees who seek help for acute emotional and mental health problems may be confused and worried about the nature of their condition and the prognosis for their recovery. They may be afraid that they are "going crazy" and will not recover or be able to return to a normal life. Employees experiencing physical symptoms, such as shortness of breath or tightness in the chest, may be afraid they have heart problems. These physical symptoms, which are often related to panic attacks or acute anxiety disorders, are often what first motivates an employee to seek help from a physician or from an emergency room. If the physician rules out the risk of a physical illness, but is concerned about the employee's acute level of distress, the physician may try to convince the employee to obtain mental health counseling and make a referral to a counselor or clinic.

On the other hand, when an employee in the process of mental health counseling has persistent physical symptoms, the therapist should make a referral to a physician to rule out other health risks. This provides an opportunity for the mental health counselor to consult with the physician and coordinate the employee's care, dispel confusion, and clear up misunderstandings about the employee's condition and prognosis for recovery. Such collaboration also prepares the employee to return to work with the support of both medical and counseling services.

Mental health and rehabilitation counselors often use cognitive approaches to treatment which are designed to help employees think about and understand what they are experiencing. Such approaches employ evidence-based, empirically validated information about identifiable and measurable improvements the employee can expect to achieve. Establishing a rational, scientific basis for mental health treatment and linking the treatment of mental health problems to an overall approach to employee health care helps dispel misunderstandings, reduce employee anxiety, and establish a firm basis for continued treatment, recovery, and the continuation of effective coping skills in the employee's workplace and personal life.

CONCLUSION

The impact of mental health problems on the well-being of both employees and employers makes it essential that, whenever possible, effective interventions address employee emotional and mental health problems before they significantly undermine job performance. The challenge for the mental health professional is to build a relationship with both the employee and the employer in which the employee sees the counselor as a treatment resource and as an ally and advocate for his or her interests, and the employer sees the mental health professional as a provider of services that help ensure the viability and productivity of the workplace.

REFERENCES

Adams, C. (1999). Effective health care: Bulletin on the effectiveness of health service interventions for decision makers (Vol. 5, No. 6). Plymouth, UK: Royal Society of Medicine Press, Latimer Trend.

Aidinoff, S., & Kahn, J. P. (1999). Occupational psychiatry and the employee assistance program. *EAPA Exchange, 29*(2), pp. 20–24.

American Psychiatric Association (1994). *Diagnostic and statistical manual of mental disorders* (4th ed.). Washington, DC: Author.

Breslau, N., Kessler, R. C., Chilcoat, H. D., Schultz, L. R., Davis, G. C., & Andreski, P. (1998). Trauma and post-traumatic stress disorder in the community: The 1996 Detroit area survey of trauma. *Archives of General Psychiatry, 55*(7), 626–632.

Brodsky, C. M. (1976). *The harassed worker.* Lexington, MA: D. C. Heath.

Carone, P. A., Kieffer, S. N., Krinsky, L. W., & Yolles, S. F. (1985). *Mental health problems of workers and their families.* New York, NY: Human Sciences Press.

Ciulla, J. B. (2000). *The working life: The promise and betrayal of modern work.* New York, NY: Times Books.

Conti, D. J., & Burton, W. N. (1995). The cost of depression in the workplace. *Behavioral healthcare tomorrow, 4*(4), 25–27.

deCarteret, J. C. (1994). Occupational stress claims: Effects on workers' compensation. *Journal of the American Association of Occupational Health Nursing, 42*(10), 494–498.

DuPont, R. L., Rice, D. P., Miller, L. S., Shiraki, S. S., Rowland, C. R., & Harwood, H. J. (1996). Economic costs of anxiety disorders. *Anxiety, 2*(4), 167–172.

Ettner, S. L., Frank, R. G., & Kessler, R. C. (1997). The impact of psychiatric disorders on labor market outcomes. *Industrial and Labor Relations Review, 51*, 64–80.

Ferry, T. S. (1990). *Safety and health management planning.* New York, NY: Van Nostrand Reinhold.

Forthofer, M. S., Markman, H. J., Cox, M., Stanley, S., & Kessler, R. C. (1996). Associations between marital distress and work loss in a national sample. *Journal of Marriage and the Family, 58*, 597–605.

Frederick, C. J. (Ed.) (1981). *Aircraft accidents: Emergency mental health problems* (DHHS Publication No. 81-956). Washington, DC: U.S. Department of Health and Human Services, Alcohol, Drug Abuse, and Mental Health Administration.

Friedman, R. J., & Framer, M. B. (1988). Early response to post-traumatic stress. *EAP Digest, 28*(6), 45–49.

Greenberg, P. E., Kessler, R. C., Nells, T. L., Finkelstein, S. N., & Berndt, E. R. (1996). *Depression in the workplace: An economic perspective.* In J.P. Feighner & W.E. Boyer (Eds.), *Selective serotonin re-uptake inhibitors: Advances in basic research and clinical practice* (2nd ed., pp. 327–363). New York, NY: Wiley.

House, J. S. (1980). *Occupational stress and the mental and physical health of factory workers.* Ann Arbor, MI: University of Michigan, Institute for Social Research.

Jacobs, D. G. (1999). Depression screening as an intervention against suicide. *Journal of Clinical Psychiatry, 60*(2), 42–45, 113–116.

Kessler, R. C., & Frank, R. G. (1997). The impact of psychiatric disorders on work loss days. *Psychological Medicine, 27*, 861–873.

Kornhauser, A. W. (1965). *Mental health of the industrial worker: A Detroit study.* New York, NY: Wiley.

Lee, C., & Slade, P. (1996). Miscarriage as a traumatic event: A review of the literature and new implications for intervention. *Journal of Psychosomatic Research, 40*(3), 235–244.

Levy, J. D. (1996, December). Employer actions can help deflect depression in the workplace. *San Antonio Business Journal,* 4.

Mataskis, A. (1994). *Post-traumatic stress disorder: A complete treatment guide.* Oakland: New Harbinger.

McLean, A. (Ed.) (1970). *Mental health and work organizations.* Chicago, IL: Rand McNally.

Mitchell, J. T. (1988a). The history, status and future of critical incident stress debriefings. *Journal of Emergency Medical Service, 13*(11), 47–52.

Mitchell, J. T. (1988b). Development and functions of a critical incident stress debriefing team. *Journal of Emergency Medical Service, 13*(12), 43–46.

Mitchell, J. T., & Everly, G. S. (1997). *Critical incident stress debriefing: Cisd: An operations manual for the prevention of traumatic stress among emergency and disaster workers.* New York, NY: Cheveron.

Moxley, D. (1997). Clinical social work in psychiatric rehabilitation. In J. R. Brandel (Ed.), *Theory and practice in clinical social work* (pp. 618–661). New York, NY: Free Press.

Murphy, S. A. (1997). Murder of a family member. *Canadian Journal of Nursing Research, 29*(4), 51–72.

Rogg, S. G., & D'Alonzo, C. A. (1965). *Emotions and the job.* Springfield: Charles C. Thomas.

Satcher, D. (1999). *Mental health: A report of the surgeon general.* U.S. Public Health Service.

Warr, P. B. (1987). *Work, unemployment, and mental health.* Oxford, UK: Clarendon.

Zisook, S., Chentsova-Dutton, Y., & Shuchter, S. R. (1998). PTSD following bereavement. *Annals of Clinical Psychiatry, 10*(4), 157–163.

CHAPTER 24

Helping People with Psychiatric Disabilities Start and Develop Consumer-Run Businesses

JOHN B. ALLEN JR. AND BARBARA GRANGER

INTRODUCTION

Getting back to work is very important to people with psychiatric disabilities; however, unemployment continues to be quite high (Anthony, Howell, & Danley, 1984; Blankertz & Robinson, 1996). Surveys of people with disabilities continue to support their interest in getting back to work (Harris & Associates, 1998; Rogers, Danley, & Anthony, 1992). The federal government has been promoting employment for people with disabilities through a variety of policy initiatives, namely the 1990 Americans with Disabilities Act; recent Social Security Work Incentives amendments; supported employment policy under amendments to the Rehabilitation Act; recent Welfare to Work policies; and recent activities of President Clinton's National Task Force on Employment of Adults with Disabilities. Supportive services developed to help people find employment have most often been provided through supported employment programs offering individual placement with job coaches or transitional employment with short-term employment experiences.

Employment experiences for people with disabilities are often assumed to be finding jobs working for others. However, entrepreneurial ventures also provide valuable employment opportunities for people with disabilities. Federal policy promoting self-employment (Arnold, 1996; Montana University, 1995; Rehabilitation Services Administration (RSA), 1998) has been complemented by the development of the Disabled Businesspersons Association (1999) and the emergence of agency-run and consumer-run entrepreneurial businesses (Granger & Baron, 1993; Warner & Polak, 1993).

While there are many peer support organizations (Furlong-Norman, 1988; Yaskin, 1992; Zinman, Howie the Harp, & Budd, 1987), few consumer-run entrepreneurial businesses were

JOHN B. ALLEN JR. • Director, Bureau of Recipient Affairs Office of Mental Health, Albany, NY.
BARBARA GRANGER • The Matrix Center at Horizon House, Inc., Philadelphia, Pennsylvania.

found in a national survey of entrepreneurial businesses employing people with psychiatric disabilities (Granger & Baron, 1993). Despite this, consumer-run entrepreneurial businesses appear to be a promising way to provide alternative employment experiences and career development opportunities (Allen & Granger, 1997; Engels, 1994; Friesen & Viti, 1994). While human services practitioners are educated and trained in the social services field, if they are provided with some added resources and guidance they can be an important force in promoting the employment of people with psychiatric disabilities by assisting their clients in starting up a business, whether with a group or with an individual interested in self-employment.

CONSUMER-RUN ENTREPRENEURIAL BUSINESS DEFINED

Consumer-run entrepreneurial businesses are those that: (1) produce a product or service for sale to people or organizations in the community; (2) provide employment opportunities for people with disabilities; and (3) are owned and/or managed by people with disabilities. Here are two examples of current consumer-run entrepreneurial businesses: Wyman Way Co-op and INCube.

Wyman Way Co-op, initiated with the assistance of a community mental health center in 1984, is a non-profit 501(c)3 small business which provides employment opportunities. Wyman Way Co-op has 60–65 employees with a history of mental illness who work part-time or full-time. The business receives less than about 15% of its income from government, generating the majority of its operating budget from business activities. Business activities include contracts for grounds keeping, cleaning, building maintenance and repair, the sale of organic produce, and a woodworking business which produces Adirondack porch and deck furniture. The community mental health agency which assisted in the Co-op's founding 15 years ago has for the past three years contracted with the Co-op to provide job-coaching services for the agency's clients. Over the years Wyman Way Co-op has built a strong working Board of Directors with half of the membership people with disabilities and half community leaders. The Wyman Way business manager reports that these community leaders have provided substantial expertise through technical assistance and training to the Board and staff of the Co-op in business planning and development (Gray, 1999). Wyman Way Co-op has received state and national recognition for its efforts in assisting people in their recovery from mental illness.

INCube, Inc., located in New York City, was founded in 1988 by a partnership of people with psychiatric disabilities and concerned professionals. Their mission has been to heighten access to mainstream entrepreneurial business development resources. INCube is a technical assistance agency supplying marketplace resources, legal and accounting services, and management consultation services to people with psychiatric disabilities who wish to start their own businesses. These services include linking people with state vocational rehabilitation systems and assisting them with decisions about Social Security work incentives. INCube has facilitated the start up of about 300 businesses and service projects, including: a national vending business for office machinery; an alcohol-free night club; Courage Communications, a pay phone business; Quality of Life, a CB radio network; three graphic design firms; a photography business for weddings, theatrical portfolios, and commercial ventures; a fashion and retail design firm; a public education consultation business teaching African American and Native American cultures in the public schools; and a variety of maintenance, food service, manufacturing, and retail businesses (Kravitz, 1999; Willwerth, 1999). Recently INCube staff have provided consultation and training to practitioners in understanding their role in providing knowledge about and supporting people in considering self-employment and entrepreneurship as their employment goal.

Currently, the greatest challenge for INCube, Inc. has been the need to keep up with very fast growth while maintaining quality—increasing excellence in the services and the help they provide people in starting up their own businesses. INCube staff have maintained a clarity of the values its founders visioned that personal freedom can grow from access to property ownership, which can generate self-sufficiency for people traditionally left without resources due to illness, discrimination, and poverty. That is to say, INCube Inc. must be a good business in order to teach others about starting up and maintaining a good business.

ISSUES FOR CONSUMER-RUN ENTREPRENEURIAL BUSINESSES

A number of human service practitioners have been called upon to help start businesses as a support to their clients and as a part of the agency mission. Practitioners need to consider the opportunities for empowerment for their clients, the types of individual supports that may be needed, and decisions about management style for such a business venture.

Empowerment Opportunities

In addition to a paycheck, consumer-run entrepreneurial businesses can provide valuable learning opportunities for people with a history of mental illness. These learning experiences include:

1. participation in the research and decision-making through business planning;
2. participation in the routine decisions concerning business practices and business growth decisions;
3. increased skills in peer support through coworker experiences (Granger & Gill, 2000);
4. employment experience for a résumé focused on strengths, rather than a gap in employment;
5. opportunity for advancement from production into supervisory and management positions;
6. sufficient income from employment to increase personal choices (i.e., housing options, transportation, health care providers, education, or leisure opportunities);
7. development of specific technical skills to increase employability in the broader community;
8. experience with decision-making about accommodations (Granger & Gill, 2000);
9. experience with managing recovery decisions and employment responsibilities (Granger & Gill, 2000); and
10. Sufficient business development and management skills to increase the potential to start one's own business.

At the same time, however, there are challenges for developers and managers of consumer-run businesses that may be beyond those faced in a traditional business. Added supports may be needed for individual employees and it may be useful to develop a management style that reflects both the peer support and mutual support expected of a peer-run organization.

Individual Supports

Individual employees in consumer-run businesses may need added support to build self-esteem, self-confidence, and specific skills enhancing their ability to contribute to decision-making and ongoing business activities. An entrepreneurial business flourishes when each person brings his or her individual perspective and skills *assertively* to the business agenda. Allen and Granger (1997) have suggested a teaching approach of "Guided Discovery" to assist people in learning research and problem-solving skills. Furthermore, employees may need individual assistance in managing their Supplemental Security Income (SSI)/Social Security Disability Income (SSDI) and public health benefits in ways that do not put them at risk given needed treatments or medications, hospitalizations, and other health care needs. It may take a number of years before a consumer-run business can generate the capability to offer private health benefits that could replace public benefits. The primary challenge for the business manager in providing support is to do so in a way that meets both the mission of need for employee support and need for a healthy business to maintain quality service or products for customers. Business managers may not be able to provide individual supports in addition to their responsibilities for the business. Collaboration with an off-site employment support program and/or a peer employment support group can provide an important service for both the employee with support needs and the business manager.

Management Style

Managers of consumer-run entrepreneurial businesses need to consider their management style; that is, their approaches to leadership and decision-making given the potential for power differences in any organization. Howie the Harp (1994) refers to this issue as maintaining a "delicate balance," given the nature of hierarchies. A cooperative approach to business management complements the management style of other peer-run organizations (Chamberlin, 1994; Yaskin, 1992; Zinman et al., 1987).

Individuals coming into the business as employees may have little to no experience in cooperative decision-making. The National Cooperative Business Association in Washington, DC, which represents over 47,000 cooperative businesses, provides training and technical assistance for those who would like to start a cooperative style business. Participating in a consumer-run business is more than a job, but is also a responsibility to the business as a whole organization. A cooperative management approach can be successful when there is clarity in and consensus agreement about all the procedures related to participation and decision-making in the business: personnel issues such as procedures for hiring and firing of production or management employees, financial issues such as setting wages and benefits, bidding for contracts, investment policies, and use of outside technical or management assistance. The primary challenge to management decision-making is the dual mission of the business of being both a profit-making entrepreneurial venture, as well as a place for compassionate peer support.

Planning A Consumer-Run Business

Business planning is crucial to a successful consumer-run business, as with any business. This includes product/service selection, financial planning, and management planning. Product/service selection includes choosing a type of product or service based on the interest, skills, and resources of the business participants and on marketing, testing, and developing a viable product or service to respond to customer demand. Financial planning involves development of an accurately projected investment and cash flow needs assessment balanced against realistic estimates of sales and public support revenues over time. Management planning involves the selection of an appropriate corporate structure which formalizes the business leadership and participation options.

The skills needed for successful business planning are not usually found in social service organizations. However, there is considerable technical assistance available locally where new businesses are usually a welcome contribution to the community (Friesen & Viti, 1994; Warner & Polak, 1993). Technical assistance is often available from the following business planning resources: SCORE—The Service Corps of Retired Executives; the Small Business Development Center Programs of the U.S. Small Business Administration; national associations of the product or service to be developed (The Directory of Associations can be found in local libraries); local public and private business development organizations such as the Chamber of Commerce, managers of Enterprise Zones and Community Block Grants; and local banks may have a technical assistance service for new business development. Another important source of business experience may also be found on an organization's Board of Directors, as well as with those individuals who are interested in starting up the business.

Mission Clarification

Before a group of business planners seeks outside help, it is important to clarify the business mission and the values supporting the business's mission. This will serve as a base for assessing decision-making choices throughout the planning process. A consumer-run entrepreneurial business by definition incorporates two major mission areas: (1) an entrepreneurial venture, and (2) a consumer-run venture. The entrepreneurial venture reflects a mission committing the business to: providing a competitive product or service for public consumption, and managing business finances efficiently to make a profit. A consumer-run venture reflects a mission committing the business to: providing real job opportunities for people with career potential, and participation and/or ownership of the business. The two missions can be both complementary and conflicting. The missions are complementary when, for example, increased contract opportunities or higher sales cause the business to grow thus providing more job opportunities and potential for career development. However, the two missions could cause conflict if personnel policies do not ensure an adequate workforce available to keep up with contract deadlines and customer satisfaction. Commitment to continuous reflection on and resolution of issues as they relate to the dual missions of a consumer-run entrepreneurial business can facilitate and promote successful business planning.

CREATING A SOUND BUSINESS PLAN

Importance of the Business Plan

Business managers who had started up agency and consumer-run entrepreneurial businesses to provide job opportunities for people with psychiatric disabilities reported through a national survey that if they could start all over again, they would do a much better job of advance planning (Granger & Baron, 1996). The Maryland state mental health office in collaboration with the state office for vocational rehabilitation developed a training program for people with disabilities on how to develop a business plan. People with disabilities who had completed the training program and had developed a business plan could then work with vocational rehabilitation for assistance in starting up the proposed business. Much of the following guidance about business plan development is based on expertise from this training program.

A formal organization or business plan serves a number of purposes for a business, whether as a start-up activity or for an established business. Most people think of a business plan as the principal financial planning tool for a business, but equally important is the framework for development that a business plan provides any organization. The research that is required to prepare a solid business plan helps management or the entrepreneur focus and clarify the development process, as well as present a comprehensive plan for outside agents, such as shareholders, banks, philanthropists, or investors—potential readers of a business plan. Most importantly, the business plan presents a benchmark for measuring actual business performance, which should be measured and reviewed as the business develops.

Every organization, including non-profit, needs to create a business plan that can be easily communicated between everyone associated with it so that everyone not only shares the same organizational vision, but has the map to help everyone in the organization arrive at the same destination. This is a relatively simple concept. Yet for many organizations the business plan may only be in the thoughts of the founder, president, or executive director. This method of creating a business plan can be successful only if a small number of people are involved, and the person with the plan is willing to continually communicate the details as needed. Unfortunately, this makes everyone in the organization dependant on a single individual for important decisions. Only rarely are business failures or poor decisions the result of too much planning; almost universally they can be traced to management ego (Sloma, 1977). Most people would instantly say that an organization with a profit has to be a success, but it is not a profit that makes an organization always a success. For example, many organizations have monies owed to them. However, if those funds cannot be collected when needed, a lack of cash in the bank on payday may cause the organization to fail, even if on paper the organization is generating a huge profit. The larger the organization or more decentralized, the more important it is for everyone in it to have a clear map of the path that will take the organization to success. In addition, any organization needing financing will almost always need a sound business plan. The business plan is like the road map to success.

Most people are familiar with the basic concepts of short- and long-range planning. A business plan uses elements from those concepts and adds research that will assist the organization in making business decisions. Most begin with business short-term strategic plans which outline actions to be taken and often include time-lines for completion of essential tasks. A business plan can use that information, and can add to it information about the industry (the business and trends associated with it), market (customers or users of services), and competition (other organizations providing the same or similar services or products). Furthermore, in order to know where to locate a business or service, it is important to know where other similar organizations are located so that the planned business is not the one to saturate (over-crowd) the market.

Elements of the Successful Plan

A successful business plan will identify the strengths and weaknesses of an organization compared with others like it. Knowing an organization's strengths can provide a clear path to business opportunities. Knowledge of the organization's weaknesses can identify challenges the organization needs to improve upon or simply avoid. A well-presented business plan will differ from business to business and should clearly explain the business, the market, and projections for the future (Seglin, 1990). The Maryland Mental Hygiene Administration has become a leader in helping people with disabilities think about operating businesses by partnering with SCORE. Training is being provided to individuals and leaders and others interested in operating a consumer-run business, including the essential elements of a business plan: an introduction/summary of the plan; organizational background; service/product identification; market analysis and strategy; operational strategy; personnel planning; financial projects and statements; and a method for evaluating business performance. Those who might read the business plan include people involved in planning and managing the business and those who might invest in the business. The plan should be comprehensive and communicate as if the reader has no knowledge of the organization or industry. A sound plan will convince a reader that the organization will be successful because of the planners' understanding of the business's place in the market. In addition to the value of the business plan itself, the organizational experience of preparing a business plan can provide assistance to the organization in understanding its mission, competition, and strategies. The process of researching, analyzing, and justifying organizational decisions can provide a solid footing on which to build success. A written business plan is just a step along the path for realization of the ultimate goal—a successful business.

Organizational Background in Planning

In preparing the business plan the organization should be clear on its mission, vision statement, and goals. The organization's own history should be presented in the plan identifying how the organization was created, funded, managed, and whether the organization's objectives have been met. A summary of the organization's achievements and performance (awards, innovations, market share, and finances) should provide a clear background of the organization. This process should enable the business planners to begin to identify the organization's strengths and weaknesses as they further develop the plan. Organizations and businesses should be dynamic and always be changing to meet new demands, so identification of any changes and the rationale behind them will assist in identifying trends. If an organization is static, analysis will identify the weaknesses and opportunities that the organization will have before it.

The simple goal of most organizations is to generate profit or funding. However, the business plan should further identify the ultimate goals of the organization by identifying its values which will govern the operation and guide relationships with customers, employees, the local community, and other stakeholders. The goals should ultimately identify clearly the organization's reason for existing, its mission in creating goods or services for a particular customer group. This will provide the management and planners with the basis for identifying markets, competitive advantages and disadvantages, uniqueness, and strategies. Goals should be specific, measurable, realistic, and achievable. They will serve with the history of the organization as benchmarks by which future growth, utilization, profitability, and efficiency can be evaluated. The ultimate goal of the written business plan is to provide, like an architect's plan, a blueprint for success.

Selecting a Product or Service

Selecting the product or service for a business needs to include a discussion that balances both a full assessment of the resources available among the people who wish to start a business and an assessment of the potential customers who would buy the business's product or service. Business resources include everyone's interests, skills, and connections. Before the group selects any specific product or service, there should be *tests* and small starts to confirm the product or service selection. For example, if a bakery or restaurant business is planned, then the business planners might try catering some events to a friendly organization.

The marketplace for prospective customers must also be included in the selection process. A marketing plan is part of the development of a business plan. National associations concerned with almost any product or service being considered can provide marketing information. Furthermore, there is a national association to assist catalog sales business—The National Association of Direct Marketers. Part of market planning is to gauge the pricing of the products or services under consideration. These estimates need to include a realistic estimate of production costs, balanced against the competition. A marketing plan can provide important information for the overall financial plan.

Market Analysis

The business plan must include an analysis of both customer need and a sales plan based on prospective customers. When a business plan identifies the services or products that the business will provide or produce, the plan should clearly identify how these products or services meet a specific need (called market niche). A product or service that fails to address a customer need will always fail. Products or services that are also identical to others that have existed before with no additional benefit may also be doomed to failure. Understanding this will help an organization to describe in the business plan what makes its product or service unique.

Business planners can find assistance with guidelines for market analysis through courses and materials offered by Small Business Development Centers located at area colleges and universities. After identifying the product or service, the next step to success is carrying out a thorough market analysis. This involves knowing the market niche and researching the size, segments, trends, and competition that exist for the product or services. A comprehensive understanding of the competition will become invaluable in differentiating the proposed product or services from others in the market. Locations, hours of operation, current customers, services provided, pricing, and advertising/promotion are critical to creating the market share for the proposed business (number of individuals buying or using the proposed products or services as compared with the competition). One major fast food chain found that by locating near its larger competitor, it could take advantage of the extensive marketing of its competitor by simply underpricing them and providing higher quality. Knowing the competition for every organization is critical to success and avoidance of making the same mistakes that have been previously made by others.

Knowing which potential customers will value the product or service makes researching the size of the market easy. Demographics can be developed on the customer base (which is simply learning as much as can be gleaned about potential customers). Once the habits of customers have been identified, understanding how to reach them becomes much easier. As an example, if potential customers read the newspaper daily, then a newspaper ad might be a very cost-effective way to advertise; however, if the customer base is illiterate, any newspaper ad, no matter how cheap, would be a potential waste. The methods used to reach potential customers is called a sales plan and would include advertising, public relations, promotion, fund-raising (non-profits), direct selling, and other methods based on the habits of potential customers. The market or sales plan should also identify methods the organization will use to differentiate itself from its competition. These may include product benefit, proximity of location to customers, pricing, quality, or other things that have been previously identified as making this product or service unique.

Operational Strategy

Another important part of the overall business plan for any successful business or organization is having a detailed implementation or operational plan. Implementation strategies clearly define the process and milestones that will need to be accomplished. There are a number of methods that can be used to present the operational strategy including GANTT and PERT charting, flow charts, or simply narrative. However the implementation strategies are presented, the plan should provide a clear set of detail-oriented action steps that the business will take. Time-lines, potential suppliers, funding mechanisms, distribution, service activities, manufacturing, and transportation should be detailed with a rationale provided for each element. It is this rationale that will ultimately guide management in making decisions regarding actual implementation progress.

Personnel Planning

The largest single expense category in operating most businesses or organizations is payroll. A good business plan should identify which areas of experience and expertise for its employees are needed for the success of the organization. An objective review of the skills of current individuals associated with the project will ultimately lead to training or recruitment as a method of having available the necessary skills base. The best plans will clearly identify (1) all the skills the organization needs to be successful, (2) the employees who currently have those skills that will assist the organization, and (3) the ways that recruitment and training will be done to bring needed skills to the business. One common mistake made by many organizations is reliance upon the team preparing the plan for its total skills need. In the event of an illness, or a simple thing like an auto accident, the organization is left without the skills it needs. Planning for turnover in employees is also part of creating a sound business plan.

Financial Projections and Statements

Financial planning involves the development of a feasibility study to project the flow of capital needed, income expected, and expenses anticipated given the type of business selected and any market planning that supports the projections in the plan. Technical assistance is available through the variety of resources listed above to assist small business planners with financial planning. The financial planning section of the business plan can be used as a decision-making tool by local banks and others who might invest in the business to determine whether or not they will invest in the business.

Keeping detailed accounting records is a necessary part of every business and organization. Preparing the financial plan for the organization is often overlooked. In preparing the business plan, detailed budgets, sales projections, income statements, profit and loss statements, and return on investment are most commonly provided. Financial advisors and accountants can help the entrepreneur or business manager clearly understand each of these projections. These projections will provide the basis for establishing and looking at common accounting ratios for understanding the health of the business. These ratios can then not only be used to look at the individual business, but can also be evaluated against industry norms to establish a clear picture of organization health.

In looking at business or organization health, most individuals will think that funding, profit, or a balanced budget is the answer to success. Cash flow and available cash are the real keys for organization survival. Most business and organizational failures are the result of a negative or poor cash flow. Cash flow is simply the amount of money coming into the business on any given day and the bills that business must pay. A negative cash flow means the business or organization is paying out on any given day more cash than it is receiving, while a positive cash flow means the organization is receiving more cash than it is paying out. Accountants simply call the difference between cash in and cash out during a given period of time as the net cash flow. Planning for a positive cashflow involves forecasting or predicting all significant cash intake from sales, services provided, loans, and interest and then analyzing in detail the timing of payments to employees (wages), taxes, suppliers, interest, and loans.

Evaluating Business Performance

A well-defined business plan will provide the benchmarks and basis for ongoing evaluation of business performance. This is often where independent advisors on an organization's Board of Directors can play a valuable role tracking progress and in using their external knowledge and expertise. Often management will wish to seek other advisors to play the role of "devil's advocate" in reviewing performance as the causes of success and failure, which may be self-evident especially to an outsider (Uris, 1976).

Each element of a business plan should be quantified and evaluated against actual performance. As simple as it seems, questions such as why, how, why only and why not, will provide clues for understanding root causes of success or failure in the individual elements of the plan. A successful business will continue to ask these questions to understand its strengths and weaknesses. Each area of the operation should be evaluated including: finances, sales, products (or services), operations, management, personnel, and costs.

In addition, industry challenges should be reviewed to identify changes or trends, competition should be analyzed, new technologies examined along with changing market, social and economic factors that may have an impact on the future direction of the organization (Naisbitt, 1984). The objective should be to build a clear picture of the current status of organization, both good and bad. Key issues can then be analyzed to create future strategy which will enhance strengths, minimize challenges, and identify new opportunities (Oxenfeldt, 1979).

Business Life Cycles and Consumer-Run Businesses

In planning any business, and particularly consumer-run businesses, the need to plan for change is imperative. Building a business around a single individual or group of individuals can become a death knell of the business should something happen to that core. Also, businesses and their products or services, like people, have a life cycle which includes: creation, growth, maintenance, and a decline phase. In each phase of the business and product service life cycle, a different focus of management is needed.

Planning for change can take many different routes. In many organizations it takes the form of cross education of workers, but often leaves out management. In consumer-run businesses, the ability to involve members in all decision-making provides an ideal method of planning for and supporting change. Members can be exposed to all aspects of running the business and trained in decision-making processes, which can prepare members to assume new roles as people leave the organization. Key individuals often do not include their functions in this process, which leaves the organization vulnerable when they leave or something happens to them. For the organization to survive longer, planning for this change as a part of overall change is imperative.

In thinking about top management changes, one needs to remember the business life cycle. Starting an organization takes great entrepreneurial skill. The growth phase relies heavily on marketing. The maintenance phase extensively uses skills in administration and finance. The decline phase requires someone with knowledge of consolidation or rebirth through planning new products and processes. Each phase requires a concentration on a particular style of leadership and ability. Planning to bring the right type of leader in at the right time is critical to long-term survival. In large businesses, the opportunities for an individual company to maintain all leadership types is a given, but in a small business, the founders may not be the ideal people or have the skills to successfully guide the organization through subsequent phases.

Each phase of business development typically requires different strategies in the payment of wages and investment as well. At the start of a new business, members and founders might be willing to take a share in the potential future earnings since the business may not initially support them. During the maintenance phase, most organizations begin investing heavily in research and development activities to find new opportunities or products. At this phase, investors typically want to see a return on their investments. For consumer-run businesses, financial decisions over time may concern sensitive issues about, for example, pay rates, benefit packages, or business cutbacks or expansion. These need to be addressed openly, with clear consensus about these decisions to avoid unnecessary conflicts.

SUMMARY

Starting a consumer-run entrepreneurial business is challenging and can be very rewarding for the individuals involved. Joining the entrepreneurial business community is yet another approach to genuine community integration—the focus is on creating a productive business and jobs in the community. Planning is the key to success. Planning needs to include clarification of the business's mission, financial planning, product/service marketing, assessment of management style and employee development, and support policies. A consumer-run entrepreneurial business, like any peer-run organization, needs to be concerned with issues of power, authority, and responsibility in the organization and the relationships between individuals and the group as a whole. Practitioners who provide services to people with psychiatric disabilities can work creatively during the business planning process by facilitating access to planning resources and heightening awareness of the kinds of questions that will be important to developing a successful business.

REFERENCES

Allen, J. B., & Granger, B. (1997) Consumer-run entrepreneurial businesses: Issues and opportunities. In D. Moxley, C. Mowbray, C. Jasper, & L. Howel (Eds.), *Consumers as providers in psychiatric rehabilitation: models, applications and first person accounts.* Columbia, MD: International Association of Psychosocial Rehabilitation Services.

Anthony, W. A., Howell, J., & Danley, K. (1984) The vocational rehabilitation of the psychiatrically disabled. In M. Mirabi (Ed.), *The chronically mentally ill: Research and services.* Jamaica, NH: SP Medical and Scientific Books.

Arnold, N. L. (1996). *Self-employment in vocational rehabilitation: Building on lessons from rural America* (Monograph of the Research and Training Center on Rural Rehabilitation Services). Missoula, MT: University of Montana.

Blankertz, L., & Robinson, S. (1996). Adding a vocational focus to mental health rehabilitation. *Psychiatric services, 47,* 333–349.

Chamberlin, J. (1994). Direct democracy as a form of program governance. In Howie the Harp & S. Zinman (Eds.), *Reaching across II: Maintaining our roots/The challenge of growth.* Sacramento, CA: California Network of Mental Health Clients.

Disabled Businesspersons Association (1999). *DBA: Advisor Newsletter, 5* (1). San Diego, CA: SDSU–Interwork Institute.

Engels, P. (1994) Starting and running your own business. In Howie the Harp & S. Zinman (Eds.), *Reaching across II: Maintaining our roots/The challenge of growth.* Sacramento, CA: California Network of Mental Health Clients.

Friesen, M., & Viti, F. (1994). *"Group Hallucinations"—Overcoming disbelief: Yes you can start a community business.* Toronto, Canada: Consumer Survivor Business Council of Ontario, National Network for Mental Health.

Furlong-Norman, K. (Ed.) (1988). Consumer/ex-patient initiatives (Special Issue). *Community Support Network News* Boston University, Center for Psychiatric Rehabilitation.

Granger, B., & Baron, R. (1993). *A national survey of agency-sponsored entrepreneurial businesses employing individuals with long-term mental illness: Final report.* Philadelphia, PA: Matrix Research Institute.

Granger, B., & Baron, R. (1996) Agency sponsored entrepreneurial businesses that employ individuals with psychiatric disabilities. *Journal of Vocational Rehabilitation, 6*(2), 185–196.

Granger, B., & Gill, P. (2000, Spring). Strategies for assisting people with psychiatric disabilities in understanding how to assert their ADA rights, arrange job accommodations and solve problems through peer support. *Psychiatric Rehabilitation Skills, 4*(1), 120–135.

Gray, P. (1999). Personal interview with business manager of Wyman Way Coop, November 29.

Harris, L., & Associates (1998). *The 1998 N.O.D./Harris Survey of Americans with Disabilities.* Washington, DC: The National Organizations on Disability.

Howie the Harp (1994). A crazy folks' guide to reasonable accommodation. In Howie the Harp & S. Zinman (Eds.), *Reaching across II: Maintaining our roots/The challenge of growth.* Sacramento, CA: California Network of Mental Health Clients.

Howie the Harp, & S. Zinman (Eds.) (1994). *Reaching across II: Maintaining our roots/The challenge of growth.* Sacramento, CA: California Network of Mental Health Clients.

Kravitz, M. (1999). Personal interview with Executive Director of INCube, Inc., November 29.

Montana University Rural Institute on Disabilities (1995). Self employment. *Rural Facts* (newsletter), April.

Naisbitt, J. (1982). *Megatrends,* Warner Books, New York, NY.

Oxenfeldt, A. R. (1979). *Cost–benefit analysis for executive decision making.* AMACOM, Washington, D.C.

Rehabilitation Services Administration (RSA) (1998). *Self employment* (Information Memorandum, RSA-IM-98-16, July 7).

Rogers S., Danley, K., & Anthony, W. A. (1992). *Survey of client preferences for vocational and educational services.* Boston, MA: Boston University, Center for Psychiatric Rehabilitation.

Seglin, J. L. (1990). *Financing your small business.* New York, NY: McGraw-Hill.

Sloma, R. S. (1977). *No-nonsense management—A general manager's primer.* New York, NY: Macmillan.

Uris, A. (1976). *The executive deskbook.* New York, NY: Van Nostrand Reinhold.

Warner, R., & Polak, P. (1993). An economic development approach to the mentally ill in the community. Boulder, CO: Mental Health Center of Boulder County.

Willwerth, J. (1999). Working their way back: Drugs and therapy help, but many mentally ill also need social rehabilitation. Here's how it succeeds. *Time Magazine,* November 22, 70–71.

Yaskin, J. C. (Ed.) (1992). *Nuts and bolts: A technical assistance guide for mental health consumer/survivor self-help groups.* Philadelphia, PA: National Mental Health Consumer Self-Help Clearinghouse/Project SHARE.

Zinman, S. (1987). Issues of Power. In Zinman, S., Howie the Harp, & Budd, S. (Eds.), *Reaching across: Mental health clients helping each other.* Sacramento, CA: California Network of Mental Health Clients.

Zinman, S., Howie the Harp, & Budd, S. (Eds.) (1987). *Reaching across: Mental health clients helping each other.* Sacramento, CA: California Network of Mental Health Clients.

RESPONDING TO REHABILITATION, MENTAL HEALTH, AND EMPLOYMENT NEEDS

The nine chapters that comprise this section of the *Sourcebook* illustrate the broad spectrum of populations that can benefit from an integrated approach to rehabilitation and mental health service delivery that focus on the achievement of employment as an outcome. The chapters address a diversity of populations and the authors of each chapter focus on a particular group that requires employment and addresses how rehabilitation and mental health service can be combined to facilitate practical outcomes that are relevant to employment.

In Chapter 25, Manela and his colleagues discuss the critical transition from high school to adult life and the specific challenges secondary students with special needs must face when they undertake such a transition. The authors of this chapter highlight an important observation that echoes through all of the chapters: employment cannot be easily isolated from the total life space of individuals and the achievement of employment outcomes must occur within a matrix of supports that ultimately improve the quality of life of recipients. The authors, experienced school social workers, show how employment is addressed within a total plan that is designed to facilitate successful transition and subsequent service provision.

Chapter 26 focuses on the integration of services for people who are deaf and hard of hearing. In this chapter Pray shows how mental health and rehabilitation services are combined with employment opportunities within the context of a community support strategy. She shows how the strengths of the deaf community can facilitate positive outcomes for this particular group. Likewise, in Chapter 27, Baer focuses on the supported employment of people coping with serious mental illness. Baer reviews different models of support and shows how people with psychiatric disabilities can benefit from an array of supports that facilitate their entry into employment and their subsequent successful job performance.

In Chapter 28 Crimando addresses the employment needs of people coping with physical disabilities. He offers an in-depth perspective on physical disability and grounds his discussion in contemporary rehabilitation theory about the functional nature of disability. The author builds his guidelines for the integration of rehabilitation and mental health services on this theoretical perspective, which offers readers practical strategies for the organization of services. In Chapter 29, Van der Tuin addresses the mental health and rehabilitation needs of immigrants. This author builds her approach to service delivery on a theoretical understanding of immigration and links her recommendations to the practical challenges immigrants face in finding employment while trying to accommodate a new and complex cultural situation. Van der Tuin illustrates how the process of immigration can create considerable stress for newcomers and she shows how the integration of mental health, rehabilitation, and social services can help them to accommodate to the new culture, and to help them secure employment as an immediate and critical outcome of service.

Hyduk and Kustowski address the employment needs of people coping with HIV and AIDS in Chapter 30. This is an exciting chapter because of its optimism based on an analysis of HIV and AIDS within a socio-medical context. The authors show how changes in societal attitudes and law as well as innovations in medical treatment combined with self-help and mental health services can help people to re-enter the workforce and/or sustain their careers and work. Like all of the chapters in this section, the authors illustrate the importance of the integration of rehabilitation and mental health services and, in the case of HIV and AIDS, the inclusion of medical care to the achievement of employment outcomes.

In Chapter 31, Moore examines the transition from welfare to work, a timely and current issue in the field of mental health and rehabilitation practice. The author analyzes the legal requirements of Temporary Assistance for Needy Families (TANF) and juxtaposes these requirements against many of the mental health needs faced by people with long-term dependency on welfare assistance. Moore identifies many mental health challenges and offers practical guidelines for integrating services to facilitate not only transition from welfare to work but long-term adjustment to employment, as well. Weisz and Black, authors of Chapter 32, analyze the mental health and rehabilitation issues that practitioners must address when they work with women. The authors analyze the dynamics of gender and illustrate the many different issues women face that range from responsibility for household and family to the experience of sexual harassment, domestic violence, and victimization. The authors offer practical guidelines for how mental health and rehabilitation services can be modified to facilitate the employment of women.

In the final chapter of this section Pallone and Hennessy focus on rehabilitation services for criminal offenders. Their thorough review of this field and their critical analysis of mental health, social, and rehabilitation services ultimately distinguishes between what offenders need and what they want. The authors recognize the challenge of helping people to want assistance, which indicates how important the development of rehabilitative readiness is to the achievement of successful outcomes.

These nine chapters communicate the broad scope of rehabilitation and mental health practice. The content of these chapters demonstrate how different practitioners frame theoretical perspectives, and how they operationalize principles of practice in actual service situations with people who face specific social issues, ones that create very serious mental health, rehabilitative, and employment challenges.

CHAPTER 25

Planning and Supporting the Transition of Secondary School Students from School to Adult Life

ROGER W. MANELA, PAMELA K. MANELA,
AND GERALYN L. JANECZKO

The change from the life of a high school student to a more independent adult life after graduation is one of the most important transitions for a student with a disability. It heralds a shift in responsibility from school and parents to the student himself or herself, and it marks a change in support services from those provided by the school to those provided by community-based agencies to help with independent living, work, and post-secondary education. Planning for this transition must take account of each student's unique needs, abilities, interests, family, and social situation (Janeczko, Kasander, Randall, Summers, & Wunderlich 1995). When students with disabilities graduate from high school, they and their families may require a bridge between the services provided by the school system and community-based services to help the graduate succeed after he or she finishes high school. Transition planning provides such a bridge by defining a structured path to adulthood that helps the graduating student with a disability live more independently, find and keep a satisfying job, continue with education and training, and obtain needed support (Pierangelo & Crane, 1997).

THE TRANSITION FROM SCHOOL
TO ADULT LIFE

Graduating from high school can be exciting, but it also raises a number of issues and questions about what comes next, whether or not the graduate is adequately prepared for the future, the continuing role of parents, and the steps the student must take to ensure the transition to adulthood is successful. The student and his or her parents have to make important decisions about personal care, living arrangements, employment, social situations, and

ROGER W. MANELA • Detroit Public Schools, Detroit, Michigan.
PAMELA K. MANELA AND GERALYN L. JANECZKO • Southfield Public Schools, Southfield, Michigan.

finances. Before graduation, the school can help guide and support the student. After graduation, the student will need to be more independent and will have to work with new professionals, master new skills, and learn a lot of new information (Lenz, 1992). If these responsibilities confront students and parents all at once, they can be overwhelming. Therefore, it is important for the student, parents, the school, and community-based service agencies to begin planning early for the student's transition to adulthood (Storms, De Stafano, & O'Leary, 1996). If transition planning is to ensure that students with disabilities prepare during their high school years for life as adults, then it should begin as early as possible to progressively build skills and transfer responsibility to the student.

PARTICIPANTS IN THE TRANSITION PLANNING PROCESS

Each participant brings a unique set of concerns, specialized information, and a specific perspective to the transition planning process. Transition planning emphasizes coordination of services to provide students with specific skills for daily living and to address the more general quality of life issues facing the student entering adulthood.

The School

The school is required by the Individuals with Disabilities Education Act (IDEA) to initiate a transition planning process for all students with disabilities (Ward, 1999). The transition plans that emerge from this process are individualized and specific for each student and are mandated as part of the Individualized Education Plan (IEP) developed for the student while he or she is in school. Through a process of "transition life planning" (TLP), the school helps students with disabilities and their parents map out various paths the student could follow and choose the most appropriate path for achieving the student's individual goals in a variety of areas of adult life. The transition plan takes the student through his or her high school years and orients the student toward moving from the security and structure of school to embrace the risks and opportunities of adult life (De Stefano & Winking, 1996). Developing a Transition Life Plan is a different activity than developing the IEP, and it is often more effective when it takes place separately from, but is coordinated with, the IEP process (Copenhaver, 1995).

The school reviews the transition plan each year and the planning team can reconvene to consider changes to the plan that reflect in the student's current needs. The school also reviews the student's educational performance and works with students and parents to help the student make appropriate educational progress. As part of this process, the school encourages the family to help their child participate more independently at home and in community activities. The school also provides information to parents and students about helpful agencies and programs in the community.

The Student

TLP is mandated to begin when a student with a disability reaches the age of 16, but it should be introduced and considered at IEPs of students age 14 or younger. Often, the success of a transition plan depends on developing and implementing plans for future employment and independent living as early as possible. This is especially true for students with severe disabilities and for those who are likely to drop out of school before graduation (Parshall, 1998). The more serious the student's disability, the earlier transition planning should begin. Even when students stay in school beyond age 18, they can benefit from beginning to plan their transition to adulthood early (Charner et al., 1995).

An important outcome of transition planning is empowering the family and student to do their own case management and to become advocates for their interests. One way to facilitate this is by helping them get involved in advocacy and policy-advisory bodies. Such involvement can motivate and equip parents and students to more fully participate in the TLP process (NICHCT, 1999). It can also arm parents and students with information and ideas they can use to more fully examine the suggestions and decisions of professional service providers. While this may be seen as challenging their authority or questioning their expertise by some professional service providers, informed and proactive parents and students enrich the transition planning process and force all participants in the planning process to think hard about their plans and decisions, justify their conclusions, and provide services which students and their parents understand and with which they are comfortable.

It is essential for the student to be an active participant in the development of his or her transition plan. If the student does not participate in TLP meetings, give opinions, and have the objectives he or she wants to achieve included in the transition plan, then the student probably will not embrace or follow the plan (McGahee-Kovac, 1995). When a student does not attend the transition planning meeting, the public education agency must make every effort to elicit student preferences and ensure that they are considered. This can be difficult, and it is much easier to make sure students attend and participate in developing their transition plans. Without their participation, it is difficult to help students learn to advocate for themselves and take control of their future (Children's Defense Fund, 1989). The transition planning meeting gives students a chance to discuss their interests, abilities, strengths, and weaknesses. By showing and discussing portfolios of their accomplishments and awards at the TLP meeting, students can learn to identify and describe their areas of strength, competence, and achievement (Kimeldorf, 1994). As students gain real-world experience, transition planning meetings give them a chance to ask questions and clarify their understanding of what lies ahead. Transition planning meetings also give students a chance to air feelings, express concerns, and share their changing ideas with the transition team (Curtis & Dezelsky, 1995). TLP gives students a chance to assess their academic and job readiness skills, develop a personal "map" of their goals, and pursue the activities that will help them reach their objectives (Parnell, 1995).

Some young people, who find it difficult to develop informed and realistic plans, may need to develop their planning and decision-making skills. Their parents can help by giving them increasing levels of responsibility for planning and implementing decisions that affect their lives. The school can help by providing students with training in decision-making and by supporting parents, as they give their children opportunities to make and implement meaningful decisions (Van Reusen, Bos, Schumaker, & Deshler, 1994). Through a process of progressively increasing responsibility both in school and at home, students with disabilities can learn to manage their own lives, coordinate the services they need, take ownership of the goals they set, and accept the choices they make.

After the student with a disability graduates from high school, the school system is not usually responsible for providing continuing educational or support services, although in some states a student with a disability may be eligible for educational and support services from the public education agency until he or she reaches a certain age (through the 21st year under federal mandates, and beyond in some states; for example, through the 26th year in Michigan). When things do not turn out as planned for the graduate, the school may still play a part in helping restart the planning process and redefine a viable path for the transition to independent living. While such continued involvement by the school is not usual, in some cases it can help ensure that planned services and activities continue to meet the graduate's changing needs and circumstances.

Parents

Parental input to transition planning is particularly important, because the whole family goes through a transition when a family member with a disability graduates from high school and enters adulthood. The school is responsible for notifying parents about transition planning meetings and informing them about the purpose of the meeting (Detroit Public Schools, 1999). The parent should know that the student will be invited to the TLP meeting and that specific agencies in the community which could help the student after graduation from high school will also be invited to send representatives to the meeting.

Parents can help plan for what their son or daughter will do after graduation by regularly communicating with the school about their child and sharing information with teachers, counselors, school social workers, and others who will be involved in the planning process. Parents can also invite or request that representatives from various agencies, such as vocational rehabilitation or mental health, attend transition planning meetings, particularly if a student is already working with these agencies.

Parents can prepare for transition planning meetings by consulting and working with advocacy groups where they can collect information, learn about their rights and options, share experiences, ask for help, and give help to others (Huff, 1994). School social workers sometimes need to encourage parents to do this by helping them navigate among service agencies and support groups and by making referrals and giving parents specific information about how to identify and contact individual advisors and advocates who may be particularly helpful.

Parents should collect as much information as possible from the service agencies with which their child may need to work. By contacting a variety of different people and organizations and collecting information that can enrich the transition planning process, parents can help ensure that their child has a number of options to consider in developing his or her transition plan. Parents also can help by compiling a record of their child's developmental history. Letters and notes from meetings with professional service providers, copies of medical records and reports, and the results of tests and evaluations are all important. Parents should keep notes on the date, time, and content of their contacts with service providers, noting with whom they spoke, what was discussed, and saving any literature that was provided. Parents also may want to write down their reflections about conversations with their child and about their meetings with professional service providers, and they should be sure to keep notes and save reports from IEP and TLP meetings. As their database grows, parents will need to develop a system for filing and keeping track of important documents. It is a good idea for parents to collect and organize this information early, and the school social worker may be able to help them develop a filing system.

Some parents of students with disabilities may face both emotional and cultural barriers that make it especially difficult for them to "let go" of their children. These parents may resist participating in the transition planning process because it forces them to come to terms with the emotional reality of their child's growing need for independence. School social workers may have to spend considerable time working with these parents before they are ready to accept the idea that eventually their child will have to live on his or her own. School social workers should identify parents who are reluctant or apprehensive about their child's independence early, and they should begin to work with these parents on this issue as soon as possible, because parents who are reluctant to help their child develop independence can derail the whole transition planning process (Allen-Meares, Washington, & Welsh, 1999). Softening parental resistance and getting parents involved in the process of transition planning can help them adjust to the fact that, eventually, their child will have to get along without them.

Indicators of parental acceptance of their child's growing independence can be seen in shifts in the values, beliefs, and language that characterize relations between parent and child. When ideas and terms such as "care for" are replaced by "work with" and when "tell" gives way to "ask," it indicates that parents have begun to replace dominating judgmental postures with listening and suggesting. As parents make these kinds of changes in how they view and relate to their children with disabilities, they will find it easier to focus on their child's unique interests and talents and avoid comparisons with children who are not disabled. The more parents focus on their child's strengths and address possibilities for their child, the easier it will be to include their child in family decision-making and allow their child some latitude to take risks and gain the experience necessary to enter adulthood with confidence (Wehmeyer, 1955).

For many parents, this will be a giant emotional step, and they will need a great deal of understanding, encouragement, and support from the school social worker and other helping professionals. One way to help is for the school social worker, special needs teachers, vocational specialists, and school counselors to behave in ways that reinforce relating to the child in terms of his or her strengths rather than in terms of the disability. This is especially important during TLP and IEP meetings. School staff also should be sensitive to the fact that some parents may themselves have a disability or other limitations that need appropriate interventions. Some parents may be involved in mutually dependent relationships with their children in which the children both obtain care from the parent and provide care to the parent. In such a situation the parent must develop a greater degree of independence before he or she is fully able to help the child become more independent.

Service Agencies

Service agencies that are likely to provide transition services should be invited to attend meetings at which those services are considered. Agency representatives attending such meetings should share information about their agencies, provide guidance in selecting appropriate programs, explain eligibility requirements, and make referrals to other agencies. Examples of community-based and public agencies that provide relevant adult services include the Vocational Rehabilitation Service, the Department of Mental Health/Mental Retardation, the Commission for the Blind, the Division for the Hearing Impaired, the Department of Human Services, and the State Employment Commission.

When interacting with a student with a disability, agency representatives should use techniques designed to help the student actively participate in the transition planning process. Asking about the student's strengths and needs; identifying what the student wants to improve; highlighting goals for school and work; discovering how the student learns best; and inquiring about hobbies and leisure activities all help the student share his or her thoughts and desires for the future. The approach should be positive, stressing what the student can do, not focusing on limitations. It is important to give the student plenty of time to think and respond. Agency representatives should encourage the student to ask questions. They should summarize points for the student, keep eye contact, and use humor where appropriate (Faas, 1980). The attitude and approach of agency representatives are crucial. Agencies should seek as much information as possible from the student's teachers and from support staff who have been working closely with the student. Discussion of policies, practices, and plans should focus on meeting the needs of the student, not those of the agency.

Involvement of agency representatives in the transition planning process will keep them and their agencies up to date with the student's progress and changing needs. By the time the student with a disability graduates from high school, the agencies that will work with the student after graduation should know him or her, and the student should know about the agencies with which he or she will work. This ensures that both student and agency are positioned to help make the transition from school-based to community-based services a smooth one.

If agency representatives do not attend transition planning meetings, then the school should solicit their input by arranging a joint planning session with them, sharing a copy of the student's IEP and transition plan with the agency (with parent and student approval), and encouraging parents and student to meet with the agency. One way to promote contact with community-based agencies is for the school to host a "transition open house" for parents and students, at which different agency representatives can make brief presentations, provide descriptive literature about their agencies and programs, and explain referral and application procedures. This gives parents and students a chance to network and ask agency representatives how their agency would help them deal with specific issues. It also gives recipients of services a chance to speak to agency representatives and ask questions that help them get a realistic picture about the transition process.

THE SPECTRUM OF DISABILITIES AND THE CONTINUUM OF NEEDS

Disabilities that qualify for educational accommodations may be emotional, cognitive, or physical. Impairment may be limited to a specific learning disability or involve multiple areas of functioning. Some disabilities may compromise an individual's ability to care for himself or herself and may keep a person from engaging in typical patterns of communication and interaction (American Psychiatric Association, 1994). Others may not impair a person's ability to live and function independently. The disability may be the result of congenital problems, an illness, or an injury. It may impair vision, speech, or hearing, and some students may suffer from a combination of disabilities. But, regardless of the nature and extent of their problems, all students with disabilities need to learn to manage their personal care, complete their education, find a satisfying and rewarding job, and make full use of community resources. Some students may be able to participate more independently and more completely in the community than others, but all are entitled to the transition services necessary to help them make full use of their abilities in the least restrictive and most independent manner possible when they leave school. To participate effectively in the adult world, students with disabilities will have to learn to communicate with others, develop and maintain satisfying social and emotional relationships, and meet the challenges and responsibilities of independent living.

COMPONENTS OF TRANSITION PLANS

Each student's TLP must take account of the student's specific disability and unique individual needs for services, accommodations, and support. The transition planning process should provide an opportunity to explore the student's current level of functioning, and it should define a path that leads to effective functioning in the adult world.

The TLP should not just list service options in each major area of adult living. It should specifically delineate a coordinated set of experiences and activities in each area that frames an outcome-oriented plan designed to help the student acquire the knowledge and develop the abilities necessary for a smooth transition from high school to adult living (National Center for Research in Vocational Education (NCRVE), 1993). Planned activities and experiences should help the student learn to manage self-care and develop independent living skills. They should start the student on a program to build skills in vocational evaluation, job finding, and job retention. They should help the student plan for post-secondary education. And, they should equip the student to deal with a range of issues that he or she may face in forming adult social and emotional relationships. The TLP should engage the student in these activities during the high school years and describe how the student can continue to learn and develop his or her skills after graduation (Henley, Ramsey, & Algozzini, 1993).

Table 25-1 highlights the kinds of questions the transition team should ask when developing such plans. Table 25-2 specifies some of the issues to consider in answering these questions. Table 25-3 suggests some of the activities students can undertake to smooth the transition to independent adult living.

TABLE **25-1.** **Transition Planning Questions in Critical Life Domains**

Home living	Where and with whom will the student live as an adult?
	Will the student continue to live with the family?
	Does the student want to live alone or with roommates?
	Does the student want to live in an apartment?
	How much independence and self-supervision will the student enjoy?
	How much economic freedom will the student have?
	How will home and community life be integrated?
Employment	What career path does the student wish to pursue?
	What kinds of work interest the student?
	What realistic opportunities does the student have for a job?
	Has the student received training in competitive skills?
	Does the student need more schooling and training?
	Where will the student continue needed education and training?
	Has the student done any type of volunteer work?
	Does the student know how to conduct a job search?
	What support services are available to enable the student to maintain employment?
Leisure/ recreation	How does the student use leisure time?
	What are the opportunities for leisure activities?
	Can the student afford leisure and recreation activities?
Community participation	Does the student have a driver's license?
	Does the student use public transportation?
	Does the student know where key services are located in the community?
	Does the student participate in service organizations, clubs, religious organizations?
	Is the student able to access service agencies on his or her own?
	Does the student do his or her own shopping, banking, use of medical/dental services?

TABLE 25-2. Topics to Consider in Planning the Transition to Adult Living

Adult living

Living arrangements	With family Supervised group	Independent living Residential placement	Foster care Shared living	Host home Local or distant
Relationships	Individual counseling Family counseling Crisis counseling	Genetic counseling Support groups Caring for others	Visiting family Guardianship Respite care	Sexuality Church Wills and trusts
Self-care	Household mgt Social skills Selection /care Dressing & grooming	Personal hygiene Family planning Drugs & alcohol Meal planning & prep	Time mgt Sex education Medication Safety/health.	Shopping Money mgt Clothes Fitness Eating

School and work

Vocational & post-secondary education	Career awareness On-the-job training Vocational rehabilitation	Career exploration Voc-tech training Community colleges	Work-study 2 + 2 programs Universities	Work experience Home study Continuing ed.
Job placement	Competitive employment	Supported employment	Apprenticeship	Volunteer work
Income & financial support	Earned income Public assistance	Unearned income Social Security (SSI)	Food stamps Trust income	Insurance Tax deductions
Workplace communication	Expressing needs & desires Understanding instructions	Interactions with peers, employers, supervisors Using telephone, computer, internet		

Community and civic participation

Community	Mobility, access, independence Transportation: public & private Family car/driver, car pooling Vehicle: car, bike, wheelchair	Planning to meet transportation needs Transport for the Disabled Reimbursement to others for transportation costs Specialized, adaptive, & modified vehicles		
Consumerism	Retail stores Fair treatment	Food shopping Counting costs	Restaurants Post Office	Health & beauty Banking
Citizenship & advocacy	Identification card Neighborhood assoc. Civic interactions	Selective service Advocacy for self Reciprocal relationships	Obeying laws Legal services	Voting
Medical services	Accessing medical, dental, hospital care Specialized care		Insurance & paying for health care Equipment purchase & maintenance	

Social and leisure activities

Social relationships	Friendships & socialization Acquaintances & friends	Levels of friendship Reciprocal relationships	Friendships with peers Friends outside school	
Leisure & fitness	Solo recreation Non-credit classes Personal fitness	Recreation with others Adult education Individual sports	Social clubs Church groups Team sports	Hobbies Scouts & camps Health clubs

Preparing for Independent Living

In preparing for independent living, students with disabilities will need to master a variety of self-care skills. They will have to manage their personal hygiene and grooming, dress appropriately for different situations, care for their health, and seek medical and dental care when they need it. If they need to take medications, they should be able to manage timing and dosage. Living on their own will require them to plan a nutritious diet, shop for healthy food, and prepare appetizing meals. Living on one's own also entails finding affordable and comfortable

TABLE 25-3. Activities That Facilitate the Transition to Adult Living

Adult living				
Living arrangements	Review a lease Look at "for rent" ads Learn maintenance skills	Visit an apartment for rent Visit a group home List criteria for supported living	Explore campus living Explore living needs Learn indep. living skills	
Self-Care	Cook dinner once a week Buy stamps & send mail Make own health/grooming appointments	Develop personal budget Do own laundry & go to cleaner	Shop for groceries Develop hygiene plan Begin to use daily planner	
School and work				
Vocational & post-secondary education	Visit technology center Visit university Develop portfolio	Take a class in welding Visit community college Complete $ aid packet	Take a class in electronics Take vocational aptitude test Complete interest inventory	
Academic skills	Demonstrate math skills	Learn to use calculator	Determine personal learning style	
Assessment	Take job service test Do intake at Voc. Rehab. agency	Develop work samples	Complete interest inventory	
Job placement	Shadow 2 businesses Complete work samples Interview a worker	Attend career days Take career class Apply to 3 businesses	Volunteer for 2 work experiences Tour supported employment Enroll in summer work program	
Income & financial support	Identify financial needs Set up savings plan	Apply for SSI Apply for Pell Grant	Check eligibility for $ aid Open a bank account	
Community participation				
Transportation	Take Driver's Education Investigate cost of a car	Obtain driver's license Find a ride share partner	Get liability insurance Learn schedule & ride bus	
Consumerism	Locate stores	Compare prices	Shop for bargains	Practice resisting sales pitches
Civic involvement	Visit pub, library & obtain card	Register & vote	Register for selective service	
Legal & advocacy	Plan legal needs Learn legal rights	Find legal resources Obtain legal advisor	Ask legal questions Identify advocacy groups	Practice seeking legal help Learn about wills/trusts
Medical services	Describe medical needs Ask medical questions	Locate medical services Compare service costs	Apply for medicaid & insurance Prepare medical information file	
Social, religious, and leisure activities				
Social relationships	Demonstrate social skills: with co-workers, with supervisor, on a date, with family Determine needs, preferences and options for a counselor Find a mentor			
Religious & spiritual	Select and attend a church Contact a religious advisor	Join church youth group Learn religious traditions	Sing in church choir Discuss moral/spiritual values	
Leisure & fitness	Identify recreation options	Visit 3 recreation sites	Join a team	Attend a school dance

housing and doing routine household chores and maintenance tasks. Transportation is also important. Students with disabilities planning to live on their own should be able to read a map, locate desired destinations, and find the best routes for getting where they want to go. Before they graduate from high school, students with disabilities should learn to understand and interpret the routes and time schedules of public transportation and practice how to negotiate the streets of their community via public transportation. Students who plan to have a vehicle of their own will have to get training and experience in its use, obtain a driver's license, learn and obey the traffic laws, and plan for the cost of gasoline, parking, and maintaining their vehicle. They should also practice finding their way to and from unfamiliar locations, first with an experienced driver, and later on their own.

As young adults on their own, students with disabilities will have to manage their finances, live within a budget, set up a bank account, shop wisely, and save for large purchases. They will have to learn how to protect their earnings and how to keep from being taken advantage of by those who seek to dupe or swindle them. Some students with disabilities may qualify for government sponsored programs of supplemental income support, and some may be beneficiaries of trust funds or other sources of income. They may need to learn how to select and work with a lawyer and financial advisor.

Living in the community entails participating in its civic life, and if students with disabilities are to be fully enfranchised members of the community, they will need to learn how to follow social and political issues, register to vote, and take part in elections. They also will need to learn their rights and how to connect with organizations that can help them secure the services and support to which they are entitled.

Participating in the social life of the community includes making friends, joining social and recreational organizations, pursuing educational opportunities, attending cultural events, and making use of leisure and recreational resources. In developing their social skills, students with disabilities will need to learn how to manage different kinds of social interactions and engage in the give-and-take of different kinds of social relationships. This requires learning about various kinds and levels of friendship and learning to handle a range of emotions and a variety of social situations.

Students with disabilities also should learn about male and female sex roles, discuss what it means to be a man or a woman, explore issues about dating and safe sex, examine how to handle emotional relationships, and learn something about the complexities of love and marriage. While mastery of a full repertoire of social skills can take the better part of a lifetime, students with disabilities should be exposed to and have a chance to discuss these issues before they graduate from high school. Participation in sex education programs can help them learn about the personal, social, and health consequences of sexual activity, their sexual rights, their responsibilities, what is entailed in having a baby, and what it takes to be a good parent.

Students with disabilities also need to consider how they will participate in the religious life of the community. Most will have received their moral, spiritual, and religious educations in their families. Their transition plans should address how they can pursue the spiritual and religious aspects of their lives when they are living independently and perhaps at some distance from other family members. Consideration should be given to how to select and maintain a relationship with a religious or spiritual advisor, how to participate in continuing religious education, how to join groups such as a church choir, and how to get involved in church-sponsored social and recreational activities.

The TLP should address all of these issues with an awareness that the extent to which a student with a disability masters the full range of skills necessary for living as an independent adult will depend in part on the nature and extent of the student's disability, in part on the learning opportunities, accommodations, and support that can be provided, and in part on the extent to which the TLP provides a plan the student can and will follow. Some students with disabilities will be able to master independent living tasks with few problems, while others will require some accommodations and support if they are to live independently in the community. And, some students with disabilities may require extensive support and the kind of supervision that may best be provided in a group home or supported living setting.

Whatever the level of independence a student with a disability is able to achieve, all students with disabilities will need education and experience to help them learn, practice, and master the skills necessary for living on their own in the adult world. And, they will need much of this education and experience before they graduate from high school. The transition plan should specify a coordinated set of activities and experiences which is feasible to provide and which ensures that students with disabilities have an opportunity to develop the life skills they will need to live as independently as possible as adults in the community. Ideally, their high school will have programs and support staff that can help with the necessary life-skill education and hands-on experiences students with disabilities will need. However, if the school cannot provide the necessary education and experiences, then the transition planning team should plan to use other programs and resources in the community to provide these services.

Vocational and Career Preparation

School work seldom resembles work on the job, and students with disabilities who do not obtain job training and career orientation in high school are not likely to be prepared for a job or career when they graduate. The success of students with disabilities in the world of work will be largely determined by whether or not they develop and follow a plan that prepares them for success at a job they both want and are capable of performing. An effective TLP balances student occupational preferences with student abilities and the need for on-the-job support and workplace adaptations. Such a transition plan will orient the student and his or her parents to the requirements of various kinds of occupations and careers and help them choose wisely and prepare adequately for the student's occupation.

A key part of such a plan can be a graduated program of work exploration, job preparation, and work experience. Such a program should begin as early as possible to combine academic preparation with pre-vocational orientation and employability training. As the student progresses through high school, he or she should have an opportunity to explore a range of occupational choices and rotate through a variety of work experiences. These work experiences should be appropriate to the student's interests and abilities and should conform with child labor laws designed to protect young people from exploitation and from dangerous occupations. They also should take account of union agreements and employer concerns about worker safety and employer liability.

Some students with disabilities will be able to perform effectively in a wide range of jobs. Others will need accommodations and support in the workplace. And, some may only be able to perform effectively in closely supervised, highly supported, or sheltered work settings. However, all students with disabilities should have an opportunity to explore a range of occupational options. It is important for each student to get experience with the kinds of jobs he or she is likely to work at after graduating from high school. The key to making a work experience program effective for students with disabilities is having a skilled vocational education professional on staff in the school who can match student needs, abilities, and preferences with appropriate jobs at work sites where employers are able and willing to provide students with meaningful work experience and job training. When a match between student and employer is made, the employer and school should sign a formal agreement which specifies the contribution and responsibilities of both parties.

By the junior year in high school, students with disabilities who have successfully completed pre-vocational and employability classes may be ready to participate in community-based vocational instruction or in cooperative employment or work-study programs. Participation in these kinds of programs is often promoted by the school, but the details are usually worked out between the student and the employer. In these programs, students attend classes during the regular school day and work on the job after school. Employers compensate students for their work, and sometimes students also earn school credit for their work experience.

Job shadowing is another way students with disabilities can gain experience with different occupations. By following an experienced worker and observing what he or she does during a typical day on the job, students who do not perform a job themselves have an opportunity to gain direct exposure to what the job entails. This also gives students a chance to discuss the job with a worker skilled at performing it.

Some school districts provide vocational education in specialized vocational and technical training centers. Students usually enter these "Voc-Tech" programs after they have successfully completed their second year in high school and have demonstrated a satisfactory level of academic proficiency in the core academic skills necessary to succeed in the vocational training program. Students with disabilities can enter Voc-Tech programs if they have mastered the academic prerequisites, but many Voc-Tech programs have not been designed with students with disabilities specifically in mind, and they may not have support staff who are specially trained to work with students with disabilities. Some school districts will be able to make such support staff available for students with disabilities in Voc-Tech programs; others may be able to make program adaptations to facilitate the success of students with disabilities. Some students with disabilities will have little trouble succeeding in Voc-Tech programs; others will find the demands of such programs overwhelming. The key to success for all students with disabilities will be finding the appropriate match between a student's interests and abilities and a program's offerings (Schilling, Schwallie-Giddis, & Giddis, 1995).

Programs of individualized on-the-job vocational training for students with disabilities may be worked out between the school and the employer during a student's senior year. Such programs can coordinate work experience and vocational training during the school day with classroom schedules and activities. Students in such programs may earn school credit for their on-the-job training experiences (NCRVE, 1993). In some school districts, students with disabilities who have not completed vocational training before they graduate from high school may continue their training in a program coordinated between the employer and the school and administered through the school district's adult education program (Martin & Serich, 1995). Vocational education and training in such a program can be integrated with supplementary classroom education. The Vocational Rehabilitation Agency may also be able to help by providing a job coach to facilitate the transition from school to work for disabled students over the age of 18. All of the pre-vocational, employability training, and work experience options available through the school should be considered in a TLP designed to help students with disabilities approach the world of work. Such a plan will be able to best address how the student will meet the special needs imposed by his or her disability, and it will define effective ways for the student to pursue the occupation or career of his or her choice.

Job coaches who are specially trained to help young adults adjust to a new job and an unfamiliar workplace can be especially helpful when students with disabilities first start a new job (Olson, 1998). In addition, mentors can help students with disabilities discuss and work through various issues in the community, in school, and at the workplace. Mentor programs, which link a student with an experienced adult, can provide students with disabilities role models, ongoing support, and a positive presence in their lives. Mentors can offer young people guidance by patiently listening to their problems and concerns, offering advice without judging, and making constructive suggestions about how to resolve conflicts and make choices. It is important to engage mentors involved with the student in the transition planning process.

Motivational activities for students with disabilities are also important and can help students realize the importance of learning the academic, vocational, and life skills they will need. By supplementing their academic and job skill training with training in interpersonal skills, negotiation skills, and conflict resolution skills, students with disabilities can learn how to work effectively on a team and better meet the multi-faceted requirements of today's jobs (Parshall, 1998).

Preparing for Post-Secondary Education

Some students with disabilities will be interested in continuing their education and training after high school. They will need to evaluate their motivation, abilities, and willingness to devote the time and effort it takes to succeed at the demanding levels of work required by post-secondary education (National Center for Educational Statistics, 1997). The TLP for students with disabilities wishing to pursue educational options after graduation from high school should address the student's educational plans early, so the student's special education teacher and school social worker can work with the high school counselor to ensure that the student takes the courses colleges and other post-secondary educational institutions will require. Guidance counselors also should make sure that students with disabilities learn about Tech-prep and other programs that coordinate academic and technical training in the high school with continued education at a community college.

Students with disabilities who embark on post-secondary education should focus on finishing the programs they select. The goal of attending a school after graduating from high school is not just to be admitted; it is to successfully achieve the student's educational objectives and graduate. If the student plans to attend a four-year college, the first two years of general education requirements will probably be the most challenging. Students with disabilities who are not prepared to do well at a four-year college should use a community college to complete as many of the most difficult general education courses as possible, and they should use the community college's remedial programs to make up any educational deficiencies. If successful, students may be able to transfer credits to a four-year college program later (Hershey, Silverberg, Owens, & Husley, 1993). The education of students with special needs may take longer than parents and students expect, and it may not follow the same path as the education of a student's friends who do not have special needs (William T. Grant Foundation, 1988). Parents and support staff need to be both encouraging and realistic about these issues.

Some students with disabilities, who want to pursue post-secondary education, may enter the labor force and work for a while after they graduate from high school. They should plan for this eventuality by identifying work-related interests and starting to acquire work-related skills while in high school. Students who take vocational education courses along with their college preparatory courses in high school are more likely to find better opportunities in the labor force when they graduate than students who pursue only a college preparatory program (Hanley-Maxwell & Collet-Klingenberg, 1997). It usually is best to balance job-related and academic skills and experiences, and students with disabilities getting ready for college or other post-secondary educational options need to sharpen both their job skills and their study skills. Even students who are sure that they will continue with some form of post-secondary education can benefit from contacting the Vocational Rehabilitation Agency and taking advantage of its vocational assessment, pre-employment training, and job placement services (Lerman & Pouncy, 1990).

Students with disabilities should also consider post-secondary vocational preparation in addition to, or instead of, college. A two-year vocational degree which requires students to take only those technical courses relevant to a selected occupation or a certificate program which offers primarily hands-on courses can equip a student with a disability for a job that can provide both economic independence and personal satisfaction. And, the student can still pursue a college degree, either full-time or part-time, while working.

It is important for students with disabilities to find out what types of accommodations and supports are available at the school they plan to attend, whether or not these services and supports meet the student's particular needs, what documentation of the student's disability the school requires, how many students with similar problems attend the school, and if there are specialists on staff who are trained to work with students who have special needs. Before finally deciding which school to attend, it is a good idea for the student to visit the school while it is in session. Some community colleges and technical schools provide a full range of support services for students with disabilities and have specialized programs that include vocational training along with their college-level courses. These schools usually have an office or counselor devoted to special student services. Students with disabilities should seek information and assistance from such a counselor during the application process and arrange for continuing support during school.

At a TLP meeting, the student with a disability planning to seek post-secondary education should practice describing his or her disability and discussing how it might affect the student's educational plans. Support staff should help the student highlight areas of strength and identify potential areas of challenge. They also should suggest appropriate accommodations and help the student role-play and practice how he or she will ask for needed accommodations and support. As part of the TLP process, support staff should encourage parents to begin discussions with their child about his or her continuing educational goals and needs for accommodations. Once post-secondary school begins, the student should meet with instructors, disclose the nature of his or her disability, and become familiar with the instructor's procedures and policies for handling the need for accommodations (Wallace & Kaufman, 1986).

COORDINATING TRANSITION SERVICES

The complex nature and long-term implications of the transition from high school to adult life make it imperative that school, family, and agency collaborate and coordinate their activities. One way to ensure that all parties interested in smoothing the transition from school to adulthood for students with disabilities work together is to develop a coordinated set of transition activities while the student is in high school that ensure that everything planned at school, at home, in the community, and in conjunction with various agencies is coordinated to facilitate a smooth transition for the student from secondary school to life as an adult.

Without such coordination, services may be provided piecemeal, there may be duplication of services, and important services may not be provided at all, making it difficult for a young person in the midst of the transition to adulthood to get the services he or she needs, especially if those services were not planned and implemented in a coordinated manner before the student graduated from high school.

CONCLUSION

Planning and implementing the transition from secondary school to independent adulthood should focus on equipping young adults with disabilities to manage and be responsible for their lives. Transition life plans which define the path a young person with a disability can follow toward this end are "person centered" and change as the experience and circumstances of the student change, but they always focus on helping the student become his or her own case manager and advocate.

While some people with disabilities may require more support than others, all transition plans should address how students with disabilities can get the information, skills, and experience they need. Service providers and family members involved in the transition process should focus on empowering students with disabilities to fully participate in the key decisions in their lives. To do this, they must help the student develop confidence and skill in expressing his or her needs, interests, and preferences. This entails helping students with disabilities find their own voices, not speaking for them.

The most effective transition plans are developed and implemented early and are fully supported by the student, the school, the family, and by community agencies. Effective transition plans address multiple areas of adult living: self-care, employment, education, and social participation, equipping students with disabilities to meet the detailed requirements of everyday living while enabling them to take responsible control of their lives.

REFERENCES

Allen-Meares, P., Washington, R. O., & Welsh, B. (1999). *Social work services in schools.* Englewood Cliffs, NJ: Prentice-Hall.

American Psychiatric Association (1994). *Diagnostic and statistical manual of mental disorders* (DSM IV) (4th ed.). Washington, DC: Author.

Charner, I., et al. (1995). Reforms of the school-to-work transition: Findings, implications, and challenges, *Phi Delta Kappa,* September, *40,* 58–60.

Children's Defense Fund (1989). *Numbers that add up to educational rights for children with disabilities,* Washington, DC: Author.

Copenhaver, J. (1995). *Section 504: An educator's primer: What teachers and administrators need to know about implementing accommodations for eligible individuals with disabilities,* Logan, UT: Mountain Plains Regional Center.

Curtis, E., & Dezelsky, M. (1995). *It's my life: Preference-based planning for self-directed goal meeting.* Salt Lake City, UT: New Hats.

De Stefano, L., & Winking, D. (1996). *Incorporating transition into the IEP: Manual and resource guide.* Springfield, IL: Illinois State Board of Education.

Detroit Public Schools (1999). *Special education referral handbook for parents* (Form 1109 Rev). Detroit, MI: Author.

Faas, L. A. (1980). *Children with learning problems: A handbook for teachers.* Boston, MA: Houghton Mifflin.

Hanley-Maxwell, C., & Collet-Klingenberg, L. (1997). Curricular choices related to work: Restructuring curricula for improved work outcomes. In P. Wehman & J. Kregel (Eds.), *Functional curriculum for elementary, middle, and secondary age students with special needs,* Austin, TX: PRO-ED.

Henley, M., Ramsey, R., & Algozzini, R. (1993). *Characteristics of and strategies for teaching students with mild disabilities*. Needham Heights, MA: Allyn & Bacon.

Hershey, A., Silverberg, M., Owens, T., & Husley, L. (1998). *Focus for the future: The final report of the National Tech-Prep Evaluation*. Princeton, NJ: Mathematica.

Huff, B. (1994). *Transition: A handbook for parents, students, and advocates*. Irvine, CA: Irvine United School District.

Janeczko, G., Kasander, T., Randall, J., Summers, J., & Wunderlich, K. (1995). *Transition life planning: A handbook for parents*. Waterford, MI: Oakland County Schools.

Kimeldorf, M. (1994). *A teacher's guide to creating portfolios for success in school, work, and life*. Minneapolis, MN: Free Spirit.

Lenz, K. (1992). *Educational alternatives for students with learning disabilities*. New York, NY: Springer-Verlag.

Lerman, R., & Pouncy, H. (1990, Fall). The compelling case for youth apprenticeships. *The Public Interest* (No 101), pp. 62–77.

Martin, J., & Serich, M. (1995). *Pre-apprentice "basic skills" training*. Grand Blanc, MI: Jack Martin.

McGahee-Kovac, M. (1995). *A student's guide to the IEP*. Washington, DC: National Information Center for Children and Youth with Disabilities, NICHCY.

National Center for Education Statistics (1997). *Compendium: Post-secondary persistence and attainment: Findings from the Condition of Education 1997*. Washington, DC: U.S. Department of Education, Office of Educational Research and Improvement.

National Center for Research in Vocational Education (NCRVE) (1993). *School-to-work facts*. Berkeley, CA: University of California, Author.

National Information Center for Children and Youth with Disabilities (1999). *Technical assistance guide: Helping students develop their IEPs*. Washington, DC: NICHCY.

Olson, L. (1998). *The school to work revolution*. Reading, MA: Perseus Books.

Parnell, D. (1995). *Why do I have to learn this? Teaching the way people learn best*. Waco, TX: Center for Occupational Research and Development.

Parshall, L. (1998). *Special education outcomes*, Lansing, MI: Michigan Department of Education, Office of Special Education Services.

Pierangelo, R., & Crane, R. (1997). *Complete guide to special education services: Ready to use help and materials for successful transitions from school to adulthood*. New York, NY: Center for Applied Research in Education and Prentice-Hall.

Schilling, D., Schwallie-Giddis, P., & Giddis, J. (1995). *Preparing teens for the world of work: A school-to-work transition guide for counselors, teachers, and career specialists*. Spring Valley, CA: Inner Choice.

Storms, J., De Stafano, L., & O'Leary, E. (1996). Individuals with Disabilities Act: Transition requirements, a guide for states, districts, schools, and families. Logan, UT: Western Regional Resource Center & National Transition Network, Mountain Plains Regional Center.

Van Reusen, A. K., Bos, C. S., Schumaker, J. B., & Deshler, D. D. (1994). The self-advocacy strategy for education and transition planning. Lawrence, KS: Edge Enterprises.

Wallace, G., & Kaufman J. M. (1986). *Teaching students with learning & behavior problems*. Columbus, OH: Merrill.

Ward, L. B. (1999). *Building a school to career system: Comprehensive guidance for a new millennium*. Seminar materials presented to Detroit Public Schools, May 12–14. Montgomery, AL: Montgomery Public Schools.

Wehmeyer, M. (1955). *Whose future is it anyway? A student directed planning program*. Arlington, TX: The Arc.

William T. Grant Foundation, Commission on Work, Family, and Citizenship (1988). *The forgotten half: Non-college youth in America*. Washington, DC: Author.

CHAPTER 26

Mental Health and Community Support Strategies for Fostering Employment of People Who Are Deaf and Hard of Hearing

Janet L. Pray

EMPLOYMENT OF DEAF AND HARD OF HEARING PEOPLE

Employment Rates and Relationship to Educational Level

There are data reporting significantly higher rates of unemployment and underemployment among deaf and hard of hearing people compared with the hearing population. An early document produced by the A.G. Bell Association for the Deaf and The American University Development Education and Training Research Institute in Washington, DC, reported on a review of the literature related to employment prior to 1968:

> We might summarize the most relevant findings in the literature on employment of the deaf as follows. The rate of unemployment among the deaf is reported to be much higher than among the hearing population. Compared to the distribution of the total labor force, the employed deaf are basically concentrated in skilled and semi-skilled occupations (Atelsek, 1968, p. 17).

Of relevance to professionals concerned with employability of deaf and hard of hearing persons[1] is the additional finding in the literature review:

> Employers of the deaf appear almost consistently to be satisfied with their deaf workers' job performance, rating it as average or superior largely because of the deaf worker's conscientiousness on the job, his punctuality, low absenteeism, and concentration on the work at hand (Atelsek, 1968, p. 18).

---

[1]Because there are no universally accepted distinctions between persons considered to be deaf and those considered to be hard of hearing, except where a report or study makes such a distinction, the author will use the inclusive phrase "deaf and hard of hearing."

Janet L. Pray • Gallaudet University Department of Social Work, Washington, D.C.

More recent studies continue to show a higher rate of unemployment among deaf and hard of hearing persons. Macleod-Gallinger (1992) reported on a survey of the graduates of 26 educational programs for deaf students in 21 states conducted by the National Technical Institute for the Deaf as part of the Secondary School Graduate Follow-up Program for the Deaf. Of 2,001 respondents, 1,406 were one year post-secondary school and 595 10 years post-secondary school. After one year, of the 52% participating in the labor force,[2] slightly more than half (53%) were unemployed. This contrasted with 79% of hearing secondary school graduates participating in the labor force with an unemployment rate of 8%. After 10 years, 81% of the deaf graduates were in the labor force with a 15% unemployment rate. Comparison figures for hearing graduates were more than 78% in the labor force and an unemployment rate of approximately 6%. The study also revealed that deaf persons had lower incomes than hearing cohorts of the same age. Another important finding was that among deaf persons who had some college education, the unemployment rate was lower, the percentage in white-collar jobs was higher, and weekly earnings were higher than for those who did not continue education beyond high school. For those deaf persons who completed a bachelor's degree the percentages were even better in the same three areas.

Interestingly, Christiansen and Barnartt (1987) report that there was a brief period when deaf men had a move favorable labor participation rate and unemployment rate than hearing men.

> In the early 1970's the labor force participation rate for deaf men was higher, and the unemployment rate lower, than for their hearing counterparts.... Recent data show that, for both deaf and hearing men, the labor force participating rate decreased, and the unemployment rate increased, during the 1970's. However, it is apparent that deaf men experienced a more unfavorable change than did hearing men.... By 1977 ... While the labor force participation rate for deaf and hearing women was about the same, deaf women experienced a significantly higher unemployment rate than their hearing peers (Christiansen & Barnartt, 1987, p. 173).

Racial and Ethnic Minorities

There is considerable evidence that persons with disabilities who are members of racial and ethnic minorities suffer disproportionately from unemployment and underemployment (American Council on Education and the Education Commission of the States, 1988; President's Committee on Employment of the Handicapped, 1986; Thorne, 1988). In 1990 a national conference was called to "continue to explore means of eliminating and reducing existing barriers to employment, educational opportunities, and rehabilitative services" for minority persons with disabilities (Douglas, 1991, pp. v & vi). Richard Douglas, Executive Director of the President's Committee on Employment of People with Disabilities, wrote in the Preface to the conference proceedings that the high unemployment rate of minority persons with disabilities is "startling" (Douglas, 1991, p. v).

Persons with disabilities who are members of a racial or ethnic minority group have lower educational levels than persons with disabilities who are non-minorities. The significance of education relative to employment is that persons with disabilities with higher educational levels are more likely to be in the workforce (President's Committee on Employment of the Handicapped, 1985). Although the report of the study conducted at the

---

[2]Labor force participation includes those who are employed or who are unemployed and actively seeking work; persons who are not actively seeking work are not considered unemployed.

National Technical Institute for the Deaf, cited above (Macleod-Gallinger, 1992), did not examine data for non-white respondents, the study did find the same correlation between educational attainment of deaf persons and rate of employment. Christiansen and Barnartt (1987, p. 177) found that:

> ...among both males and females, unemployment rates for non-white deaf persons in the United States have traditionally been higher than for their white colleagues.... In addition to experiencing higher unemployment rates, non-white deaf people have traditionally been found in lower status occupations than white deaf persons.

Deaf and Hard of Hearing People with Additional Disabilities

It can be argued that since deaf and hard of hearing people are at a disadvantage in employment and people with disabilities are also at a disadvantage, then those who are deaf/hard of hearing and have another disability are likely to be additionally challenged when seeking employment. Among the most challenging are the "traditionally underserved deaf." Historically various terms have been used to describe this group of deaf people: "low functioning, low achieving, hearing-impaired developmentally delayed, severely handicapped deaf, and disadvantaged deaf" (Dowhoser & Long, 1992, p. 1).

Traditionally underserved persons who are deaf are seen as possessing the following characteristics:

1. unable to use written English or English speech/speechreading to convey ideas effectively;
2. minimal ability to communicate using sign language;
3. require long-term support for successful employment;
4. possess reading and math achievement levels at no more than third-grade level;
5. exhibit inappropriate and/or deficient social skills; and
6. need support to live independently (Larew, Long, & Mittal, 1992–93, p. 14).

This list makes it clear that there are multiple areas for intervention in order to enhance the prospects for successful employment.

Deaf people who have visual problems, or are blind, are another group who face particular challenges in the employment arena. Deaf persons with the genetic condition Usher's Syndrome, typically begin to experience progressive vision loss in adolescence or early adulthood and they may ultimately become blind. It is not within the scope of this chapter to identify and discuss every disability except to observe that deaf persons may experience the same range of disabilities as their hearing counterparts. When they do, there are additional considerations with respect to vocational planning.

Nelipovich and Naegele (1989) identify major consequences of misdiagnosis of persons who are deaf and blind and also make a strong case for appropriate employment: "Misdiagnosis, particularly of mental retardation or mental illness, is highly likely and often occurs when standard measures are administered and interpreted by professionals without sufficient knowledge of and exposure to the implications of the disabilities involved" (p. 17). Because of the difficulties imposed by the dual sensory disability, the client may warrant referral for counseling related to social and emotional functioning. Nelipovich and Naegele further note that "One of the most substantial contributions a rehabilitation counselor can make, which affects the client's overall mental and physical adjustment, is the placement of the individual in a job that is well suited to his or her abilities and interests" (p. 19).

MENTAL HEALTH ISSUES

Historically, deaf and hard of hearing people have had limited access to mental health services. Even as we enter the new millennium the need for mental health services greatly exceeds the availability of professionals with the knowledge and skills to work with the diverse populations of people who are deaf or hard of hearing. The problems in mental health service delivery are many, but this discussion limits its focus to issues that have a direct relationship to obtaining and maintaining employment. In a national survey of agencies serving deaf clients, Danek (1988) found that the greatest gap in the rehabilitation area was the availability of personnel to provide mental health services. Loera (1994) found that most rehabilitation counselors for the deaf surveyed by the Center on Deafness at the Western Pennsylvania School for the Deaf identified majors problems with accessibility of mental health services:

> Center on Deafness at the Western Pennsylvania School for the Deaf conducted a survey of Pennsylvania Rehabilitation Counselors for the Deaf (RCD). The survey gathered information on the counselors' perceptions of mental health service needs for hearing-impaired clients of the Office of Vocational Rehabilitation. With a 75 percent response rate to the survey, representing a caseload of over 1000 Pennsylvania deaf clients annually, at least 17 percent of the clients were considered to have mental health problems and 12 percent had confirmed mental health diagnoses. Seventy-five percent of the counselors cited major problems with the inaccessibility of mental health services (p. 156).

In a national survey of professionals, Bullis and Reiman (1989) found that the ability to access and use mental health services were among 10 "critical transition skills" for deaf adolescents and young adults.

Deaf People with Chronic Mental Illness

This is a population of people who have conditions such as schizophrenia, bipolar disorder, and borderline personality. They often experience repeated hospitalizations, reside in or are in need of a supervised group living situation, require long-term supportive counseling, monitoring of medication, and vocational rehabilitation (VR) services. Many of these individuals also have characteristics associated with traditionally underserved deaf. Loera's (1994) experience at the Western Pennsylvania School for the Deaf was that "referrals to the Center on Deafness mental health program include many persons who have a history of rehabilitation failures and chronic mental health or adjustment problems" (p. 157). Clearly, then, there was an identified need for mental health services which could effectively address employment-related mental health problems.

Among the many gaps in the mental health delivery system is a lack of professionals who are culturally competent to work with this population, including having the appropriate communication skills. These skills include the ability to communicate in American Sign Language (ASL), and knowledge of visual gestural methods for communicating with deaf persons who themselves are not skilled in ASL, an other sign system, or English. There are also inadequate numbers of qualified interpreters for situations in which an interpreter might be an alternative when there is no mental health professional available with the required communication skills.

Traditionally Underserved Deaf Adults

A survey of service providers in the Pacific Northwest (Mathay & LaFayette, 1990) found that 90% of the "hearing impaired" population served by mental health agencies were low achieving, as were 41% of those served by VR counselors. Low achieving was defined as having one or more of the following characteristics: reading and language skills below fourth-grade level; deficiency in independent living skills; may not be considered eligible for VR supported services for reasons such as being considered unemployable; and may not be eligible for Developmental Disability (DD) supported services for reasons such as IQ level above DD limits. The mental health service providers surveyed identified the obstacles faced by low achieving deaf persons as: few independent living skills, undeveloped social skills, lack of interpreters, information deprivation, education deprivation, lack of job placement services, low motivation, substance abuse, lack of supported living programs, and lack of long-term support services.

Interviews with the service providers revealed frustration with the low success rate of working with this population, concerns about the high risk of unsatisfactory employment outcomes, and yet a "sense of commitment to this population" (Mathay & LaFayette, 1990, p. 32). There was consensus that "a networking system among agencies would be a valuable tool to begin an organized approach to resolving the dilemma experienced by low achieving deaf persons" (p. 32).

Late Deafened Adults

This group includes persons who, because of illness, injury, and sometimes unknown causes, become deaf or hard of hearing in adulthood. Frequently, the acquired hearing loss has effects upon family and social relationships and self-esteem, and requires adaptation in the workplace or even consideration of an employment change (Pray, 1996). For late deafened adults, communication usually presents major difficulties and mental health professionals often are not prepared to communicate, or work effectively, with such persons. If people who become deaf as adults decide to learn sign language then they are likely to choose a sign system that follows English word order (such as Pidgin Signed English or Manually Coded English) in contrast with ASL which has its own grammar and syntax, quite different from English. They may also be interested in assistive listening devices (ALDs) that will enhance their residual hearing and speechreading/lipreading abilities.

Deaf–Blind Adults

Deaf people who develop vision loss or become blind as adults may need mental health services because of adjustment issues: adjusting to the double disability, dealing with the possibility of having to consider an employment or career change, changed interpersonal relationships, etc. Few mental health settings are prepared to respond to the communication needs that might be for tactile signing (fingerspelling and signing into the hands of the person who cannot see), or sitting in close proximity to the mental health professional in order to be able to see the signing, or providing a close vision interpreter (an interpreter who sits directly in front of and close to the person).

In addition to the concern about the extent of the service provider's knowledge of the issues facing deaf–blind people, there are many transference and countertransference issues that must be addressed. What feelings, for example, are generated by the atypical physical closeness between client and professional? How does the professional deal with her or his personal reactions to the severity of the client's condition and is it possible to employ strengths and empowerment models?

CREATIVE PARTNERSHIPS FOR EMPOWERMENT

Historical Perspectives

Hancock (1981) observed that for many years the state VR office was the only place a deaf person could find professionals fluent in sign language. As a result, deaf people brought many concerns to the VR counselor that otherwise would more appropriately belong in a mental health setting. This occurred even though most of the VR counselors did not have the education and training to provide mental health services. The phenomenon is eloquent testimony to the centrality of effective communication, even in the absence of formal credentials in the area of need. Late in the 1970s, Professor Arlene Gavin in the School of Social Work and Community Planning at the University of Maryland recognized the need for master's level social workers who were deaf to be prepared for addressing the mental health needs of deaf clients in the VR system. Her concern was validated when she surveyed VR agencies who indicated interest in hiring deaf and hard of hearing social workers. She received 5 years of funding from the Office of Rehabilitation Services to create a center in the School to prepare deaf and hard of hearing social workers to work in the area of VR. In the late 1970s and early 1980s that was the only program preparing social workers for this specialization. Unfortunately, lack of funds and Professor Gavin's retirement marked the end of a program whose vision was consistent with the theme of this volume: integration of employment, rehabilitation, and mental health services.

Cross-Cultural Issues in the Deaf Community

The initial challenge in developing effective strategies for addressing unemployment and underemployment of deaf and hard of hearing people is to understand the diversity that exists within these two groups. Some of that diversity was addressed earlier in the chapter when discussing the types of deaf people who experience the greatest difficulty in employment and populations of deaf people who may be seeking and receiving mental health services. Appropriate services cannot be provided if the populations to be served and the distinct needs of each are not well understood (Pray, 1995).

CULTURALLY DEAF IDENTITY.   Service providers need to know that among deaf persons who have been deaf since birth or early childhood there are many who identify themselves not as disabled but as members of a linguistic and cultural minority distinguished by their use of ASL and their pride in their Deaf heritage. This is particularly true in families with many generations of Deaf people (Padden, 1980; Padden & Humphries, 1990; Stokoe, 1980). Those who identify with Deaf culture use a capital "D" to distinguish themselves from those who consider deafness to be a disability. Padden (1980) also points out that cultural identification, not degree or severity of hearing loss, is the determining factor for membership in Deaf culture.

DEAFNESS AS DISABILITY.   Other deaf people, particularly those who become deaf as adults or late in life, do not identify with Deaf culture and are more likely to describe themselves as having a disability. As noted earlier, if they decided to learn sign language it is likely to be a sign system other than ASL and follows English word order. Older adults are unlikely to learn sign language at all and are also inclined to be interested in assistive technology and speechreading/lipreading. Growing numbers of persons who become deaf as adults have obtained cochlear implants which usually enhance their ability to process speech.

Hurwitz (1991, p. 4) wrote that:

> There is a growing concern about how individuals who are hard of hearing, or who are losing their hearing in later years, may require special assistance with their unique needs. Many regular VR counselors and RCD's [rehabilitation counselors for deaf] are unfamiliar with the communication needs of hard of hearing clients. These clients can be expected not to know any sign language and may not want to be categorized with other clients who are deaf. Special care must be taken to address their unique needs. To name a few, comprehensive audiological examinations must be provided for all hard of hearing clients experiencing difficulty due to, progressive hearing loss. Retraining programs with emphasis on communication skill development must be provided for these hard of hearing clients whose vocational skills are inadequate due to progressive hearing loss.... .Assistive devices, including TDD's, assistive listening systems (e.g., FM system, loop system, ultra red system) and visual warning systems (e.g., smoke alarms, telephone lights)must be provided for deaf and hard of hearing clients to assure successful employment.

HARD OF HEARING. Although there is no clearcut definition of "hard of hearing," nor specific decibel loss on an audiogram, generally speaking a hard of hearing person has usable hearing and may benefit from hearing aid use and other assistive technology such as that described by Hurwitz (1991). The cultural identifications made by hard of hearing people vary greatly and include identifying with the culturally Deaf community, striving to be part of the hearing community, identifying as hard of hearing, or feeling as though they do not "fit" comfortably with any of these groups.

Creating a Culturally Affirmative Environment in the Service Delivery System and in the Workplace

According to Long, Long, and Ouellette (1993), persons who are deaf and members of racial and ethnic minority groups have not benefited from service delivery systems either because they do not access them or, even if they do access them, they are poorly served "due to prejudices, stereotypes, pre-conceived notions, paternalism, and/or lack of awareness or sensitivity to their needs" (p. 241). They stress the importance of aggressive efforts to recruit strong leadership and role models who are deaf and hard of hearing from racial and ethnic minority groups for VR programs. With their increased presence, cross-cultural issues can be better identified and addressed. This author would add that such leadership is of critical importance in the mental health, social service, and all delivery systems.

Long, Long, and Oullette (1993) further note that the National Black Deaf Advocates and the National Hispanic Council of the Deaf and Hard of Hearing have been influential advocates for greater cultural sensitivity. Organizations such as these are excellent models of self-empowerment (Lee, 1994).

Campbell (1991) proposes strategies for maintenance of employment for minority persons with disabilities. These strategies are not specific to persons who are deaf but are suggested here as having relevance for employers of minority deaf persons. The strategies include a multicultural employment self-analysis, hiring a cultural broker, and providing cross-cultural training. The goal of the employment self-analysis is to achieve a multicultural environment in which diversity is embraced. Campbell proposes a series of questions employers can ask themselves. These include whether there are special recruitment efforts to hire minority individuals with disabilities, whether the efforts are voluntary, whether there are minority persons with disabilities in the organization, the extent to which the work environment is "primed" to incorporate minority persons within the organization, among many others.

The cultural broker is conceptualized as a person knowledgeable about diverse cultures, their values, and symbols and serves as an intermediary among the various cultures represented in the employment setting as they seek to adapt and adjust to each other. The concept was developed originally for educational settings (Gentemann & Whitehead, 1983).

Campbell (1991) also emphasizes the importance of cross-cultural training in the workplace related to both disability and cultural diversity. The two-fold goal of training is to convey the competence and self-sufficiency of employees with disabilities as well as achieving respect for diverse cultures.

Since Hispanics are becoming the largest minority population in the United States, Suazo (1991) stresses the importance of paying particular attention to the culture and values of Hispanic persons with disabilities in the workplace. Douglas (1991) cites Census data as showing that "one working age Hispanic adult in twelve has a disability" (p. v), a statistic that underscores Suazo's recommendation. Similar needs for American Indians are identified by Joe (1991).

Speaking from the perspective of California, which has a large Asian/Pacific population, Woo (1991) cites barriers to employment of Asian/Pacific persons with disabilities and proposes a plan to address them:

> Barriers to success include difficulties in cultural transitioning; family systems differences; language differences; lack of culturally relevant assessment tools, rehabilitation techniques and services; differences in cultural values, beliefs, and behaviors; inadequate service delivery systems, inadequate cultural sensitivity training; and a lack of linguistically appropriate staff (p. 64).

Woo (1991) proposed a 13-point plan to overcome cultural and language barriers, including encouraging Asian/Pacific community groups to organize and demand culturally sensitive and bilingual services, conduct research and disseminate information to better understand the cultural differences, train and employ more bilingual Asian/Pacific professionals, work with employers to encourage a more culturally diverse and inviting environment, and develop a service delivery system that is more culturally sensitive.

A SYSTEMS APPROACH TO INTEGRATED SERVICES

Drawing from a systems approach to family therapy, Harvey (1994), a psychologist, emphasizes the importance of including all the relevant systems when working with the deaf client who is receiving mental health services and services from a VR counselor. Harvey notes:

> From the vantage point of the RCD, his or her interventions influence and are influenced by, the individual, family, and clinician. These members comprise the relevant system. The RCD's intervention will be noticed by these members, and thus will influence all of them in some way. As a result, the client, family, and clinician will, in turn, influence the RCD's interventions. Similarly, from the vantage point of the clinician, his or her interventions influence, and are influenced by the individual, family, and RCD. In both of these cases, the RCD and the clinician must take into account the context, the relevant system, that includes the other in order to effectively promote change. Simply put, they must work in close collaboration with each other (pp. 190–191).

Social workers will recognize this approach as consistent with systems theory as applied in social work practice and taught in schools of social work throughout the country (see, for example, Kirst-Ashman & Hull, 1999).

Belknap, Korwin, and Long (1995) challenge the traditional VR model and hold it responsible for unemployment and underemployment of deaf people:

> The reported lag in employment rates for deaf people occurs despite intervention and assistance from the state-federal vocational rehabilitation (VR) services system. This is likely due to the predominant model of placement utilized by VR counselors which focuses on consumers preparing for and obtaining employment without giving adequate attention to job retention and career mobility issues. This lack of attention to post-employment service needs has resulted in unemployment and underemployment. A need exists to revisit the traditional approach of job placement used with deaf people, including those who possess additional disabilities or who possess limited functioning skills (pp. 21–22).... If problems arise at the worksite, the job placement specialist, the counselor, or both may not be informed because that individual's relationship with the employer is limited in nature. The specialist or counselor often does not have an in-depth knowledge of the details of the employee's responsibilities or the company's performance expectations, policies, and procedures, and is, therefore, not perceived as a viable resource to assist the employer with resolving work concerns. Performance problems by the deaf employee can therefore escalate to the point of termination or resignation without further contact with the rehabilitation professionals by either the employee or employer, despite the theoretical availability of postemployment services (p. 28).

In the proposed new model the job coach for deaf persons must provide the same services as those for persons with other disabilities (which they identify as including "task analysis, performance evaluation, intensive skill training for the employee, development and implementation of behavior management strategies, mental health support, employer negotiation related to work tolerance and schedule adjustments, and disability awareness training" (p. 29)) and must include, in addition,

> ...fluency in all forms of manual communication, knowledge of deafness and the psychosocial implications of hearing loss, sensitivity to cultural issues, familiarity with community services, and awareness of adaptive technology options. The goal of the model is to enhance the assimilation and success of deaf employees in competitive work environments. Unlike many supported employment settings for severely disabled persons, this model assumes that the need for job coaching assistance will diminish as the employee's overall skills and independence are developed, accessibility issues have been addressed, and workplace accommodations are securely in place (p. 29).

Like Belknap, Korwin, and Long (1995), Muth (1995) notes the important role of job coaches. "In 1986, the amendments to the Rehabilitation Act of 1973, defined supported employment for consumers with severe disabilities (including deafness) and required that states provide these individuals with the services necessary to maintain employment" (Muth, 1995, p. 13). This led to the creation of job coaches, originally for persons with mental retardation, and, subsequent to the Reauthorization of the Rehabilitation Act in 1992 and increased emphasis on persons with disabilities considered to be the most severe, the role of job coaches expanded. Among these disabilities are traumatic brain injury (Goodall, Groah, Sherron, Kreutzer, & Wehman, 1991) and mental illness (Furlong, Jonikas, Cook, Hathaway, & Goode, 1994). Currently for a deaf consumer,

> common duties of a Job Coach may include: performing job analysis, job development, job placement, sign language interpreting, conducting family meetings, teaching the consumer to use public transportation, report writing, market analysis, training employers, trouble-shooting on the job, conflict resolution, teaching a sign language course to employees, informal counseling, arranging medical appointments, communicating with state and federal agencies, and community education (Muth, 1995, p. 14).

Muth notes that the literature shows a lack of persons with training to be job coaches and further indicates that of the 10 higher education institutions in the Baltimore–Washington, DC, area with sign language courses and/or "career paths in the area of deafness," none provides specific preparation for job coaching. "A 1989 Statewide Needs Assessment conducted in the Baltimore–Washington Metropolitan area, reported that three of the top five identified employment needs of deaf individuals were: Job Coaching, job placement, supported employment" (p. 17).

Barker (1988) stresses that coordination between the VR and mental health systems helps the consumer remain in the community, maintain a closer relationship with business and industry, and the mental health expertise helps the VR process.

ROLE OF SUPPORTED HOUSING AND SUPPORTED EMPLOYMENT

The concept of supported employment began with persons with mental retardation and later expanded to other disabilities. Anthony and Blanch (1987) noted that supported employment is based in vocational intervention characterized by competitive employment in integrated settings with on-job and off-job site support for as long and intensively as needed to ensure success in the workplace. Schauer (1988) noted the importance of empowerment of consumers and their participation in decision-making regarding their treatment, consistent with strengths and empowerment perspectives in social work (Gutierrez, Parsons, & Cox, 1998; Lee, 1994; Saleebey, 1997;). Schauer also noted that "Case management has become extremely critical in serving deaf persons with mental illness because of the multiplicity of their needs and the inaccessibility of programs…" (p. 23). She cites the need for professionals fluent in sign language and the psychosocial aspects of deafness, TTYs, flashing lights, and the like.

The characteristics of an effective systemic approach to services for diverse groups of deaf and hard of hearing people designed to ensure employment and maintenance of employment are summarized as follows:

1. Services are tailored to meet individual needs taking into consideration the particular deaf or hard of hearing identity of the person.
2. Communications needs, preferences, and abilities of the deaf or hard of hearing person are accommodated by service providers.
3. Services are culturally competent in relation to race, ethnicity, and other diverse characteristics.
4. The deaf or hard of hearing consumer who has more than one disability is viewed as an integrated whole and services provided accordingly.
5. Mental health, vocational (including job coaching), and other services are coordinated by a case manager.
6. Strengths and empowerment perspectives that maximize self-sufficiency and self-actualization underpin intervention plans.
7. The deaf or hard of hearing consumer is actively involved in the planning process.
8. The employer is included as a member of the team and education/training is provided by the service delivery system as needed to ensure an accepting, affirming, and supportive environment that encourages success in the workplace.
9. The service delivery system remains involved with the deaf or hard hearing consumer and with the employer until such time as a consistently satisfactory level of performance is achieved in employment and long-term supportive services continue if needed to maintain satisfactory job performance.

REFERENCES

American Council on Education and the Education Commission of the States (1988). *A report on the Commission on Minority Participation in Education and American Life: One-third of a nation.* Washington, DC: American Council on Education.

Anthony, W. A., & Blanch, R. (1987). Supported employment for persons who are psychiatrically disabled: A historical and conceptual perspective. *Psychosocial Rehabilitation Journal, 11,* 5–23.

Atelsek, F. (1968). *Assessing the attitudes of industry hiring personnel toward employment of deaf applicants.* Washington, DC: A. G. Bell Association for the Deaf.

Barker, J. T. (1988). Coordination of efforts between vocational rehabilitation and mental health systems. In L. G. Perlman & G. F. Austin, *Rehabilitation of persons with long-term mental illness in the 1990's: A report of the 12th Mary E. Switzer memorial seminar.* Alexandria, VA: National Rehabilitation Association.

Belknap, P., Korwin, K. A., & Long, N. (1995). Job coaching: A means to reduce unemployment and underemployment in the deaf community. *Journal of the American Deafness and Rehabilitation Association, 28*(4), 21–38.

Bullis, M., & Reiman, J. W. (1989). Survey of professional opinion on critical transition skills for adolescents and young adults who are deaf. *Rehabilitation Counseling Bulletin, 32*(3), 231–242.

Campbell, L. R. (1991). Enhancing diversity: A multicultural employment perspective. In S. Walker, F. Z. Belgrave, R. W. Nicholls, & K. A. Turner (Eds.), *Future frontiers in the employment of minority persons with disabilities.* Proceedings of the National Conference co-sponsored by The President's Committee on Employment of People with Disabilities and Howard University Research and Training Center for Access to Rehabilitation and Economic Opportunity.

Christiansen, J. B., & Barnartt, S. N. (1987). The silent minority: The socioeconomic status of deaf people. In P. C. Higgins & J. E. Nash, *Understanding deafness socially.* Springfield, IL: Charles C. Thomas.

Danek, M. (1988). Deafness rehabilitation needs and competencies: Results of a survey. In D. Watson, G. Long, M. Taff-Watson, & M. Harvey (Eds.), *Two decades of excellence: A foundation for the future* (pp. 183–193) (American Deafness and Rehabilitation Association Monograph 14). Myersville, MD: ADARA.

Douglas, R. (1991). Preface. In S. Walker, F. Z. Belgrave, R. W. Nicholls, & K. A. Turner, (Eds.), *Future frontiers in the employment of minority persons with disabilities.* Proceedings of the National Conference co-sponsored by The President's Committee on Employment of People with Disabilities and Howard University Research and Training Center for Access to Rehabilitation and Economic Opportunity.

Dowhower, D. D., & Long, N. M. (1992). What is traditionally underserved? *NIURTC Bulletin, 1*(1), 1.

Furlong, M., Jonikas, J. A., Cook, J. A., Hathaway, L., & Goode, S. L. (1994). *Providing mental health services: Job coaching and ongoing support for persons with severe mental illness.* Chicago, IL: Thresholds National Research and Training Center on Rehabilitation and Mental Illness.

Gentemann, K. M., & Whitehead, T. L. (1983). The cultural broker concept in bicultural education. *Journal of Negro Education, 52*(2),118–129.

Goodall, P., Groah, C., Sherron, P., Kreutzer, J., & Wehman, P. (1991). *Supported employment for individuals with traumatic brain injury: A guide for service providers.* Richmond, VA: Virginia Commonwealth University Rehabilitation Research and Training Center.

Gutierrez, L. M., Parsons, R. J., & Cox, E. O. (Eds.) (1998). *Empowerment in social work practice: A sourcebook.* Pacific Grove, CA: Cole.

Hancock, J. (1981). Vocational rehabilitation services: The point of entry. *Proceedings of the Region X conference on mental health services for deaf and hearing impaired people.* Regional Resource Center on Deafness, Western Oregon State College, Monmouth, OR.

Harvey, M. A. (1994). Systemic rehabilitation. In R. C. Nowell & L. E. Marshak (Eds.), *Understanding deafness and the rehabilitation process.* Needham, MA: Allyn & Bacon.

Hurwitz, T. A. (1991). Quality of communication services for deaf and hard of hearing clients: Currents issues and future directions. *Journal of the American Deafness and Rehabilitation Association, 25*(1), 1–7.

Joe, J. (1991). Vocational rehabilitation and the American Indian: Where is the innovation? In S. Walker, F. Z. Belgrave, R. W. Nicholls, & K. A. Turner (Eds.), *Future frontiers in the employment of minority persons with disabilities.* Proceedings of the National Conference co-sponsored by The President's Committee on Employment of People with Disabilities and Howard University Research and Training Center for Access to Rehabilitation and Economic Opportunity.

Kirst-Ashman, K. K., & Hull, G. F., Jr. (1999). *Understanding generalist practice.* Chicago IL: Nelson-Hall.

Larew, S. J., Long, G., & Mittal, N. (1992–1993). Identifying independent living skills needs of traditionally underserved persons who are deaf. *Journal of the American Deafness and Rehabilitation Association, 26*(3), 13–21.

Lee, J. A. B. (1994). *The empowerment approach to social work practice.* New York, NY: Columbia University Press.

Loera, P. A. (1994). The use and application of cognitive–behavioral psychotherapy with deaf persons. In R. C. Nowell & L. E. Marshak (Eds.), *Understanding deafness and the rehabilitation process.* Needham, MA: Allyn & Bacon.

Long, G., Long, N. M., & Ouellette, S. (1993). *Habilitation and rehabilitation of persons who are deaf: A conundrum.* Springfield, IL: Charles C. Thomas.

Macleod-Gallinger, J. (1992). Employment attainment of deaf adults one and ten years after graduation from high school. *Journal of the American Deafness and Rehabilitation Association, 25*(4), 1–10.

Mathay, GA., & LaFayette, R. H. (1990). Low achieving deaf adults: An interview survey of service providers. *Journal of the American Deafness and Rehabilitation Association, 24*(1), 23–32.

Muth, P. (1995). Assessing the need for a job coaching curriculum in the Baltimore–Washington area. *Journal of the American Deafness and Rehabilitation Association, 28*(4), 13–20.

Nelipovich, M., & Naegele (1989). The rehabilitation process for persons who are deaf and blind. *Dimensions: Visually impaired persons with multiple disabilities* (Selected papers from the *Journal of Visual Impairment and Blindness*). New York, NY: American Federation for the Blind.

Padden, C. (1980). The deaf community and the culture of deaf people. In C. Baker & R. Battison (Eds.), *Sign language and the deaf community* (pp. 89–103). Silver Spring, MD: National Association of the Deaf.

Padden, C., & Humphries, T. (1990). *Deaf in America: Voices from a culture.* Cambridge, MA: Harvard University Press.

Pray, J. L. (1995). Social work. In R. R. Myers (Ed.), *Standards of care for the delivery of mental health services to deaf and hard of hearing Persons.* Silver Spring, MD: National Association of the Deaf.

Pray, J. L. (1996). Psychosocial aspects of adult aural rehabilitation. In M. J. Moseley & S. J. Bally (Eds.), *Integrated approaches to adult aural rehabilitation.* Washington, DC: Gallaudet Press.

President's Committee on Employment of the Handicapped (1985). *Black adults with disabilities: A statistical report drawn from Census Bureau data* (Shipping list No. 85–1133P; Item 766; MC#86–7133, SuDoc #1.10:B56). Washington, DC: Author.

President's Committee on Employment of the Handicapped (1986). *Out of the job market* (ERIC Document Reproduction Service No. ED 288 312). Washington, DC: Author.

Saleebey, D. (Ed.) (1997). *The strengths perspective in social work practice.* New York, NY: Longman.

Schauer, C. (1988) Review and comments. In L. G. Perlman & G. F. Austin. *Rehabilitation of persons with long-term mental illness in the 1990's: A report of the Twelfth Mary E. Switzer memorial seminar.* Alexandria, VA: National Rehabilitation Association.

Stokoe, W. C. (1980). *Sign and culture: A reader for students of American sign language.* Silver Spring, MD: Linstok Press.

Suazo, A. (1991). Hispanics with disabilities in the labor force: A window of opportunity. In S. Walker, F. Z. Belgrave, R. W. Nicholls, & K. A. Turner (Eds.), *Future frontiers in the employment of minority persons with disabilities.* Proceedings of the National Conference co-sponsored by The President's Committee on Employment of People with Disabilities and Howard University Research and Training Center for Access to Rehabilitation and Economic Opportunity.

Thorne, C. V. (1988). Effective approaches to education and economic independence for Black Americans with disabilities: A response. In S. Walker et al. (Eds.), *Equal to the challenge: Perspectives, problems, and strategies in the rehabilitation of the nonwhite disabled.* Proceedings of the National Conference on the Howard University Model to Improve Rehabilitation Services to Minority Populations with Handicapping Conditions. Washington, DC: Howard University, School of Education, The Center for the Study of Handicapped Children and Youth.

Woo, A. H. (1991). The employment of Asian/Pacific minority persons with disabilities. In S. Walker, F. Z. Belgrave, R. W. Nicholls, & K. A. Turner, (Eds.), *Future frontiers in the employment of minority persons with disabilities.* Proceedings of the National Conference co-sponsored by The President's Committee on Employment of People with Disabilities and Howard University Research and Training Center for Access to Rehabilitation and Economic Opportunity.

CHAPTER 27

Supporting the Employment of People with Serious Mental Illness

ROBERT BAER

In previous chapters readers have been acquainted with the critical role that employment plays for persons with serious mental illness in advancing their quality of life. This chapter describes supported employment as an option for persons with serious mental illness. The first section, Models of Supported Employment, examines individual and group models of employment where supports are provided on site. Legal Definitions of Supported Employment acquaints the reader with how supported employment has been written into the law for persons with serious mental illness. The third section, Characteristics of Effective Supported Employment Programs, identifies some general principles that should be considered in the selection and development of supported employment programs for persons with serious mental illness. Supported Employment Process outlines the sequence of activities that make up supported employment programs. Finally, Adapting Supported Employment Approaches addresses some issues related to applying traditional supported employment approaches to persons with serious mental illness and how mental health practitioners can address these issues. The objectives of this chapter are for the reader to be able to:

1. Describe five models of supported employment
2. Describe the legal definition of supported employment and supported employment services
3. Identify characteristics of effective supported employment programs
4. Discuss the four stages of supported employment

BACKGROUND

Approximately 1.5 million Americans suffer from serious mental illness. They currently comprise 18% of federal and state rehabilitation clients and represent the second largest population served by this system. Until recently, competitive employment has not been considered

ROBERT BAER • Outreach Center for Innovation in Transition and Employment, Kent State University, Kent, Ohio.

a viable option for them. Vocational services, if any, have been typically provided in day treatment programs, activity centers, and sheltered work settings on the assumption that persons with serious mental illness needed to be symptom-free before entering employment (Simmons, Selleck, Steele, & Sepetuac, 1993). Additionally, rehabilitation and Social Security programs have lacked parity for their treatment and financial support, and have often penalized those entering employment with the loss of benefits and health care. These barriers to employment have persisted in spite of research showing better management of symptoms while working and greater stress related to being unemployed.

Supported employment services stressing community integration and consumer empowerment began to emerge in the mid-1980s as a viable alternative for this population (Simmons et al., 1993). Early supported employment programs for persons with serious mental illness included transitional work programs, client-employing businesses, and the "Choose–Get–Keep" model of supported employment (Simmons et al., 1993). Transitional work programs stressed the importance of developing work skills and coping strategies in a series of temporary jobs and shared some therapeutic orientation with hospital work programs. Client-employing businesses, such as earlier day activity and sheltered work programs, emphasized the approach of developing supportive environments for persons with serious mental illness and bringing in competitive work. The "Choose–Get–Keep" model of supported employment focused on individual supported employment placement and shared some characteristics of earlier job club and peer support models.

As supported employment evolved for persons with serious mental illness, general agreement emerged among researchers that the employment support needs of individuals with serious mental illness were different from the support needs of persons with developmental disabilities. Shafer, Middaugh, Rubin, and Jones (1998) reported that "a common criticism of supported employment had been its primary orientation toward individual experiencing cognitive or physical limitations" (p. 63). Bond (1992) suggested that supported employment for persons with serious mental illness could be better characterized as "place and support" rather than "place and train." Researchers generally agreed that persons with serious mental illness required more supportive interventions than training interventions (Shafer et al., 1998).

MODELS OF SUPPORTED EMPLOYMENT

Researchers have emphasized that supported employment for persons with serious mental illness represents a range of orientations and theories (Shafer et al., 1998). Slotting any supported employment program into a given model may therefore be difficult. Some popular models that researchers have identified in the supported employment literature included:

1. Enclaves—employ a group of three to eight individuals who were placed in a business by a human service agency to work as a group. Either a human service agency worker supervised the enclave or a supervisor assigned to the group by the business.

2. Mobile work crews—three to eight persons with disabilities were established as a work crew by a human service agency typically to provide janitorial or landscaping services at various sites. In this model, the human service agency that obtained contracts from community businesses to provide ongoing services typically paid the mobile work crew.

3. The dispersed group or cluster—employed up to eight persons to work within the same company with a supervisor from a human service agency or the business. In this model the individuals were dispersed throughout the business and the employees were hired by the business and paid competitive wages.

4. Entrepreneurial models—employed both groups and individuals by establishing businesses with the help of supports. These included businesses set up by human service agencies to employ both persons with disabilities and persons with expertise in the business and individual businesses established with supports.

5. Individual models—characterized by a four-step process that included: (a) the individual profile, (b) job development and placement, (c) job training and support, and (d) extended services. Danley and Anthony (1987) adapted individual models of supported employment to the needs of persons with serious mental illness by developing the Choose–Get–Keep model that focuses on individual progress rather than staff activities.

6. Transitional employment—persons with serious mental illness are placed in a series of temporary job placements in competitive work settings with ongoing supports. These jobs are designed sequentially to lead up to permanent job placement. The Thresholds programs used this approach before moving to an individual placement model (Cook & Razzano, 1992).

LEGAL DEFINITIONS OF SUPPORTED EMPLOYMENT

Supported employment was funded in the Rehabilitation Act of 1986 to help persons with severe disabilities who could not be served through traditional rehabilitation programs and was included as a vocational rehabilitation service in the Rehabilitation Act of 1992. Legislation defined it in the Rehabilitation Act Amendments of 1992 as:

> 18(A) The term "supported employment" means competitive work in integrated work settings for individuals with the most severe disabilities—
>
>   (i)   (I) for whom competitive employment has not traditionally occurred;
>   (II) for whom competitive employment has been interrupted or intermittent as a result of a severe disability; and
>   (ii) who, because of the nature and severity of their disability, need intensive supported employment services or extended services in order to perform such work.
> (B) Such term includes transitional employment for persons who are individuals with the most severe disabilities due to mental illness (29 U.S.C. 706(18)).

Supported employment services were described in the Rehabilitation Act Amendments of 1992 as including: (1) job development and placement, (2) time-limited services, and (3) extended services. The Rehabilitation Act Amendments of 1992 viewed time-limited services as training and support services to an individual with a severe disability until employment is stabilized. According to this legislation, extended services cannot be paid for with vocational rehabilitation (VR) funding. Extended services must be funded by other agencies or through natural supports. Extended services may include services provided by a human service agency, community organizations, family, friend, the employer, or by the consumer. The amendments further define extended or ongoing services as:

> 1. Provided to individuals with the most severe disabilities
> 2. Provided, at a minimum, twice monthly:
>   —to make an assessment, regarding the employment situation, at the worksite of each such individual in supported employment, or under special circumstances, especially at the request of the client, off site; and
>   —based on the assessment, to provide for the coordination or provision of specific intervention services, at or away from the worksite, that are needed to maintain employment stability; and

3. Consisting of:
   —a particularized assessment supplementary to the comprehensive assessment;
   —the provision of skilled job trainers who accompany the individual for intensive job skill training at the worksite;
   —job development and placement;
   —social skills training
   —regular observation or supervision of the individual;
   —follow-up services, such as regular contact with the employers, the individuals, the parents, family members, guardians, advocates, and other authorized representatives of the individuals, and other suitable professional and informed advisors, in order to reinforce and stabilize the job placement;
   —facilitation of natural supports at the workplace
   —any other services identified (P.L. 102–569, 106 Stat. 4354)

Legislators included the Rehabilitation Act Amendments of 1998 as part of the Workforce Investment Act (WIA) and did not change the definition of supported employment. However, the WIA did introduce some new provisions pertinent to persons with serious mental illness including: (1) expansion of the exercise of informed choice, (2) presumptive eligibility for individuals who are Supplemental Security Income (SSI) or Social Security Disability Income (SSDI) recipients, (3) including telecommuting, self-employment, and small business operations as legitimate employment outcomes, and (4) requiring trial work experiences before determining the individual cannot benefit from VR services (P.L. 105–220).

CHARACTERISTICS OF EFFECTIVE SUPPORTED EMPLOYMENT PROGRAMS

Supported employment research has identified a number of characteristics of supported employment programs that have been highly correlated with employee tenure, productivity, earnings, and employer and employee satisfaction (Shafer et al., 1998). These include:

1. accelerated placement;
2. career-focus and career recovery approaches;
3. self-determination and consumer ownership;
4. ecological services and supports;
5. peer support mechanisms;
6. responsive and integrated service provision; and
7. ongoing supports and support building.

Research by Bond (1992) reported significantly better employment outcomes for participants who bypassed pre-vocational activities. Accelerated individuals retained employment for a longer period than did participants who participated in sequential and graduated activities leading to employment. Bond (1992) questioned the use of the "Choose–Get–Keep" models where the "Choose" phase was extended for use individuals with serious mental illness. However, other researchers emphasized that the strength of the "Choose–Get–Keep" model was the focus on client choice and self-determination that was missing in many traditional "Place–Train" models (Shafer et al., 1998).

Research related to supported employment programs for persons with serious mental illness suggests that services that are individualized and focused on career recovery show better job retention and employee satisfaction (Anthony, Cohen, & Farkas, 1990; Shafer et al., 1998). The concept of career recovery embraces a strength-based approach that views the individual in what Anthony described as a "deeply personal" way. In this process, the individual changes by living a "satisfying, hopeful, and contributing life." This concept of career recovery draws heavily on Super, Thompson, Lindeman, & Myer's (1981) definition of career:

> The sequence of major positions occupied by a person throughout his preoccupational, occupational, and post occupational life: includes work-related roles such as those of student, employee, and pensioner, together with complementary avocational, familial and civic roles. Careers exist only as people pursue them, they are person-centered.

Self-determination/consumer control is a third characteristic of effective supported employment programs for persons with serious mental illness. Research shows that involvement in the process of supported employment is a significant predictor of placement success, job tenure, and employee satisfaction (Baer, Martonyi, Simmons, Flexer, & Goebel, 1994). It is important because participants need to feel ownership of the outcomes—ownership that comes from determining their own goals, choosing their own providers, and determining their own methods of support. Additionally, persons with serious mental illness need to feel ownership of the rehabilitation system itself by being employed and placed in positions of *real* power. Through ownership comes responsibility and through responsibility comes the ability to assume the roles of student, employee, family member, and life participant

Ecological approaches have emerged as a fourth characteristic of effective supported employment programs. These types of supported employment programs address the interdependence of social, leisure, work, and residential environments when persons with serious mental illness become employed (Baer, Goebel, & Flexer, 1993; Szymanski, Hershenson, Enright, & Ettinger, 1996). Ecological practitioners recognize the fact that supported employment cannot change one aspect of a person's life without changing others. Lack of social relationships and leisure activities with working peers can be a serious hindrance to work stability, as can poor living conditions and lack of transportation. Ecological approaches also stress the importance of interagency collaboration, family involvement, and natural supports.

Peer support mechanisms are a fifth characteristic of effective supported employment programs. Peer support models address the concern that persons with serious mental illness are often lonely, disempowered, and reluctant to use formal mental health services. Peer support provides them with the opportunity for individual and group empowerment through socialization and self-help activities, collective advocacy, and control of the programs that are providing services (Shafer et al., 1998; Stroul, 1993).

Responsiveness is a sixth characteristic of effective programs. Research has shown that programs that can respond quickly to employer and employee concerns show significantly better tenure outcomes and more efficient allocation of resources. Supported employment providers need to be alert and responsive to all employee needs and act before a problem requires major interventions such as hospitalization or termination of employment (Cook & Razzano, 1992).

SUPPORTED EMPLOYMENT PROCESS

Supported employment models for persons with serious mental illness may vary in approach, but generally they follow a similar sequence of activities of: (1) assessment, (2) job development, (3) job placement, (4) job training and support, and (5) extended services. Supported employment service providers often face the daunting task of patching together a variety of service providers and funding streams to put all these components into place.

The Assessment Phase

In this phase the supported employment provider initiates collaboration with the individual, families, friends, and human service professionals to identify supports and service needs. An ecological approach to assessment defines supports and service needs, not only in the area of employment, but also in the areas of independent living and community participation. Proponents of independent living models assert that dependence on professionals should be avoided whenever possible by identifying services and supports that are the least intrusive. The following list includes some types of assessments that may be useful for specific individuals (Clark & Patton, 1997):

- Interest inventories (computer and written)
- Employability skills inventories
- Personal-futures planning
- Structured situational (home, community, work) assessments
- Structured interviews
- Social histories
- Adaptive behavior inventories
- Life skills inventories
- Aptitude tests
- Personality scales
- Social skills inventories
- Vocational skills assessments
- Professional assessments (e.g., psychology, medical, vision, speech, mobility)
- College entrance examinations
- Assessment of technology needs
- Career portfolios

Care must be used in selection of standardized assessment instruments and in presentation of their findings. Assessment information should be: (1) valid for the individual being tested, (2) related to actual and desired student environments, (3) understandable, and (4) focused on individual strengths. Research shows that standardized assessment procedures often lack validity for persons with disabilities because they do not consider the effects of supports, technology, and training on student performance (Menchetti & Piland, 1998). Hagner and Dileo (1993) point out that standardized assessment procedures may have little use for persons with severe disabilities, since they lack the pressures, cues, sights, and sounds of the environments in which they will perform.

Because supported employment is by definition non-exclusionary, it is important to conduct assessments that are not designed to screen out individuals from employment. Functional assessments examine the functional abilities of the individual in the context of what is required by the environment where the skill is to be performed (Parent, Unger, & Inge, 1997). The supported employment provider can then identify gaps between what the person with serious mental illness can do and what the environment requires. The services and supports that bridge this gap become the "supported" component of supported employment. Functional assessments are, by definition, contextual, so they should be performed in a variety of environments. Consequently, supported employment providers need access to a variety of worksites to provide consumers job shadowing, situational assessment, and community work experience opportunities.

The Planning Phase

Depending on the type and degree of disability, persons with serious mental illness may benefit from person-centered planning, career planning, or both. Planning approaches emphasizing *person-centered planning* have been used primarily for individuals who have difficulty developing career goals due to the extent of their disability or due to a difficulty in expressing preferences (Menchetti & Piland, 1998). While typically used with individuals with severe disabilities, they may also benefit persons with milder disabilities who have no goals or direction (Rojewski, 1993). Person-centered planning approaches typically involve a facilitator, a recorder, the individual, and various family, friends, peers, and coworkers who work together to answer questions regarding the person's history, dreams, nightmares, relationships, abilities, and plan of action. Person-centered planning approaches include:

1. Personal Futures Planning—a type of person-centered planning that involves dreaming, describing, and doing with the family and their support system (Mount & Zwernick, 1988).
2. Life-Style Planning—a form of person-centered planning that describes future goals and defines the steps needed to reach them (O'Brien, 1987).
3. Making Action Plans (MAP)—a form of person-centered planning that asks eight questions regarding the individuals history, dreams, nightmares, talents, and needs (Vandercook, York, & Forest, 1989).

Career planning approaches can be effective for persons with serious mental illness who can respond to more detailed instructions. These career-planning approaches may be used in conjunction with a peer support group or job club where persons with serious mental illness can support each other in planning their future. Career planning approaches tend to be more comprehensive and systematic than person-centered planning approaches. They include:

1. What Color is My Parachute—an eclectic approach that provides an overview of career development and some useful exercises and examples related to identifying interests, researching jobs, developing résumés, and conducting interviews (Bolles, 1995).
2. The Career Maturity Index along with the Career Development Inventory—a developmental approach that can direct counseling (or use of a computerized DISCOVER program) to address competencies in the areas of student, leisurite, citizen, worker, and homemaker (Crites, 1978).
3. The Self-Directed Search—an approach that identifies six personality types and matches them with six matching categories of jobs (Holland, 1985).

Consumers, with the support of friends and family members, should be prepared and supported in taking an active role in: (1) identifying employment goals, (2) choosing supports, and (3) identifying ideal job characteristics. Consumers, friends, and family members should also be prepared to provide ideas about potential job sources and support providers in their network of friends. The agency representative should be prepared to support consumer decisions, commit agency resources, and facilitate a positive planning atmosphere.

The Job Development and Placement Phase

In this phase the supported employment provider uses the vocational profile and planning information to develop a set of consumer-focused job search activities. The job developer's role must suit the needs of the individual, developing as little dependence on professional supports as possible while maintaining effectiveness. Some individuals may play a very active role in their job search while others may require more direct intervention. In either case, the jobs developed must be based on the career path, interests, and needs of the individual with serious mental illness.

The development and use of natural supports in job development and placement is critical, especially in mental health programs where professional supports and resources are extremely limited. Individual, family, and community networks give the job developer leads and support options that cannot be developed with agency resources alone. Additionally, the involvement of individual, family, and community networks engenders commitment and support by persons involved in obtaining and maintaining employment.

The job developer also needs to network with employers and help consumers represent themselves in terms of what they can contribute. Job searches need to be individualized, but simultaneously, job developers must be aware of labor market needs and employer concerns. Establishing employer networks can be described as a process that involves networking, listening, negotiating, and supporting employers (Baer et al., 1994). The job developer develops networks through a community job market screening that includes: (1) research on job market trends, (2) a review of classified ads, (3) meetings with representatives of Chambers of Commerce and employer groups, and (4) consultation with local job developers and employment specialists. The job developer needs to take time to listen and understand the organizational culture and how it is likely to affect the employment of a person with a serious mental illness (Parent et al., 1997). The job developer negotiates a job with an employer by suggesting how the employee with a serious mental illness can meet the employer's needs (Hagner & Dileo, 1993). Finally, the job developer supports the employer by viewing the employer as a customer of supported employment (Brooke, Wehman, Inge, & Parent, 1997).

Job accommodations are an important aspect of job development. For persons with serious mental illness, job accommodations are often needed in the form of job restructuring. Job restructuring can include: carved jobs, negotiated jobs, or created jobs (Callahan & Garner, 1997). Job carving refers to the process of removing certain job responsibilities and, in some instances, the addition of other responsibilities to tailor the job to the capability of the person with a serious mental illness. Negotiated jobs refers to the process of identifying employer job duties for which no existing job description exists and negotiating the creation of a job suited to the consumer. Job creation refers to the process of identifying a new service that may benefit the employer. Flippo, Gibson, and Brooke (1997) identify thirteen steps to follow in job restructuring:

- Listen to employer needs
- Study job descriptions
- Conduct job analysis
- Observe work routine
- Interview employers
- Interview coworkers
- Spend time in various departments
- Take written notes
- Do a work culture analysis
- Determine needs
- Put proposals together
- Discuss the proposal with the employer
- Set interview(s) or a time for the employer to meet the applicant

The job interview may be conducted in several ways. The job developer and the consumer should determine: (1) whether the job developer should accompany the consumer to the interview, (2) how the job developer will prepare the individual for the interview, and (3) how the consumer will be supported in getting to the interview. Generally, interviewees should be prepared to say how they can help the employer, what kind of persons they are, and why they should be hired. The individual should also be prepared to decide whether to accept a job offer, taking into consideration factors such as work environment, wages, benefits, transportation, and impact on Social Security benefits (Owens, 1999).

The job developer should be prepared to discuss the impact of supported employment on the benefits that a person with serious mental illness is receiving. This may be a complex process if the individual is living in subsidized housing, receiving food stamps, Social Security, and Medicaid benefits. The individual, and often the family, depend on these benefits and fear their loss. The job developer should therefore be prepared to provide or obtain an extensive benefit analysis to ensure that needed supports remain in place. The Social Security Administration has developed some work incentives that have been strengthened over the years to reward and encourage SSDI, SSI, and Medicaid beneficiaries. These include deductions for impairment related work expenses (IRWEs), Plans to Achieve Self-Support (PASS), and Student Earned Income Exclusion. Persons with serious mental illness typically receive SSI payments that decline only one dollar for every two earned after earned income, IRWE, and PASS deductions.

The Job Training and Support Phase

Once a job has been accepted the supported employment provider implements the job training and support plan. Typically, a job coach or employment specialist provides supported employment job-site training, but occasionally a coworker or even a family member may provide it. Job-site training typically follows a sequence of steps (Inge, 1997) including:

- Job duty analysis
- Task analysis of each job duty
- Identification of natural supports
- Identification of natural cues
- Development of an instructional plan
- Application of assistive technology
- Negotiating changes in job duties as needed
- Development of a fading plan

The job duty analysis is conducted before the individual starts working. Often supported employment specialists arrange to work in a job for several days to conduct this analysis. A job duty analysis includes: (1) an analysis of the environments where jobs are to be performed, (2) determination of essential and non-essential job functions, and (3) establishing a work routine. A typical entry in a job duty list would state the time frame (e.g., 7:00–7:30 a.m.) and a description of the job duty (e.g., photocopy work in "In Box").

Once job environments, duties, and routines are determined, individual job duties are broken down into steps known as a task analysis. The makeup and size of the steps in the task analysis are determined by the needs of the individual. A typical task analysis for photocopying might look as follows:

- Place jobs to the left of the copier
- Clear table to the right of the copier

- Place the first job in the copier feeder face up
- Select the number of copies requested on the post-it note
- Remove the post-it note
- Press the start button
- Remove and stack copies on the table to the right of the copier
- Place originals neatly on the stack of copies

For persons with serious mental illness, it is important to analyze both work and non-work aspects of the job. This includes routines such as arriving to work, coffee breaks, lunch breaks, and leaving work, and also non-routine activities such as birthday parties, office parties, and staff meetings. Additionally, it may be necessary to look at other training responsibilities related to: appropriate dress and hygiene; accepting criticism; coping with stressors; and getting to work on time.

Workplace supports and natural cues are important considerations in the development of job-site training. Workplace supports are those supports that are available to all employees such as orientation and training, car-pooling, employee assistance programs, and eating with coworkers. Natural cues are ways that typical employees are signaled to move to the next job, job breaks, or work activities. Supported employment providers need to use these supports whenever possible to avoid excessive cue dependency and stigmatization of the employee with serious mental illness.

Once job duties, tasks, workplace supports, and natural cues are identified, the supported employment provider develops an instructional plan. An important consideration in the development of this plan is the need to individualize supports according to the preferences and needs of the supported employee. This is particularly true for persons with serious mental illness who often find the presence of job trainers as stigmatizing but cannot maintain a job without them. The best approach to this problem is to provide as many choices regarding job supports as possible without seriously compromising the supports needed by the employee. Assistive technology and self-management approaches can be a good support choice for persons with serious mental illness who need help in managing problems with attention, sequencing, or work pace. The use of timers, assignment boards, flow charts, recorded prompts, picture lists, or self-reinforcement strategies may lessen dependence on job trainers and help during the phase-out period.

Upon completion of the instruction plan and the application of assistive technologies, the supported employment provider needs to develop a plan for fading of the job trainer. At this stage of supported employment the person moves into extended (or follow-along) services. These terms refer to any ongoing support services needed to maintain an individual in supported employment after the fading out of the job trainer. Extended services include: (1) periodic monitoring of work performance, (2) crisis intervention, (3) periodic monitoring of social integration, (4) support training for employers and coworkers, (5) retraining of previously learned skills, (6) training of new skills, and (7) general problem-solving. As with job training, extended support providers will need to address the need for employment-specific supports, as well as personal supports such as housing, financial, leisure activity, and transportation.

The transition to extended services occurs after the fading of the job trainer. This has been described by Brook et al. (1997) as a seven-step process that includes:

1. Discussion of the fading schedule with the individual and the supervisor
2. Agreement on a day to begin fading the job trainer
3. Informing the individual and coworkers of plans to leave the job site and how long

4. Giving the individual and the supervisor a telephone number where the job trainer can be reached.
5. Leaving for 1–2 hours for the first fading session.
6. Monitoring performance for periods when the trainer is absent
7. Gradually increasing time off the site

Often, the job trainer and the person providing extended services are different persons. This requires considerable attention to collaboration throughout the job training process and communication during and following transition. The trainer and extended service provider should be involved in all planning for the individual to ensure that instructional methods and expectations are consistent.

A CASE STUDY IN SUPPORTED EMPLOYMENT

Frank was a person with serious mental illness who came to our agency seeking employment. He was diagnosed as having paranoid schizophrenia while he was in the military serving in Germany. He was referred to the program by his mental health counselor who felt that Frank was withdrawing and suffering serious self-esteem issues as a result of having no work and living at home with his family.

After assessment, it was determined that Frank had a supportive family, some close friends, and an interest in outdoor work. He was initially resistant to the idea of working because he was afraid of losing his Social Security and Veterans benefits. However, after discussion it was determined that Frank was interested in working outdoors both as a means of reducing stress and as a way of building his body.

An interdisciplinary team was formed to develop a plan for employment. The team included key players from all environments including Frank, his family, his counselor/case manager, VR services, a representative of a community college, and mental health vocational staff. The team's supported employment plan included seven critical components:

1. Assessment of job interests and benefit concerns by the mental health vocational staff
2. Opening a case with VR services by the counselor/case manager
3. Job tryouts as part of an existing mobile work crew with VR work adjustment funding
4. Vocational training in landscaping from the community college with VR support
5. Job development through the community college career services and job club program
6. Job and self-management training and job restructuring through VR services
7. Ongoing support from case management and agency staff.

Through careful benefits analysis, it was possible to maintain Frank's eligibility for SSI and Medicaid by starting him on the mobile work crew at 20 hours per week. This job tryout phase was not time-limited, to allow Frank time to decide whether to proceed with employment and a landscaping career. Frank was also enrolled in the local vocational landscaping training program, which also provided career counseling and job clubs.

After an eight-month period of working with the mobile work crew, the team was able to determine that his support needs included: (1) schedule adjustments to allow for work absences related to psychiatric flare-ups, (2) coworker mentoring to help Frank understand the work culture, (3) mobile job support to help Frank deal with job stressors and delusional thinking, (4) family support services to assist the family getting Frank to work, and (5) case management services to help Frank deal with budgeting, service, housing, and leisure time issues.

Frank decided that he would be willing to seek work with the help of these supports. It was determined that Frank would play a major role in his own job search by participating in the community college job club with non-disabled peers. With the help of the job club facilitator, Frank was able to develop job search skills and a résumé. He agreed to make at least five contacts per week with the help of the facilitator. Frank quickly located possible jobs and was successful in his third interview.

After being offered the job, Frank (with coaching by the counselor) requested a reasonable accommodation in the form of allowing for absences related to periodic medical concerns. He reported that he would still be able to do the job by working additional hours the weeks following his absence. After some negotiation, it was agreed to schedule Frank for 32 hours per week. This allowed him to work up to an additional eight hours per week following periods of medical leave.

Frank's case manager did a benefit analysis and determined that Frank could work for two years without losing his benefits, if he set up a Social Security PASS and deducted IRWE. The case manager also set up a meeting with Frank and the employer to discuss a plan to enlist a coworker to help Frank become part of the work culture.

Frank completed a job analysis with the help of his mobile job supporter and his duties were broken down and scheduled for each of his landscaping jobs. A "Pocket Elephant" was used to help Frank stay on schedule and avoid long periods of rumination. This device played key instructions to Frank each hour. Job duties were outlined in a pocket guide that could be used to remind Frank of key steps in each job duty. Initially, the job trainer/supporter observed Frank to ensure that job training was proceeding as anticipated. Once Frank became comfortable with the job and using his assistive technology, the mobile job supporter negotiated a fade-out period. However, the mobile job supporter emphasized that he would be available at any time that Frank or the employer needed help. Additionally, the mobile job supporter stated he would make regular contacts to ensure that both Frank and the employer were satisfied.

As Frank began earning money, the case manager met with him to set up a financial plan. Frank's interests began expanding as a result of a growing network of community contacts and money to participate in leisure activities. He also began expressing interests about moving away from home. The case manager started the process of assessing leisure and residential environments and the areas that Frank would need support. Frank's career continued to develop over the years with the ongoing assistance of his support team who were able to quickly respond to career changes and mental status concerns.

ADAPTING SUPPORTED EMPLOYMENT TO THE NEEDS OF PERSONS WITH SERIOUS MENTAL ILLNESS

Research suggests that the concept of "fading" may be of questionable value to persons with serious mental illness (Cook & Razanno, 1992; Shafer et al., 1998). They note that individuals with mental illness typically require a higher level of follow-along services, with more frequent periods of intense support (Shafer et al., 1998). Ongoing support is perhaps the most difficult characteristic to address in supported employment for persons with serious mental illness. Typically, mental health programs have been extremely limited in professional resources relative to providing ongoing support. Effective programs have supplemented professional supports with family, peer, employer, and community supports. Effective supported employment programs are therefore support-building, not simply support-providing. Supported employment approaches for persons with serious mental illness need two additional kinds of flexibility: (1) support lasting as long as the consumer desires and (2) delivery of services in a way that consumers can fade in and out of the program, as needed (Cook & Razzano, 1992).

A second limitation of supported employment as applied to persons with serious mental illness relates to the process of choosing to work. Most supported employment models assume that consumers have made a choice to work. This may not be true for the person with serious mental illness for whom the establishment of the choice to work is a significant component of the rehabilitation process (Danley & Anthony, 1987). Traditional supported employment models may address assessing the needs, preferences, and interests of consumers, but they typically do not address psychosocial issues related to the decision to re-enter the world of work.

A third concern in applying supported employment to persons with severe mental illness relates to the stigmatizing effects of having a job coach. A program serving persons with severe mental illness will need to provide job support as unobtrusively as possible, using coworker supports, self-management strategies, and assistive technology approaches whenever possible. When job coaches are utilized, they need to minimize their visibility, avoid development of consumer dependency, and understand the dampening effect their presence may have on social interaction between the consumer and coworkers.

Facilitating the readiness of consumers for supported employment is a significant issue for mental health practitioners. They need to teach the social skills specific ecological environments require using modeling, role-playing, and feedback. It may also be important to teach consumers to initiate and respond to work requests (e.g., requesting work, responding to criticism) and to initiate and respond to non-work related social interaction (e.g., greetings, teasing, asking questions about coworkers' families) (Chadsey & Shelden, 1998).

Mental health practitioners should also address work environment issues before placement. This could include teaching coworkers to initiate or respond socially to the consumers, train social skills, or be employee advocates. The practitioner may also ask several coworkers to develop a plan to socially integrate the new employee and for coworkers with similar interests to do things with the consumer. To facilitate integration, the practitioner may also need to target jobs that are shared or similar to those held by coworkers, build in tasks that overlap or intersect with coworkers, develop schedules for social times, and use work culture and rituals as opportunities for interaction (Chadsey & Shelden, 1998).

CONCLUSION

Supported employment for persons with serious mental illness is a relatively new concept that encompasses a variety of models, philosophies, and orientations. Increasingly, supported employment services for persons with serious mental illness have become differentiated from programs serving other disability groups with greater emphasis on long-term support and less on job training. Six models of supported employment continue to be used for persons with serious mental illness including: (1) enclaves, (2) mobile work crews, (3) dispersed groups or clusters, (4) entrepreneurial models, (5) individual models, and (6) transitional employment. Supported employment is a service recognized and funded by

VR and now includes: (1) assessment, (2) job development, (3) job placement, (4) job training and support, and (5) extended services.

A number of best practices have been discussed in this chapter. They include: (1) accelerated placement, (2) career-focus and career recovery approaches, (3) self-determination and consumer ownership, (4) ecological services and supports, (5) peer support mechanisms, (6) responsive and integrated service provision, and (7) ongoing supports and support building. The challenge for supported employment providers will be to implement these best practices for persons with serious mental illness who need more flexible and intense levels of extended services.

REFERENCES

Anthony, W. A., Cohen, M., & Farkas, M. (1990). *Psychiatric rehabilitation*, Baltimore, MD: University Park Press

Anthony, W. A., Howell, M., & Danley, R. (1984). Vocational rehabilitation for the psychiatrically disabled. In M. Mirabi (Ed.), *The chronically mentally ill: Research and services* (pp. 215–237). Jamaica, NY: Medical and Scientific Books.

Baer, R., Goebel, G., & Flexer, R. W. (1993). An interdisciplinary team approach to rehabilitation. In R.W. Flexer & P.L. Solomon (Eds.), *Psychiatric rehabilitation in practice*. Boston, MA: Butterworth-Heinemann.

Baer, R., Martonyi, E., Simmons, T., Flexer, R. W., & Goebel, G. W. (1994). Employer collaboration: A tri-lateral group process model. *Journal of Rehabilitation Administration 18*(3), 151–163.

Bolles, R. N. (1995). *What color is my parachute? A practical manual for job hunters and career changers*. Berkely, CA: Ten Speed Press.

Bond, G. (1992). Vocational rehabilitation. In R.P. Liberman (Ed.), *Handbook of psychiatric rehabilitation*. New York, NY: Macmillan.

Brooke, V., Wehman, P., Inge, K., & Parent, W. (1997). Supported employment: A customer-driven approach. In V. Brooke, K. Inge, A. Armstrong, & P. Wehman (Eds.), *Support employment handbook: A customer-driven approach for persons with significant disabilities*. Richmond, VA: Virginia Commonwealth University.

Callahan, M. J., & Garner, J. B. (1997). *Keys to the workplace: Skills and supports for people with disabilities*. Baltimore, MD: Brookes.

Chadsey, J. G., & Shelden, D. (1998). Moving toward social inclusion in employment and postsecondary settings. In F.R. Rusch & J. Chadsey (Eds.), *Beyond high school: Transition from school to work*. Belmont, CA: Wadsworth.

Clark, G. M., & Kolstoe, O. P. (1995). *Career development and transition education for adolescents with disabilities* (2nd ed.). Needham, MA: Allyn & Bacon.

Clark, G. M., & Patton, J. R. (1997). *Transition planning inventory: Administration and resource guide*. Austin, TX: PRO-ED.

Cook, J. A., & Razzano (1992). Natural vocational supports for persons with severe mental illness: Thresholds supported competitive employment program. In L. Stein (Ed.), *Innovative community mental health programs* (pp. 23–41). San Francisco, CA: Jossey-Bass.

Crites, J. (1978). *Theory and research handbook for the career maturity inventory*. Monterey, CA: McGraw-Hill.

Danley, K., & Anthony, W. (1987). The choose-get-keep model. *American Rehabilitation, 13*(4), 6–9.

Flippo, K., Gibson, K., & Brooke, V. (1997). Job development: The path to careers. In V. Brooke, K. Inge, A. Armstrong, & P. Wehman (Eds.), *Support employment handbook: A customer-driven approach for persons with significant disabilities*. Richmond, VA: Virginia Commonwealth University.

Hagner, D., & Dileo, D. (1993). *Working together: Workplace culture, supported employment, and persons with disabilities*. Cambridge, MA. Brookline Books.

Holland, J. L. (1985). *Making vocational choices: A theory of vocational personalities and work environments*. Englewood Cliffs, NJ: Prentice-Hall.

Inge, K. (1997). Job site training. In V. Brooke, K. Inge, A. Armstrong, & P. Wehman (Eds.), *Support employment handbook: A customer-driven approach for persons with significant disabilities*. Richmond, VA: Virginia Commonwealth University.

Menchetti, B., & Piland, V. C. (1998). A person-centered approach to vocational evaluation and career planning. In F.R. Rusch & J. Chadsey (Eds.), *Beyond high school: Transition from school to work*. Belmont, CA: Wadsworth.

Mount, B., & Zwernick (1988). *It's never too early, it's never too late: A booklet about personal futures planning* (Publication No. 421-88-109). St. Paul, MN: Governor's Planning Council on Developmental Disabilities.

O'Brien, J. (1987). A guide to life-style planning: Using the activities catalogue to integrate services and natural support system. In G. T. Bellamy & B. Wilcox (Eds.), *A comprehensive guide to the activities catalogue: An alternative curriculum for youth and adults with severe disabilities.* Baltimore, MD: Paul H. Brookes.

Owens, D. M. (1999). *Supported employment: A training manual for consumers, families, and service providers.* Columbus, OH: Ohio Rehabilitation Services Commission.

Parent, W., Unger, D., & Inge, K. (1997). Customer profile. In V. Brooke, K. Inge, A. Armstrong, & P. Wehman (Eds.), *Support employment handbook: A customer-driven approach for persons with significant disabilities.* Richmond, VA: Virginia Commonwealth University.

Rojewski, J. W. (1993). Theoretical structure of career maturity for rural adolescents with learning disabilities. *Career Development for Exceptional Individuals, 16*(1), 39–52.

Shafer, M. S., Middaugh, A., Rubin, M., & Jones, R. (1998). *Career recovery: Best practices in the vocational rehabilitation of persons with serious mental illness.* St. Augustine, FL: Training Resource Network.

Simmons, T. J., Selleck, V., Steele, R. B., & Sepetauc, F. (1993). Supports and rehabilitation for employment. In R. W. Flexer & P. L. Solomon (Eds.), *Psychiatric rehabilitation in practice.* Boston, MA: Butterworth-Heinemann.

Stroul, B. A. (1993) Rehabilitation in community support systems. In R. W. Flexer & P. L. Solomon (Eds.), *Psychiatric rehabilitation in practice.* Boston, MA: Butterworth-Heinemann.

Super, D., Thompson, A., Lindeman, R., & Myer, R. (1981). *A career development inventory.* Palo Alto, CA: Consulting Psychological Press.

Szymanski, E. M., Hershenson, D. B., Enright, M. S., & Ettinger, J. (1996). Career development theories, constructs, and research: Implications for people with disabilities. In E. M. Szymanski & R. M. Parker (Eds.), *Work and disability: Issues and strategies in career development and job placement* (pp. 79–126). Austin, TX: PRO-ED.

Vandercook, T., York, J., & Forest, M. (1989). The McGill Action Planning System (MAPS): A strategy for building the vision. *Journal of the Association for Persons with Severe Handicaps, 14*(3), 205–215.

CHAPTER 28

Addressing the Employment Needs of Persons with Physical Disabilities

Implications for Rehabilitation and Mental Health Service Workers

WILLIAM CRIMANDO

In 1873, Dostoevsky wrote, "Originality and the feeling of one's own dignity are achieved only through work and struggle" (cited in Lee, 1999). The need to be engaged in meaningful activity, whether for survival, self-esteem, or self-transcendence, is nearly as old as humankind itself. Similarly, President Clinton (cited in Rasco, 1996, p. 10) said, "I do not believe we can repair the basic fabric of society until all people who are willing to work have work. Work organizes life. It gives structure and discipline to life." Thus, work is an "organizing principle" by which we perceive, think about, and plan our activities.

According to the U.S. Census Bureau (1997), approximately one American in five has some kind of disability, and one in 10 has a severe disability. Using data from a October 1994–January 1995 survey, the Census Bureau goes on to state that in the prime employable years (21–64), 82% of people without disability had a job or business, while 77% of those with a non-severe disability, and only 26% of persons with severe disability held employment. Furthermore, the 1990 census tables (U.S. Census Bureau, 1999) give these data about civilian, non-institutionalized persons between the ages of 16 and 64: (1) 10.4% have a work disability, mobility limitation, or self-care limitation, with 8.2% having a work disability; (2) 24.3–31.2% of those with a work disability live below the poverty level; (3) 39.3% of those with a work disability are in the labor force, while only 34.1% are employed.

This chapter is an examination of the mental health implications of physical disability, especially as they relate to return-to-work, new employment, and career directions for persons with physical disabilities. The integration of rehabilitation and mental health practices will be

WILLIAM CRIMANDO • Rehabilitation Administration and Services Program, Rehabilitation Institute, Southern Illinois University, Carbondale, Illinois.

discussed in an analysis of factors that must be addressed; these factors will be presented in a framework that includes biological, psychological, environmental, and cultural influences. The rehabilitation and mental health processes of comprehensive assessment, planning, environmental support and design, mobility enhancement, and development/support of employment opportunities are discussed. This chapter cannot be, nor is it meant to be, a comprehensive and exhaustive discussion of the issues raised. It is hoped, however, that the reader will gain an appreciation of the complexity of employment needs of persons with physical disabilities, as well as the strategies suggested for managing that complexity.

A BIO-PSYCHOLOGICAL–SOCIAL–ENVIRONMENTAL–CULTURAL FRAMEWORK FOR PHYSICAL DISABILITIES

A definition of physical disability is, at first glance, simple, but it becomes complicated when one examines the factors that may influence disability. A person is considered to have a disability if she or he has difficulty performing certain functions—such as seeing, hearing, walking, and climbing stairs—or has difficulty performing activities of daily living or certain social roles. A severe disability is the inability to perform these functions without assistance (U.S. Census Bureau, 1997) from a device or another person. Finally, in the consideration for eligibility to receive vocational rehabilitation services, the impairment must be long-lasting and must constitute a substantial impediment to employment (Department of Rehabilitation Education and Research, University of Arkansas, 1994). Falvo (1991) identified 13 types of disorders and discussed the major disabling conditions associated (Table 28-1). But as the definition suggests, the presence of the condition does not necessarily constitute disability, unless the person's ability to perform certain life functions has been limited. Thus, a person who has experienced myocardial infarction and bypass surgery, but returns to work and daily living at full functioning, would not be considered disabled.

The "biological definition" of disability, constituted by the physical impairment, must then be viewed within larger contexts, the psychological, environmental—both social and physical—and cultural factors that influence disability. Figure 28-1 demonstrates the interaction of these factors. Psychological and environmental factors influence the impairment directly, and are influenced themselves by cultural factors.

Psychological Context

The psychological context consists of beliefs, feelings, and opinions the person with impairment has about him or herself, the impairment, and living with the impairment. Thus, it includes what would be considered self-concept or self-image, the manner in which a person perceives him or herself (Fitts, 1965). Self-concept is important because it influences our behavior. A person with a disability and a positive self-concept may be said to be adjusting well to the disability, while another's poor adjustment is likely associated with a negative self-image. Shontz (1977) discussed six principles relating disability with psychological adjustment. Among them were these, which he termed "confutative principles," because they confute commonly held beliefs:

1. Psychological reactions to physical disability are not uniformly disturbing and do not necessarily result in maladjustment. Conversely, psychological reactions to removal

TABLE **28-1.** **Examples of Disabling Conditions**

Type of disorder	Examples of disabling conditions
Cardiovascular	Hypertension Arteriosclerosis Congestive Heart Failure Coronary Artery Disease
Respiratory	Emphysema Asthma Occupational Lung Diseases Cystic Fibrosis
Renal and Urinary Tract	Polycystic Kidney Disease Renal Failure
Endocrine	Diabetes Mellitus Hypothyroidism
Gastrointestinal	Peptic Ulcers Irritable Bowel Syndrome Hernia Pancreatitis
Musculoskeletal and Connective Tissue	Rheumatoid Arthritis Systemic Lupus Erythematosus Ankylosing Spondylitis Carpal Tunnel Syndrome Amputation
Nervous System	Traumatic Brain Injury Cerebrovascular Accident Cerebral Palsy Epilepsy Spinal Cord Injuries Multiple Sclerosis
Hearing	Conductive Hearing Impairments Sensorineural Hearing Impairments Ménière's Disease
Visual	Refractive Errors Macular Degeneration Retinitis Pigmentosa
Dermatologic	Burns Allergic Reactions Herpes Zoster
Cancers	Carcinoma Sarcoma Melanoma Lymphoma Leukemia
Blood and Immune System	Sickle Cell Anemia Hemophilia Human Immunodeficiency Virus Spectrum
Substance Use	Addictions Cirrhosis

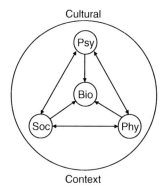

FIGURE 28-1. A bio-psychological–social–environmental–cultural framework for physical disabilities.

of disability are not necessarily pleasant nor do they automatically lead to improved adjustment.

2. Favorable or unfavorable reactions to disabilities are not related in simple ways to their physical properties.

3. Disability itself is only one of all factors that affect the life situation of a person with a disability, and its influence is often relatively minor.

Shontz's assertions show the importance of treating each person with a disability as an individual, with her or his unique profile of physical, psychological, and emotional traits, interests, needs, goals, problems, and passions. These should all be considered in providing services leading to employment outcomes.

How a person reacts to disability and the environment, and makes plans for the future, may depend upon the stage of adaptation he or she is in. It is suggested (cf. Livneh, 1991a) that everyone goes through a series of predictable stages in adapting to disability; a number of models have been proposed describing what the stages are and how people progress through them. Livneh (1991a) examined existing models and proposed a unified approach, which made 18 assumptions, including these: (1) while most people experience most of the stages, not all people experience all the stages; (2) the stages may fluctuate or overlap with each other; (3) while there is a "theoretically ordered sequence of stages" (p. 113), it is possible to become stuck in a stage, to regress to an earlier stage, and to skip over stages; and (4) not everyone reaches "final adjustment" (p. 114). These five stages comprise Livneh's (1991a) model:

1. Initial impact: Immediately following the onset of the disabling condition, the person experiences protective psychic shock, followed by panic, as he or she is "exposed … to converging and painful sensations associated with the traumatic event" (p. 117).

2. Defense mobilization: Following initial impact, the person displays two overlapping substages—bargaining and denial. Bargaining involves attempts by the individual to negotiate with God for reversal of the disability. Bargaining is accompanied by the person's expectation of full recovery. Denial also includes expectancy of recovery but, in this case, because the disability does not exist, rather than a cure from God.

3. Initial realization: During the third stage, the individual experiences brief mourning for the lost body part or function, longer lasting depression, and internalized anger, guilt, or self-blame.

4. Retaliation: Retaliation is characterized by a rebellion against the turn of events, and against weakness and perceived dependency on others. Retaliation may take the form of externalized anger and hostility toward caregivers, significant others, objects, and environmental conditions.

5. Reintegration: Three substages comprise the reintegration stage. The first is acknowledgment of the permanency of the disability and its implication. This is followed by emotional acceptance of the disability and, ultimately, final adjustment. Livneh suggests this final stage is characterized by vocational and social integration into the outside world, as the individual has reconciled the disability and implications for future goals and plans.

Finally, Livneh avers that each stage has its own idiosyncratic affective, cognitive, and behavioral correlates, as well as ways the individual is more likely to expend energy.

Ultimately the affective, cognitive, and behavioral correlates of the particular stage a person is in should influence how services are planned and implemented. Persons with disability differ in their reactions to and acceptance of disability (Livneh, 1982; Shontz, 1977; Wright, 1960), and the degree of acceptance may influence decisions to apply for rehabilitation services, which services to seek, and the success of those services. While it would be meaningless to give a formula or cookbook approach for choosing strategies (e.g., for a person at "X" stage, do "A" and "B."), Livneh (1991b) provides some guides: he suggests that the choice of method depends on the client's needs, the degree of psychosocial impact, the onset and progression of the disability, the support system of the client, the mental health practitioner's mastery of methods, and so on. He further suggests that practitioners should adopt a flexible and eclectic approach when working with persons with disabilities. Accordingly, Livneh (1991b) has reviewed the literature and listed techniques from the insight therapies (e.g., client-centered and Gestalt therapies) for those in the earlier stages of adaptation, when the individual is involved in bringing the disability and its consequences into awareness. For those in later stages, when the person begins to do something about the disability and life thereafter, strategies may be chosen from the cognitive–behavioral therapies (e.g., behavioral, rational-emotive, and reality therapies).

Self-efficacy beliefs (Bandura, 1982), or self-competence beliefs also play an important role in the psychological context, and they demonstrate the influence of other contexts. Self-efficacy beliefs are the expectations that one can actually do something. Hackett and Betz (1981) asserted that self-efficacy was influential in our achievement, career decisions, and adjustment behaviors. The self-image is affected by environmental and cultural factors. Tuttle (1984) suggested that a sense of self-competence and the perceptions of others are critical factors in an individual's self-concept. Furthermore, each culture has a "body ideal" against which we tend to measure our own and others' bodies (cf. Livneh, 1982). The closer our bodies are to the ideal, the more likely it will be that we will hold positive self-images.

Environmental Context

Two entities comprise the environmental context: the social environment and the physical environment. Shontz (1977) suggested that environmental factors are at least as important as internal states of persons who have disabilities in determining psychological reactions to disability. Lewin (1935) asserted that behavior is a function of the person and the environment. Parker and Schaller (1996) suggested that interactions between the person (P)

and the environment (*E*) were equally important, so that a mathematical representation would read

$$B = f(P, E, P \times E)$$

where *B* is the behavior and *f* means "function of." As an example, Parker and Schaller suggest worker values—a personal factor—and employer values—an environmental factor—act individually to influence career and job choice; they also interact since there may be a reciprocal relationship between worker and employer values.

SOCIAL ENVIRONMENT.   The social environment, consisting of the behaviors and attitudes of those around us, is so important that Oliver (1983) distinguished "impairment," an individual limitation, and "disability," a socially imposed restriction. For example, "spread" (Kutner, cited in Marinelli & Dell Orto, 1991; Thoreson & Kerr, 1978; Wright, 1960) describes a phenomenon in which negative characteristics are attributed to those with disabilities through generalization or "halo effect." That is, frequently when encountering those with a specific physical disability, people generalize the disability to unrelated physical, mental, or emotional characteristics. Thus persons with disabilities are frequently perceived as less intelligent, less sociable, or less stable than the non-disabled, or functionally limited in ways that have nothing to do with their disabilities. As a second example, a person who has HIV/AIDS but who maintains a healthy lifestyle and is free of secondary opportunistic infection may still be perceived not only as disabled but contagious, and thus shunned.

Livneh (1982) attempted to classify the causal literature, both theoretical and empirical, on sources of attitudes toward disability. Livneh suggested that there were 10 categories of sources:

1. *Sociocultural conditioning* resulting from social and cultural norms and expectations. Examples in this category were emphasis on personal appearance and athletic prowess, delineation of the "sick role" phenomenon, and the status degradation attached to disability.
2. *Childhood influences* resulting from child-rearing practices and early parental influences.
3. *Psychodynamic mechanisms* including unconscious psychological processes related to childhood experiences. These included a requirement of mourning for the loss of functioning, unresolved conflict over scopophilia, associating responsibility with etiology, and guilt of being non-disabled.
4. *Disability as a punishment for sin*, that sin being either a personally committed act or ancestral wrong.
5. *Anxiety-provoking unstructured situations* arising from the "newness" of experience with persons with disability. The anxiety stems from both affective and cognitive unpreparedness.
6. *Aesthetic aversion* or the feelings of repulsion and discomfort triggered by the sight of a person with a visible disability.
7. *Threats to body-image integrity* stemming from the incongruence between the reality of the person with disability and the expectations for a "normal" body. This category included reawakening of the castration anxiety, anxiety about becoming disabled, and fear of contamination.
8. *Minority group comparability*, negative stereotypic reactions triggered by the marginality of persons with disabilities.

9. *Disability as a reminder of death*, suggesting that the loss of functioning constitutes the death of a body part which is integrally associated with the ego.
10. *Prejudice-inviting behaviors* of persons with disabilities themselves, such as acting dependent, fearful, insecure or inferior, and not speaking out positively about their rights, interests, and concerns.

Livneh (1982) also suggested that attitudes toward disability were influenced by disability-related factors (e.g., level of severity, degree of visibility, and body part affected), demographic (e.g., sex, age, and educational level), and personality (e.g., ethnocentrism, self-insight, and ambiguity tolerance) variables in the "beholder." Finally, in a series of studies, Bordieri and Drehmer reported that both employers and graduate business students' attitudes toward disabilities, manifested in their stated willingness to hire a person with a disability, may be influenced by attribution for the disability. That is, they professed less favorable tendencies if the disability was thought to have internal causes (i.e., the person caused the disability by his or her own behavior) than if the disability was thought to be externally caused (cf. Bordieri & Drehmer, 1986, 1987; Bordieri, Drehmer, & Comninel, 1988).

The 20th Institute on Rehabilitation Issues (IRI, 1993) demonstrates the interaction of personal factors and social environment factors (Figure 28-2). A person with a disability presents a number of personal factors such as job skills, attitudes and values toward working, employment history, and what he or she has gained through rehabilitation services. These influence how that person acts toward the environment. Depending on the specific configuration of personal factors, the individual will seek and gain employment, or not, and will thus participate in and contribute to the place of employment and the local economy. These may affect employers' attitudes toward persons with disabilities, as exposure to positive models (Beattie, Anderson, & Antonak, 1997) and positive experience (Amsel & Fichten, 1988; Maras & Brown, 1996) with persons with disability have both been shown to improve attitudes, in limited research. The individual's behavior will also have a marginal effect on the local economy and labor market. These will, in turn, influence the amount of employment opportunities for persons with disabilities. In theory, a strong labor market and a strong economy mean that more persons with disabilities are employed; the inverse would also be true. This is the "queue theory" of labor markets (Adams, Krislov, & Lairson, 1972), which states that during strong economies—when unemployment is low—"marginalized" persons are more likely to be considered for employment than during weak economies. A better economy may also result in better services for persons with disabilities.

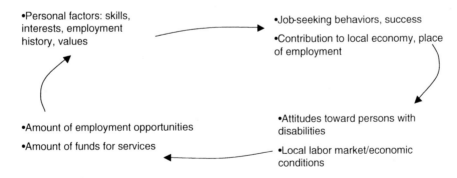

FIGURE 28-2. A person × environment diagram for community attitudes and persons with disabilities.

PHYSICAL ENVIRONMENTAL.   The physical environment consists of the physical surroundings of the person with the disability—the home, neighborhood, community, and workplace. The physical world presents certain barriers which interact with a disabling condition to create disability; without those barriers the disability technically would not exist. For example, we receive much of our information from visual cues, such as traffic signage and signals, body language, and facial expressions. A person who was blind would be limited in her or his ability to receive information visually, and thus would have a disability. But, if that person was able to receive the exact same information from redundant auditory, kinesthetic, or tactile cues, the disability would be mitigated. Similarly, a person whose ability to climb stairs was limited by orthopedic or stamina problems would not be disabled if she or he never encountered stairs. Shontz (1977) averred that environmental barriers reinforce the message often communicated to persons with disabilities that they are inferior.

Cultural Context

Schein (1987) suggests that culture consists of elements at three levels. The most fundamental of these levels are a people's basic assumptions about the nature of human nature, activity, and relationships, the nature of reality, time and space, and its relationship to the environment. At the next level are a people's values, while at the top level are its language, technology, art, rituals, and visible and audible behavior patterns. While it would seem that the most fundamental level—the basic assumptions—would be highly individualized, these elements, as well as elements of the second and top levels, are often shared by people who share a common background. Thus, we can speak of the African American culture, the Hispanic culture, the deaf culture, organizational culture, and so on.

Culture shapes human behavior which, in turn, shapes culture. When the norms, values, and rules of a society are followed, those cultural elements are strengthened and propagated. A subgroup within a society may become dominant when its cultural elements are accepted by, or forced upon, the whole society. When people of another culture follow a different set of norms, values, and rules, they are either enculturated—that is, they adapt to the host culture—or their norms, values, and rules are assimilated into the host culture, thus changing it. Marginalized people, such as those from minority and disability backgrounds, are often marginalized because of their "differentness" and the divergence of elements of their cultures from the dominant culture. They are forced to either become enculturated, or they are treated as "second class citizens" by society.

Culture affects the biological, psychological, and environmental contexts of disability: there is certainly evidence of cultural differences in infant mortality, nutrition, availability of adequate health care, incidence of certain diseases and disabling conditions (biological context). Arnold (cited in Smart & Smart, 1991) wrote that "cultural elements such as language, family roles, gender roles and beliefs and acculturative stress can play a significant role in the etiology, symptom manifestation, and rehabilitation treatment of disabilities" (p. 358). Smart and Smart (1991) identified five cultural factors influencing the acceptance of disability (psychological context) among Mexican Americans: a familial, cohesive, protective society; stoic attitudes toward life in general; well-defined gender roles; religious views; and reliance on physical labor. There are cultural differences in the "body ideal," and the status degradation attached to disability (cf. Livneh, 1982); these are part of the social environment. There are certainly cultural differences in architecture and the use of space (physical environment). The empowerment of persons with disability and other marginalized people requires major shifts in the cultural paradigm (Morrison & Finkelstein, 1993).

INTEGRATION OF REHABILITATION AND
MENTAL HEALTH SERVICES

To effectively address the employment needs of persons with disabilities requires the integration of a number of rehabilitation and mental health services. The case process—from intake to employment—needs the active voice of many different professionals. This is frequently seen in the use of the interdisciplinary team, with its core of rehabilitation and mental health professionals, and the consumer her or himself, but frequently joined by other medical, technology, and community partners. The interdisciplinary team is important not only because of the specialized knowledge and services each member "brings to the table," but because it forms the network necessary to support the consumer throughout the implementation of the rehabilitation plan and thereafter into employment.

The consumer is an important player on the interdisciplinary team. Wright (1980) explains:

> All people have a right to self-determination insofar as they are capable of responsible judgments; people should make their own decisions, set their own goals, and decide how they should achieve those goals. This does not mean that the rehabilitationist must assume a passive role or be totally nondirective. Active intervention by the rehabilitation counselor helps the client make decisions by providing needed information, by fostering the development of self-confidence, and by facilitating problem solving (p. 11).

This suggests both the right of the consumer to be on the interdisciplinary team, and the way that right should be implemented. That is, professional members of the team, whether rehabilitation counselors or mental health personnel, must walk a line between non-intervention and over-intervention. Moxley and Daeschlein (1997) describe the properties of a consumer-driven case management system, one which fully incorporates input from the consumer. These properties take the form of five questions:

1. Does the person possess an active voice; is this voice encouraged, heard and taken seriously; and does this voice determine the purpose and direction of human services?
2. Does the person exercise control over outcomes and the strategies used to achieve these outcomes?
3. Is there a valuing of meaningful choices from among real substantive alternatives?
4. Can the person readily and safely engage in dissent, and does dissent result in the freedom to rectify what has created dissatisfaction?
5. Does the system protect the reputation of the people it serves, and, perhaps more importantly, even venerate people, their histories, and the barriers they have experienced in their life journeys (pp. 113–114)?

As this section will demonstrate, every part of the rehabilitation process is interdisciplinary, from assessment and planning—involving the consumer, vocational evaluator, rehabilitation counselor, and so on—to provision of assistive technologies—introducing the assistive technology professional—and finally to placement, which brings the employer to the partnership. As will also be demonstrated, all activities should be planned and viewed from within the bio-psychological–social–environmental–cultural framework discussed earlier.

Comprehensive Assessment

Assessment is the process of identifying the discrepancy between consumer needs and the capacity of the consumer, his or her social network, and the mental health/rehabilitation provider network to meet those needs (Moxley, 1989). Given the bio-psychological–environmental–cultural framework through which disabilities must be viewed, assessment necessarily is a holistic, comprehensive, interdisciplinary process.

Assessment is, first, holistic. Each aspect of biological, psychological, and social functioning should be addressed, if only to rule out its importance. Parker and Schaller (1996) suggest that an ecological assessment model, consisting of assessment of the person (*P*), environment (*E*), and interactions between the person and environment may be the most appropriate strategy for vocationally assessing persons with severe disability. Personal factors include cultural identity, health, functional capacity, goals, interests, aptitudes, aspirations, and interpersonal skills. Environmental factors include economic conditions, family and social variables, environmental barriers, availability of training and transportation, and employer attitudes.

Assessment is comprehensive: a wide variety of sources should be used in determining needs. Moxley (1989) identifies six data collection strategies for use in consumer needs assessment:

1. Verbal description provided by the consumer
2. Collateral information provided by the consumer's social network
3. Direct observation of the consumer's environment
4. Information collected by previous service providers
5. Review of agency records
6. Vocational, educational, medical, physical, and psychological testing

Finally, assessment is interdisciplinary. Individual cases may require the temporary services of a wide variety of professionals to collect the necessary data: doctors, psychiatrists, substance abuse counselors, vocational evaluators, work hardening specialists, and assistive technology professionals are among these. The consumer is also involved in assessment: Farley, Bolton, and Parkerson (1992) provide limited support for the suggestion that client involvement in the vocational assessment process enhances career development outcomes of that process. They found that consumers who were involved in the process had significantly higher levels of vocational self-awareness and vocational decision-making ability than those who were not involved. There was a third effect: a decrease in career indecisiveness, although it only "approached significance ($p = 0.07$)" (Farley et al., 1992, p. 151).

The assessment process, however, may be vulnerable to cultural factors, factors that may lessen the reliability and validity of results. For example, Smart and Smart (1992) suggested that vocational assessment strategies requiring introspection may be uncomfortable and unfamiliar for some with Hispanic American backgrounds. The writings of Atkins (1988) and Alston and McCowan (1994) suggest a "negative Pygmalion effect," whereby African Americans may perform poorly because of the racism and low performance expectations of rehabilitation staff. Lack of appropriate norms makes testing culturally different persons troublesome (Fouad, 1993).

Planning

The immediate result of assessment is the development of a comprehensive client service and support plan. Developing an effective plan requires the active participation of the interdisciplinary team, including the consumer. Moxley (1989) identified five characteristics of service plans that highlight the importance of the plan: (1) they are work plans and plans for division of labor; (2) they are, by nature, participatory, facilitating the building of commitment by members of the interdisciplinary team; (3) they provide accountability; (4) they serve as guidance systems for case managers; and (5) well-written plans provide a means by which they can be evaluated, especially in the impact of services on consumer needs.

Crimando and Riggar (1996) identified seven categories of community resources offering a variety of services. A holistic, comprehensive assessment may uncover a need in any of these areas:

1. *Health and diagnostic programs* provide diagnostic, restorative, and therapeutic psychological and medical services.
2. *Social service programs* provide family, financial, and protective services.
3. *Legal services* offer help in protecting legal and civil rights.
4. *Vocational and employment programs* assist in identifying and seeking appropriate employment and employment training.
5. *Rehabilitation programs* offer case management, vocational, diagnostic, and therapeutic services, among others, depending on the particular vendor.
6. *Educational programs* train and educate consumers.
7. *Human services* are miscellaneous services such as housing, community disaster, and financial counseling.

Care should be taken not to assume a need unless there is evidence to support that assumption. Take, for example, "counseling" as a service need. Shontz's (1977) assertion that disability itself is only one of all factors that affect the life situation of a person with a disability, and its influence is often relatively minor should be a warning against the automatic assumption that all persons with disability need counseling. As a matter of fact, in reference to this assumption, Lenny (1993) retorted, "while disabled people may need political action, self-help groups, community work, social programmes and the like, *they unequivocally do not need counselling* [emphasis in the original]" (p. 233). When counseling is supported by assessment evidence, Lenny (1993) suggests that it be from "person-centered" theories that do not (1) make any assumptions about how people adjust to their disabilities, (2) impose meaning on situations, or (3) put labels on people.

Once needs are assessed and services identified, a service provider must be identified. Crimando (1996) presents a number of questions that might be asked when identifying and selecting community service providers. Among the questions are these: What is the nature of the funding? What constraints in service provision does the organization face? What linkages or service agreements does the organization have to meet special needs? What experience does the staff have in working with a specific population? Are program facilities accessible to consumers? Does the organization have an acceptable number of successful outcomes, and do those outcomes match organizational goals and objectives, as well as professional standards?

Assistive Technologies and Environmental Support

The Technology-related Assistance for Individuals with Disabilities Act of 1988 defines assistive technology as "any item, piece of equipment, or product system, whether acquired commercially or off the shelf, modified or customized, that increases, maintains, or improves functional capabilities of individuals with disabilities" (Cook & Hussey, 1995, p. 5). Assistive technologies, and other devices and modifications made to the environment to increase or improve employment options or functions of daily living are a major part of the rehabilitation of persons with physical disabilities.

The rehabilitation team must treat each request or need for assistive technology individually, since there is no such thing as an "off the shelf disability." Each person's functional capacities will be different, and his or her profile unique. Although some devices are produced in quantity, they must be customized for each user. The "customized assistive technology service delivery process" is described by Cook and Hussey (1995):

1. Referral and Intake: The consumer identifies the need for technology, and a referral is made to an assistive technology professional (ATP). The ATP collects basic data to decide whether a match exists between the consumer's need and the type of service he or she (the ATP) can provide.
2. Initial Evaluation: The consumer's technology needs are described in more detail, using a thorough evaluation of the consumer's language, cognitive, physical, and sensory skills. Potential devices are selected and tried out; the ATP notes modifications that need to be made.
3. Recommendation and Report: Evaluation results are summarized in a written report, including recommendations for technology based on the consensus of the ATP, consumer, and any other person involved in the referral and evaluation processes.
4. Implementation: The equipment is fabricated, or ordered and modified, and delivered to the consumer, who receives training on its use.
5. Follow-up: The ATP provides routine repair and maintenance as needed, and makes sure that the goals of the referral have been met, and that the consumer is satisfied with results.
6. Follow-along: Regular contact is made with the consumer to identify the need for further intervention.

Thus, the roles of all members of the rehabilitation team, especially the consumer, are important.

ASSISTIVE TECHNOLOGIES. Assistive technology enhances an individual's ability to perform basic life functions—such as ambulating, dressing, eating, and performing self-care—as well as providing a means of achieving greater levels of independence and employment (Crimando, 1997). Shontz's (1977) assertion that psychological reactions to removal of disability are not necessarily pleasant nor do they automatically lead to improved adjustment must be kept in mind here: the individual's reaction to technology is unique, and may not be favorable. A wheelchair may be freeing to some and limiting to others. The attitudes of others toward the technology may also need to be addressed. For example, in a study (cf. "Some view accommodations," 1999) conducted by Adrienne Colella, a professor of management at Texas A&M University, many workers perceived accommodations for colleagues with disabilities as unfair under certain conditions. This was especially true when the accommodations were perceived as giving the worker an unfair advantage. Thus, environmental support in these cases may have to include intervention in the social environment by providing "awareness of disability" training to workplace colleagues, and continual monitoring of attitudes of the person with disability and her or his colleagues toward accommodations.

Examples of devices include these:

1. Prosthetics: Prosthetic devices replace a body part or function (Crimando, 1997). Augmentative communication devices (speech prostheses), for example, are designed for those whose disability results in diminished communication ability.

2. Orthotics: Orthotic devices augment an existing function; leg and hip braces are examples.

3. Adaptive computing: Adaptive computing devices are designed for those whose impairment limits their finger dexterity, vision, hearing, and so on, such that they cannot use standard computer equipment or software. These devices include input aids (e.g., head sticks and sip-and-puff switches), alternate input devices (virtual keyboards), and alternate output devices (e.g., voice synthesizers and braille printers).

4. Wheelchairs and mobility devices: According to Puckett (1996), new designs and materials have changed the functionality and appearance of wheelchairs and other mobility devices. They range from versatile motorized scooters for persons who can ambulate, to full-size power-base wheelchairs that can be operated by any kind of control (joystick, chin, head, foot, and breath), and can accept specialized seating systems for persons with decubiti, certain spinal cord injuries, and scoliosis.

WORKPLACE ACCOMMODATIONS.   Since 1973, with the passage of the Rehabilitation Act (P.L. 93–112), the concept "reasonable accommodation" of the worksite has become an important issue in the business and rehabilitation communities (Crimando, 1997), and even more so with the passage in 1990 of the Americans with Disabilities Act (P.L. 101–336). A reasonable modification is the modification of a job, worksite, employment practice, and so on, that allows an otherwise qualified handicapped person to hold a job, as long as that modification does not impose a financial hardship on an employer or potential employer. Puckett (1996) identifies the goal of worksite modification: "maximiz[ing] the individual's functional capability and independence, in the safest and most cost-efficient manner possible" (p. 172). Workplace accommodations may include use of the assistive technologies discussed above, as well as "high tech" electronic environmental control units and robotics. It may also include architectural modification to remove barriers (e.g., ramping steps, widening doorways, and installing elevators), job modification and restructuring (i.e., minimizing or eliminating non-essential tasks), and changing employment practices (e.g., modifying work schedules, changing employment testing procedures and screening practices, and training supervisors to work with persons with disabilities). There is a widely held assertion in rehabilitation that 80% of job accommodations cost $500 or less. Berkeley Planning Associates (1982) surveyed accommodations in private sector employment and found that about 50% of those accommodations studied cost nothing, while 30% cost less than $500. An additional 10% cost between $500 and $2,000. However, Moore and Crimando (1995) suggest that those figures "may pale in some instances when compared to a complete job analysis [study] to identify 'essential' elements of jobs. Furthermore, other numerous costs go toward modifying selection or hiring procedures" (p. 245). Rehabilitation and mental health workers should be prepared to work with employers in (1) minimizing the cost of worksite modification, (2) identifying resources that can be used to offset the cost of modification, and (3) providing training and consultation to human resources units and supervisors on working with people with disabilities.

ERGONOMICS.   Ergonomics is the study of human performance and the application of human factors to the design of technological systems (Olsen, 1999). Its goal is to enhance productivity, safety, convenience, and quality of life. Ergonomics includes models and theories of human performance, design and analytical methodology, human–computer interface issues, environmental and work design, and physical and mental workload assessment (Olsen, 1999). Ergonomics has received its greatest recent attention in its applications to workplace health and safety, particularly in connection with carpal tunnel syndrome, repetitive strain injuries, and cumulative trauma disorders. While the focus of ergonomics is in design for injury prevention, its principles are equally useful for preventing re-injury in persons with disability, and making work easier to do for such persons.

EXPANDING EMPLOYMENT OPPORTUNITIES FOR PERSONS WITH PHYSICAL DISABILITIES

The quintessential mark of success in the rehabilitation process is meaningful employment for the consumer. The word "meaningful" suggests that the job gives meaning and purpose to life—echoing the remarks of Dostoevsky and Clinton cited at the beginning of this chapter—and provides not only a way to meet survival needs, but also a sense of satisfaction with life. The state of employment opportunities for persons with disabilities is a "good news–bad news" situation. The good news is that more persons with disabilities are employed, making more money than ever before, and in more types of employment than ever before. This subsection will highlight some of the more innovative and exciting efforts. The bad news is that even in these times of remarkably low unemployment, persons with minority background—such as those with disabilities—still suffer from astounding levels of unemployment and underemployment. As demonstrated at the beginning of this chapter, nearly two thirds of persons with disabilities aged 16–64 are unemployed, in spite of the Americans with Disabilities Act, the Job Training Partnership Act, the School-to-Work Act, and all the other formal and informal efforts of federal, state, and local governments, as well as private citizens and businesses described in this subsection.

Advances in Job Development

The recent advances in job development and placement have come from updating and modification of older programs or concepts. The monograph *Effective employment strategies for individuals with disabilities* (Pacinelli & Dew, 1996) describes numerous model programs, the most exciting of which include job creation initiatives, self-employment programs, and expansion of "temp" services.

This decade has seen an expansion and modification of traditional job creation strategies. The Office of Vocational Administration, Commonwealth of Pennsylvania (OVA, 1996) and the Ohio Rehabilitation Services Commission (ORSC, 1996) have undertaken job creation programs in which jobs in expanding industries are "traded" for equipment. That is, businesses planning or undergoing expansion are given "access to (and eventually ownership of) needed industrial equipment in exchange for job slots for a negotiated time period. If the employer meets its commitments, ownership of the equipment is transferred to the employer at the conclusion of the negotiated time period" (p. 200). Program guidelines of the Pennsylvania program include these: (1) only fixed assets can be purchased; no buildings, rolling stock, inventory, computers, or software can be included; (2) each slot must be for a full-time job at a minimum of $6.00/hr; health benefits must be included in the fringe package; (3) the company must provide a minimum of 10%–20% of the equity required for the expansion and secure the participation of another financial entity, so that the entire equity package provided exceeds 50%; and (4) it must be a true expansion rather than a delayed start-up or equipment upgrade. In connection to their job creation program, ORSC (1996) reports 82% of participants with disabilities being satisfied with their jobs, while 84% of employers reported an increase in productivity, 63% reported increased profits, and 84% cited increased sales. Nearly all stated "they would use OVA to help fill future vacancies" (p. 122).

Self-employment, in general, is one of the fastest growing employment options for persons with disability (Silvestri, 1991), although its use as a strategy for enhancing vocational outcomes in the state–federal vocational rehabilitation (VR) system has not grown (Arnold, Seekins, & Ravesloot, 1995). Self-employment was enhanced as a VR strategy in 1936, with the passage of the Randolph–Sheppard Act, which authorized business enterprises for persons who are blind or visually impaired. These took the form of vending stands in federal buildings and installations that would be owned and operated, exclusively, by persons with visual impairments. In a recent study, Arnold et al. (1995) found that from just 0.53% to 7.34% (mean = 2.3%) of the employment outcomes reported by state VR agencies during the period studied could be attributed to self-employment. VR counselors in rural states tended to both use the strategy more often and view the strategy more favorably than their urban counterparts. Current self-employment initiatives (cf. Rural Institute on Disabilities, Missoula, MT et al., 1996) include a procurement service project which helps business owners with disabilities procure government contract and the Disability Community Small Business Development Center in Ann Arbor, Michigan, which provides business counseling. Furthermore, Arnold et al. (1995) list 118 different types of businesses that were developed by consumers in the state–federal system.

According to a recent study by the National Association of Temporary and Staffing Services, the staffing industry generated $72 billion in revenue in 1998, with $59 billion attributable to temporary help services (Poe, 1999). However, until recently this industry has not experienced much success accommodating persons with disabilities, since they usually require that an applicant have personal transportation and a telephone, while the timed tests and computerized application procedures used by many staffing agencies often limit and exclude qualified persons with disabilities (Full Citizenship, Inc., 1996). This lack of success has begun to change with programs such as Project Reach Out (Full Citizenship, Inc., 1996), Goodwill Temporary Services (Drury, 1998), and Peak Performers Inc. (Showalter, 1997). The latter two are temporary employment services specializing in serving persons with disabilities, while Project Reach Out is a "bridge between Adia Temporary Services, a nationwide employment service ... and prospective employees with disabilities" (Full Citizenship Inc., 1996, p. 150). Central to their strategy are no or low-cost accommodations made for job seekers which include extended time on tests, assistance in reading tests or writing answers, assistance in preparing computerized applications, and even waiving tests that are either not pertinent to the job sought or ones that may to too susceptible to test anxiety. The program also arranges job sharing for persons who may not be able to meet a full-time schedule, or those whose medical benefits need to be protected. Among the benefits cited by the project are increased consumer satisfaction due to the number of choices the consumer is allowed to have; and increased employer satisfaction, arising from the project's willingness to provide follow-along services to ease the transition. Another benefit is that, through temporary services, persons with disability may gain access to permanent positions. Temporary employment services certainly bear watching as a potential source of employment outcomes.

Sheltered and Supported Work

An employment model that, since the late 1980s, has become increasingly popular is the supported employment model (Wehman, Kreutzer, Wood, Morton, & Sherron, 1988). Although the primary disability classification of supported employment participants is mental retardation (Wehman, Revell, & Kregel, 1998), it has also been used to promote employment opportunities for persons with physical disabilities such as traumatic brain injury, sensory impairments, and assorted orthopedic conditions. According to Preston, Ulicny, and Evans (1992), the supported employment model emphasizes these components:

1. On-site job evaluation and training with attention to environmental modification and the use of job coaches or trainers
2. An integrated interdisciplinary team for problem-solving
3. A fading approach to job support
4. Education of the employer and coworkers concerning employee special needs
5. Follow-up to investigate and ensure durability of outcomes

There has been substantial research support for use of the model, as it has been associated with increases in hourly wages and vocational options (Wehman et al. 1989), job retention rates (Wehman et al., 1990), consumer satisfaction (Test, Hinson, Solow, & Kuel, 1993), and improvements in employer perceptions (Kregel & Unger, 1993). Support for the model remains strong today, although in a cost–benefit comparison of supported employment and a traditional group placement model, Clark, Xie, Becker, and Drake (1998) found no significant differences in costs or benefits over the short run (less than 18 months). However, the authors suggested that longer term studies might show significant differences between them and, curiously, concluded that supported employment is "likely to be most beneficial from a societal or governmental perspective when ... substituted for ... other rehabilitative services" (p. 32). Similarly, in a cost efficiency study, Coker and Valley (1995) found that, in the short run at start-up, supported employment is nearly three times more costly to operate than group off-site and traditional sheltered workshop models of placement. They contend, however, that supported employment has the potential to become more cost efficient over time, while there are no data to suggest that traditional sheltered employment will do likewise. These studies highlight the continuing strong philosophical support for supported employment, even while empirical support is equivocal.

Certainly not a new model, but one which has grown in popularity in recent years, affirmative industries (DuRand, 1978) offer a cross between traditional sheltered employment and an entrepreneurial competitive employment atmosphere. Affirmative industry models offer the unique feature of "employ[ing] a mix of individuals with and without disabilities to produce goods or services. The business is formost intended to be a profitable enterprise that relies on a workforce primarily consisting of persons with disabilities" (Coker, Osgood, & Clouse, 1995, p. 7). The Institute for Community Inclusion (ICI, 1999) lists the common features of affirmative industries: employment vendors develop business ventures, assuming the responsibility for capital investment and ongoing operations. These vendors can include any for-profit or non-profit firm, although the affirmative industry itself must be developed as a profit venture. The ICI (1999) also lists advantages and disadvantages of affirmative industries. Advantages include:

1. Can develop creative business options based on interests of consumers
2. Is advantageous in rural areas where job options may be limited
3. Can serve well people who require intensive supports
4. Potential to redesign jobs and find creative ways to include all people in employment

These are potential disadvantages:

1. Typically low wages and few benefits
2. Limited opportunities for community participation and social integration
3. Potential for conflict between business operations and rehabilitation goals

4. Starting and managing a business is often very time-intensive
5. Two out of every three new business fail, often due to lack of financial resources, and most businesses lose money during the first three years of operation

Coker et al. (1995) compared four models of employment for persons with disabilities: traditional sheltered work, sheltered enclaves (involving small groups of persons with disabilities employed at a host business that primarily hires non-disabled persons), supported employment, and affirmative industry. They found that job satisfaction among employees was significantly higher for the three latter models than for sheltered employment. They also found that both gross and net income were significantly higher for the supported employment and affirmative industry models than the other two; the difference between supported employment and affirmative industry was non-significant. However, Coker et al. (1995) warned that average incomes for all four models were below the poverty level.

Telecommuting

Telecommuting is the use of personal computers, telephones, fax machines, and electronic mail—usually in the person's home—to receive, send, and perform work assignments (Crimando & Godley, 1985). Grantham and Nichols (1994–1995) estimated that about 4.3 million persons perform at least part of their work assignments—in skilled, professional, and managerial jobs—as telecommuters. Its use to improve the employment opportunities of persons with disabilities is apparent, in that telecommuting would allow someone who was otherwise homebound to secure and hold employment. Crimando and Godley (1985) warned, however, that rehabilitation workers must watch that telecommuting did not become a way to further isolate persons with disabilities from the workplace.

SUMMARY AND IMPLICATIONS

The bio–psychological–social–environmental-cultural framework for physical disabilities suggests that one must look well beyond the physical characteristics of disabling conditions, that disability is likely to be the result of a complex of physical, psychological, environmental, and cultural characteristics. But how is one, especially the new rehabilitation or mental health practitioner, to have a full understanding of all the factors that may enter into assessing, planning with, and placing not just one consumer, but a whole caseload? And what of the veteran mental health professional who has not previously considered all the complexities of working with persons with severe physical disabilities?

Minimally, pre-service curricula should include coursework in the medical, psychosocial, and vocational aspects of physical disabilities. Programs accredited by the Council on Rehabilitation Education (CORE) are required to offer such courses. This is addressed elsewhere in this book. But the same type of course or training should be available on an in-service basis, to address the needs of mental health professionals who are unfamiliar with rehabilitation content and practices. Such courses would help them incorporate the theory and practices discussed above into their own practice.

These courses should not require mere memorization of facts about disabling conditions; there are just too many of them. Rather, they should accomplish three goals:

1. Expose the student to the biological, psychological, environmental, and cultural factors, *and their interactions*, that may exacerbate or moderate disability.

2. Provide the student with a general problem-solving strategy for making case decisions based on functional ability and limits, interests, and social supports, viewed within the framework presented herein. Such a strategy might include identifying questions to ask in intake, needs assessment strategies, identifying and selecting community resources, and ensuring consumer input. Students should also be taught how to work with, and make the best of, the interdisciplinary team.

3. Teach the student how best to use the resources available on disability and rehabilitation. These would certainly include medical encyclopedias and dictionaries, the *Encyclopedia of Disability and Rehabilitation* (Dell Orto & Marinelli, 1995), and desk references on pharmacology. This might also include the expanding body of information available on the Internet, including such sources as Abledata (http://www.abledata.com/index.htm), Job Accommodations Network (http://janweb.icdi.wvu. edu/), MedLine (http://www.medportal.com/medline.html), and the University of Kansas Internet Resources on Disability (http://www.sped.ukans.edu/disabilities/). A number of client advocacy and peer self-help groups also maintain web pages such as Deaf World and Alcoholics Anonymous. The information on these pages would tend to be of a more subjective, personal nature.

Mental health practitioners should also become keen, but critical consumers of the professional literature that abounds in mental health, rehabilitation, social work, education, rehabilitation engineering, and medicine. This will allow them to keep abreast of the latest advances in those areas, especially in assistive technology, assessment, and job development and placement Practitioners should be able to glean the best of the research related to the disabilities of their consumers without being misled by faulty research methods and specious logic. They should become adept at consulting the literature and making decisions based on the best knowledge available.

Finally, to facilitate the integration of rehabilitation and mental health services, practitioners should become advocates for their consumers and their systems. Advocacy suggests that one "gives voice" to one party at the expense of others. Clearly, practitioners should be advocates for their consumers when it comes to consumer civil rights and privileges. Practitioners should advocate with employers to expand career opportunities for persons with disabilities. They should advocate to remove environmental barriers, whether they are attitudinal in nature or physical. They should advocate for their systems with the community, the legislature, and funding agencies. However, they should also know when to give up the role of advocate. Those who are too caught up in the role of advocate may fail to listen—to their consumers when they express needs and desires. Practitioner–advocates may also fail to listen to other members of the interdisciplinary team, as those members advocate for their positions. We form the interdisciplinary team to ensure we have the expertise to develop a plan that will meet the needs of the consumer, and to "grow" the support system that will follow the consumer along toward their career and life goals. When our advocacy role leads us to ignore or dismiss the input of the team, we risk losing that expertise and support.

REFERENCES

Adams, A. V., Krislov, J., & Lairson, D. R. (1972). Plantwide seniority, black employment, and employer affirmative action. *Industrial and Labor Relations Review, 26*, 686–690.

Alston, R., & McCowan, C. (1994). Aptitude assessment and African–American clients: The interplay between culture and psychometrics in rehabilitation. *Journal of Rehabilitation, 60*(1), 41–46.

Amsel, R., & Fichten, C. S. (1988). Effects of contact on thoughts about interaction with students who have a disability. *Journal of Rehabilitation, 54*(1), 61–65.

Arnold, N. L., Seekins, T., & Ravesloot, C. (1995). Self-employment as a vocational rehabilitation employment outcome in rural and urban areas. *Rehabilitation Counseling Bulletin, 39*, 94–106.

Atkins, B. (1988). An asset-oriented approach to cross-cultural issues: Blacks in rehabilitation. *Journal of Applied Rehabilitation Counseling, 19*(4), 45–49.

Bandura, A. (1982). Self-efficacy mechanism in human agency. *American Psychologist, 37*, 122–147.

Beattie, J. R., Anderson, R. J., & Antonak, R. F. (1997). Modifying attitudes of prospective educators toward students with disabilities and their integration into regular classrooms. *Journal of Psychology, 131*, 245–259.

Berkeley Planning Associates (1982). *A study of recommendations provided to handicapped employees by federal contractors* (Contract No. J-9-E-1-009). Berkeley, CA: Author.

Bordieri, J. E., & Drehmer, D. E. (1986). Hiring decisions for disabled workers: Looking at the cause. *Journal of Applied Social Psychology, 16*, 197–208.

Bordieri, J. E., & Drehmer, D. E. (1987). Attribution of responsibility and predicted social acceptance of disabled workers. *Rehabilitation Counseling Bulletin, 30*, 218–226.

Bordieri, J. E., Drehmer, D. E., & Comninel, M. E. (1988). Attribution of responsibility and hiring recommendations for job applicants with low back pain. *Rehabilitation Counseling Bulletin, 32*, 140–148.

Clark, R. E., Xie, H., Becker, D. R., & Drake, R. E. (1998). Benefits and costs of supported employment from three perspectives. *The Journal of Behavioral Health Services & Research, 25*(1), 22–34.

Coker, C. C., Osgood, K., & Clouse, K. R. (1995). *A comparison of job satisfaction of four different employment models for persons with disabilities.* Menomonie: University of Wisconsin–Stout, Rehabilitation Research and Training Center.

Coker, C. C., & Valley, J. (1995). Costing employment models. *Journal of Rehabilitation Administration, 19*, 199–213.

Cook, A. M., & Hussey, S. M. (1995). *Assistive technologies: Principles and practice.* St. Louis, MO: Mosby.

Crimando, W. (1996). Case management implications. In W. Crimando & T. F. Riggar (Eds.), *Utilizing community resources: An overview of human services* (pp. 7–17). Delray Beach, FL: St. Lucie.

Crimando, W. (1997). Role of technology: Engineering and computers. In D. R. Maki & T. F. Riggar (Eds.), *Rehabilitation counseling: Profession and practice* (pp. 234–245). New York, NY: Springer.

Crimando, W., & Godley, S. H. (1985) The computer's potential in enhancing employment opportunities of persons with disabilities. *Rehabilitation Counseling Bulletin, 28*, 275–282.

Dell Orto, A. E., & Marinelli, R. P. (Eds.) (1995). *Encyclopedia of disability and rehabilitation.* New York, NY: Simon & Schuster/Macmillan.

Department of Rehabilitation Education and Research, University of Arkansas (1994). *Disability handbook* (2nd ed.). Fayetteville, AK: Author.

Drury, T. (1998, December 14). Goodwill launches temp service. *Business First.* Abstract retrieved October 1, 1999 from Proquest Direct electronic database.

DuRand, J. (1978). *The affirmative industry.* St. Paul, MN: Minnesota Diversified Press.

Falvo, D. R. (1991). *Medical and psychosocial aspects of chronic illness and disability.* Gaithersburg, MD: Aspen.

Farley, R. C., Bolton, B., & Parkerson, S. (1992). Effects of client involvement in assessment on vocational development. *Rehabilitation Counseling Bulletin, 35*, 146–153.

Fitts, W. H. (1965). *Manual: Tennessee self-concept scale.* Nashville, TN: Counselor Recordings and Tests.

Fouad, N. (1993). Cross-cultural vocational assessment. *Career Development Quarterly, 42*, 4–13.

Full Citizenship, Inc. (1996). Jammin' with the big boys: Accessing temporary employment services—Project Reach Out. In R. N. Pacinelli & D. W. Dew (Eds.), *Effective employment strategies for individuals with disabilities. Proceedings of the 1996 National Employment Conference* (pp. 149–154). Washington, DC: George Washington University Regional Rehabilitation Continuing Education Program.

Grantham, C. E., & Nichols, L. D. (1994–1995, Winter). Learning to manage at a distance. *Public Manager*, 31–34.

Hackett, G., & Betts, N. E. (1981). A self-efficacy approach to the career development of women. *Journal of Vocational Behavior, 18*, 326–329.

Institute for Community Inclusion (1999, September 20). *Employment and employment-related services* [On-line]. Available Internet: http://web1.tch.harvard.edu/ici/publications/fulltext/mti_guide/mti-html/ section4emp.html.

Lee, T. R. (1999, January 4). Love and work in early adulthood: News reference. *PENpages: College of Agricultural Sciences* [On-line]. Available Internet: http://www.penpages.psu.edu/reference/28507/285071599. html.

Lenny, J. (1993). Do disabled people need counseling? In J. Swain, V. Finkelstein, S. French, & M. Oliver (Eds.), *Disabling barriers—enabling environments* (pp. 233–240). London, UK: Sage.

Lewin, K. (1935). *A dynamic theory of personality: Selected papers.* New York, NY: McGraw-Hill.

Livneh, H. (1982). On the origins of negative attitudes toward people with disabilities. *Rehabilitation Literature, 43*, 338–347.

Livneh, H. (1991a). A unified approach to existing models of adaptation to disability: A model of adaptation. In R. P. Marinelli & A. E. Dell Orto (Eds.), *The psychological & social impact of disability* (pp. 111–138). New York, NY: Springer.

Livneh, H. (1991b). A unified approach to existing models of adaptation to disability: Intervention strategies. In R. P. Marinelli & A. E. Dell Orto (Eds.), *The psychological & social impact of disability* (pp. 241–248). New York, NY: Springer.

Maras, P., & Brown, R. (1996). Effects of contact on children's attitudes toward disability: A longitudinal study. *Journal of Applied Social Psychology, 26*, 211–213.

Marinelli, R. P., & Dell Orto, A. E. (Eds.) (1991). *The psychological & social impact of disability*. New York, NY: Springer.

Moore, T. J., & Crimando, W. (1995). Attitudes toward Title I of the Americans with Disabilities Act. *Rehabilitation Counseling Bulletin, 38*, 232–247.

Morrison, E., & Finkelstein, V. (1993). Broken arts and cultural repair: The role of culture in the empowerment of disabled people. In J. Swain, V. Finkelstein, S. French, & M. Oliver (Eds.), *Disabling barriers—enabling environments* (pp. 122–127). London, UK: Sage.

Moxley, D. P., (1989). *The practice of case management*. Newbury, Park, CA: Sage.

Moxley, D. P., & Daeschlein, M. (1995). Properties of consumer driven forms of case management. In D. P. Moxley (Ed.), *Case management by design: Reflections on principles and practice* (pp. 111–133). Chicago, IL: Nelson-Hall.

Office of Vocational Administration, Commonwealth of Pennsylvania (1996). Seating VR at the economic development table. In R. N. Pacinelli & D. W. Dew (Eds.), *Effective employment strategies for individuals with disabilities. Proceedings of the 1996 National Employment Conference* (pp. 122–123). Washington, DC: George Washington University Regional Rehabilitation Continuing Education Program.

Ohio Rehabilitation Services Commission (1996). The governor's initiative: Trading equipment for jobs. In R. N. Pacinelli & D. W. Dew (Eds.), *Effective employment strategies for individuals with disabilities. Proceedings of the 1996 National Employment Conference* (pp. 200–202). Washington, DC: George Washington University Regional Rehabilitation Continuing Education Program.

Oliver, M. (1983). *Social work with disabled people*. London, UK: Macmillan.

Olsen, E. (1999, August 27). *Definitions important to human factors & ergonomics* [On-line]. Available Internet: http://www.geocities.com/CapeCanaveral/4316/links.html.

Pacinelli, R. N., & Dew, D. W. (Eds.) (1996). *Effective employment strategies for individuals with disabilities. Proceedings of the 1996 National Employment Conference*. Washington, DC: George Washington University Regional Rehabilitation Continuing Education Program.

Parker, R. M., & Schaller, J. L. (1996). Issues in vocational assessment and disability. In E. M. Szymanski & R. M. Parker (Eds.), *Work and disability: Issues and strategies in career development and job placement* (pp. 127–164). Austin, TX: Pro-Ed.

Poe, S. (1999, September 9). Temporary work agencies growing as economy booms. *Austin American Statesman*. Retrieved October 1, 1999 from Proquest Direct electronic database.

Preston, B., Ulicny, G., & Evans, R. (1992). Vocational placement outcomes using a transitional job coaching model with persons with severe acquired brain injury. *Rehabilitation Counseling Bulletin, 35*, 230–239.

Puckett, F. D. (1996). Rehabilitation engineering/technology services. In W. Crimando & T. F. Riggar (Eds.), *Utilizing community resources: An overview of human services* (pp. 167–176). Delray Beach, FL: St. Lucie.

Rasco, C. H. (1996). Keynote address: Effective employment strategies for individuals with disabilities. In R. N. Pacinelli & D. W. Dew (Eds.), *Effective employment strategies for individuals with disabilities. Proceedings of the 1996 National Employment Conference* (pp. 9–15). Washington, DC: George Washington University Regional Rehabilitation Continuing Education Program.

Rural Institute on Disabilities, Missoula, MT, Disability Community Small Business Development Center, Ann Arbor, MI, & Pennsylvania Office of Vocational Rehabilitation, New Castle (1996). Self-employment and economic development: Innovative strategies for these times and the future. In R. N. Pacinelli & D. W. Dew (Eds.), *Effective employment strategies for individuals with disabilities. Proceedings of the 1996 National Employment Conference* (pp. 202–206). Washington, DC: George Washington University Regional Rehabilitation Continuing Education Program.

Schein, E. H. (1987). *Organizational culture and leadership: A dynamic view*. San Francisco, CA: Jossey-Bass.

Shontz, F. C. (1977). Six principles relating disability and psychological adjustment. *Rehabilitation Psychology, 24*, 207–210.

Showalter, K. (1997, December 19). Nonprofit exec spreads word of finding work for disabled. *Business First*. Abstract retrieved October 1, 1999 from Proquest Direct electronic database.

Silvestri, G. T. (1991, Spring). Who are the self-employed? Employment profiles and recent trends. *Occupational Outlook Quarterly*, 26–36.

Smart, J. F., & Smart, D. W. (1991). Acceptance of disability and the Mexican–American culture. *Rehabilitation Counseling Bulletin, 34*, 357–367.

Smart, J. F., & Smart, D. W. (1992). Curriculum changes in multicultural rehabilitation. *Rehabilitation Education, 6*, 105–122.

Some view accommodations as unfair (1995, September). *HR Magazine*, 30–31.

Test, D., Hinson, K., Solow, J., & Keul, P. (1993). Job satisfaction of persons in supported employment. *Education and Training in Mental Retardation, 28*(1), 38–46.

Thoreson, R. W., & Kerr, B. A. (1978). The stigmatizing aspects of severe disability: Strategies for change. *Journal of Applied Rehabilitation Counseling, 9*(2), 21–25.

Tuttle, D. W. (1984). *Self-esteem and adjusting with blindness: The process of responding to life's demands.* Springfield, IL: Charles C. Thomas.

U.S. Census Bureau (1997, December). *Census Brief.* Washington, DC: Author.

U.S. Census Bureau (1999). *Disability: 1990 census table 1: U.S. totals* [On-line]. Available Internet: http://www.census.gov/hhes/www/disable/census/tables/tablus.html.

Wehman, P., Kreutzer, J., West, M., Sherron, P. D., Zasler, N. D., Groah, C. H., Stonnington, H. H., Burns, C. T., & Sale, P. R. (1990). Return to work for persons with traumatic brain injury: A supported employment approach. *Archives of Physical Medicine and Rehabilitation, 71*, 1047–1052.

Wehman, P., Kreutzer, J., Wood, W., Morton, M. V., & Sherron, P. (1988). Supported work model for persons with TBI: Toward job placement and retention. *Rehabilitation Counseling Bulletin, 31*, 298–312.

Wehman, P., Kreutzer, J., Wood, W., Stonnington, H., Diambra, J., & Morton, M. V. (1989). Helping traumatically brain injured patients return to work with support employment: Three case studies. *Archives of Physical Medicine and Rehabilitation, 70*, 109–113.

Wehman, P., Revell, G., & Kregel, J. (1998, Spring). Supported employment: A decade of rapid growth and impact. *American Rehabilitation, 24*(1), 31–42.

Wright, B. A. (1960). *Physical disability: A psychological approach.* New York, NY: Harper & Row.

Wright, G. N. (1980). *Total rehabilitation.* Boston MA: Little, Brown.

CHAPTER 29

Meeting the Employment and Mental Health Needs of Immigrants

Noelle Van der Tuin

INTRODUCTION

"As the USA is more involved in the world, the world is more involved in the USA" (Rumbaut, 1994, p. 588). Changes in the face of immigration during the past decades translate into a more urgent need for people of every human service field to work between cultures. Mental health rehabilitation and employment specialists must learn to look at the complexity of immigration situations in order to find the best employment links for individuals who have left everything familiar for a new life in the United States.

This chapter begins with a description of immigration from a policy perspective. It will identify several factors that combine to affect employment prospects for immigrants. The various aspects of immigration are then brought together in a hypothetical scenario that involves an ideal level of human service involvement. The chapter will continue with an exploration of the human service challenges posed by immigration and will conclude with the implications of immigration in employment rehabilitation for newcomers to the United States.

IMMIGRATION BASICS

The increasing communications and ease of travel throughout the world manifests into microcosms growing in every U.S. urban center. Their growth began with increases in legal immigration at the end of World War II and moved forward with mass migrations of displaced people with few marketable skills (Hurst, 1998, pp. 5–6).

There were 660,477 people who lawfully immigrated to the United States in the fiscal year of 1998 (Immigration and Naturalization Service Annual Report, 1999). Some arrived after long periods of planning and preparation, and others arrived with only the clothes on their back as a result of displacement by natural disasters or war. The United States attracts seekers of the "land of the free and the home of the brave," where anyone willing to work hard will succeed. Of course, along with willingness to work hard, any newcomer must arrive and

---

Noelle Van der Tuin • Migrant Health Promotion, Progresso, Texas

face culture shock, learn anew how to function in society, and face anti-immigrant sentiment and legislation. Immigration is not as simple as coming to strike it rich in the land of promise. The following section explains several (but not all) categories of immigration and the legal situations that surround them.

Immigration status is a designation that the Immigration and Naturalization Service (INS) assigns newcomers who will live in the United States. This does not include people with non-immigration visas, such as temporary workers or people with specialized trades (performers, artists, etc.), fiancés, or tourists (The Immigration Law Center, 1996). Those people receive visas that do not include long-term residency or immigration. Every immigrant who arrives in the United States enters with a status, except for undocumented immigrants, or people who enter "without inspection" by a U.S. immigration official. Immigration status can be separated into three major categories ranging from temporary to permanent.

Temporary Immigration Status

The INS offers refuge, asylum, parole, or temporary protective status to people who have survived displacement due to instability in their home countries. People with the above status designations are allowed to remain in the United States until conditions change in their countries which would facilitate their safe return. Work authorization is granted along with each of these status designations. After one year with one of the above temporary status designations, a person may be eligible to apply for legal permanent residence. However, since criminal activity and some political group affiliations may render people "removable" (deportable), some people opt to keep temporary status designations instead of calling attention to themselves at the INS.

Semi-Permanent Immigration Status

Legal permanent residents (LPRs) can be former asylees, parolees, refugees, or holders of temporary protective status; or they can come to the United States through employment-sponsored immigration, family-based immigration, or the acquisition of a Diversity Visa. When an immigration visa is granted, and a person gains the status of LPR, she or he receives an Alien Resident Card (known as a "Greencard"). The Greencard allows a newcomer to work and live in the United States as long as she or he does not engage in criminal activity or faciliatate terrorism. It is a necessary stepping-stone for naturalization (the transition to citizenship).

For employment-sponsored immigration, an employer will arrange for a newcomer's immigration before that immigrant arrives in the United States. As employment specialists will seldom, if ever, handle this type of immigration, it will not be discussed in this section.

Family-based immigration accounted for 72% of legal immigration in 1998, and occurs in two ways (INS Annual Report, 1999). LPRs can create a petition for an immediate family member's immigration. LPRs may only petition the INS for the immigration of a spouse, unmarried child, or a parent, and in any case must wait for the family member's priority date to become current for immigration. The priority date is the date a petition is processed and approved by the INS, and people awaiting a visa must wait until people from their region or country with priority dates before theirs, receive visas. Depending on a person's country of origin and priority date, a visa might be available immediately or may be years away. U.S. citizens (USCs) can petition for immediate family members without waiting for the priority date to become current. Furthermore, USCs can petition the INS for the immigration of siblings and fiancées.

Another way to gain LPR status is to win the "Diversity Lottery," which accounted for 7% of all legal immigration in 1998 (INS Annual Report, 1999). The INS created this lottery system to offer more chances for immigration to people from countries with characteristically low numbers of immigrants (INA II (1)(203)). The Attorney General determines those countries. In 1998, 45,499 immigrants gained LPR status through the Diversity Visa (INS Annual Report, 1999).

Permanent Immigration Status

After five years of status as an LPR, a person can apply for naturalization as long as she or he has shown good moral standing and a clean criminal record. Naturalization requires a test of citizenship (which evaluates a person's knowledge of government systems), an interview in English, and a pledge of allegiance. Once naturalized, an immigrant is a citizen, and can enjoy the most important of right of a USC—the right to vote.

Absence of Immigration Status

People without an assigned status from the INS are known as "illegal immigrants" or "undocumented immigrants." The latter term is more appropriate, as the term "illegal" strips newcomers of their dignity and humanity. Since undocumented immigrants do not have a designated status by the INS, they are not permitted to work. If the INS discovers them working, the worker can be deported and the employer fined $10,000 per undocumented worker through the Employer Sanctions Program. Undocumented immigrants face many challenges, such as finding equitable employment, unionizing, or even getting a telephone number, lease, or bank account. However, this chapter will exclude the undocumented immigrants as potential clients because they cannot lawfully work, and an employment specialist cannot lawfully aid them in the acquisition of paid employment.

Immigration is not only a function of the INS and its policy. Social policy also takes its toll on new immigrants. The government refuses most public assistance to immigrants who have not worked for 40 quarters (10 years) in the United States. This policy aims to discourage people from coming to the United States who might depend on the social welfare system. Unfortunately, this exclusion ignores the difficulty of moving to another country, working toward legal status and independence, and still grappling with sustained work and acculturation.

THE IMMIGRATION BUNDLE AND ITS INTERACTION WITH EMPLOYMENT

After understanding the categories and legal requirements of immigration, it is important to address the Immigration Bundle (Figure 29-1). The Immigration Bundle is a complex group of factors which affect an immigrant's acclimatization to the United States, and ultimately her or his employment. Together, the factors included in the Bundle may impede the acquisition of meaningful employment or may enhance it. The following section describes a cross-section of the Immigration Bundle and how each aspect relates to employment.

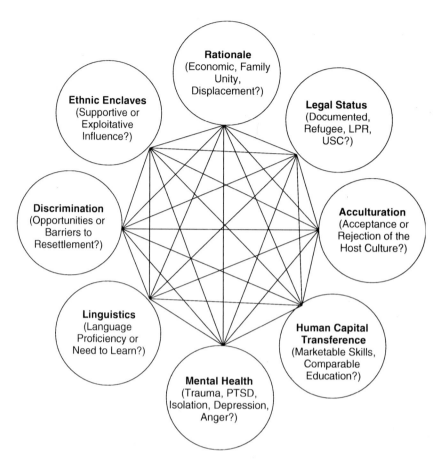

FIGURE 29-1. The Immigration Bundle.

Rationale

One aspect of the Immigration Bundle is the rationale for migration, and therefore the manner in which a newcomer enters the United States. Hurst (1998, p. 7) divides the motivating factors for immigration into economic, social (family-based), cultural (for increased ethnic diversity), and moral (promoting human rights) categories. A person who immigrates for economic reasons through employment-sponsored immigration may have the means and time to learn English, prepare culturally, and even seek education acceptable in the United States in her or his chosen field of employment before arriving.

The above situations shows one extreme in terms of preparation for life in the United States. Between these extremes are the people who have come to the United States to join family members and people who gain a Diversity Visa and come for enhanced opportunities. In the event of family-based immigration, a family sponsor must guarantee that the immigrating family members will not become a public charge. For this reason, people who join their families in the United States may not have to work right away. They may have the opportunity to go to school and prepare to compete in the labor force first.

Economically motivated immigrants often envision themselves leaving their own country and plan accordingly. Conversely, asylees or refugees generally have no time to prepare for employment in the United States. In such circumstances, physical survival is more of a priority than gathering diplomas and résumés. Often, these people do not want to leave their own countries, but cannot stay, for whatever reason. It is important to note that these people did not choose the United States. Rather, it was one of the few options available once they realized that a continuation of their lives in their own country was not possible. These people might come to the United States with only the clothes on their backs, and have neither the documentation nor the linguistic skills to compete with U.S. nationals for jobs. In any event, immigration works as a function of the losses and gains expected by any individual who emigrates from another country (Hurst, 1998, pp. 11–13).

An employment specialist can examine the reasons for emigration to find clues about vocational readiness and preparation for work in the United States.

Acculturation and Language Use

Acculturation is defined best as a multi-faceted process in which age, intent of immigration, religious beliefs, kinship structure, academic achievement and persistance, career decision, income/education level, and years of residence shape the adaptation of a newcomer to the host culture (Miranda & Umhoefer, 1998). Acculturation does not mean assimilation. While acculturation deals with navigating the two cultures and reconciling the differences between them, assimilation suggests the rejection of one's own culture in favor of the mainstream culture in the host region. No individual should completely reject her or his own culture, but there must be a give and take of culture, otherwise life will be more difficult for the newcomer and all of her or his contacts. Acculturation, in this text, is a bidimensional process as Ruelas Atkinson and Ramos-Sanchez (1998) described in their article about counselor helping models, acculturation level, and perceived counselor credibility. These authors measured not only the acculturation to U.S. culture (acquisition of the skills necessary to thrive in U.S. mainstream culture), but also the enculturation (the extent to which participants put aside their own birth culture). This chapter deals with acculturation, rather than enculturation, because adaptation to mainstream culture is of interest to the substance of this work, and enculturation is an unnecessary process, unrelated to the benefits of acculturation (Ruelas et al., 1998).

Acculturation and language use, combined, are the best predictors of career self-efficacy of Latinos according to Miranda and Umhoefer (1998). Acculturation is also associated with the modification of career plans by Asian American students (Park & Harrison, 1995). While language, employment, education, family roles, and sociopolitical/immigration status all impact the rate of acculturation (Miranda & Umhoefer, 1998; Thomas-Presswood, 1998, pp. 461–464), acculturation also influences the rate of language acquisition, employment, family roles, etc. (Park & Harrison, 1995). This bidirectional influence of acculturation and other features of the Immigration Bundle weigh heavily on the employment outlook for immigrants in the United States.

An example of the successful acculturation and language acquisition involves a past client. One year ago, a woman from an African nation arrived at a shelter which provides legal aid and social services for asylum-seekers. Her case took approximately nine months, and she spent the entirety of her time at the shelter taking English lessons, talking with volunteers about mainstream culture, and starting to build a résumé. In her home country, she would not have had the need to work, nor would the cultural norms have affirmed her right to work. She had never used a washing machine until she arrived in the United States, and she had little access to any form of technology. Within one year of her arrival, she gained computing skills, cultural prowess, and a job as a hostess in a major restaurant chain. During the year of transition, that client nurtured relationships with her fellow ex-patriots and actively participated in events and activities associated with her region of Africa. Some may not consider her work as a hostess meaningful, but this job gave her the stability and independence to rebuild her life. Owing in great part to her willingness to learn about culture in the United States, she was able to navigate in a new cultural world without losing the close ties with her fellow ex-patriates.

At the other end of the spectrum, we can note the case of a man, an LPR from a Caribbean nation who has lived in ethnic enclaves for the past 30 years. This man, a hard worker and trained kitchen manager, moved from one ethnic enclave to a new one in another state. Although he has 12 years experience managing a kitchen, he has little hope of finding equivalent work in his new state. This is due to his poor English proficiency and his discomfort in the mainstream culture. He is accustomed to the informal business networking that worked in his home country and old enclave, but is neither accustomed to nor comfortable with a job application in Spanish or English. In addition to that discomfort, this man has great difficulty finding a work environment in which he will be able to communicate completely in his own language. Employment is not impossible for this man, but it is much more difficult for his employment specialist to link him with employers because he has, in large part, rejected mainstream culture.

A person's acculturation level may also highlight other mental health concerns. During the acculturation process it is natural to experience isolation, withdrawal from the host culture, withdrawal from one's own culture, changing family relations, and all manner of stress associated with acclimatizing one's value system to a new environment. Employment can either serve as a tool for accelerated acculturation and stability, or it can serve as an added stressor that makes the entire process more difficult. Employment specialists can learn much about clients and their prospects from their acculturation or refusal to acculturate. That information can be useful in linking them with more or less mainstream work.

Ethnic Enclaves

Ethnic enclaves are a weighty component in the Immigration Bundle. They create a sense of community in which newcomers can ease into mainstream culture. Everything a family might need is accessible in a culturally familiar manner within the enclaves. There, newcomers work together, shop in stores that carry familiar brand names, see doctors who speak their language, and even visit their families with the help of multilingual travel agencies.

Ethnic enclaves can be instrumental in helping newcomers find work. In San Diego, many household workers (involved in housekeeping and gardening) are immigrants from Mexico, Central America, and South America. The majority of these household workers live in ethnic enclaves. When a new immigrant arrives in the ethnic enclave, a more established worker may pass on some of the more troublesome employers or worksites to her or him. As the new immigrant gains experience and language skills, she or he will find other, preferable employers, and may then pass on the troublesome employers to another newcomer (Mattingly, 1999). In this process the ethnic enclave surrounds a newcomer to the United States with employment opportunities and support in an environment that is familiar to the newcomer. The enclaves also provide many resources (such as classes in English as a second language, public health programs, etc.) for those who are interested in accelerated acculturation and eventual competition in the mainstream job market.

The ethnic enclaves have as much potential to hinder meaningful employment as to facilitate it. They are the perfect place for exploitation. Employers can pay undocumented (or unacculturated, documented) workers very little while capitalizing on cultural and linguistic isolation. They may use the enclave as a safe haven to subject workers to threats of INS raids and block unionization by keeping employees away from the mainstream culture and language (Harris, 1995, pp. 137–139). In short, ethnic enclaves create a familiar cultural island for newcomers, but also may relegate them to sweatshops.

Mental Health Concerns Associated with Immigration

Another aspect of the Immigration Bundle involves mental health concerns, which may effect the employment, functioning, and acculturation of a newcomer at any point in her or his new life.

Asylees, refugees, and people with temporary protective status face the challenging and sometimes debilitating effects of post-traumatic stress disorder (PTSD). These people spend their nights re-living the tragedies of war, genocide, and flight instead of sleeping. By morning, they are exhausted and still plagued with memories they try to ignore. With every loud or sudden noise, they might face a memory trigger or anxiety attack or unexpected violence. People with traumatic immigration histories must work through their experiences and find a way to stop hoarding, start sleeping normally, and start a "normal life." Needless to say, a job can either help them or hinder their progress in dealing with PTSD.

For many of the asylees with whom the author interacts, a job is a reason to go to bed at night and wake up in the morning. Many clients brim with pride when they return to the organization that helped them acquire asylum status and work authorization. They tell past caseworkers how they can barely recognize the people they were before they worked because their jobs kept their minds from being idle and helped them move on to independence.

Other mental health concerns that may face immigrants in their journey to establish their new lives in the United States are isolation and depression. Isolation may take place in a linguistic or cultural manner. While teaching English as a second language (ESL) to Mexican and Czech automotive executives and their wives, the author noted that the wives of the executives were not connected to their ethnic enclaves because of class differences. They were isolated in communities which did not recognize them, and they had no social preparation for participation in the activities of other women in the communities. They watched their children make friends and their husbands immerse themselves in their work, but the wives seemed to give up hope of breaking into the community and its activities. In situations like those, the wives showed signs of depression, and sometimes signs of substance abuse.

Smith and Edmonston (1997) state that a larger proportion of immigrants (higher than that of natives of the Unites States) have jobs that require higher education. Public sentiment lends a contradictory image to newcomers. Several months ago, a local union president told an organizer of naturalization information seminars that the naturalization of immigrant laborers in his local union chapter was not important. He explained that all the jobs there were high-level jobs, too specialized for an immigrant, and required higher-skilled workers. Many employers, like the president of this local union chapter, do not consider the possibility that the education and meaningful experiences of workers from different parts of the world will be a boon to their businesses, or that foreign-born employees may be as educated (or more educated) than their native counterparts. This may force workers into menial labor jobs instead of bolstering the educational efforts and employability of immigrant workers.

With employers that disregard potential employees solely on the basis of immigration, immigrants end up bearing the psychological scars of intolerance. Many immigrants internalize the oppressive behavior of employers, resulting in depression. Other immigrants harbor anger for the discriminatory treatment they face. Paradoxically, immigrant workers often have more marketable skills than their native-born counterparts, but have been led to believe their skills are less useful because they accompany an accent.

The dramatic change that takes place for newcomers is tremendous. Employment can either provide stability, social networks, and a firm base for acculturation; or it can become an added stressor and impediment to successful acculturation. In either event, immigrants can benefit from the careful consideration of their strengths and vulnerabilities with the assistance of employment specialists from a mental health standpoint.

Human Capital

Another aspect of the Immigration Bundle is the degree to which human capital transfers to the host environment. As Hurst (1998, p. 185) asserts in his book about immigrants in the U.S. labor market, even immigrants with the same levels of education as U.S. natives may face barriers to employment and economic well-being because their human capital does not transfer easily to the American market (Hurst, 1998, pp. 11–13).

In some instances, human capital can transfer without much difficulty. For example, some Tibetan Buddhist monks passed through the United States on the way to Canada. They were seeking political asylum there. These monks did not have conventionally marketable skills, but sought creative ways to sustain themselves without compromising their traditions or beliefs and therefore transferred their human capital effectively. These monks combined traditional, cultural expressions with the practicality of life in the United States by creating Mandalas for some communities and museums. Mandalas are intricate designs of loose sand on a flat surface which are created to be destroyed later as a testament to the impermanence of form. For the monks, this was a skill that helped them on their journey financially, allowed them to teach others about Buddhist traditions, and fit with their skills and desires.

In some events, poor transference of human capital interacts with other aspects of the Immigration Bundle to make employment almost impossible. This can be observed most clearly when newcomers come from an agricultural background in a developing or underdeveloped nation. Many people arrive in the United States without the privilege of even a basic education. They may know about agricultural techniques in their own countries, but often do not have knowledge of the more mechanized agricultural work. Some end up in sweatshops or in exploitative harvesting jobs, all because they lacked the skills valued in the U.S. labor market. These people possess skills which were imperative in their own regions, but that are poorly suited to employment in their new community. This is poor transference of human capital as one aspect of the Immigration Bundle, which combines with public sentiment, language, and education to form barriers for many newcomers.

DRAWING TOGETHER THE
IMMIGRATION BUNDLE

This section draws the separate pieces of the immigration bundles together, offering one hypothetical Immigration Bundle. This immigration and social service experience includes public sentiment in favor of (or at least not against) immigration, as well as an immigrant's reactions to a dramatic change in environment. Although employment specialists are not likely to have the necessary resources for this eventuality or the time to address every aspect of the Bundle at once, this example should serve as a potential service example for employment specialists and their organizations.

Tsering, an immigrant, has arrived in the United States. She has come to an urban center in which several ethnic enclaves are close together and accessible through good public transportation. Tsering has joined other émigrés from her home country in the city, and they helped her find a place to live. She is glad to have "won" her Diversity Visa, but is worried about how she will go on living in the United States when all her savings are gone. She is overwhelmed by the noises of a strange city, the signs she can barely read in English, and the isolation she feels because she cannot seem to do anything for herself in this new city. Fortunately, her friends are aware of a multi-cultural agency that helps immigrants throughout their acclimatization to life in the United States.

Tsering, with a pep talk from her friends in her new neighborhood, finds her way to a local satellite of The World, a multi-cultural human services organization. The World offers satellites in almost every ethnic enclave in the city, and has a central gathering place easily accessible to the majority of those enclaves through public transportation. In the satellite of The World, Tsering walks along a wall with literature on several topics. Under the picture of a doctor, she easily finds a list of doctors in the area that speak her language. She notices that all the pamphlets in other colors have similar lists in other languages. She collects information about doctors, the various programs of The World, and community events that appeal to her before approaching the reception desk.

At the reception desk of The World, Tsering sees her flag among others under plastic on the counter. She is certain the receptionist will not speak her language, and so she points to it. The receptionist smiles and tells Tsering that she should go down the hall and find the office door with that flag on it. She walks down the hall, which opens up to a large common room. All around the room are doors with different flags. People in the common room are grouped in little pockets. Many people speak in languages Tsering does not recognize, and a few groups of people are speaking in English.

In the office with her nation's flag, Tsering talks to someone in her own language about the possibility of finding work in the new community. The first questions the cultural liaison at The World asks are, "What kinds of things do you like to do? What kind of job would make you most happy?" Tsering, feeling more comfortable after seeing this concern for her interests, is able to think of several activities she enjoys. She tells the liaison that she filled out the Diversity Visa application with an image in her mind of working as a nurse. She tells the liaison that she feels silly saying this, because she studied business in her three years of college at home, and most of her work experience was in bookkeeping.

The liaison looks over Tsering's transcripts and résumé, and talks with Tsering about her English proficiency and desire to go on to finish college in the United States. The two discuss the layout of the city and the trades that many people from Tsering's country practice, as well as Tsering's adjustment to the city and social connections that Tsering has or would like to make. After an hour, the liaison summarizes what she understands as Tsering's priorities. Tsering offers feedback and ranks these priorities.

During the days that follow, Tsering attends meetings at The World's central office. At every office, she arrives to find that the liaison from her satellite office has shared her priorities with the other workers. First, she visits the employment office with a résumè she made before coming to the United States. The employment specialist tells her about jobs for which she qualifies, and points out that one of the jobs in the employment program is bookkeeping in a clinic near Tsering's apartment. Tsering takes information about that job, and also about a food service job at another nearby hospital. She is worried about English classes, and how she will schedule them around a work schedule.

At the ESL office in The World, Tsering receives a list of all the ESL classes available at the central office and the many satellites. She finds that there is a satellite near each medical center, and both of them offer ESL classes during the mornings, afternoons, and evenings.

Tsering schedules and attends interviews at both medical centers after some coaching from the liaison at the satellite nearest her. She finds that the medical centers are familiar with The World, and they seem less worried than Tsering about her English (which is sufficient for basic communication, but is not yet at a level that is suitable for business). Both employers offer her employment, and each suggests that she tell her final decision to the employment specialist at The World's central office. She talks to her liaison, and returns to the employment office to tell the specialist she would rather take the food service job. She says that she will be around the hospital more with that job, and not stuck in an office. It is also close to a satellite where she can take ESL in order to study for the TOEFL (Test of English as a Foreign Language). That way, if she passes the TOEFL, she can study nursing at the university level. The employment specialist congratulates her on a good choice and calls the employer and Tsering's cultural liaison to set up Tsering's training.

The cultural liaison from The World accompanies Tsering to her first day of training. After Tsering fills out the tax forms at the hospital, the liaison and her new employer introduce her to María. María presents herself as Tsering's Buddy. Tsering and María, the liaison explains, will work together until Tsering feels comfortable enough to work alone. And after they start working separately, they will still meet daily to talk about work, English, transportation, or any concerns Tsering has about working and living in the new city. María explains that she started working a year ago, and that her Buddy helped her keep a steady job and go to ESL classes at the same time. María and Tsering work the same shift, and start walking to the nearby satellite of The World for ESL classes after work.

During Tsering's first year in the United States, she and María spend a good deal of time together. Tsering learns her job in a matter of weeks, and studies for her English classes. She meets weekly with her boss and daily with María to receive feedback on her work, and in turn she offers feedback to the employment program at The World. At first, Tsering is disappointed that she and María do not speak the same language, but after a few weeks pass, she notices that she is able to communicate better in English than she thought. She notices that her friends from her home country stay together and never practice their English. Those friends all work at the same place, assembling parts for flashlights, and complain that they cannot compete for the jobs of U.S. natives. She feels she will be able to compete.

In time, Tsering passes the TOEFL test, sends her transcripts from college to be evaluated, and starts taking classes at a community college to become a nurse's aide. By the time this happens, she has developed a good relationship with her employer, and starts another shift in order to take the classes she needs. She has kept in touch with The World, often attending the social events associated with her country and parties hosted by the ESL classes (particularly enjoying the party held for her when she passed the TOEFL). After starting her new shift at the hospital, her boss and The World introduce her to Abdullah, who will be her Buddy for the next several months. She is proud when she calls María to tell her about her new experiences as a "Big Buddy."

Tsering's experience with The World has provided her with the ability to work and study at the same time. This is very important, as she learned to compete in an English-speaking environment while at the same time supporting herself financially. By working full-time,

Tsering was able to secure benefits at work. The World helped Tsering maintain contact and close ties with her fellow expatriates through social programs; at the same time the ESL classes and María facilitated her acculturation to mainstream culture in the United States. The World also helped Tsering find doctors, counselors, and lawyers that could speak her language and could attend to her in a culturally familiar way. Tsering is satisfied that The World has helped her become part of the greater society without sacrificing her own cultural identity. She feels The World is always at work to teach people in the community about immigrants and their rights, and at the same time it helps her excel in her new environment.

EMPLOYMENT OF NEWCOMERS AS A
HUMAN SERVICE CHALLENGE

In the hypothetical case of the previous section, The World offered comprehensive help to Tsering as she looked for a job that would sustain her. The employment specialist and cultural liaison worked with a variety of departments of The World to facilitate Tsering's acclimatization to her host culture. The complexity of the Immigration Bundle is the most difficult challenge that any employment specialist will face while working with newcomers. The following are special issues to which an employment specialist must remain vigilant in the process of assisting newcomers to the United States.

Ethnic Enclaves as a Human Service Challenge

Employment in ethnic enclaves is very convenient and may seem preferable to more stressful, mainstream employment. However, too much involvement in the ethnic enclave may turn any job into a sheltered workshop. These workshops use a controlled environment to give people something to produce (Murphy & Rogan, 1995, p. 5). Unfortunately, sheltered workshops often perpetuate isolation and ignore self-determinism (Murphy & Rogan, 1995, p. 5). In this respect, many businesses in ethnic enclaves, especially those dubbed "sweat-shops," work in a similar way to sheltered workshops. They provide a pre-arranged niche of work in which employees will not have to learn English or acculturate, essentially sorting employees of certain ethnic groups into different industries (Harris, 1995, pp. 137–139). Because of language barriers and lack of exposure to the labor movement, working immigrants may be vulnerable to exploitation. In some instances, employers may hold exposure of the worker to the INS as a threat, even to LPRs who may not understand their rights as residents (Mattingly, 1999). In other events, employers in ethnic enclaves may profit from ethnic and linguistic isolation to prevent the organization of workers (Harris, 1995, pp. 137–139). Employment specialists must recognize the potential for exploitation within the ethnic enclaves, and must remain vigilant about employers who actively recruit workers from the enclaves.

Linguistics as a Human Service Challenge

Another challenge for employment specialists might be a language barrier. Multi-lingual work is a difficult and costly matter for any organization. Often, an agency must choose between recruiting multi-lingual workers, using multi-lingual paraprofessionals as interpreters, hiring translators, or asking clients to provide their own translation (Le-Doux & Stephens, 1992). Multi-lingual human service workers may not be easily recruited depending on a person's ethnic group and acculturation level. For instance, Asian Americans and Pacific Islanders who have not fully acculturated to the United States generally opt for more conventional careers instead of the social careers such as vocational training and social work (Park & Harrison, 1995). In these circumstances, culturally and linguistically accommodating employment facilitation might be a serious challenge. Many ethnic enclaves in the author's area show a trend in which agencies bring in paraprofessionals to translate for specialists and their clients. In this circumstance, confidentiality and accuracy of translation cannot be guaranteed, and paraprofessionals may edit translations and therefore skew the direction and feeling of the interaction. Paraprofessionals, however, often serve as good liaisons between cultures as well as languages. The hiring of professional translators ensures accurate translation and eliminates editing, but is very costly and time-consuming. The last, and most problematic strategy for translation requires clients to seek out their own translators, which often results in the use of children as translators. Often, immigrant families discover that children acculturate and learn new languages more quickly than adults. As a result of missing school and play to translate for (and on some levels "take care" of) their parents, children and parents experience a role-reversal, and parents run the risk of becoming complacent in their discipline while children shoulder the burden of speaking and acting for the family. Every agency must create its own strategy surrounding the handling of translation and cultural facilitation. Whatever the agency's stance, employment specialists must also be prepared to take the situations of immigrant clients into consideration in order to make the most appropriate choice for translation.

Transportation as a Human Service Challenge

In addition to ethnic enclaves and language concerns, transportation might be a significant issue of concern for immigrants which an employment specialist must address. Clients who reside in ethnic enclaves run a high probability of facing residential segregation, according to Preston, McLafferty, and Liu (1998). These authors identify the combined impact of long commuting time, comparatively low wages, and a difficult (and costly) job search as a hindrance to meaningful employment for newcomers to the United States. Families without reliable transportation may bear the absence of a commuter, may not have access to childcare along the transportation route, and may live too far away from profitable employment prospects (Mattingly, 1999). The employment specialist must handle these issues when linking clients with employers. Otherwise, the client might not be able to sustain a troublesome commute (and therefore a troublesome job) for very long.

Psychological Support as a Human Service Goal

Dignity is an essential, but often ignored issue for immigrants as they look for employment in the United States. Amidst the influx of "undesirable" immigrants—or unskilled workers from developing countries—the need for social services and Social Security Insurance payments has increased since World War II (Hurst, 1998, pp. 5–6). This reality, in addition to the growth of ethnic enclaves, tends to create tension between groups of different cultures and manifests itself as anti-immigrant sentiment (Hurst, 1998, p. 6). Many employers and even unions complain that newcomers freeze unskilled U.S. natives out of the labor market, although research on the subject finds little evidence of this (Harris, 1995, pp. 194–196; Smith & Edmonston, 1997, p. 7). In fact, Harris (1995, pp. 194–196) and Smith and Edmonston (1997, pp. 4–5) report that immigration results in gains for domestic residents on an economic level, only effecting the wages of U.S.-born high school drop-outs by 5%. Although a high proportion of immigrants (higher than U.S. nationals) has employment that requires higher education (Smith & Edmonston, 1997, p. 8), the transfer of human capital remains a barrier for meaningful employment of immigrants (Hurst, 1998, p. 185). Employment specialists must work as liaisons between potential employers and the entire immigrant community to combat the inaccurate assumptions of immigrants' impact on the economy and also the internalization of public sentiment by newcomers that need work. The employment specialists have a duty to assert themselves and the interests of their clients in the face of such assumptions, and must ensure that each client is treated with the dignity that any human deserves.

As with any other population, employment is much more complicated than creating a link between an employer and employee. Employment specialists must prepare themselves to deal with continuing employment issues and support after the hiring date.

IMPLICATIONS FOR HUMAN SERVICE WORK

The ideal human service organization for immigrants will provide employment linkage as well as services which address as many of the aspects of the Immigration Bundle as possible. It should offer culturally accommodating help without fostering isolation. It should remain involved in the employment process until other aspects of the Immigration Bundle cease to be stressors. It should help newcomers compete in the mainstream job market with confidence and cultural ease. And, most importantly, it should center around the immigrant and her or his interests and dreams. This section addresses manners in which human service organizations can put all of these important parts of immigration and acculturation together.

The Council of Europe Directorate of Social and Economic Affairs (1995, pp. 41–48, 71–77) presented two model programs for employment preparation for immigrant women. Both programs centered around immigrant women in Germany, one dealing with Turkish women and the other with Moroccan women. These programs offered training in literacy, reducing social isolation, interacting with social service organizations and institutions, adjusting to different roles in a new country, and networking. The main focus throughout the training sessions revolved around self-confidence, independence, and assertiveness. These two programs, although providing class situations instead of individual-centered plans, offered training that addressed several aspects of the Immigration Bundle at the same time. The programs linked women with employment after the training session was complete. They each carried out follow-up after different lengths of time to see the effectiveness of long-term employment of participants. The comprehensiveness of the programs in Germany forms a strong foundation for any vocational program or employment facilitation. However, they were not strong in some other areas of employment facilitation.

After the training programs that dealt with multiple aspects of the Immigration Bundle, the participants in the model programs worked together in jobs arranged by the organizations. No evidence could be found that the organizers of the German programs worked to link the immigrant women with jobs to which they aspired. As Kregel (1998, pp. 72–75) asserts, plans for employment should revolve around a client's individual interests and goals. Unger, Parent,

Gibson, and Kane-Johnston (1998, pp. 185–192) assign seven steps for creating workplace support. These include the determination of the client's needs and preferences, a brainstorm of possible options, assessment of job and community supports, identification of the client's choices, strategies for accessibility of supports, evaluation of the supports' effectiveness, and arrangements for ongoing mentorship. The most important part of these steps toward employment is validation of the client's determination and importance. Without that acknowledgment of the client's will, an employment specialist is simply processing people.

Another important factor in the planning stages of employment facilitation is the cultural accommodation of the employment specialist to the individual client. One might imagine that each culture has its own defining features, and that cultural norms apply across the entire culture. However, as in the population of U.S. nationals, each individual defines herself or himself differently. Miranda and Umhoefer (1998) identify acculturation (not enculturation) and language use as the two best predictors of career self-efficacy for Latinos. The same authors follow that conclusion with a reminder that counseling must reflect the cultural learning and adaptation of the individual within the new culture as well as the ability of each individual to learn, use, and develop instrumental skills. Ruelas and colleagues (1998) further warn that "counselors need to be aware that ethnic self-identification in and of itself does not represent one's adherence to cultural attitudes and behaviors." Employment specialists must heed these reminders to consider each client as an individual with her or his own personality characteristics. By avoiding generalizations, employment specialists will best understand the situation of each person and her/his employment goals.

The role of the employment specialist continues beyond the planning stage when that specialist creates links to employment. The seven-step process of employment facilitation presented by Unger and colleagues (1998, pp. 185–192) highlights the specialist's role in a client's adaptation to the workplace. The same authors go on to emphasize that the involvement of the employment specialist is important in the job-site training process and as a facilitator (not simply the provider) of employment services. In their framework of employment facilitation, the specialist is just as active as the client in forging a place for the client within the workplace. In the context of immigration work, this might include facilitation of job training and intensive vocabulary training. At the same time, an employment specialist would help the client identify resources such as childcare and transportation while the client settles in to her or his new job.

The employment specialist is not alone in creating a healthy and nurturing workplace for the client. Floyd (1994, pp. 6–11) suggests continued work by the employment specialist and client on self-esteem and stress reduction after employment is established, while the employer concentrates on issues that might help the worker acclimatize to her or his new job. With immigrant clients, the employer could introduce the Buddy system, as in the example with Tsering, or could use small-group or "team" work to draw the newcomer into the rhythm of the workplace. Whatever the method for introducing the immigrant worker into the workplace, the employer, as much as the employment specialist and client, should engage in frequent evaluation and feedback. Such feedback will assist the client and employer to overcome cultural differences before they become issues of conflict. It will facilitate a better understanding of the cultural adaptation on both sides, and will reduce further stress that might result from unclear assumptions about cultural norms or work habits.

In a partnership between newcomers to the United States, employment specialists, and employers, everyone should be involved in decreasing stressors. The client is in charge of mastering a job and acclimatizing to a new environment. At the same time, the employment specialist works on strengthening the resources that will address all possible aspects of the

Immigration Bundle that might serve as a hindrance to employment (child care, transportation, cultural isolation, etc.). An employer is also at work arranging stress prevention programs, offering feedback, and considering the needs of the newcomers along with the senior employees.

The employment specialist, in short, carries out the same basic function with immigrants as with any other population. The goal is the acquisition of meaningful employment with the added bundle of immigration issues in tow. Immigration is a complex issue that spans every aspect of a newcomer's life. An employment specialist or social service worker can be the link to a solution for multiple immigration issues at one time. If the employment specialist takes the time to learn about the special circumstances and acculturation of each client, then employment can be the stabilizing factor in a confusing and new life.

REFERENCES

Council of Europe Directorate of Social and Economic Affairs (1995). *Immigrant women and integration: Community relations.* Croton-on-Hudson, NY: Author.

Floyd, M. (1994). Mental health at work conference. In M. Floyd, M. Povall, & G. Watson (Eds.), *Mental health at work* (pp. 1–11). Bristol, PA: Rehabilitation Resource Centre.

Harris, N. (1995). *The new untouchables: Immigration and the new world worker.* New York, NY: I.B. Tauris.

Hurst, M. E. (1998). *The assimilation of immigrants in the U.S. labor market: Employment and labor force turnover.* New York, NY: Garland.

Kregel, J. (1998). Developing a career path: Application of person-centered planning. In P. Wehman & J. Kregel (Eds.), *More than a job: Securing satisfying careers for people with disabilities* (pp. 71–92). Baltimore, MD: Paul H. Brookes.

Le-Doux, C., & Stephens, K. S. (1992). Refugee and immigrant social service delivery: Critical management issues. In A. S. Ryan (Ed.), *Social work with immigrants and refugees* (pp. 31–45). Binghamton, NY: Haworth Press.

Mattingly, D. J. (1999). Job search, social networks, and local labor-market dynamics: The case of paid household work in San Diego. *Urban Geography, 2*(1), 46–74.

Miranda, A. O., & Umhoefer, D. L. (1998). Acculturation, language use, and demographic variables as predictors of the career self-efficacy of Latino career counseling clients. *Journal of Multicultural Counseling and Development, 26,* 39–51.

Murphy, S. T., & Rogan, P. M. (1995). *Closing the shop: Conversion from sheltered to integrated work.* Baltimore, MD: Paul H. Brookes.

Park, S. E., & Harrison, A. A. (1995). Career-related interests and values, perceived control, and acculturation of Asian–American and Caucasian–American college students. *Journal of Applied Social Psychology, 25*(13), 1184–1203.

Preston, V. S., McLafferty, S., & Liu, X. F. (1998). Geographical barriers to employment for American-born and immigrant workers. *Urban Studies, 35*(3), 529–545.

Ruelas, S. R., Atkinson, D. R., & Ramos-Sanchez, L. (1998). Counselor helping model, participant ethnicity and acculturation level, and perceived counselor credibility. *Journal of Counseling Psychology, 5*(1), 98–103.

Rumbaut, R. G. (1994). Origins and destinies: Immigration to the United States since World War II. *Sociological Forum, 9*(4), 583–621.

Smith, J. P., & Edmonston, B. (Eds.) (1997). *The new Americans: Economic, demographic, and fiscal effects of immigration.* Washington, DC: National Academy Press.

Thomas-Presswood, T. N. (1998). The impact of acculturation on the adjustment of immigrant families. In R. A. Javier, & W. G. Herron (Eds.), *Personality Development and Psychotherapy in our Diverse Society* (pp. 451–464). Dunmore, PA: Jason Aronson.

Unger, D. D., Parent, W. S., Gibson, K. E., & Kane-Johnston, K. (1998). Maximizing community and workplace supports: Defining the role of the employment specialist. In P. Wehman & J. Kregel (Eds.), *More than a job: Securing satisfying careers for people with disabilities* (pp. 183–224). Baltimore, MD: Paul H. Brookes.

United States Department of Justice, Immigration and Naturalization Service. (1999). Annual Report: Legal Immigration, Fiscal Year 1998. [On-line]. Available: *http://www.immigration.gov/graphics/publicaffairs/newsrels/98Legal.pdf*

CHAPTER 30

Helping People Coping with HIV and AIDS Manage Employment

CHRISTINE HYDUK AND KATHY KUSTOWSKI

INTRODUCTION

When HIV was first identified in the United States between 1983 and 1984 (Kalichman, 1998), seropositive status was considered a death sentence. Population groups affected by HIV included primarily white gay males and injecting drug users. In the early years of the spread of HIV, there were no medications to stop progression of the virus and the subsequent development of AIDS. An individual diagnosed HIV positive experienced a steady and rapid decline. The individual's life, let alone career, was suddenly cut short. The initial preoccupation was the fear that anyone close to him/her, including spouse, lover, friends, people at church, even health care professionals, would discover they too had HIV/AIDS. Fear included the perceived negative repercussions that could follow the disclosure. Reactions of significant others could involve leaving the individual out of fear of contracting the virus or AIDS, or ostracizing the individual through judgment of how the individual contracted HIV/AIDS. Fear also included discriminatory practices such as the individual losing his/her housing or job with no legal recourse. Another primary focus for the individual became preparing for his/her own death, given that the disease progression even granted the time to accomplish such preparation.

The approval of AZT in 1987 (Klosinski, 1992) provided more time for individuals to plan their much shortened lives. The medication did not help individuals return to work. The majority of persons diagnosed with HIV were eligible for disability benefits, which did enable them to somewhat enjoy the time they had left.

With the advent of combination antiretroviral therapy in 1995 (reverse transciptase inhibitors and protease inhibitors or highly active antiretroviral therapy (HAART)) and thus an even longer lifespan, HIV/AIDS is now recognized as more of a chronic illness (Mukand, Startkeson, & Melvin, 1991; Rabkin, 1998, p. xi; Sebesta & LaPlante, 1996). The change in disease progression from terminal illness to chronic illness enables individuals the opportunity to address many issues not previously considered relevant. One major issue is that of

CHRISTINE HYDUK • Marygrove College Department of Social Work, Detroit, Michigan.   KATHY KUSTOWSKI • Visiting Nurses Association of Southeast Michigan, Detroit, Michigan.

employment: either remaining employed; returning to work if previously employed; or even starting a new career for those who have worked before or for those who had never worked.

> Work and career are important and defining aspects of many persons' lives and represent one of the most important of life's goals and adult roles. Work supports feelings of worth, provides an important component of identity, is a source of social support, and provides financial independence. One of the first role losses that the PWHIV may experience is that of being a full-time worker (Hoffman, 1996, p. 116).

This chapter begins with important background information on the disabling aspects of HIV/AIDS related to employment. This information includes a synopsis of the disabling social, emotional/psychological, and physical/cognitive aspects of the illness related to work. The focus then shifts to rehabilitation issues with specific focus on community and social service supports for successful rehabilitation. Discussion also identifies policy, employee, personal, and service provider barriers to support. Community-based case examples serve to highlight key issues, supports, and barriers to supports. Joe is a long-term survivor diagnosed with HIV in 1986. Joe's occupation is as a minister. Paul is a 50-year-old long-term survivor diagnosed HIV seropositive in 1990. Prior to his diagnosis, Paul was an electrician. The chapter concludes with a discussion of preliminary support components to help HIV/AIDS individuals successfully manage employment issues.

BEHAVIORAL HEALTH ISSUES

Emotional/Psychological Aspects of Illness

For the career or job-oriented individual employed prior to the onset of the diagnosis or symptoms of HIV/AIDS, the inability to work due to physical and behavioral manifestations can be quite devastating. Loss of employment can affect the individual's self-worth and thus negatively affect self-esteem (Hoffman, 1997).

Loss of employment can also result in anxiety as the individual faces the prospect of being unable to afford to live in his/her accustomed lifestyle. HIV seropositive individuals can also experience more severe depression and anxiety (George, 1989; Hoffman, 1997; Kassel, 1991; O'Dowd, Natali, Orr, & McKegney, 1991 as cited in Kalichman, 1998). "The most common psychiatric diagnosis in this population is adjustment disorder, with features of anxiety and/or depression" (O'Dowd & Zofnass, 1991, p. 202). In the cases of Joe and Paul, both encountered problems with emotional distress related to adjustment to their physical problems, with Paul suffering from anxiety and Joe from depression. These individuals sometimes also experience paranoid thoughts that somehow people are trying to find out about their HIV status through misinterpreted co-worker comments or questions. Thus, how the individual perceives his/her work environment is framed through the fear of disclosure of HIV status or the diagnosis of AIDS.

Social Aspects of Illness

An individual's discovery of seropositve HIV status can increase his/her fear of someone finding out at work and the possible discriminatory practices resulting from the negative societal stigma associated with HIV/AIDS. According to Allport (1979) there are five types of negative action that can be a result of prejudice, one of which is discrimination:

> Here the prejudiced person makes detrimental distinctions of an active sort. He undertakes to exclude all members of the group in question from certain types of employment, from residential housing,

political rights, educational or recreational opportunities, churches, hospitials, or from some other social privileges (Allport, 1979, pp. 14–15).

Discrimination becomes one more obstacle that the HIV positive individual must face (Senak, 1996, p. 81). The stigma associated with AIDS originates from societal perceptions that AIDS leads to steady deterioration and death and that individuals who pass on the virus already belong to negatively viewed groups—gay men and injecting drug users (Herek & Capitanio, 1983; Herek & Glunt, 1988 as cited in Hoffman, 1996, p. 34). Associated with these beliefs is the thought that these individuals knowingly participated in behaviors that resulted in AIDS, such as sex or drugs, therefore they lost their right to *not* be discriminated against (Senak, 1996, p. 81).

Negative consequences can include: co-worker avoidance, reduced work responsibilities, and even loss of employment (Kalichman, 1998). At a more subtle level, discrimination can be operationalized through a hostile work environment (Hoffman, 1996). The individual's fear of discrimination can result in withdrawl from work relationships and subsequent isolation (Crandall & Coleman, 1992, as cited in Kalichman, 1998). Joe feared being thrown out of the church and therefore hid his HIV status from his pastor (supervisor). The fears were somewhat realized when Joe experienced stigma in his place of employment (the church), as certain members of the congregation did not share his pastor's support of his AIDS diagnosis or his gay lifestyle.

Loss of employment remains a very real fear for those who have HIV/AIDS. The financial loss is substantial, as individuals' primary source of income shifts from employment to entitlement programs (Massagli, Weissman, Seage, & Epstein, 1994). With loss of employment comes not only loss of income, but loss of health insurance and other types of insurance (Nussbaum, 1991, as cited in Hoffman, 1996). For those with HIV/AIDS, obtaining and retaining life and health insurance is a major problematic issue (Kassel, 1991). For many with HIV or AIDS, unemployment is directly related to lack of insurance or loss of insurance (Hoffman, 1996; Kass, Munoz, Chen, Zucconi, Bing, & Hennessey, 1994).

As a result of alleged discriminatory practices in the workplace, HIV/AIDS cases comprise the largest category of the Equal Opportunity Employment Commission (EEOC) filed lawsuits (AIDS Policy and Law, 1995, as cited in Hoffman, 1997). According to Hoffman (1997),

> ... review of the basis for employment discrimination in these cases shows several themes beginning with the most common: (1) firing (or not hiring) an employee based on HIV status; (2) inequities in access to medical benefits including lower lifetime caps on HIV care; (3) refusal to make appropriate accomodations (e.g. flexible work schedule; switching to a less desirable job); (4) violation of confidentiality; and (5) condoning a hostile work environment (pp. 180–181).

More subtle forms of discrimination can include actions such as isolating the individual with HIV or AIDS from other workers or the public. These actions make the individual with HIV or AIDS feel uncomfortable, thus pushing him or her to quit the job (Senak, 1996). The severe stigma of HIV, its impact on the workplace, and the subsequent employment difficulties cannot be minimized even with the establishment of current employment laws (Hoffman, 1996, 1997; Kassel, 1991; O'Dell, Levinson, & Riggs, 1996, as cited in Hoffman, 1997).

Physical and Health Aspects of Illness

Individuals with HIV/AIDS experience a multitude of infections and illnesses which, in turn, cause many physical and neurological symptoms. Table 30-1 summarizes the physical

TABLE 30-1. **Physical and Neurological Complications and Symptoms Associated with HIV/AIDS and Their Influence on Work**

Pulmonary	Rheumatological	Neuromuscular	Neuropsychological
Physical conditions by complication type			
Pneumonias, tuberculosis	Arthritis	Peripheral neuropathies	Mild Neurocognitive disorder
Karposi's sarcoma Non-Hodgkin's lymphoma myopathies, arthralgias	Fibromyalgia		HIV-associated dementia
Physical symptoms associated with complication type			
Fatigue	Joint problems	Pain, numbness	Limitations in processing information quickly
Breathing problems	Walking problems	Burning, tingling	Attention problems
Poor endurance	Pain	Motor skill problems	Problems learning new information
	Fatigue	Motor weakness problems	Problems recalling new information
			Impaired language-naming/ fluency[a]
			Psychomotor slowing[a]
			Affective changes[a]

(Hoffman, 1996, p. 14; Hoffman, 1997, pp. 171–172).
[a]Specific to HIV-associated dementia.

and neurological complications along with the resulting symptoms. Additional symptoms associated with symptomatic HIV infection include: night sweats, fever, fatigue and weight loss; enlarging lymph nodes; problems of the skin and mucous membrane including "herpes, shingles, thrush, canker sores, human papillomavirus, and oral hairy leukoplakia" (Hoffman, 1996, p. 14). Any of these conditions can be the cause of periods of malaise, lethargy, weakness, and problems with eating (O'Connor, 1997, p. 38). The potential fatigue, as well as the physical and cognitive impairment caused by these conditions, can create multiple challenges for these individuals in the work environment. Both Joe and Paul experienced physical difficulties related to AIDS. Joe suffered from such physical conditions such as CMV retinitis (visual deterioration), peripheral neuropathy, and wasting syndrome. At one point he even lapsed into a coma for three days. Paul experienced a MAC (mycobacterium avium complex) infection and excessive loss of strength and weight.

In addition, the nature of the disease progression is unpredictable, with physical and cognitive functional impairment fluctuating throughout the course of the disease. In the cases of Joe and Paul, both initially were very ill in the beginning stages of AIDS, but with medication and physical and occupational therapy they improved to almost their previous level of functioning. Given the uncertainty of disease progression, individuals may experience difficulty in making future plans. This was true of Paul, an electrician, who expressed concern about how long he could remain at his current level of functioning. Some individuals may discover that, while previously they were too ill to work and thus went on disability, they have currently returned to a level of health permitting them to return to work (Hoffman, 1997). This was the case for Joe and Paul. Other individuals, who may never have worked and were receiving disability for the illness, may find that they are now able to work, but lack job skills. For others, their illness may have progressed to where the person is not able to work full-time but not ill enough to be considered disabled.

As the disease progresses and functional impairment increases, full-time labor participation decreases (Sebesta & LaPlante, 1996). Individuals with AIDS who hold jobs that do not require physical labor or that do require increased mental effort are more likely to be employed (Massagli et al., 1994). Individuals "... whose work requires high physical exertion, and who have less control over the pace of work, are more likely to have to withdraw from employment" (Yelin, Greenblatt, Hollander, & McMaster, 1991, as cited in Adam & Sears, 1996, p. 121). As a minister, Joe did not experience the physical demands that Paul did as an electrician. Paul had to give up the electrician trade and thus his previous job. Examples of non-physical jobs include: executive positions, administrative positions, managerial positions, service industry positions, and clerical/administrative support positions (Sebesta & LaPlante, 1996, pp. 9–10).

For someone who is HIV positive or who has AIDS, an additional challenge involves medication compliance, given the complex regimen of medications needed to treat the disease. The individual must maintain a medication schedule that involves taking certain medications at specific times, with or without food. Individuals will vary in their ability to tolerate potential side-effects. Both Joe and Paul work part-time because of the fatigue and the side-effects associated with the many medications. Others may be unable to afford the high medication costs.

"Fundamental power inequalities structure the workplace, laying grounds for generosity and creativity, or for harassment, humiliation or dismissal" (Adam & Sears, 1996, p.118). Employed individuals learning their HIV positive status for the first time must struggle with the demands of work, while facing the emotions associated with discovering they have HIV. Anxiety centers on hiding the diagnosis for fear that a colleague will find out about their HIV status. Associated with this fear of discovery is the additional fear that they will be fired as a result of the employer learning of their diagnosis. This anxiety may affect the individual's ability to concentrate, thus negatively influencing work performance.

Many individuals with HIV face a lack of support from colleagues. Joe and Paul shared supportive supervisors in their prospective places of employment. Joe's pastor provided encouragement for him to write sermons and present them to the congregation, while Paul's supervisor at the gift shop allowed him flex-time to address his physical needs. According to Herek & Capitano (1993) as cited in Kalichman (1998) "... 20% would avoid an infected co-worker" (p. 214). The primary determinant of AIDS phobia is homophobia (Nelkin, 1987; Triplet & Sugarman, 1987, as cited in Adams & Sears, 1996).

Disclosure is a constant consideration that looms over the individual on a daily basis. This becomes an even greater concern when the person becomes symptomatic and cannot hide his/her illness. At this time, the individual with HIV or AIDS can no longer conceal the multiple bathroom trips due to diarrhea, the increased use of sick time, or the increased requests for time off for medical appointments. Thus, the individual may be forced to talk with the employer about his/her diagnosis and workplace issues. The result can be discriminatory acts which include: "... reduced responsibilities, isolation from co-workers and the public, or termination" (Kalichman, 1998, p. 221). Joe, the minister, disclosed his diagnosis to the congregation in the hope of educating the parishioners on AIDS and increasing their acceptance of him as a gay individual with AIDS. Many accepted him and some did not. While

TABLE 30-2. Summary of Issues for Successful Employment of Individuals with
AIDS

Physical/health	Disease—here-and-now focus
	New diagnosis versus long-term survivor
	Disease progression history
	Physical/functional limitations
Emotional/psychological	Coping ability
	Emotional status—severity of symptoms
Work	Employment history—never worked, re-entry into workforce, type of work
	Individual's view of employment—meaning to him/her
	Work environment support—administrative, co-worker, benefits

HIV-infected individuals in all occupations face potential discrimination, "HIV-positive teachers, hairstylists, cooks, food servers, sales clerks, receptionists, and other service providers are among the most likely to endure employment discrimination" (Kalichman, 1998, p. 222).

In order to address workplace issues around HIV and AIDS, companies need specific workplace AIDS policies (Adams & Sears, 1996, p. 126). Yet most companies rely on the Americans with Disabilities Act (ADA) policies rather than specific AIDS policies, with over 50% of companies larger than 100 employees likely to have AIDS policies compared with 33% of companies smaller than 100 employees (Green, 1998). According to Masi (1990), as cited in Adams & Sears (1996), an ideal AIDS policy would include: "... specific education about HIV transmission at work, an approach that treats AIDS like other chronic illnesses, a commitment to supporting people with HIV as long as possible in their jobs, and general AIDS education" (p. 127).

Table 30-2 summarizes the physical/health issues, emotional/psychological issues, and work issues for successful employment of individuals with AIDS.

REHABILITATION ISSUES

Community and Social Service Supports

Having addressed the social, emotional/psychological, and physical/cognitive aspects of the illness related to work, the next issue becomes one of determining current community/societal and social service supports to create the opportunity for successful employment.

LAWS AND STATUTES.   Laws and statues that protect an individual's rights and defend against discrimination serve to increase the chances of succeeding in a work environment. The ADA was signed into law on July 26,1990, by President George Bush and became law on July 26, 1991 (Hoffman, 1996). This federal law covers anyone who develops "... any mental or physical impairment which limits life time activity ... including contagious and infectious diseases" (Marcus, 1989, as cited in Mukand et al., 1991, p. 16). Protection under this Act applies whether an HIV-infected person is or is not symptomatic. In the case of John, a program assistant in a medical center, this protection resulted in enabling John to talk to his supervisor about flexing his time so that he could keep his medical appointments and work around those periods when he was not feeling very well. Arrangements also could be made for him to work at home for the day or part of the day.

The Rehabilitation Act of 1973 (29 U.S.C. 706 et seq.) "... defines the condition of being handicapped as a 'mental or physical impairment which substantially limits one or more of such person's major life activities' and prohibits discrimination" (Yesner, 1982, as cited in Mukand et al., 1991, p. 15). In 1987, the U.S. Supreme Court found that "other communicable diseases, including AIDS were considered a handicap" (Mukand et al., 1991, p. 15). This federal act applies to federal government issues around employee rights, federal program and activities participation, and federally affiliated private business treatment of employees (Michigan Protection & Service, 1998, p. 9). State laws can mirror federal laws in their protection of individuals with disabilities, including those diagnosed with AIDS. An example of this in Michigan is the Persons with Disabilities Civil Rights Act 220 of 1976 (Michigan Handicapper's Civil Rights Act-MHCRA, 37.1101–37.1103), which covers issues similar to The Rehabilitation Act of 1973.

Other acts concentrate on community supports around housing. The Fair Housing Act Amendment (42 U.S.C. 3601.16) invokes equal rights in the purchase, sale, and rental of housing. The Act "... does not apply to landlords who rent four or fewer units and live in the building themselves, nor to persons who sell their own home without a real estate broker" (Michigan Protection & Service, 1998, p. 9). In the case of James, this amendment did not prove helpful. James lived in the basement of his brother-in-law's home. James needed to find another place to live as he feared that if his brother-in-law found out he was HIV positive, he would get kicked out of the basement and have no where to live. He had not yet worked consistently to know if he could afford to independently pay rent. He felt trapped, resulting in fear which interfered with his ability to concentrate at work.

A recent employment-centered law includes the Ticket to Work and Work Incentives Improvement Act of 1999 (Public Law 106–170). President Clinton signed this Act into law on December 17, 1999 (to view the complete Act go to http://frwebgate.access.gpo.gov). The Act provides supports for disabled individuals to return to work. The Act includes extension of the grace period for receipt of social security during the trial work period from 36 to 60 months starting in 2001. During this period, an individual can apply for reinstatement and still be eligible for benefits for up to 6 months during the reinstatement review. Even if individual is denied reinstatement, he/she is not required to pay back the benefits to the Social Security Administration. In addition, individuals receiving Medicare can work during a nine-month work trial period and still receive Medicare coverage. If the individual continues to work after the trial period, then he/she can receive Medicare Part A for an additional 39 months starting October 1, 2000. This law also addresses Medigap coverage by allowing disabled Medigap beneficiaries to suspend their premiums and benefits if they become covered under a group health insurance plan for an employer with 20 or more employees. If the beneficiary loses his/her group health insurance, then Medigap insurers must automatically reinstate the beneficiary, provided the beneficiary notifies the Medigap insurer within 90 days of loss of the insurance (Franzoi, 2000). In helping anyone with HIV/AIDS enter or re-enter the workforce, one needs to be aware that, in general, anti-discrimination laws do not typically apply to private membership clubs, religious organizations, and American Indian tribes.

When dealing with employers around disclosure, the individual with HIV/AIDS must consider why an employer needs to know the diagnosis. The client needs to know if the medical papers can be completed by the physician without disclosing the diagnosis. The laws may help to protect the HIV/AIDS employee from obvious forms of discrimination, but not from more subtle forms of discrimination that could be difficult to prove yet could result in increased stress.

CONFIDENTIALITY LAWS. Confidentiality laws also help HIV infected individuals be successful in the workplace. "The confidentiality of an individual's HIV status is protected by a wall of legislation that makes disclosure an offense punishable by hefty fines or imprisonment" (Burkett, 1995, pp. 206–207). For example, the state of Michigan has a statute MCL333.5131 that protects an individual's HIV status. Violating an individual's HIV status is a misdemeanor punishable by up to a year in jail and/or up to a $5,000 fine. It can also be a civil cause of action. A person whose confidentiality has been breached can sue for his/her actual damages or $1,000, whichever is greater, per violation, plus costs and reasonable legal fees. In addition, the employer of a person who violates this law can also be held liable, unless the employer had taken reasonable precautions to prevent such a breach (Department of Community Health, HIV/AIDS Prevention and Intervention Section, 1998).

BENEFITS. The Social Security Administration (SSA) provides economic support to disabled individuals, including those diagnosed with AIDS through Social Security Disability Insurance (SSDI) and Social Security Income (SSI). Both Joe and Paul applied for and received SSDI, which is a monthly amount based on employee earnings. While a support for some, the guidelines for eligibility stipulate that "patients must have made payroll contributions, then prove their inability to work for a continuous period of 12 months..." (Mukand et al., 1991). The SSA also specifies that the inability to work includes the inability to do "substantial work" and defines this monetarily, with an individual making $500.00 a month in earnings representing "substantial work" (SSA, 1995). SSI is also a monthly income for individuals who have not worked long enough to qualify for SSDI or who receive a low SSDI monthly income (SSA, 1995).

The federal government provides health insurance for disabled people through the Medicare program. Individuals qualify for Medicare after receiving SSDI for a period of 24 months. "Medicare helps pay for hospital and hospice care, lab tests, home health care, and other medical services" (SSA, 1995). While a support for some, it is a barrier for others because of the 24-month receipt of SSDI eligibility factor. Joe and Paul also applied for and received Medicare. Joe also received private insurance though his church had helped pay for medical expenses.

State administered programs also support those with AIDS. Medicaid is an example of such a program, whereby individuals receiving SSI may be eligible for Medicaid. Medicaid coverage varies by state but can include: inpatient and outpatient care, hospice care, private nursing care, and prescription drug coverage (SSA, 1995). The food stamp program is also a state-run program. Individuals receiving SSI may also be eligible for food stamps. The amount varies from state to state.

THERAPEUTIC SUPPORTS. Kalichman addresses three types of supports important for those with HIV/AIDS. These include emotional support, informational support, and instrumental support. Emotional support includes supports designed to help the individual cope with the different emotional reactions associated with HIV/AIDS, including "... shock ... relief ... anger ... guilt ... decreased self-esteem ... loss of identity ... loss of sense of security ... loss of personal control ... fear ... sadness and depressed mood ... obsessions and compulsions … (and) … positive adjustment" (George, 1989, pp. 70–73). Individual emotion-focused coping includes "… selective ignoring, wishful thinking, blaming others, focusing on the positive, distancing, avoidance, and acceptance …" (Kalichman, 1998, p. 258). Still others include denial, distraction, and escape (Kalichman, 1998, p. 268). For the HIV/AIDS individual, work can be a form of distraction that is lost when employment is discontinued.

Sources of emotional support can include different types of therapy. Psychotherapy is useful to help the individual deal with emotional and psychological issues such as addressing meaning and purpose in life (Kassel, 1991). Individual and group psychotherapy are viable options (Kalichman, 1998; Kassel, 1991). Psychotherapy models include psychodynamic perspectives, humanistic client-centered, cognitive–behavioral (Kalichman, 1998). Behavioral interventions, designed to target stress and pain management, can include hypnosis, biofeedback, and behavioral medicine techniques (Kassel, 1991, p. 238). Because of the fluctuating nature of the disease progression and the subsequent emotional and physical precariousness, crisis intervention becomes an extremely important therapeutic support (Kalichman, 1998). Sources of emotional support also can include psychopharmacological interventions (Kalichman, 1998; Kassel, 1991).

Paul and Joe each received individual therapy to help them with various emotional issues. For Paul, therapy centered around the anxiety and depression about the uncertainty of the disease progression and its impact on his ability to make future plans. Therapy also focused on Paul's present contributions. For Joe, therapy emphasized his unstable physical condition and its impact on his ability to function physically. Other therapeutic issues included relationships, disclosure, family, and living and dying.

Additional resources to help provide emotional support should focus on developing or expanding the individual's support network (Kassel, 1991). Community resources include support groups, volunteer programs, and hospice services (Kalichman, 1998). Support groups can play a vital role in helping those with HIV/AIDS gain knowledge, decrease isolation, learn shared problem-solving skills, and vent emotions in an accepting environment (Hoffman, 1996). Paul received emotional support through his participation in social events sponsored by agencies that provide services to those with HIV/AIDS and his weekly attendance at his church which has a ministry for helping people living with HIV/AIDS.

Emotional supports are even more critical if informal support provided by family is limited. Paul's family lives out-of-state and provides support through frequent telephone contact. Joe's family provides mixed support. His parents live out-of-state, but provide support such as visits when needed. His siblings offer mixed support, with not all of this siblings being supportive.

Informational support relates to problem-focused coping. "Examples of illness-related problem-focused coping include seeking information about the disease, calling others for help, and seeking medical advice and effective treatment" (Kalichman, 1998, p. 258). Other examples include "… lifestyle changes and social activism (Kalichman, 1998, p. 265). This type of coping is also called active confrontation (Solano et al., 1993, as cited in Mulder, Antoni, Duivenvoorden, Kaufmann, & Goodkin, 1995) or "active cognitive behavioral coping" (Hoffman, 1996, p. 62). Joe exhibited problem-focused coping by his disclosure of his AIDS status and gay lifestyle as well as through his advocacy with church policies. Paul demonstrated this coping style by seeking out the latest information on treatments and attending education sessions that focus on staying healthy. He also closely followed his medical regime which gave him a sense of control over AIDS. Informational support also involves providing the individual with up-to-date information on HIV/AIDS and/or providing the resources to obtain the updated information.

TABLE 30-3. Summary of Supports for Successful Employment of Individuals
with AIDS

Social Service supports	Laws and statutes on discrimination and confidentiality
Benefits	SSD, SSI, Medicare, Medicaid, Food Stamp Program
Therapeutic supports	Counseling interventions
	Individual and group psychotherapy—psychodynamic, client-centered, cognitive–behavioral
	Crisis intervention
	Psychopharmacology
	Case management
Community resources	Support groups, volunteer programs, hospice services
	HIV/AIDS agencies
	Homemaker services, respite services, visiting nurse services
	Transportation, housing services, legal services
	Home delivered meals
	Political advocacy—gaps in support
	Research

Instrumental support focuses on providing assistance with the activities of daily living. This type of support allows individuals the opportunity to channel their energies to other activites, including employment. Examples of community support services designed to enhance daily activities include homemaker services, respite services, visiting nurses, transportation services, housing services, legal services, civil rights, and meals on wheels (Zlotnik, 1987, p. 7). Joe's instrumental support services included a housekeeper who cleaned his home and grocery shopped. He also received home-delivered hot meals five days a week. A summary of social service, therapeutic, and community resource supports is presented in Table 30-3.

Barriers to Supports

SUPPORTIVE WORK ENVIRONMENTS.   According to Hoffman (1997) the existing literature fails to show how many employers are addressing supportive work environments for individuals with HIV. "Reasonable accommodations for persons with HIV disease include offering flexible hours, allowing time off for medical appointments, reducing travel requirements, working at home, or implementing HIV awareness training for employees to improve the workplace environment" (Pranschke & Wright, 1995, as cited in Hoffman, 1997, p. 181). Fortunately, Joe and Paul both had supportive employers. Paul's employer allowed him flextime to work afternoons and evenings and avoid mornings which were physically his worst time of the day. Joe's employer, his pastor, modeled acceptance of Joe's gay lifestyle and AIDS status, thus providing an example and expectation for members of the congregation. Green (1998) cites 1996 Centers for Disease Control statistics which indicate that 43% of worksites with over 50 employees have workplace policies that include individuals with HIV/AIDS, although only 16% of the worksites offer employee education on HIV/AIDS. Education of employers and employees is critical for creating a supportive work environment.

> Education is the first line of defense against the epidemic of HIV-related stigma Even brief education programs can successfully reduce negative attitudes toward HIV/AIDS and remove unfounded fears of contracting HIV infection (Bliwise et al., 1991; Gallop, Taerk et al., 1992; Riley & Greene, 1993, as cited in Kalichman, 1998, p. 232)

PSYCHOSOCIAL CHARACTERISTICS OF PERSONS WITH HIV/AIDS. Multiple psychosocial factors influence an individual's ability to work. Injecting drug users, regardless of race or gender, have the lowest educational attainment, lowest income, and highest unemployment rate (Diaz et al., 1994, as cited in Hoffman, 1997). Hoffman (1997) includes a collection of factors that can potentially impact employment including: mode of HIV infection, sexual orientation, parenting of an HIV-positive child, caring for an HIV-positive spouse or partner, limited access to resources such as transportation, and race/ethnicity.

Other relevant variables previously discussed involve the emotional/psychological and physical problems that can arise from disease progression. An issue related to the emotional/ psychological and physical problems of the illness is the multiple side-effects of the medications used to help treat these problems. These side-effects can hinder rehabilitation efforts (O'Dowd & Zofnass, 1991). Neurological/cognitive impairment can also promote unemployment (Heaton et al., 1994, as cited in Hoffman, 1997). Miller (1987), as cited in Kassel (1991), states that persons who have the most difficult time adjusting to HIV/AIDS are those with minimal and/or conflicted family ties, low acceptance by peers, inadequate housing, and those who blame their past behavior for acquiring the disease (p. 223). Poor adjustment to HIV/AIDS can lead to problems with employment.

Gender and racial/ethnic group status can act as barriers to accessing supports. Men and women access different social spheres of support, with men including partners and family, and women including friends, along with partners and family (Smith & Rapkin, 1996, as cited in Kalichman, 1998). Racial and ethnic minority groups already face discrimination and exclusion because of prejudicial attitudes against them. As a result of discrimination and ostracism, racial and ethnic groups suffer from a lack of access to medical, legal, and social services (Kassel, 1991). Cultural mores and language difficulties also add to the potential lack of service accessibility for these vulnerable groups (Kassel, 1991).

Creating supports for disenfranchised, vulnerable individuals will require the social worker to embrace multiple roles including "... resource broker, counselor, client advocate, educator, and political activist ..." (Coleman & Sharp, 1991, p. 359). Social workers must help overcome resource shortages including housing, substance abuse treatment facilities, long-term care facilities, mental health facilities, hospices, and employees willing help those with HIV or AIDS (Mukand et al., 1991).

Social workers will need to strive toward understanding the differences in how HIV/AIDS effects women versus men around work issues. Women with HIV/AIDS, many of whom are also members of minority groups, are often the primary source of emotional and financial support for their families (Kassel, 1991). Childcare resources become critical to provide supports for women seeking new employment or maintaining continued employment. Career-oriented HIV seropositive women face a multitude of issues similar to men, including "... loss of identity, loss of future goals, and fear of disclosure and judgement about their HIV status (Rosen & Blank, 1992). Many women choose the job of homemaker. The social worker needs to understand and advocate for a broader explanation of work that includes the job of homemaker (Hoffman, 1996).

Social workers must also work toward achieving cultural competency in understanding how HIV/AIDS impacts racial and ethnic groups and how they view the context of work. The current literature lacks a focus on how HIV/AIDS affects work for certain racial and ethnic groups. The literature does emphasize how different racial and ethnic groups, such as African Americans, Latinos, Haitians, and Asian and Pacific Islanders perceive HIV/AIDS and the practice implications (Medrano & Klopner, 1992). Table 30-4 presents a summary of the work environment and psychosocial barriers to successful employment of individuals with AIDS.

TABLE 30-4. Summary of Barriers to Successful Employment of Individuals with AIDS

Work environment	Supportive or non-supportive work environment
Psychosocial characteristics	Gender, ethnicity, HIV transmission
	Substance abuse history
	Personal support system
	Previous psychiatric history
	Access to community resources
	Transportation
	Stable housing
	Side-effects of medication
	Neurological/cognitive impairments

SUPPORT COMPONENTS

Social workers can play a critical role in helping those who are HIV positive or who are living with AIDS with vocational rehabilitation to help them channel their work skills (Kalichman, 1998). In order to work effectively with HIV/AIDS individuals on employment issues, the human service worker needs to address the multiple issues, barriers, and supports. Best practice support components have been developed for individuals with other chronic conditions such as multiple sclerosis, serious mental illness, and developmental disability. An integrated summary of these support services provides important information for establishing an initial framework of intervention components for those with AIDS addressing work issues. This focus is relevant in light of the fact that AIDS is now considered a chronic illness.

A primary component of supports for these chronic conditions includes an empowerment-based or strengths-based focus. Characteristics representative of an empowerment-based perspective include: client participation in the care plan (Jacobson, 1996); client self-determination (Sands & Doll, 1996); client informed decision-making (Roberts, Becker, & Seay, 1997); and family involvement in the care plan (Freedman & Boyer, 2000; Hassiotis, 1996).

An additional component of supports includes service provider structural characteristics. These include an emphasis on: service integration (Jacobson, 1996; Roy, 1991); comprehensive services (Lam & Rosenheck, 1999); and service coordination and collaboration (Bouras & Szymanski, 1997). Service providers carried out their services in community-based service centers (DiFabio, Soderberg, Choi, Hansen, & Schapiro, 1998; Mary, 1998) or non-centered home-based services (Ardito, Botuck, Freeman, & Levy, 1997). Another important characteristic of supports included the emphasis on the use of multidisciplinary teams (DiFabio et al., 1998) or interdisciplinary teams (Bouras & Szymanski, 1997; Hassiotis, 1996).

Other characteristics serve to describe the necessary knowledge areas for the human service worker in assisting individuals with chronic illness or disability, including an understanding of: the disability and entitlements (Ardito et al., 1997; Miller & Keys, 1996); service system navigation (Freeman & Boyer, 2000); social justice (Jacobson, Malloy, Cheney, & Cormier, 1998; Mary, 1998); how to change public attitudes about disability (Jacobson, 1996; Miller & Keys, 1996); cultural competency (Hassiotis, 1996); and community outreach (Lam & Rosenheck, 1999; Miller & Keys, 1996). Human service workers also need to have a comprehensive picture of the physical and, especially, the emotional/mental health needs of individuals with a chronic disability (Buchanan & Lewis, 1997; Kraft, Freal, & Coryell,

1986). Additional worker skills include understanding the long-term nature of the care needed (Hustad, Hekking, & Niederman, 1999; McNair & Swartz, 1997; Roberts, Becker, & Seay, 1997) and the importance of setting and meeting short-term and long-term goals (Abdul-Hamid, Stansfeld, & Wykes, 1998; Carlo, Pubpion, & Fisher, 1997). Finally, human service workers need to understand the importance of addressing the vocational/employment needs and supports for individuals with chronic disabilites (Jackson, Purnell, & Anderson, 1996; Kraft et al., 1986; Malloy, Cheney, & Gail, 1998; McNair & Swartz, 1997).

CONCLUSION

While it is beyond the scope of this chapter to develop a detailed intervention model, a summary of support components for other chronic illnesses and disabilities provides an initial frame of reference for identifying key supports for individuals with HIV/AIDS. From identifying these components it becomes clear that for those who are HIV positive or who have AIDS, managing employment is only one of many issues that require understanding and support. Human service workers cannot separate work issues from these other issues.

Issues and barriers such as physical or health issues, emotional or psychological issues, work issues, and psychosocial characteristics can help human service workers develop a comprehensive assessment of the HIV/AIDS individual seeking their assistance. The human service worker needs to understand how the issue of employment fits with the other issues facing an individual with HIV/AIDS.

Reviewing the literature on other chronic conditions suggests that empowerment-oriented practice may also be the best approach in working with these individuals. Because work or employment is just one of many issues facing the HIV/AIDS individual, human service providers must emphasize interdisciplinary service coordination and collaboration. Without this effort, service efficiency and effectiveness could be compromised, resulting in gaps in services. Accessibility to services is also a key intervention component. Human service workers must also embrace a sense of social justice to overcome service barriers and to change attitudes—public and employer—about HIV/AIDS as a disability. The complex nature of HIV/AIDS points to the need for specialized case management.

An evaluation of HIV/AIDS service models that help HIV/AIDS individuals manage employment is indicated. Are community-based centers better able to assist HIV/AIDS individuals manage employment issues as compared with non-centered home-based services? What are the differences in emphasis in these two settings? What are their areas of strength and weakness in providing case management services? If there are differences, should a more collaborative model be developed and evaluated? Presently, there are more questions than answers. Yet one thing is clear: the face of AIDS has changed from a terminal illness to a chronic disability. Along with this change comes the need to help individuals accomplish important life tasks such as work.

REFERENCES

Abdul-Hamid, W., Stansfeld, S., & Wykes, T. (1998). The homeless clients of a community psychiatric nursing service in inner London: 2. Referral process and main intervention. *International Journal of Social Psychiatry, 44*(3), 164–169. Retrieved May 9, 2000, from WilsonSelect database (#BSSI99036836.ISSN: 0020–7640) on the World Wide Web: http://firstsearch.oclc.org.

Adam, B., & Sears, A. (1996). *Experiencing HIV, personal, family, and work relationships.* New York, NY: Columbia University Press.

Allport, G. (1979). *The nature of prejudice.* Reading, MA: Addison-Wesley.

Ardito, M., Botuck, S., Freeman, S., & Levy, J. (1997). Delivering home-based case management to families with children with mental retardation and developmental disability [Abstract]. *Journal of Case Management, 6*(2), 56–61. Retrieved May 9, 2000, from Medline, #97476441 on the World Wide Web: http://firstsearch.oclc.org.

Buchanan, R., & Lewis, K. (1997). Services that nursing facilities should provide to residents with multiple sclerosis: A survey of health professionals [Abstract]. R*ehabilitative Nursing, 22*(2), 67–72. Retrieved May 9, 2000 from Medline, #97265060 on the World Wide Web: http://firstsearch.oclc.org.

Burkett, E. (1995). *The gravest show on earth.* New York, NY: Picador.

Coleman, E., & Sharp, J. (1991). AIDS and the social work role. In J. Mukand (Ed.), *Rehabilitation for patients with HIV disease* (pp. 359–369). New York, NY: McGraw-Hill.

Department of Community Health, HIV/AIDS Prevention and Intervention Section (1998). *Case manager certification training resources.*

Difabio, R., Soderberg, J., M., Choi, T., Hansen, C., & Schapiro, R. (1998). Extended outpatient rehabilitation: Its influence on symptom frequency, fatigue, and functional status for person's with progressive multiple sclerosis [Abstract]. *Archives of Physical Medical Rehabilitation, 79*(2), 141–146. Retrieved May 9, 2000, from Medline, #88134269 on the World Wide Web: http://firstsearch.oclc.org.

Franzoi, L. (2000, February 14). *Ask the expert: Returning to work—Post-social security.* Retrieved February 26, 2000, on the World Wide Web: http://www.thebody.com/cgi/work_ans/619Ret.html.

Freedman, R., & Boyer, N. (2000). The power to choose: Supports for families caring for individuals with developmental disabilities [Abstract]. *Health and Social Work, 25*(1), 59–68. Retrieved May 9, 2000, from Medline, #20154194 on the World Wide Web: http://firstsearch.oclc.org.

George, H. (1989). Counselling people with AIDS, their lovers, friends, and relations. In J. Green & A. McCreamer (Eds.), *Counseling in HIV infection and AIDS* (pp. 69–87). Oxford, UK: Blackwell Scientific.

Green, J. (1998). Employers learn to live with AIDS. *Human Resource Magazine, 43,* 96–101. Retrieved May 9, 2000, from WilsonSelect database (#BBPI99020233.ISSN: 1047–3149) on the World Wide Web: http://firstsearch.oclc.org.

Hassiotis, A. (1996). Clinical examples of cross-cultural work in a community learning disability service. *International Journal of Social Psychiatry, 42,* 318–327. Retrieved May 9, 2000, from WilsonSelect database (#BSSI97011797.ISSN: 0020–7640) on the World Wide Web: http://firstsearch.oclc.org.

Hoffman, M. (1996). *Counseling clients with HIV disease: Assessment, intervention, and prevention.* New York, NY: Guilford.

Hoffman, M. (1997). HIV disease and work: Effect on individual, workplace, and interpersonal contacts. *Journal of Vocational Behavior, 51,* 163–201.

Jackson, R., Purnell, D., & Anderson, S. (1996). The clubhouse model of community support of adults with mental illness: An emerging opportunity for social work education. *Journal of Social Work Education, 32,* 173–180. Retrieved May 9, 2000, from WilsonSelect database (#BEDI96018017. ISSN: 1043–7797) on the World Wide Web: http://firstsearch.oclc.org.

Jacobson, J. (1996). Rehabilitation services for people with mental retardation and psychiatric disabilities: Dilemmas and solutions for public policy. *Journal of Rehabilitation, 62,* 11–22. Retrieved May 9, 2000, from WilsonSelect database (#BSSI96024477.ISSN: 022–4154) on the World Wide Web: http://firstsearch.oclc.org.

Kalichman, S. (1998). *Understanding AIDS: Advances in research and treatment* (2nd ed.). Washington, DC: American Psychological Association.

Kass, N., Munoz, A., Chen, B., Zucconi, S., Bing, E., & Hennessey, M. (1994). Changes in employment, insurance, and income in relation to HIV states and disease progression. *Journal of Acquired Immune Deficiency Syndromes, 7,* 86–91.

Kassel, P. (1991). Psychological and neuropsychological dimensions of HIV illness. In J. Mukand (Ed.), *Rehabilitation for patients with HIV disease* (pp. 217–240). New York, NY: McGraw Hill.

Klosinski (1992). AIDS education and primary prevention. In H. Land (Ed.), *AIDS: A complete guide to psychosocial intervention* (pp. 13–23). Milwaukee, WI: Family Service America.

Kraft, G., Freal, J., & Coryell, J. (1986). Disability, disease duration, and rehabilitation service needs in multiple sclerosis: Patient perspectives [Abstract]. *Archives of Physical Medical Rehabilitation, 67*(3), 164–168. Retrieved May 9, 2000, from Medline, #86158194 on the World Wide Web: http://firstsearch.oclc.org.

Lam, J., & Rosenheck, R. (1999). Social support and service use among homeless persons with serious mental illness. *International Journal of Social Psychiatry, 45*(1), 13–28. Retrieved May 9, 2000, from WilsonSelect database (#BSSI99014839.ISSN: 0020–7640) on the World Wide Web: http://firstsearch.oclc.org.

Malloy, J., M., Cheney, D., & Gail. M. (1998). Interagency collaboration and the transition to adulthood for students with emotional or behavioral disabilities. *Education and Treatment of Children, 21*(3), 303–320. Retrieved May 9, 2000, from WilsonSelect database (#BEDI99005224. ISSN: 0748–8491) on the World Wide Web: http://firstsearch.oclc.org.

Mary, N. (1998). Social work and the support model of services for people with developmental disabilities. *Journal of Social Work Education, 34*(2), 247–260. Retrieved May 9, 2000, from WilsonSelect database (#BEDI98016665. ISSN: 1043–7797) on the World Wide Web: http://firstsearch.oclc.org.

Massagli, M., Weisman, J., Seage, G., & Epstein, A. (1994). Correlates of employment after AIDS diagnosis in a Boston Health Study. *American Journal of Public Health, 84*, 1976–1981.

McNair, J., & Swartz, S. (1997). Local church support to individuals with developmental disability. *Education and Training in Mental Retardation and Developmental Disabilities, 32*(4), 302–312. Retrieved May 9, 2000, from WilsonSelect database (#BEDI98014762. ISSN: 1079–3917) on the World Wide Web: http://firstsearch.oclc.org.

Medrano, L., & Klopner, C. (1992). AIDS and people of color. In H. Land (Ed.), *AIDS: A complete guide to psychosocial intervention* (pp. 117–136). Milwaukee, WI: Family Service America.

Michigan Protection & Service (1998, February). *Your rights in Michigan: Legal rights of people who are HIV+ or living with AIDS* (Revised) (Available from the Michigan Protection & Service, 106 W. Allegan, Suite 300, Lansing, MI 48933–1706, Toll Free 1–800–288–5923.)

Miller, A., & Keys, C. (1996). Awareness, action, and collaboration: How the self-advocacy movement is empowering for persons with developmental disabilities. *Mental Retardation, 36*, 312–319. Retrieved May 9, 2000, from WilsonSelect database (#BEDI96028359.ISSN: 0047–6754) on the World Wide Web: http://firstsearch.oclc.org

Mukand, J., Starkeson, E., & Melvin, J. (1991). Public policy issues for the rehabilitation of patients with HIV-related disability. In J. Mukand (Ed.), *Rehabilitation for patients with HIV disease* (pp. 1–17). New York, NY: McGraw-Hill.

Mulder, C., Antoni, M., Duivenvoorden, H., Kaufmann, R., & Goodkin, K. (1995). Active confrontational coping predicts decreased clinical progression over a one-year period in HIV-infected homosexual men. *Journal of Psychosomatic Research, 39*(8), 957–965.

O'Conner, M. (Ed.) (1997). *Treating the psychological consequences of HIV.* San Francisco, CA: Jossey-Bass.

O'Dowd, M., & Zofnass, J. (1991). Neuropsychiatric and psychosocial factors in the rehabilitation of patients with AIDS. In J. Mukand (Ed.), *Rehabilitation for patients with HIV disease* (pp. 199–215). New York, NY: McGrawHill.

Rabkin, J. (1998). Forward to the second edition. In S. Kalichman (Ed.), *Understanding AIDS: Advances in research and treatment* (2nd ed. pp. xi–xii). Washington, DC: American Psychological Association.

Roberts, G., Becker, H., & Seay, P. (1997). A process for measuring adoption of innovation with the supports paradigm. *Journal of the Association for Persons with Severe Handicaps, 22*, 109–118. Retrieved May 9, 2000, from WilsonSelect database (#BEDI97028745. ISSN: 0749–1425) on the World Wide Web: http://firstsearch.oclc.org

Rosen, D., & Blank, W. (1992). Women and HIV. In H. Land (Ed.), *AIDS: A complete guide to psychosocial intervention* (pp. 141–151). Milwaukee, WI: Family Service America.

Roy, C. (1991). An integrated community and hospital service for adults with physical disability: Two years experience [Abstract]. *New Zealand Medical Journal, 194*(919), 382–384. Retrieved May 9, 2000, from Medline, #92019224 on the World Wide Web: http://firstsearch.oclc.org.

Sands, D., & Doll, B. (1996). Fostering self-determination is a developmental task. *Journal of Special Education, 30*, 58–76. Retrieved May 9, 2000, from WilsonSelect database (#BEDI96012131.ISSN: 022–4669) on the World Wide Web: http://firstsearch.oclc.org

Sebesta, D., & LaPlante, M. (1996). *HIV/AIDS, disability, and employment* (Disability Statistics Report (9)). Washington, DC: U.S. Department of Education, National Institute on Disability and Rehabilitation Research.

Senak, M. (1996). *HIV, AIDS, and the law: A guide to our rights and challenges.* New York, NY: Insight Books.

Social Security Administration (1995, May). *Social security benefits for people living with HIV/AIDS: Fact sheet* (SSA Publication No. 05–10019, May 1995). Washington, DC: U.S. Government Printing Office.

Zlotnik, J. (1987). *AIDS: Helping families cope. Recommendations for meeting the psychosocial needs of persons with AIDS and their families* (Report to the National Institute of Mental Health).

CHAPTER 31

Responding to Mental Health Concerns of People Transitioning from Welfare to Work

Ernestine Moore

INTRODUCTION

Jane Brown is the 46-year-old mother of three children, aged 16, 18, and 20 years. She has relied on public assistance on and off for 12 years. She applied for public assistance two months after the children's father abandoned the family. During the 12 years she has relied on public assistance, she participated in several work readiness and job training programs, obtained jobs and after working six months to a year, was "laid off." Each lay off generated and reinforced a sense of worthlessness and inability to provide for her children. She became so depressed that she had to receive inpatient treatment approximately three years ago. She has not sought or been encouraged to seek employment since her discharge. Her welfare caseworker has included her in the "hard to serve" category. She is being screened for permanent exemption from the Temporary Assistance for Needy Families (TANF) work requirements despite the fact that her disability is not severe enough to qualify for Supplemental Security Income (SSI) benefits. She has been referred for SSI twice and has been found ineligible. At present she is receiving no services designed to assist her in the transition to work.

The history of welfare policy in the United States, beginning with general relief granted by the localities or the states and progressing to federal welfare policy (Aid to Families with Dependent Children (AFDC)), shows a movement away from a policy supporting and encouraging widowed or abandoned mothers staying home to take care of their children to a policy requiring participation in work or work preparation activities for all recipients as a condition of eligibility to receive public assistance. This historical shift will be discussed in greater detail in the next section.

This chapter explores the contemporary welfare policy focus on work as applied to persons coping with mental health issues. Specifically, we will review and discuss how the

---

Ernestine Moore • Wayne State University School of Social Work, Detroit, Michigan.

policies help and/or hinder persons coping with mental health issues secure and/or maintain employment. That review will also include a review and discussion of other public policies, such as SSI, Welfare to Work Grants, Workforce Investment Act, Section 504 of the Rehabilitation Act of 1973, the Americans With Disabilities Act of 1990 (ADA), civil rights protection, and the Final Rule: TANF Program, the administrative rules for the implementation of the law that took effect October 1, 1999, to ensure that persons with mental health issues receive the supports necessary to maximize their abilities to secure productive employment and be assured of continued public welfare support where their earnings do not meet their family's full needs. Finally, we will review and discuss how mental health and rehabilitation issues can be addressed, within the context of PRWORA work requirements, to ensure successful transitions from welfare to work.

The findings leading to the passage of the PRWORA included that the number of recipients had tripled since 1965; more than two thirds of the recipients were children; and 89% of those children lived in homes without fathers (PRWORA, 1996).

In 1996, Olson and Pavetti reported that, based on their review of the current literature 90% of welfare recipients experienced at least one of the following barriers to employment: low basic skills, substance abuse, depression, a child with a chronic illness or disability, or a physical health condition themselves (Olson & Pavetti, 1996).

Some commentators argue that persons with mental illnesses and developmental disabilities should be exempt from all work requirements, while others argue vehemently that to do so subjects persons with mental health issues to lesser access to the benefits of work and lesser personal fulfillment (Kramer, 1998). The author supports the latter approach while recognizing that there are some people with developmental disabilities and mental illnesses who cannot secure and maintain private employment owing to the nature and severity of their disabilities. Jane Brown must be given an opportunity to function in the work world and know that she will not be abandoned by the public welfare system or the mental health system, and will receive full support and encouragement to achieve as much as she is capable of achieving. She is representative of many women receiving TANF. In two years, her youngest child will reach 18 years of age and her eligibility for TANF will end. She has been found ineligible for SSI. Thus, unless her condition becomes more disabling, she will be without public assistance since most states do not provide benefits to single adults not awaiting SSI eligibility determination. With the clock ticking, she requires immediate, concentrated support services not deferral and/or permanent exemption. Securing and maintaining productive employment for her and others similarly challenged is as much the welfare system's and, ultimately, society's challenge to overcome as it is a challenge to the individual recipient with mental health issues.

WELFARE WORK REQUIREMENTS

A discussion of contemporary welfare to work policies and practices necessitates a historical review of welfare policies and practices. Welfare to families in the United States began as a program of the localities, then the joint purview of the localities and the states, and finally of the federal government and the states with the passage of the Social Security Act of 1935 (Bell, 1965). As stated above, the welfare policy framework has shifted from one providing economic support so that widowed and abandoned mothers could stay home and raise their children to one that has encouraged, supported, and required participation in job training/job preparation activities and ultimately work for all recipients.

This shift started in 1939 when the more deserving mothers, namely widowed, were included in the Social Security survivors' program. This inclusion of widows in the survivors' program left mostly divorced or never married mothers on the welfare rolls by the late 1940s. These mothers were perceived as less deserving of public support than widowed mothers.

The connection of work and welfare in the form of work requirements as a condition of eligibility had its earliest formal governmental support in the 1940s. States, particularly in the South, having the authority to determine who was deserving of welfare assistance, refused to extend aid to Black women arguing that they could be employed as field hands/laborers or domestic workers for which there was great demand. Their income from employment would be more than that on welfare, and thus they and their children would be better off. The 1950s saw the general public becoming more vocal with their concern that welfare was no longer available to widowed mothers, but increasingly was, in their minds, supporting mothers who were unfit because of the illegitimacy of their children. In response to the perceived "crisis in welfare," the social service amendments of 1962 provided for federal government reimbursement of an additional 25% of the state costs for administering the AFDC program if the state implemented rehabilitation programs targeted at reducing the barriers to employment for current recipients. Several states implemented counseling and employment services programs. The overall results were insignificant (Abramovitz, 1995; Trattner, 1974, 1989; Piven & Cloward, 1971).

The Work Incentive Program (WIN) was adopted in the Social Security Act amendments of 1967. Work participation became a condition of eligibility for AFDC with the 1967 amendments, and with 1971 amendments, sanctions were added for non-participation. However, the appropriations were never sufficient to serve all recipients. The WIN required states to assess current recipients in a priority order with unemployed fathers and children over 16 years of age mandated for assessment. Mothers who were already participating in job training programs under the Economic Opportunity Act (Title V), or mothers with no pre-school children who volunteered but were not in a training program, were next in order of assessment. Needless to say, there was insufficient funding to assess all recipients. Furthermore, those assessed and served did not receive the childcare, transportation, work placement, and social services supports originally contemplated in the legislation. Thus again there was disappointment in the outcomes (Abramovitz, 1995; Trattner, 1974, 1999; Piven & Cloward, 1971).

Despite limited success with the work programs attempted from 1962 until 1980, the Omnibus Budget Reconciliation Act of 1981 strengthened the AFDC work requirements and the 1988 Family Support Act, and its Jobs Opportunities and Basic Skills Training (JOBS) program, solidified the change in AFDC program policy from a support so that mothers could stay at home to raise their children to one that required work participation. These two changes laid the foundation for the PRWORA, Public Law 104-193, the law that currently governs the work requirements for recipients of TANF, the new name for AFDC.

From this historical review, the reader should be clear that the federal welfare policy has had a work focus since 1962. What is unique about PRWORA is that the included recipients are all recipients of TANF who are not included in a temporary or permanent exemption category by the states (which is capped at 20% of caseload); the states benefit from recipients securing and maintaining employment and suffer penalties if they do not achieve established work participation goals; and there is a maximum lifetime limit on receipt of federal welfare benefits, namely 60 months unless the adult in the grant is included in the 20% of average monthly caseload exemption cap. This full inclusion of all recipients, tempered with the 20% caseload exemption to allow for extenuating circumstances of the states and/or the recipients, with a "carrot and stick" approach applied to both program administrators and TANF recipients, is the one thing that appears to be making a difference in the short term. In the first full year of implementation, all states met their work participation requirements except, for the two-parent family work participation requirements. The work participation rate for two-parent families is set much higher than the one-parent family requirement (25% for one-parent families and 75% for two-parent families in 1997, respectively) (Relave, 1999).

The pertinent sections of PRWORA related to work requirements are stated here to provide the reader with the necessary background to understand the subsequent discussion. In addition, the administrative rules related to these work requirements that were effective October 1, 1999, will be discussed following the sections of PRWORA. The reader should be aware that there are several other matters addressed in PRWORA and the administrative rules implementing PRWORA that are not discussed here. Given the space limitations of this chapter, any other sections that have bearing on understanding the work requirements sections will be summarized rather than cited at the appropriate point in the discussion. The interplay of PRWORA and SSI, Welfare to Work Grants, Workforce Investment Act, Section 504 of the Rehabilitation Act of 1973, and the ADA will be discussed in the section on alleviating mental health issues in the transition from welfare to work.

Section 407(a)(7)(A) establishes the urgency to move forward on work. It states

> A state to which a grant is made shall not use any part of the grant to provide assistance to a family that includes an adult who has received assistance under any State program funded under this part attributable to funds provided by the Federal Government, for 60 months (whether or not consecutive) after the date the State program funded under this part commences, subject to this paragraph.

To reduce the harshness of this provision, it goes on to provide that

> The state may exempt a family from the application of subparagraph (A) by reason of hardship or if the family includes an individual who has been battered or subjected to extreme cruelty (Section 407(a)(7)(C)(i).

But not wanting to give the states an opportunity to overexempt and, by default, to shift from the work/self-sufficiency focus, it limits the total number of exemptions to "20% of the average monthly number of families to which assistance is provided under the State program funded under this part" (Section 407(a)(7)(C)(ii)).

The specific work requirements sections of PRWORA are

- Section 401. Purpose
  The purpose of this part is to increase the flexibility of the States in operating a program designed to—... (2) end the dependence of needy parents on government benefits by promoting job preparation, work, and marriage; ... (110 STAT. 2113, 42 USC 601).
- Section 402. Eligible States; State Plan

  (i) Conduct a program, designed to serve all political subdivisions in the State (not necessarily in a uniform manner), that provides assistance to needy families with (or expecting) children and provides parents with job preparation, work, and support services to enable them to leave the program and become self-sufficient.
  (ii) Require a parent or caretaker receiving assistance under the program to engage in work (as defined by the State) once the State determines the parent or caretaker is ready to engage in work, or once the parent or caretaker has received assistance under the program for 24 months (whether or not consecutive), whichever is earlier.
  (iii) Ensure that parents and caretakers receiving assistance under the program engage in work activities in accordance with section 407 (110 STAT. 2113, 42 USC 602).

- Section 407. Mandatory Work Requirements.
  (a)–(c) ...

(d) Work Activities Defined. As used in this section, the term "work activities" means—

(1) unsubsidized employment;

(2) subsidized private sector employment;

(3) subsidized public sector employment;

(4) work experience (including work associated with the refurbishing of publicly assisted housing) if sufficient private sector employment is not available;

(5) on-the-job training;

(6) job search and job readiness assistance;

(7) community service programs;

(8) vocational educational training (not to exceed 12 months with respect to any individual);

(9) job skills training directly related to employment;

(10) education directly related to employment, in the case of a recipient who has not received a high school diploma or a certificate of high school equivalency;

(11) satisfactory attendance at secondary school or in a course of study leading to a certificate of general equivalence, in the case of a recipient who has not completed secondary school or received such a certificate; and

(12) the provision of childcare services to an individual who is participating in a community service program (110 STAT. 2133, 42 USC 607).

Minimum work participation rates were established by the legislation. Beginning in fiscal year 1997, they are 25% of caseload and increasing 5% per fiscal year to a 50% participation rate for 2002 and thereafter for all families. Two-parent minimum work participation rates were established at 75% for fiscal years 1997 and 1998 and 90% for fiscal year 1999 and thereafter (110 STAT. 2129, 42 USC 607). These are the rates that states must meet in order to avoid monetary penalties. The rates are calculated using complex formulas stated in the legislation that are not necessary to an understanding of the topic of this chapter.

- Section 408(b) Individual Responsibility Plans

(1) Assessment.—The State agency responsible for administering the State program funded under this part shall make an initial assessment of the skills, prior work experience, and employability of each recipient of assistance under the program who—

(A) has attained 18 years of age; or

(B) has not completed high school or obtained a certificate of high school equivalence, and is not attending secondary school.

(2) Contents of Plans.—

(A) In General.—On the basis of the assessment made under subsection (a) with respect to the individual, the State agency, in consultation with the individual, may develop an individual responsibility plan for the individual, which—

(i) sets forth an employment goal for the individual and a plan for moving the individual immediately into private sector employment;

(ii) sets forth the obligations of the individual which may include a requirement that the individual attend school, maintain certain grades and attendance, keep school age children of the individual in school, immunize children, attend parenting and money management classes, or do other things that will help the individual become and remain employed in the private sector;

(iii) to the greatest extent possible is designed to move the individual into whatever private sector employment the individual is capable of handling as quickly as possible, and to increase the responsibility and amount of work the individual is to handle over time;

(iv) describes the services the State will provide the individual so that the individual will be able to obtain and keep employment in the private sector, and describe the job counseling and other services that will be provided by the State; and

(v) may require the individual to undergo appropriate substance abuse treatment (110 STAT. 2141, 42 USC 608).

These individual responsibility plans (IRPs) are to be completed within 30 days of eligibility determination.

The Final Rule: Temporary Assistance for Needy Families (TANF) Program effective October 1, 1999, addresses work requirements, time limits, state penalties, and data collection and reporting requirements. The pertinent rules for work requirements essentially reiterate the statutory requirements enumerated above. In its summary statement of the rule, the Department of Health and Human Services states

> States may define many key terms, including the activities that count as work (within the limits of the statute). By not defining these terms ourselves, we are giving States overall flexibility to design their programs in a way that will address their unique needs and circumstances (U.S. DHHS, 1998, p. 3).

The rules provide for the 20% exemption cap, which permits states, at their option, to define certain families as having hardships that preclude the adult member from engaging in the work requirements and thereby to continue federal assistance to those families after the adult member has received 60 months of assistance.

It is important to remember throughout the discussion of work requirements for recipients with mental health issues that neither the PRWORA legislation nor the Final Rule provided for categorical exemption of such persons from work requirements; but they did provide for a 20% of caseload exemption for reasons enumerated in the individual state plans and accepted by the Secretary of Health and Human Services. Thus, families whose adult care-taker experiences mental health issues that are not severe enough to qualify him or her for SSI or Social Security Disability payments, and thus change the TANF case to a "child only" case (i.e., a case where the adult is not a member or recipient of TANF funds), are still required to meet the work requirements unless there are specific individual exemptions after individual personal responsibility assessment.

As of January 1999, 24 states had exempted persons with disabilities from time limits. Many advocates argued that the states should not unilaterally exempt these families, but should differentially assess and offer services to help them become more employable (Kramer, 1999). In response to arguments from these advocates, the HHS Office of Civil Rights issued a policy guidance in August 1999 clarifying the application of civil rights laws, specifically Section 504 of the Rehabilitation Act of 1973 and Title II of the ADA, in the context of welfare reform policies and practices. In January 2001 it issued another policy guidance:

> in response to the myriad of additional questions that have been raised by State agencies, counties, serv-
> ice providers, and persons with disabilities regarding the obligations to adopt methods for administer-
> ing welfare programs to ensure equal opportunity for persons with disabilities in all aspects of a TANF
> program, including applications, assessments, work program activities, sanctions, and time limits. This
> guidance also is necessary because the Department has indicated that States may be subject to penal-
> ties if audits show that they "over-sanction", i.e., impose sanctions on individuals when sanctions are
> inappropriate (HHS Policy Guidance January 2001, www.hhs.gov./ocr/prohibition.html, p. 5).

The January 2001 Policy Guidance reiterates the legal framework governing non-discrimination in administration of federally financed programs. Specific to the administration of TANF involving persons with disabilities, it requires state, local government entities, and any other entities that receive federal funding for TANF activities to provide individualized treatment and effective and meaningful opportunity to participate in all aspects of programming offered to individuals who do not have disabilities.

The definition of "disability" is the more inclusive one found in the Americans with Disabilities Act and Section 504 of the Rehabilitation Act of 1973: "a physical or mental impairment that substantially limits one or more of the major life activities of such individual, a record of such an impairment, or being regarded as having such an impairment" (28 C.F.R. Section 35.104). This definition is different from that used for SSI and Social Security

Disability Insurance (SSDI) programs. Thus, there will be reasons why some persons will be disabled for TANF purposes, but not qualify for SSI or SSDI.

The Policy Guidance states that

> individualized treatment requires that individuals with disabilities be treated on a case-by-case basis consistent with facts and objective evidence. Individuals with disabilities may not be treated on the basis of generalizations and stereotypes. Such prohibited treatment would include denying TANF beneficiaries with disabilities access to parts of the TANF agency's program based on the stereotypical view, unsupported by any individual assessment, that people with disabilities are unable to participate in anything but the most rudimentary work activities.

In the next section we will discuss some identified mental health issues that cause barriers to employment and the application of PRWORA provisions, administrative rules, and the Policy Guidance to these situations.

MENTAL HEALTH ISSUES IN THE TRANSITION FROM WELFARE TO WORK: MAKING PRWORA WORK FOR THOSE WITH MENTAL HEALTH ISSUES

Zedlewski (1999a, p. 4) commented, "Many observers expect that, as states move further along in welfare reform and their caseloads shrink, the remaining recipients will be increasingly disadvantaged because those with fewest obstacles to work will have left the rolls first." However, the responses of TANF recipients who participated in the 1997 National Survey of America's Families (NSAF) who resided in Michigan and Wisconsin, the two states implementing welfare reform initiatives in 1994 and 1995, respectively, that had provisions consistent with those required by PRWORA, were less likely to report multiple obstacles to work than in those states implementing changes to comply with PRWORA in 1997 (Zedlewski, 1999). This result would argue against the hypothesis that those who have multiple barriers to employment would clog the caseloads as the 60-month time limit approached.

However, while many others have made similar projections, one of the significant barriers to strategy development for services to assist hard to serve welfare recipients is lack of specific data on the nature, scope, severity, and interrelationship of their personal barriers to their ability to secure and maintain work. Research in the foreseeable future will need to be refined to such an extent that this level of data is extracted using multiple methodologies.

The 1997 NSAF found that 40% of the respondents reported three obstacles to work: low education, lack of work experience, mental or physical health problems. Yet it also found that in those states with more stringent work-focused welfare provisions before PRWORA a large proportion of the respondents reported working irrespective of these obstacles. With respect to mental health issues, the NSAF found that 48% of the respondents had poor mental health or poor general health and 32% had very poor mental health. In this particular study, poor and very poor mental health were derived from the responses of TANF recipients to five questions asking them to rate their mental health in relation to anxiety, depression, loss of control, and psychological well-being. They were categorized as having poor mental health if they fell in the bottom 20% of respondents, and categorized as having very poor mental health if they fell in the bottom 10% of respondents (Zedlewski, 1999b). These data are not definitive as to the nature, scope, and severity of the mental health issues. Implementing effective strategies to move as many people with mental health issues from welfare to work requires more specific data.

Based on published studies to date, the predominant mental health issues for welfare recipients appear to be depression, bipolar disorder, post-traumatic stress disorder (generally associated with domestic violence), anxiety disorder, agoraphobia, and borderline mental retardation. The incidence of mental health issues amongst welfare recipients or former recipients reported in these studies range from 6% to 42% (Kramer, 1998, 1999; Pavetti, Olson, Nightingale, Duke, & Issacs, 1997; Zedlewski, 1999). Unfortunately, at this early stage in research on PRWORA implementation and impact, the methodological weaknesses, including differences in definitions, samples, and survey techniques, are so severe that conclusive statements are impossible.

The focus of this section is to answer this question: What is necessary to assist recipients with these mental health issues, however defined, become work ready, obtain and maintain employment? The reader is referred to other chapters for detailed discussions of mental health treatment, general rehabilitation tools, and models of employment support for persons with mental health issues. This chapter focuses on using PRWORA provisions and the Policy Guidance to accommodate the special needs of persons with mental health issues while assisting them to meet the work requirements.

People with mental health issues work every day in jobs ranging from low-skill–low-pay to highly-skilled–highly-paid. Thus, there should be no blanket assumption that TANF recipients who present with mental health issues cannot be rehabilitated sufficiently so that they can secure and maintain productive employment in the private and/or public sectors.

Assessment is an important cornerstone of individual responsibility plans and for those eligible recipients it includes the appraisal of skills, prior work experience and employability. The contents of individual responsibility plans incorporate an employment goal guiding the movement of the recipient into competitive, private sector employment, and identifies the "obligations of the individual" including school attendance and performance, school participation of children, and participation in self-management classes. The stipulations are broad enough to include other requirements the state program deems necessary for recipients entering and maintaining employment. The plan is time-sensitive and requires the movement of the person into employment quickly with the attainment of the necessary productivity and work expectations to maintain a job successfully. The plans must identify those services the state program will provide to the recipient and requires involvement in substance abuse treatment if this is necessary.

In addition to the assessment and the individual responsibility plan, PRWORA identifies a range of mandatory work requirements within Section 407. These work activities include a full spectrum of alternatives including subsidized and unsubsidized forms of employment, and some forms of vocational development including job search and job readiness assistance, vocational educational training, and education relevant to the achievement of an employment outcome. PRWORA is employment-driven and incorporates those elements of readiness and social services that are relevant to the achievement of a specific employment outcome in a time sensitive manner. Thus, recipients must develop a strong orientation to work, and must embrace the performance requirements of PRWORA.

The assessment and individual responsibility plan, on face, do not appear flexible for individuals coping with mental health issues. However, utilizing the provisions of PRWORA, a three-step model of intervention is feasible. This model incorporates: (1) mental health screening into assessment, (2) identified mental health issues as barriers that the individual responsibility plan must address through appropriate referral, services, and coordination, and (3) the use of non-subsidized employment to facilitate the readiness of those individuals coping with mental health issues. More specifically, these modifications can be incorporated into PRWORA in the following way to facilitate the responsiveness of employment for those individuals who are coping with serious mental health issues:

Step 1: *Individual Assessment.* This step involves screening the recipient for mental health issues, broadly defined, as part of the assessment required within 30 days of finding eligibility; determining the impact of the mental health issues on the recipient's capability to understand and adhere to the PRWORA requirements; determining if the recipient might have a condition that qualifies her for SSI benefits and, if so, making the appropriate referrals, assisting with application requirements and authorizing a deferral from work requirements pending determination of SSI eligibility; and determining the impact of the condition on the recipient's ability to participate in work activities as defined in PRWORA and the state plan.

Step 2: *IRPs.* This step involves, for those recipients not referred to SSI after Step 1 or for those recipients referred to SSI but who are found ineligible for benefits, the establishment of an IRP. The IRP should be tailored to alleviate the barriers to employability identified in Step 1. The state is permitted, in consultation with the recipient, to set forth the obligations of the individual and these obligations can include "or do other things that will help the individual become and remain employed in the private sector." Furthermore, IRPs should be designed "to the greatest extent possible ... to increase the responsibility and amount of work the individual is to handle over time" and "should describe the services the State will provide the individual." PRWORA list several "work activities" that are appropriate to the recipient with mental health issues: work experience, job search and job readiness assistance, subsidized private or public sector employment, and community service programs. The specific work activity and sequencing of activities should be constructed to provide for incremental successes upon which the recipient builds to achieve the final success—unsubsidized employment. Supportive mental health services should continue at the intervals necessary to assist the transition.

Step 3: *Non-subsidized Employment.* This step involves assisting the recipient in securing employment that pays a living wage without TANF or Welfare to Work subsidies. This is the most desirable work outcome. Depending on the nature and severity of the mental health issues and the duration of and skills derived from the subsidized and supported sequencing of work activities in Step 2, the recipient may or may not continue to need supportive mental health services beyond a short transition period of 30–60 days. However, these services stop only when the recipient feels comfortable.

Assuming that the mental health issues identified at the beginning of this section, namely depression, bipolar disorder, post traumatic stress disorder, agoraphobia, anxiety disorder, and mild mental retardation, are the presenting mental health issues for TANF recipients, program administrators need to know what impact those disorders have on the recipient's ability to comply with work requirements, and then establish IRPs that provide the supportive services in the dosages and in the sequencing necessary to promote success.

For example, we know that depression changes behavior, appearance, performance, and the ability to handle everyday decisions and pressures. However, 80% of all persons with depression can be treated effectively with outpatient counseling and medication (National Institutes of Health, 1997). In a PRWORA context then, the strategy would be to

1. Screen all recipients for depression and, if the screening shows a probability of depression, refer the recipient for complete evaluation, diagnosis and treatment. Depending on the nature, scope, and severity of the depression as well as the response to medication, determine the timing of inclusion in other work requirement activities.

2. Engage the recipient in work readiness activities, including specific job training, once the recipient appears to have relief of the depressive symptoms.
3. Place the recipient in a work setting with continuing support from the welfare worker, therapist, and employer once the recipient appears to have relief of the depressive symptoms.

Bipolar disorders or manic-depressive illness is marked by episodes of mania (i.e., extreme highs) and depression (i.e., sadness, hopelessness, suicidal threats) with times of normal behaviors and emotions. These disorders are treatable with medication. Unfortunately, many persons with bipolar disorders do not recognize that they have an illness and refuse treatment (National Institutes of Health, 1995). Belligerent attitudes and behaviors are strong impediments to gainful employment. If the recipient can be diagnosed and complies with medication orders, the mood swings are greatly controlled and employment is feasible. The challenge is to get compliance with medication orders. In a PRWORA context then, the strategy would be to

1. Place the recipient in a job preparation program that includes medication administering if the recipient is non-compliant. The plan should be to phase out the medication administration as the recipient grows to understand the benefits of the medication and the success symbolized in personally administering it.
2. Utilize community service programs or work experience programs to determine the "work readiness" of the recipient.
3. Progress to subsidized/unsubsidized job placements as the recipient demonstrates tolerance to the challenges in the work environment.
4. Continue to provide medication monitoring and outpatient mental health treatment services.

The author's experience as a public welfare caseworker and administrator, coupled with preliminary findings from surveys of welfare caseworkers, leads to the conclusion that to make PRWORA work for persons with mental health issues that are not severe enough to qualify them for SSI requires that the system

1. Provide public welfare caseworkers with training and tools for preliminary screening of all recipients for mental health issues, not necessarily mental health diagnoses, that might be a barrier to participation in work requirements. Public welfare caseworkers have varying educational backgrounds. They need to have the knowledge to be able to identify, with the recipient, the individual barriers to employment and methodically establish a plan to eliminate those barriers.
2. Establish an integrated, collaborative system of mental health agencies, vocational rehabilitation agencies, and local employment support agencies along with the TANF agency to more appropriately and effectively serve recipients with mental health issues. TANF agencies are not the designated mental health agencies in most states; yet a significant proportion of the TANF recipients are eligible for mental health services. Few states have created seamless systems of care between the welfare and mental health systems. The same is true of TANF agency relationships with vocational rehabilitation and employment support agencies. If the TANF agency is to be successful in assisting persons with mental health issues to secure employment, then this seamless system is necessary.
3. Develop a system of public agencies and mental health friendly private agencies as personal preparation and training sites for persons with mental health issues. Both the TANF agencies and the individual recipients need success. A few public and private agencies that understand the unique needs of persons with mental health issues in work environments are

critical to providing "safe places" in which the recipient can "practice" appropriate work behaviors and secure additional work skills, both interpersonal and technical.

CONCLUSIONS

The majority of persons with mental health issues who are receiving TANF funds and who will continue to receive TANF funds for the full 60-month lifetime limit will not be eligible for ADA protections in actual employment given the narrowing of the scope of the ADA by the U.S. Supreme Court in three decisions issued June 22, 1999. Those decisions, *Sutton* v. *United Air Lines, Inc., Murphy* v. *United Parcel Service, Inc.*, and *Albertsons, Inc.* v. *Kirkingburg*, in summary, state that where a condition is correctable by medication or other measures, then it is not a protected condition under the ADA. If the TANF recipient's condition was not correctable by medication or other measures, then he/she would be eligible for SSI/SSDI benefits and, even though receiving TANF benefits for children residing with him/her, would not be subject to the PRWORA work requirements.

TANF recipients with mental health issues can and should benefit from PRWORA's work requirements. There must be recognition of the additional supports and time needed to help them become work ready and the need to provide mental health supportive service as they transition into work environments. PRWORA provides the opportunity for these additional supports and additional time for receipt of TANF benefits. The issue is whether or not individual states want to adopt these flexibilities into their state plans or choose, as 24 of them have already, to provide a blanket exemption from work requirements for persons who present with mental health issues.

Clearly, there are lessons to be learned from the supported employment movement of the 1980s and 1990s to ensure that persons with disabilities or mental illnesses are not unilaterally judged to be "exempt" from the TANF work requirements. They are very important as applied to persons who are ineligible for SSI benefits and whose children will attain adulthood in the next three to five years, making them ineligible for TANF assistance. Many states have eliminated state or county funded public assistance for adults except as temporary bridges while SSI eligibility is being determined. Without any skills, those persons with disabilities failing to meet the SSI definition will have no source of support. With increased supports now such as substance abuse and mental health treatment, as well as job skill development, most would be able to obtain and maintain employment.

Kramer 1999 suggests that vocational rehabilitation and mental health agencies with programs—"which tolerate long duration of training and employment services not consistent with TANF's time limits"—should become cornerstones of a collaborative relationship with the TANF agency. Furthermore, she suggests that: "TANF programs that have specially trained workers or contract specialists in-house, or who co-locate with mental health, VR, or substance abuse treatment providers may increase the opportunities for collegial or team consultation on individual cases, reduce the need for formal referrals, and enhance the chances for cooperation of reluctant clients" (Kramer, 1999, p. 5).

REFERENCES

Abramovitz, M. (1992). *Regulating the lives of women: Social welfare policy from colonial times to the present.* Boston, MA: South End Press.

Abramovitz, M. (1995). Aid to families with dependent children. In *Encyclopedia of Social Work* (19th ed., pp. 183–194. Washington, DC: National Association of Social Workers.

Bell, W. (1965). *Aid to dependent children.* New York, NY: Columbia University Press.

Kramer, F. D. (1998, March). The hard-to-place: Understanding the population and strategies to serve them. *Welfare Information Network Issue Notes, 2*(5).

Kramer, F. D. (1999, January). Serving welfare recipients with disabilities. *Welfare Information Network Issue Notes, 3*(1).

Olson, K., & Pavetti, L. (1996, May 17). *Personal and family challenges to the successful transition from welfare to work* (Project report). Washington, DC: The Urban Institute.

Pavetti, L., Olson, K., Nightingale, D., Duke, A., and Issacs, J. (August 1997). Welfare-to-work options for families facing personal and family challenges: rationale and program strategies. Washington, DC: The Urban Institute.

Piven, F. F., & Cloward, R. A. (1971). *Regulating the poor: The functions of public welfare.* New York, NY: Random House.

Relave, N. (1999). Moving from welfare-to-work: An overview of work participation issues (Compiled from the WIN website). *Welfare Information Network Issue Notes, 3*(7).

Trattner, W. I. (1974). *From poor law to welfare state: A history of social welfare in America.* New York, NY: The Free Press.

Trattner, W. I. (1984). *From poor law to welfare state: A history of social welfare in America* (4th ed.). New York, NY: The Free Press.

Trattner, W. I. (1999). *From poor law to welfare state: A history of social welfare in America* (6th ed.). New York, NY: Simon & Schuster Publishing Group.

U.S. Department of Health and Human Services (1998). *Temporary assistance for needy families, 1936–1998.* Washington, DC: HHS Administration for Children and Families.

Zedlewski, S. R. (1999a). *Work activity and obstacles to work among TANF recipients* (Report No. B-2 in Series: New Federalism: National Survey of American Families). Washington, DC: The Urban Institute.

Zedlewski, S. R. (1999b). *Work-related activities and limitations of current welfare recipients.* (Report No. 99-06 in Assessing the New Federalism: An Urban Institute Program to Assess Changing Social Policies). Washington, DC: The Urban Institute.

CHAPTER 32

Mental Health and Rehabilitation Issues in the Employment of Women

ARLENE N. WEISZ AND BEVERLY M. BLACK

Women facing mental health issues must grapple with the multiple consequences of these issues as well as with the consequences of being members of the less-powerful gender in our society. Being the subordinate gender has multiple consequences for these women economically, psychologically, socially, and in terms of safety, health care, and mental health care.

GENDER ROLES

Gender roles stereotyping involves expectations about how people should behave based on gender. Gender roles stereotyping begins at birth for boys and girls and often limits people's alternatives. Parents communicate differently with their sons and daughters; both parents and teachers vary in their expectations of girls and boys (Lott, 1994). Although pre-adolescent boys tend to feel more heavily pressured by sex role stereotypes than girls do (Pogrebin, 1980), both males and females view female sex role characteristics (nurturing, supportive, emotional) as less desirable than male characteristics (powerful, courageous, strong). Research suggests that at adolescence girls tend to become more hesitant, doubtful, and afraid to trust their own perceptions (Brown & Gilligan, 1992).

Gender sex role stereotyping creates disadvantages for women in several areas. Our culture gives women the message that they must be very thin, girlish, and passive. The media is full of portrayals of women as decorative objects that active men admire or act upon (Kaschak, 1992). Many women spend a great deal of time and energy worrying about their appearances, and the goal of the perfect body contributes to mental health problems such as anorexia and bulimia. Women with mental health problems may have particular difficulties

ARLENE N. WEISZ AND BEVERLY M. BLACK • Wayne State University School of Social Work, Detroit, Michigan.

living up to the media ideals of beauty, since mental illnesses and medications used to treat them may affect women's appearances.

Numerous studies demonstrate that sex discrimination persists in the United States. Discrimination exists in areas such as health care research (coronary, AIDS) access to drug treatment facilities, salary discrimination, and sexual harassment (Landrine & Klonoff, 1997).

Sexist discrimination plays an important role in the mental health of women, regardless of how an individual woman appraises that discrimination. Landrine and Klonoff (1997) found that sexist discrimination contributes to physical and psychiatric symptoms whether women subjectively appraise sexist acts as stressful or dismiss them as inconsequential. Thus, it is not a woman's high or extreme personal subjective appraisal of or response to sexist behavior but rather the presence and frequency of that sexist behavior that is related to symptoms among women. Landrine and Klonoff (1997) also found that sexist events had an even "greater negative impact on non-feminists than on feminists, even though feminists appraised such events as more stressful and reported more of such events" (p. 118).

Landrine and Klonoff conclude that:

> non-feminists find sexist events stressful because they interpret the events as their own fault, and their appraisal ratings may increase with the degree of self-blaming entailed in the sexist discrimination. Feminists find sexist events stressful because they are inherently unfair and their appraisal ratings may increase with the degree of blatant injustice entailed in sexist discrimination. Thus, the appraisals of stressful events play a major role in the symptoms of non-feminists but no role whatsoever in the symptoms of feminists—despite feminists having higher appraisal scores (p. 118).

Landrine and Klonoff (1997) found that sexist events had an even greater negative impact on the physical and mental health of women of color than on the physical and mental health of white women. This occurred because women of color experienced sexist events more often. Landrine and Klonoff found "sexism accounted for 46% of the variance in depression among women of color and only 9% of the variance among white women" (p. 118).

ECONOMIC ISSUES

Perhaps nowhere is discrimination more evident than in the workplace. Women earn about 70% of what men earn. Women earn less than men when doing the same kind of job and with the same level of education and experience (Lott, 1994). Women of color are significantly more disadvantaged than white women. Regardless of educational level, Hispanic women earn less than African American women do; both groups earn less than white women do. For all races, women with four years of college earn less than 4% more than men with only four years of high school.

Sex discrimination in the workplace influences more than salaries. Today the discrimination is generally subtle or covert (Swim & Cohen, 1997). Employers' negative or limited responses to requests for pregnancy or maternity leave are often a sign of discrimination. Glass ceilings also prevent women's advancement to higher levels of financial remuneration and power, and glass walls limit their access to particular professional specialties and higher paying blue-collar jobs (Landrine & Klonoff, 1997). The military prohibits women from some positions—those that are often high paying and important steps for career advancement.

The influence of sex role stereotyping on older women in the workplace is especially evident. Although three quarters of women between the ages of 25 and 54 are in the labor force, only about two thirds of the women over age 54 are in the labor force. The drop off has been attributed to workplace discrimination and disruptions due to elder care responsibilities falling primarily to the responsibility of women (Doress-Worters, 1994).

Many research studies suggest that work can have salutary effects on women's health, self-esteem, and overall well-being (Thomas, 1997). Work can serve as a buffer against stress arising from other roles (Baruch, Biener, & Barnett, 1987). However, when women's employment status is incompatible with their desires concerning work, poorer physical and mental health is the result (Waldron & Herold, 1986). Thomas (1997) also found that women's work experiences are generally less satisfying than men's. The combination of high demand and low control typical of most women's employment is related to the highest levels of stress (Bowman & Stern, 1995).

What is critical is the perceived quality of the work experience, not simply an assessment of occupancy of the role of worker. It is not enough to ask women if they are employed and the nature of their tasks. To comprehend the impact of their work roles on health variables, it is also important to assess the distressing and rewarding experiences of the job.

Nationally, female-headed households make up the majority of the nation's poor (Queralt, 1996). Many women with mental health problems have so few economic and social resources that they end up homeless (Bachrach, 1988a). Because family responsibilities often interrupt their job or career tracks, women end up with lower wages and lower status jobs. Since women's jobs often require less training and carry fewer responsibilities, their employers are less willing to hold their jobs for them after absences related to mental health problems.

Women are frequently single parents, which plays a large role in keeping them in the lower socioeconomic classes. Divorced women lose income after separation, and child support still goes unpaid in many cases (Queralt, 1996). The lack of economic resources can lead to or aggravate mental health problems. A study by the Commonwealth Fund reported that poor women, single women with children, and women without social support were more likely to report depressive symptoms than other women (Collins et al., 1999).

CARE-TAKING/HOUSEHOLD RESPONSIBILITIES

Gender role stereotyping and sexist discrimination lead to additional life stressors for women. Russo (1995) identified two general types of gender-specific stressors that tend to erode women's mental health. The first are role-related stressors, including multiple role strain, role overload, and role conflict. Russo's research suggests that multiple roles require more time than women have—yet it is when these roles conflict in ways different from how they conflict for men that women's greatest stress occurs. The second type of gender-specific stressors is physical, gender-specific stressors—all forms of violence against women. Although previous studies have suggested that major life events and especially daily hassles were good predictors of psychiatric symptoms, Russo's study found that sexist discrimination was a more powerful predictor of psychiatric and physical symptoms among women than generic stress.

Women experience higher levels of generic stressful life events than men do, which plays a role in their mental health—especially depression and anxiety disorders. In addition, women experience stress differently than men. Thomas (1997) questioned over 500 women about the greatest stress in their lives. Women reported vicarious stress most prominently—from a son's divorce to a mother's terminal illness. Women clearly appear to take on the burdens of others. This is consistent with the conception of women's "sense of self" as in relation to others (Gilligan, 1982).

Most women who have male partners still end up performing the majority of the household tasks, such as cleaning, shopping, etc. and if there are children involved, they do most of the childcare (Hochschild, 1989). Some research suggests that women with chronic mental illnesses find motherhood especially stressful (Bachrach, 1988b). The stress on a woman who is struggling with mental health problems, a paid job, and household responsibilities can be intense. However, one study of women six months after discharge from psychiatric treatment noted no differences between the level of functioning and service use between women who worked and had major household responsibilities and women who worked without major household responsibilities (Goering, Cochrane, Potasznik, Wasylenki, & Lancee, 1988). This suggests a high level of resiliency according to the researchers, since many of the women were able to cope with multiple responsibilities after an acute illness.

When mothers with mental health problems and young children wish to enter a rehabilitation program or return to work, they must find suitable childcare. This can be a daunting problem for any woman. It may be especially difficult for more fragile, less assertive women, since high-quality, affordable day care is scarce. In addition, entry-level jobs that are available to women with mental health problems are often available at unconventional times, rather than the daytime hours that most day care programs offer.

Women are the majority of care-takers for sick or elderly relatives. The Commonwealth Fund report on women's health (Collins et al., 1999) reports that "nine percent, or more than nine million women, are currently caring for a sick or disabled family member, often devoting 20 hours or more to provide supportive care" (p. 3). Only 4% of men reported doing this type of care-taking. Having these responsibilities adds stress for women with mental health problems and can interfere with recovery. When women are unable to fulfill care-taking responsibilities, they often feel inadequate and guilty.

Women who have taken time out of the paid workforce to stay home and raise children may have special difficulties rejoining the paid workforce, because they feel very insecure about whether they have marketable skills. Being diagnosed with a mental illness may make these women even more insecure about their employment prospects.

VIOLENCE AGAINST WOMEN

Based on data from victims, police reports, and hospital data, the Bureau of Justice Statistics estimates that women in the United States experienced victimization by an intimate at a rate of 8 per 1,000 women between 1992 and 1996 (Greenfeld et al., 1998). The rate for men was 1 out of 1,000. The recent Commonwealth Fund report on women's health (Collins et al., 1999) reports that 39% of 2,850 women surveyed in a community sample had been victimized by violence or abuse during their lifetimes. Thirty-one percent of the sample had experienced domestic violence by a partner or spouse. Nine percent of women reported being raped or sexually assaulted during their lives. Young women are the most frequent targets of rape (Koss, Giarretto, & Wisniewski, 1987), and someone known to the victim, very often perpetrates it (Koss et al., 1987). Women are much more frequently victimized by child sexual abuse than men (Barnett, Miller-Perrin, & Perrin, 1997). Child sexual abuse is frequently associated with mental health problems for victims during adult life (Barnett et al., 1997).

Women are more vulnerable than the majority of males in our society to rape and other physical attacks, because they are usually weaker and less schooled in aggressive tactics. Therefore, homeless women with mental illnesses are especially vulnerable and exposed.

In our society, women who are lucky enough to escape victimization are usually aware of the high rates of violence against women. Fear of street crimes and home invasions causes women to be very cautious, frequently altering their behavior or dress to try to prevent being victimized (Gordon & Riger, 1991; Kasper & Aponte, 1996).

Intimate partner violence often begins during adolescence (Barnett et al., 1997) and occurs across all socioeconomic levels. However, this type of violence is more frequent among people with fewer economic resources (Collins et al., 1999; Moore, 1997). In addition to physical attacks, sexual and psychological abuse are serious problems within many relationships. Women often report that psychological abuse is more painful than physical abuse (Tolman & Bhosley, 1991).

After separating from an abusive partner, women are at high risk for serious physical violence, stalking, or murder (Wilson & Daly, 1993). Separation abuse frequently occurs at the woman's place of work. Women may avoid going to work because they know their abuser can find them there, or they may lose their jobs because of the abuser's threatening behavior.

Intimate partner violence may interfere with help-seeking due to the batterer's fears that his partner's seeking help may lead to legal problems or separations. Many battered women are ashamed to report abuse because they feel they brought it on themselves or should have been able to stop it. Women with mental health problems are particularly vulnerable to this type of shame. Women of color may hesitate to report abuse because of experiences with discrimination by criminal justice or social welfare programs. Immigrant women may fear that reporting abuse will jeopardize their stay in the United States. For all of these reasons, only 29% of the women who reported being abused in the Commonwealth Fund survey said that they had discussed the abuse they experienced with a health care professional (Collins et al., 1999). Women report only half of the intimate violence they experience to the police (Greenfeld et al., 1998).

Batterers usually control their partners' access to friends, family, and work. Therefore, battered women experience a sense of isolation that can aggravate mental health problems. Batterers often tell their victims that they are "crazy" or pathetic. Battered women, especially those with a history of mental health problems, may be afraid that no one will believe them if they talk about abuse that they are experiencing. If no one else notices the abuse or if others seem to like the batterer, then victims may doubt their own perceptions about the abuse.

It is also important to be aware that lesbian women may be experiencing violence in their intimate relationships. Research suggests that battering occurs in 17–26% of lesbian relationships (Lie, Schilit, Bush, Montagne, & Reyes, 1991). In addition, elderly women are at risk for abuse by partners or other caretakers. It is difficult to determine the rate of elder abuse because it is often hidden, but one study that interviewed a random sample of elderly reported a 2% rate of physical abuse (Pillemer & Finkelhor, 1988).

Women who have experienced violence in past or current relationships are likely to experience mental health problems because of the violence. Half of the women interviewed for the Commonwealth Fund report who reported having experienced violence or abuse also reported experiencing depressive symptoms (Collins et al., 1999). Thirty-four percent of those who had been raped or sexually assaulted said they were diagnosed as depressed by a doctor. These women also often experience high levels of anxiety. Women who had been assaulted also reported more physical health problems than did women who had not been assaulted.

Battered women and women who have been sexually assaulted often show symptoms of post-traumatic stress disorder (PTSD) (Kemp, Green, Hovanitz, & Rawlings, 1995). When clinicians are not aware of the trauma a woman has experienced, symptoms of PTSD can resemble symptoms of other mental health problems and can lead to misdiagnosis (Gondolf, 1998). Battered women in rehabilitation programs may seem extremely fearful and might appear unwilling to talk to staff, especially male staff. Consequently, they may be mislabeled as particularly resistant and uncooperative.

SEXUAL HARASSMENT

Almost all women in our society are subject to sexual harassment, such as men making comments about their bodies or inappropriate sexual overtures. This behavior can cause women to fear public situations. It is also a common problem at work, especially in male-dominated settings. Treatment providers or fellow clients might harass a woman during a treatment or rehabilitation program. Women with mental health problems may already feel vulnerable in a program or at work, and they might feel especially defenseless in the face of sexual harassment.

LESBIANS

Lesbians using rehabilitation services may experience discrimination for being female and for being gay, while lesbians of color may experience three types of discrimination. Ryan, Bradford, and Honnold (1999) studied the positive and negative contributions of being lesbian to mental health by both heterosexuals and lesbian/gay mental health providers and overall found those higher proportions of respondents noting negative contributions than positive contributions. The greatest percentage of all respondents viewed increased emotional strength as a positive contribution of being lesbian. They also viewed the potential for community and relationships and increased tolerance as positive contributions of being lesbian. Negative contributions to mental health of being lesbian include discrimination against lesbians, being uncomfortable with lesbian identity, lack of social support, and general emotional problems.

Because "coming out," that is acknowledging one's sexual orientation to self and others (Morrow, 1996), represents a shift in the individual's core identity, it may be accompanied by significant levels of emotional distress (Gonsiorek & Rudolph, 1991). This distress may include a range of psychiatric symptoms that generally disappear when the crisis resolves. However, coming out is generally associated with both positive and negative mental health effects, with somewhat more emphasis on positive effects. The positive mental health effects include decreased feelings of isolation (Murphy, 1989), higher ego strength, less depression, and higher self-esteem (Savin-Williams, 1989). Those who invest energy in keeping their sexual orientation a secret expend significant emotional energy hiding a central aspect of their identity. The emotional toll of secrecy can result in internalized shame and self-doubt.

Ryan et al.'s (1999) study found that 41% of all respondents thought that coming out improved the mental health of lesbians, while 83% of lesbians felt that this was the case. Positive attributes of coming out include improved self-esteem, increased social support, and being comfortable with lesbian identity. The most common negative effect of coming out included the lack of social support, negative emotional effects, and discrimination against lesbians. More heterosexuals than lesbians/gay respondents viewed lack of social support as a negative effect of coming out.

ISSUES IN MENTAL HEALTH TREATMENT

Gender role stereotyping that leads to sexist discrimination is also present in therapeutic interventions. The mental health professions reflect the same biases and discrimination present throughout society. Some researchers have suggested that our standards of mental health are based on male standards (Broverman, Broverman, Clarkson, & Rosenkrantz, 1970). Clinicians rarely are educated to understand that the path of women's development may differ from that of men's, which has been more frequently studied (Gilligan, 1982; Jordan, Kaplan, Miller, Stiver, & Surrey, 1991). Sometimes clinicians use constructs such as "codependency" to measure mental health without considering the unique aspects of women's development (Collins, 1993). Most therapies fail to emphasize the detrimental influence of sexism on the lives of women and assist women in learning to adapt to their environments rather than in learning to change their environments (Stout & McPhail, 1998).

Determining the causes of a woman's problem is critical, for etiology determines the choice of a solution. For example, if a social service professional believes that a woman is depressed because women are naturally more emotional than men, then perhaps antidepressants should be prescribed. However, if women are more likely to be depressed because of their inferior status in a patriarchal society, the solutions look very different and suggest major societal and political changes that cannot be addressed with medication (Stout & McPhail, 1998).

The majority of clients seeking mental health services are women, and 70% of all psychotropic medications are prescribed to women. However, men experience higher rates of mental disorders over their lifetimes than do women (Blumenthal, 1994). Women are two to three times more likely to experience depression. In the United States, one out of every seven women will be hospitalized for depression during her lifetime (Wetzel, 1994). Rates of depression are higher for women, and the differences in risk hold true for white, black, and Hispanic women and across occupations, income, and educational levels (Droppleman & Wilt, 1993). Depression remains a problem for women into the later years of life.

The American Psychological Association's task force's report by McGrath, Kietal, Strickland, and Russo (1990) refuted the myth that more women than men are diagnosed as depressed because women are more willing to talk about their feelings and more likely to seek help. Instead, they reported that women are at greater risk for depression due to social, economic, biological, and emotional factors. Stout and Mcphail (1998) contend that the problems that bring women to seek mental health services, including stress-related disorders, depression, low self-esteem, body image problems, and eating disorders, are not symptoms of mental illness. They are the result of women's experiences living with sexism.

Treatment and rehabilitation program developers often design programs without taking women's developmental needs and special responsibilities into account. Although there are more women than men diagnosed with some serious mental illnesses, there has been a lack of meaningful publication and analysis on women with serious mental illnesses (Mowbray, Herman, & Hazel, 1992). This may be because men are more highly valued by society. It is also possible that women with mental health problems display more internalizing symptoms and behaviors. Men often externalize and act-out, so that mental health programs may pay more attention to male clients (Mowbray et al., 1992). Rehabilitation programs often emphasize competitive employment skills for men while expecting women to be unemployed or working as babysitters or housekeepers (Bachrach, 1988b).

The use of mental health services among lesbians is high (Murphy, 1991). Lesbians use mental health services for a variety of concerns including relationships, family, career and job-related concerns, decisions about parenting, confusion about sexual identity, personal growth, and because of discrimination and anti-gay violence. However, lesbians at mid-life and in their elder years apparently look less toward mental health services and more to their own peer groups for support and information as their bodies age (Martin & Lyon, 1997). Older lesbians tend to find young social service providers, even young lesbians, to be insensitive to their issues (Butler & Hope, 1999). Although recent literature suggests that mental health issues related to lesbians are no longer viewed as pathological, homophobia, lack of knowledge, ambivalence, and disdain among mental health providers and agencies persists (Rudolph, 1989). Ball (1994) states that an administrator's resistance to the development of a gay- and lesbian-affirmative program is often an indirect expression of lack of knowledge or institutional denial of the specific needs of gay men and lesbians.

Although professionals may argue that lesbian clients could explore their issues in any relationship, dating, or family groups, "homosocialization"—friendships and alliances with other people like oneself—is needed. Peer socialization, and formation of support networks create a sense of belonging to a community that helps protect against decompensation during times of stress.

Few rehabilitation programs simultaneously address the problems and needs of women who are both mentally ill and lesbian. Being a member of two or more stigmatized minority groups can exacerbate psychiatric symptoms and presentations. A lesbian woman with significant mental illness has problems that affect social functioning, self-care, and self-direction, in addition to the external and internal stressors of being self-identified as a lesbian (Ball, 1994). Lesbians often must leave their rehabilitation programs to find support for their sexual and social needs. Ball states that:

> in the lesbian community, many chronically mentally ill clients report feeling awkward because of their mental illness and its related debilitating effects and if they seek counseling in a clinic that serves gay men and lesbians, they are often turned away because of their psychiatric diagnosis (pp. 109–110).

Because sexuality pervades one's mental life, lesbian clients at conventional treatment programs need a special group that can address their psychosocial totality (Ball, 1994).

The majority of the elderly are women, so women are the majority of the elderly mentally ill (Bachrach, 1988b). The special vulnerabilities of elderly people with mental illnesses, "such as inappropriate placements and increased mortality risks associated with transfer" (Bachrach, 1988b, pp. 86–87) are largely women's issues.

Workers also need to be aware that psychotropic medications affect women differently from men (Bachrach, 1988b). Some medications require different dosage schedules during different times of women's menstrual cycles (Seeman, 1988), and pregnancy is an issue in prescribing psychotropic medications.

RESPONDING TO WOMEN'S ISSUES

Women with mental health problems need rehabilitation programs that are sensitive to women's economic, safety, diagnostic, and treatment issues. First, in order to begin to work on rehabilitation, women need housing that is appropriate for their level of functioning. Pregnant women and women with children may need residential support, which is often hard for women with mental illnesses to find. Staff who assist persons diagnosed with mental illnesses in finding and maintaining employment must be careful not to assume that women wish to maintain the traditional role of staying at home to care for home and family. Although there are not necessarily large differences in the daily functioning of men and women diagnosed with serious mental illnesses (Mowbray et al., 1992), mental health and rehabilitation workers should be aware of different contexts and issues that women with mental illnesses bring with them to a rehabilitation program. Workers should be aware of ways that women's relational development may lead them to behave differently from men with mental health problems (Jordan et al., 1991). Rehabilitation program staff clearly must be aware of women's special health issues, such as pregnancy and menopause.

Assessment of Victimization

Staff members of a rehabilitation program should ask women about their current and past experiences with violence, how these experiences affect them, and how they want to handle any current violence. Workers should screen all women and should not assume that women who are upper or middle class have never experienced violence. It is important to use a screening instrument that asks detailed questions about acts of violence that were perpetrated against the woman. Asking general questions such as "have you ever been raped?" or "have you ever been a victim of domestic violence?" will not yield complete information, because many women do not label the abuse they experienced as "rape" or "domestic violence." They may believe such abuse is normal or that they deserved it. Assessment should include the development of a safety plan for women who are currently involved with or recently separated from abusive partners (Gondolf, 1998). Staff should be educated about domestic violence, and it should be included as a very relevant factor in case reviews and planning sessions.

Strengths Perspective

It is important to be proactive to protect women from sexual harassment in rehabilitation programs. Staff helping women plan for employment should also be sensitive to fears that women have about dangers on the job and travelling to and from the job.

Staff should be sensitive to the importance of relationships in many women's lives, assess women's levels of social support, and work on increasing and improving social support. Although social support can help counter sexist messages women hear and remind them of their strengths, Thomas (1997) suggests that social support should not automatically be viewed as a buffer of stress. The degree of reciprocity within supportive relationships should be assessed. Women tend to give more than they receive in many relationships, and Luchetta and Alberts' (1994) study found that disparity in levels of support given and received was associated with greater levels of depression. Both losses and benefits of women's social support networks must be assessed. Staff should be aware that women probably want and expect different things from their social networks than men expect, and they should be prepared to find out what individual women clients want (Walsh, 1994).

People who work in rehabilitation or mental health programs should not treat any women in an authoritarian manner. However, with battered women, in particular, authoritarian treatment seems to repeat the dynamics of the abuser's behavior (Gondolf, 1998). Staff should take an empowerment (Dutton, 1992) or strengths perspective approach (Saleeby, 1992) with women who have survived violence, recognizing the strength it took to survive the violence. One option in working with survivors of abuse is for staff to conduct a strengths assessment, which helps women clarify and concretize their strengths (Gondolf, 1998). It is important to understand that many women feel they love their abusers or are anxious to preserve the nuclear family for their children's sake. Staff members who insist that a woman must leave an abuser are oversimplifying a complicated situation. They may be echoing advice that the woman has already received from family and friends but has been unable or unwilling to follow. Women with diagnoses of severe mental illnesses must feel especially insecure about the prospect of breaking up a partnership.

Staff should confer with domestic violence programs' staffs to be sure they are willing and able to work effectively with women with mental health problems and then refer battered women to domestic violence programs for individual or group therapy that focuses on the effects of abuse. Workers should be sensitive to the possibility that women may be reluctant to talk in the rehabilitation program about past or current violence, especially in groups with males.

Many experts in domestic violence believe that marital therapy with violent men should not be conducted (Bograd, 1992), because the victim will be afraid to speak or may be punished later for speaking up. Batterers need group or individual treatment focused on holding them accountable for their violence.

It is important for mental health workers to educate women about the very real presence of sexist events in their lives. Feminism itself may serve as an important schema that mediates and decreases the negative impact of sexism on women and acts as a buffer to protect their physical and mental health. Feminism may be beneficial to women in the personal arena of their everyday lives and play as an important role as social support and similar resources in mediating negative impact of stressors (Landrine & Klonoff, 1997). Thus, it may be important for mental health workers to ask women if they are feminists. This question allows for an assessment of how psychological and sociological principles and variables may operate very differently depending on women's views on feminism.

Along with education, women's internalized sexism must be challenged. For example, Russo (1995) suggests women must learn to reframe the term "nag," which women often apply to themselves or other women. Women can learn to see the behavior as a positive characteristic— "hanging in there" and "persistence." Additionally, women must learn to reclaim their voice. Lott's (1994) research suggests that women's most frequent response to dealing with sexism that they encounter in everyday life is to simply ignore it (39.3% of the women). Lott found also that women frequently left the site of a sexist incident (22.1%) to avoid the interaction.

An important way for some women to overcome the effects of sexism in their lives is to become activists (Landrine & Klonoff, 1997). Activism can take many forms (including insisting on equitable relationships with partners) and serves as an effective way to keep sexism externalized and away from the personal realm. It is also critical that women find support to deal with sexism and its effects on their lives (Landrine & Klonoff, 1997). To be truly effective in countering the sexist messages inside their own heads and in the everyday world, they need people in their lives who can be counted on to remind them of their strengths, accomplishments, and potential. Rehabilitation programs can teach women assertiveness and help them learn to value many aspects of themselves rather than focusing primarily on appearances.

In discussing employment, staff should ask about women's care-taking responsibilities. They should help women weigh the importance of caring for sick or aging relatives against the potential benefits of participating in the workforce. A sensitive rehabilitation program might provide family meetings for women and their adult siblings, who might be able to increase their involvement in the care of sick or aging relatives.

If a woman is part of a couple, and there is no violence within the couple, then marital meetings that focus on helping the male partner support the woman's rehabilitation efforts by doing an equal share of housework and childcare are very important. It is difficult for many women to be assertive in negotiations about these matters, and a woman who feels stigmatized by mental illness may need even more help in asking for household equity.

For lesbians, groups that directly address a client's sexual orientation will be most effective in fostering rehabilitation. It is critical that lesbian women have the opportunity to safely explore and discuss their development of a lesbian identity. Successful resolution does not happen quickly and requires transforming a stigmatized identity into an integrated positive sense of self (Espin, 1993).

To summarize, rehabilitation programs should be sensitive to the multitude of issues accompanying women's secondary status in our society. These issues include self-esteem, economic discrimination, safety, social support, and issues accompanying discrimination against lesbians and women of color.

REFERENCES

Bachrach, L. L. (1988a). Chronically mentally ill women: An overview of service delivery issues. In L. L. Bachrach & C. C. Nadelson (Eds.), *Treating chronically mentally ill women* (pp. 1–17). Washington, DC: American Psychiatric Press.

Bachrach, L. L. (1988b). Chronically mentally ill women: Emergence and legitimation of program issues. In L. L. Bachrach & C. C. Nadelson (Eds.), *Treating chronically mentally ill women* (pp. 77–96). Washington, DC: American Psychiatric Press.

Ball, S. (1994). A group model for gay and lesbian clients with chronic mental illness. *Social Work, 39*(1), 109–115.

Barnett, O. W., Miller-Perrin, C. L., & Perrin, R. D. (1997). *Family violence across the lifespan: An introduction.* Thousand Oaks, CA: Sage.

Baruch, G., Biener, L., & Barnett, R. C. (1987). Women and gender in research on work and family stress. *American Psychologist, 42,* 130–136.

Bennett, M. B., Handel, M. H., & Pearsall, D. T. (1988). Behavioral differences between female and male hospitalized chronically mentally ill patients. In L. L. Bachrach & C. C. Nadelson (Eds.), *Treating chronically mentally ill women* (pp. 1–17). Washington, DC: American Psychiatric Press.

Blumenthal, S. J. (1994). Issues in women's mental health. *Journal of Women's Health, 3*(6), 453–458.

Bograd, M. (1992). Values in conflict: Challenges to family therapists' thinking. *Journal of Marital and Family Therapy, 18,* 245–256.

Bowman, G. D., & Stern, M. (1995). Adjustment to occupational stress: The relationship of perceived control to effectiveness of coping strategies. *Journal of Counseling Psychology, 42*(3), 294–303.

Broverman, I. K., Broverman, D. M., Clarkson, F. E., & Rosenkrantz, P. S. (1970). Sex-role stereotypes and clinical judgments of mental health. *Journal of Consulting & Clinical Psychology, 34,* 1–7.

Brown, L. M., & Gilligan, C. (1992). *Meeting at the crossroads: Women's psychology and girls' development.* Cambridge, MA: Harvard University Press.

Butler, S. S., & Hope, B. (1999). Health and well being for late middle-aged and old lesbians in a rural area. *Journal of Gay and Lesbian Social Services, 9*(4), 27–46.

Collins, B. G. (1993). Reconstruing codependency using self-in-relation theory: A feminist perspective. *Social Work 38,* 470–476.

Collins, K. S., Schoen, C., Joseph, S., Duchon, L., Simantov, E., & Yellowitz, M. (1999). *Health concerns across a woman's lifespan: The Commonwealth Fund 1998 Survey of Women's Health.* http://www.cmwf.org/programs/women/ksc_whsurvy99_332.asp.

Doress-Worters, P. B. (1994). Adding elder care to women's multiple roles: A critical review of the caregiver stress and multiple roles literatures. *Sex Roles, 31*(9/10), 597–616.

Droppleman, P. G., & Wilt, D. (1993). Women, depression, and anger. In S. P. Thomas (Ed.), *Women and anger* (pp. 209–232). New York, NY: Springer.

Dutton, M. A. (1992). *Empowering and healing battered women: A model for assessment and intervention.* New York, NY: Springer.

Espin, O. M. (1993). Issues of identity in the psychology of Latina lesbians. In L. Garents & D. Kimmel (Eds.), *Psychological perspectives on lesbian and gay male experiences* (pp. 348–363). New York, NY: Columbia University Press.

Gilligan, C. (1982). *In a different voice.* Cambridge, MA: Harvard University Press.

Goering, P., Cochrane, J., Potasznik, H., Wasylenki, D., & Lancee, W. (1988). Women and work: After psychiatric hospitalization. In L. L. Bachrach & C. C. Nadelson (Eds.), *Treating chronically mentally ill women* (pp. 45–62). Washington, DC: American Psychiatric Press.

Gondolf, E. W. (1998): *Assessing woman battering in mental health services.* Thousand Oaks, CA: Sage.

Gonsiorek, J. C., & Rudolph, J. R. (1991). Homosexual identity: Coming out and other developmental events. In J. C. Gonsiorek & J. D. Weinrich, (Eds.), *Homosexuality: Research implications for public policy* (pp. 161–176), Thousand Oaks, CA: Sage.

Gordon, M. T., & Riger, S. (1991). *The female fear: The social cost of rape.* Urbana and Chicago, IL: University of Illinois Press.

Greenfeld, L. A., Rand, M. R., Craven, D., Klaus, P. A., Perkins, C. A., Ringel, C., Warchol, G., Maston, C., & Fox, J. A. (1998). *Violence by intimates: Analysis of data on crimes by current or former spouses, boyfriends, and girlfriends.* Washington, DC: Bureau of Justice Statistics.

Hochschild, A. (1989). *The second shift.* New York, NY: Avon Books.

Jordan, J. V., Kaplan, A. G., Miller, J. B., Stiver, I. P., & Surrey, J. L. (1991). *Women's growth in connection. Writings from the Stone center.* New York, NY: Guilford.

Kaschak, E. (1992). *Engendered lives: A new psychology of women's experience.* New York, NY: Basic Books.

Kasper, B., & Aponte, C. I. (1996). Women, violence, and fear: One community's experience. *Affilia, 11*(2), 179–195.

Kemp, A., Green, B. L., Hovanitz, C., & Rawlings, E. I. (1995). Incidence and correlates of posttraumatic stress disorder in battered women: Shelter and community samples. *Journal of Interpersonal Violence, 10* (1), 45–55.

Koss, M. P., Giarretto, C. A., & Wisniewski, N. (1987). The scope of rape: Incidence and prevalence in a national sample of higher education students. *Journal of Consulting and Clinical Psychology, 55*, 162–170.

Landrine, H., & Klonoff, E. A. (1997). *Discrimination against women: Prevalence, consequences, remedies.* Thousand Oaks, CA: Sage.

Lie, G., Schilit, R., Bush, J., Montagne, M., & Reyes, L. (1991). Lesbians in currently aggressive relationships: How frequently do they report aggressive past relationships? *Violence and Victims, 6*, 121–135.

Lott, B. L. (1994). *Women's lives: Themes and variations in gender learning.* Pacific Grove, CA: Brooks/Cole.

Luchetta, T., & Alberts, J. (1994, April). *Social support disparity among adult women: Relationships to femininity and health outcomes.* Paper presented at the Society of Behavioral Medicine, Boston.

Martin, D., & Lyon, P. (1997). Old lesbians come of age. In J. White & M. C. Martinez (Eds.), *The lesbian health book* (pp. 210–219). Seattle, WA: Seal Press.

McGrath, E., Kieta, G. P., Strickland, B., & Russo, N. F. (1990). *Women and depression: Risk factors and treatment issues.* Washington, DC: American Psychological Association.

Moore, A. M. (1997). Intimate violence: Does socioeconomic status matter? In A. P. Cardarelli (Ed.), *Violence between intimate partners: Patterns, causes, and effects* (pp. 90–100). Boston, MA: Allyn & Bacon.

Morrow, D. F. (1996). Coming-out issues for adult lesbians: A group intervention. *Social Work, 41*(6), 647–656.

Mowbray, C. T., Herman, S. E., & Hazel, K. L. (1992). Gender and serious mental illness: A feminist perspective. *Psychology of Women Quarterly, 16*, 107–126.

Murphy, B. C. (1989). Lesbian couples and their parents: The effects of perceived parental attitudes on the couple. *Journal of Counseling & Development, 68*, 46–51.

Murphy, B. C. (1991). Educating mental health professionals about gay and lesbian issues. *Journal of Homosexuality, 22*(3–4), 229–246.

Pillemer, K. A., & Finkelhor, D. (1988). The prevalence of elder abuse: A random sample survey. *Gerontologist, 28*, 51–57.

Pogrebin, L. C. (1980). *Growing up free.* New York, NY: Bantam Books.

Queralt, M. (1996). *The social environment and human behavior: A diversity perspective.* Boston, MA: Allyn & Bacon.

Rudolph, J. (1989). Effects of a workshop on mental health practitioners' attitudes toward homosexuality and counseling effectiveness. *Journal of Counseling and Development, 68*(1), 81–85.

Russo, N. F. (1995). Women's mental health: Research agenda for the twenty-first century. In B. Brown, B. Kramer, P. Reiker, & C. Willie (Eds.), *Mental health, racism, and sexism* (pp. 373–396). Pittsburgh, PA: University of Pittsburgh Press.

Ryan, C. C., Bradford, J. B., & Honnold, J. A. (1999). Social workers' and counselors' understanding of lesbian needs. *Journal of Gay and Lesbian Social Services, 9*(4), 1–26.

Saleeby, D. (Ed.) (1992). *The strengths perspective in social work practice: Power in the people.* Plains, NY: Longman.

Savin-Williams, R. C. (1989). Coming out to parents and self-esteem among gay and lesbian youths. *Journal of Homosexuality, 18*(1–2), 1–35.

Seeman, M. V. (1988). Schizophrenia in women and men. In L. L. Bachrach & C. C. Nadelson (Eds.), *Treating chronically mentally ill women* (pp. 21–28). Washington, DC: American Psychiatric Press.

Stout, K., & McPhail, B. (1998). *Confronting sexism and violence against women*: A challenge for social work. New York: Longman.

Swim, J. K., & Cohen, L. L. (1997). Overt, covert, and subtle sexism: A comparison between the attitudes toward women and modern sexism scales. *Psychology of Women Quarterly, 21*, 103–118.

Thomas, S. P. (1997). Distressing aspects of women's roles, vicarious stress, and health consequences. *Issues in Mental Health Nursing, 18*, 539–557.

Tolman, R. M., & Bhosley, G. (1991). The outcome of participation in a shelter sponsored program from men who batter. In D. D. Knudsen & J. L. Miller (Eds.), *Abused and battered: Social and legal responses to family violence* (pp. 113–122). New York, NY: Aldine de Gruyer.

Waldron, I., & Herold, J. (1986). Employment, attitudes toward employment, and women's health. *Women and Health, 11*, 79–98.

Walsh, J. (1994). Gender differences in the social networks of persons with severe mental illnesses. *Affilia, 9*(3), 247–268.

Wettel, J. W. (1994). Depression: Women at risk. *Social Work in Health Care, 19*(3/4), 85–108.

Wilson, M., & Daly, M. (1993). Spousal homicide risk and estrangement. *Violence and Victims, 8*(1), 3–17.

CHAPTER 33

Rehabilitation Services for Criminal Offenders[1]

NATHANIEL J. PALLONE AND JAMES J. HENNESSY

A first priority for mental health and social service professionals in virtually any setting is to develop a reasonably accurate inventory of the "needs" of prospective clients. From such an inventory will emerge not only the design of responsive services and programs but also the criteria by which the effectiveness of those programs and services should be judged. In the case of rehabilitation services in correctional settings (jails, prisons, parole and probation agencies), however, there is a powerful intervening factor, namely cyclically vacillating public attitudes, sometimes inimical, toward the provision of services of any sort to persons who should be "punished" and not "treated."

During the latest year for which data are available, records of the Bureau of Justice Statistics (an agency of the U.S. Department of Justice with responsibility for collating data of all sorts concerning the criminal justice system), reveal that some 5.7 million people were (to use the term current in the Federal lexicon) "under correctional supervision" (Maguire & Pastore, 1999, p. 462), distributed among prisons, jails, and parole and probation agencies as depicted in Figure 33-1. In the aggregate, slightly more than 2% of the nation's population of 280 million were thus "under correctional supervision" during the year in review.

Rehabilitation services necessarily differ for offenders in confinement (prisons, with relatively stable populations of convicted felons serving sentences of specified lengths; jails, with a largely "revolving door" clientele of accused felons awaiting trial and convicted misdemeanants serving short sentences) and those at large in the community. Offenders under "community supervision" on probation or parole comprise nearly 70% of the total represented in Figure 33-1, outnumbering offenders incarcerated in state or Federal prisons as a result of felony convictions at a ratio greater than 3:1 and outnumbering the population of jails at a ratio greater than 7:1. In general, psychosocial, mental health, and educational services are provided to incarcerated offenders by employees of the correctional authority (i.e., state, county, or Federal departments of corrections), although a trend has emerged toward the "privatization" of many such services (Bowman, Hakim, & Seidenstat, 1993; Demone &

---

[1] Certain portions of this chapter have also appeared in: To punish or to treat: Substance abuse within the context of oscillating attitudes toward correctional rehabilitation, *Journal of Offender Rehabilitation, 2002, 37*(3–4), 7–19.

NATHANIEL J. PALLONE • Rutgers, The State University of New Jersey, New Brunswick, New Jersey.
JAMES J. HENNESSY • Fordham University Graduate School of Education, New York, New York.

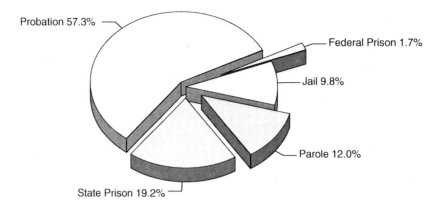

FIGURE 33-1. Persons under correctional supervision, United States. 5.7 million offenders annually in custody or on probation or parole (Data from Maguire & Pastore, *Sourcebook of Criminal Justice Statistics*, 1999, 462).

Gibelman, 1990) in much the same way that correctional institutions have long contracted with private vendors to operate food preparation services. In either case, the character (and sometimes the frequency) of mental health, educational, and rehabilitation services is determined by policies of the correctional authority, in their turn responsive to legislative and judicial instruction. In contrast, offenders under community supervision usually are served by social service or mental health agencies in the community whose policies are not controlled by the correctional authority. Generally, direct referral to relevant community agencies (including outpatient clinics at hospitals) is made by a probation or parole officer; less frequently, referral is made to community agencies or institutions under contractual relationships to serve offender clients.

Demographic disparities between the population in general and the offender population also clearly impinge upon the planning and delivery of mental health, social, and educational services. Hence, it is a matter of more than passing interest that Whites, who constituted 80% of the nation's population in the 1990 census, comprise only 60% of the correctional population depicted in Figure 33-1. Similarly, according to the 1990 census, girls and women constituted 51% of the general population, but they represent only 16% of the correctional population.

OSCILLATING ATTITUDES TOWARD CORRECTIONS

At least since the time of the Marquis di Beccaria in the 18th century, the goals of corrections have been conceded to include *rehabilitation* as well as *incapacitation, retribution*, and *deterrence* (Taylor & Brasswell, 1979), generally within the context of the principle of *proportionality* between offense and sanction traceable to the Code of Hammurabi in the 18th century BC and reinforced in the British Magna Carta three millennia later. In response to societal, political, and intellectual forces (Foucault, 1978), emphasis has of course shifted among and between these four goals over time, so that some permutations and combinations may temporarily discernibly ascend while others recede.

Penance v. Punishment: Rehabilitation as an American Tradition

Indeed, an oscillation of virtually tectonic proportions occurred not long after the founding of the American republic, when in 1787 the Quakers of Pennsylvania invented the penitentiary as an alternative to the prison, the purpose of which had historically been to punish and incapacitate. In contrast, the Quaker penitentiary was to be a place where offenders were confined to do penance through religious meditation and "spiritual exercises" and thus become "penitent" for their transgressions, in the process vowing irrevocably, with the aid of the Almighty, to forgo wrongdoing forevermore.

However much the religious–spiritual dimension which shaped the Quaker invention may have eroded, there is little question that, half a century ago, if rehabilitation did not quite stand univocally as the primary goal of corrections (American Friends Service Committee, 1971; Lindner, 1949), it surely stood alongside incapacitation, deterrence, and retribution as *primus inter pares*. Legislators and the general public alike expected, and were willing to finance, the provision of rehabilitation services of various sorts for offenders incarcerated in the nation's prisons.

Pugh v. *Locke:* **The Right of Prison Inmates to Mental Health "Care"**

A perception of rehabilitation as a primary purpose in corrections is readily inferable in the landmark decision of Federal appellate court judge Frank M. Johnson in *Pugh* v. *Locke* (1976), a case concerning the operation of the prisons of Alabama, later upheld by the U.S. Supreme Court and therefore uniformly precedental throughout the nation. In his decision, Mr. Johnson imposed a wide-ranging set of "minimum Constitutional standards for inmates" that mandated "humane" and sanitary living conditions (with strict standards imposed to address prison overcrowding), "meaningful programs" staffed by qualified personnel, and at least first-line mental health care within correctional institutions (Fowler, 1976, 1987). Over the next two decades, no fewer than 37 states were ordered by the Federal courts to meet the standards specified in *Pugh*.

Mr. Johnson had earlier issued the linchpin decisions in *Donaldson* v. *O'Connor, Wyatt* v. *Hardin*, and *Wyatt* v. *Stickney*, cases brought on behalf of patients confined in public mental hospitals. In upholding those decisions, the U.S. Supreme Court declared unequivocally that patients in mental hospitals have an absolute *right to treatment* and that to confine patients in the absence of treatment in effect constitutes involuntary imprisonment, in violation of Constitutional guarantees against deprivation of liberty without due process (Golann & Fremouw, 1976, pp. 129–185). Although he affirmed the right of inmates to mental health *care*, Mr. Johnson stopped short in *Pugh* of articulating a right to *treatment*. Instead, he ordered that prison administrators "shall identify those inmates who require mental health care within the institution and make arrangements for such care," while simultaneously ordering that there should be "routine" provision for identification of "those inmates who, by reason of psychological disturbance or mental retardation require care in facilities designed for such persons" and for the transfer of prisoners thus identified to such (presumably forensic) psychiatric installations. From the judicial perspective, "treatment" thus appears to be that form of professional intervention provided in psychiatric hospitals, while "care" is that form of intervention to be provided *in situ* for prisoners whose disorders are not severe enough to warrant hospitalization.

Pugh specifically adopts the mental health staffing ratios proposed by the Center for Correctional Psychology at the University of Alabama (Gormally, Brodsky, Clements, & Fowler, 1972), which reduce to an overall ratio of one mental health specialist for each 91 inmates—specifically: one bachelor's level mental health technician or correctional counselor for each 135 inmates; one psychologist for each 506 inmates; one social worker for each

578 inmates; one psychiatrist for each 4,048 inmates. Mr. Johnson's ruling in effect held that these personnel were required to provide "mental health care" as a sort of first-line intervention within the prisons themselves, since the most severe cases were to be transferred to appropriate mental hospital facilities.

Inventories of mental health staffing in state prisons shortly after *Pugh* provided evidence of enormous discrepancies between those standards, staff actually employed and deployed, and staffing standards promulgated by such organizations as the American Correctional Association (Pallone, Hennessy, & LaRosa, 1980). Mayer (1990), a legal scholar, has labeled the failure of correctional administrators to meet court-imposed standards an exemplar of Constitutionally impermissible "deliberate indifference." And, in view of definitive *Pugh* standards governing prison overcrowding, it is distressing to observe that, nearly a quarter century after that historic decision, the number of prisoners confined in correctional institutions exceeded the capacity of those institutions by 25% in the Federal system, 72% in California, 77% in Hawaii, 41% in Illinois, 20% in Indiana, 64% in Iowa, an astounding 230% in Massachusetts, 96% in Montana, 39% in Nebraska, 46% in New Jersey, 69% in Ohio, 51% in Pennsylvania, 55% in Virginia, 41% in Washington, and 48% in Wisconsin (Maguire & Pastore, 1999, p. 487). That the prison systems of 14 states and the Federal system itself apparently no longer perceive themselves bound by the "minimum Constitutional standards" enunciated in *Pugh* and affirmed by the highest court in the land perhaps reveals a posture for which "deliberate indifference" is too euphemistic a descriptor.

Therapeutic Nihilism: The Martinson Report and the "Nothing Works" Doctrine

However favorable to rehabilitation the prevailing ethos when the *Pugh* decision was announced, countervailing forces were beginning to emerge. Even the entertainment media entered the lists, with offender rehabilitation parodied mercilessly by director Stanley Kubrick in his 1971 film version of Anthony Burgess's *A Clockwork Orange*. With the publication of the now-famous (or perhaps infamous) Martinson Report, quasi-empirical challenges were directly mounted against the primacy of rehabilitation as a goal in corrections.

Media attention immediately surrounded publication of Martinson's report on the efficacy of rehabilitation efforts in prisons (1974) largely because the government agency that had sponsored the study on which the report was based had formally suppressed its release. In 1971, a major prisoner revolt took place at the New York state prison at Attica, ultimately claiming 43 lives. Among the "non-negotiable" demands made by leaders of the revolt were requests for increased quantity and quality in rehabilitation services; as Governor of the state, Nelson Rockefeller quickly agreed. However, there was underway at the time a major state-funded study of the effectiveness of rehabilitation programs of all sorts in correctional institutions of various sorts. Because its conclusions countered the state's capitulation to prisoners' demands, and because it constituted a "work for hire" and could thus quite legitimately be classified as "confidential," state administrators ordered that no report of the research be released. But the leaders of the revolt knew of the study and of Martinson's role as an investigator (though not the principal investigator). At their trial on varied criminal charges, they sought to mitigate responsibility by appealing to the evidence accumulated by the research team that showed rehabilitation to be relatively ineffective. The research saw the light of day only when the judge presiding in those trials ordered that the suppression be lifted. Thus it was that the "Martinson Report" (1974), published in a neo-Conservative "journal of opinion" entitled *Public Interest* rather than in a peer-reviewed scholarly journal, became almost instantly a focus of national press attention.

Martinson concluded that most offender rehabilitation regimens for adult prisoners constitute a colossal waste of professional energy and of taxpayers' money. That dire judgment was mollified somewhat in a more detailed monograph by Lipton, Martinson, and Wilks (1975)—and indeed mollified even further by Lipton (1995), the lead investigator. But a similarly pessimistic conclusion was reached by Shamsie (1982), who reviewed the research evidence on the effectiveness of rehabilitation services for juvenile offenders. Predictably, members of the professional community committed to rehabilitation in corrections sought to answer the Martinson judgments (Cullen & Gilbert, 1982; Gendreau & Ross, 1979, 1981; Glaser, 1976), often with more heat than light. As Martinson (1976) himself suggested, these responses may have issued from a sense of disbelief that "all the well-intentioned efforts of the psychiatric, psychological, and social service communities, of the medical establishment, of the prisons and the jails, and even of the schools have yielded such disappointing results."

The controversy reached even into the prestigious National Academy of Sciences (NAS), which commissioned a blue-ribbon panel to re-analyze the more than 200 studies of rehabilitation effectiveness on which the Lipton et al. conclusions were based (Sechrest, White, & Brown, 1979). But those excruciating re-analyses (Feinberg & Gramsbach, 1979) did little to gainsay the "gloomy conclusions" reached by Martinson. Instead, focusing on flaws in the research design of the 200-plus studies reviewed (especially the absence of adequate control or comparison groups), the NAS panel (Sechrest et al., 1979, p. 34) provided a fail-safe position: "The quality of the work that has been done ... militate[s] against ... a final pessimism." A further re-analysis of the original data base by British researchers similarly focused on the adequacy of the research design employed in the studies represented therein, and, like the NAS panel, avoided "a final pessimism" (Hollin, 1990, pp. 119–120).

From "Just Deserts" to "Get Tough, Hang 'em High"

Whatever the cautions against "therapeutic nihilism" (to borrow Hollin's phrase) in the scientific community, the "nothing works" proposition fueled challenges to rehabilitation as a goal in corrections launched by advocates of a "just deserts" policy (Morris, 1974; von Hirsch, 1985, 1988). That policy argues in essence that the sanction for a criminal offense must be predicated on the character of the offense, not the characteristics of the offender. Most particularly, such sanction should not be mitigated by post-offense, post-conviction considerations such as progress in a program of rehabilitation. Similarly, particularly since early release on parole had become in practice at least related to, if not contingent on, such participation, "just deserts" advocates also sought to curtail sharply parole eligibility. Such eligibility should pivot on completion of a mandatory and inflexible minimum proportion of the sentence imposed. As a minor codicil, a "just deserts" model not irrationally holds that, if psychosocial rehabilitation in correctional settings had proved dependably effective, its advantages should have been abundantly clear without the protection of equivocal statements about whether valid conclusions can or cannot be drawn from the body of evidence by resorting to recondite modes of data analysis in feverish efforts to ferret out whatever small statistical advantages may lie therein. Explicitly, then, the "just deserts" model contends that correctional institutions should, once and for all, re-define themselves as places whose purposes are to deter and incapacitate—in short, to punish in precise and inflexible fashion.

"Just deserts" policies found substantial support in the Federal Congress. In a series of measures enacted with bipartisan support—epitomized by the Criminal Sentencing Reform Act (CSRA) of 1981, cosponsored in the Senate by Ted Kennedy and Strom Thurmond, as unlikely a pair of political bedfellows as can be imagined—the Congress remolded the Federal correctional system in the "get tough" direction. The pivots in CSRA (1) mandate that offenders convicted of certain offenses be sentenced to incarceration, thus removing substantial discretion in sentencing previously ceded to judges, and (2) require that an offender serve a "mandatory minimum" portion of his/her sentence before becoming eligible for parole. Federal prisoners constitute but a small minority of the correctional population of the nation, so CSRA does not directly affect a majority of offenders under correctional supervision. But Federal legislation often achieves its principal effects indirectly, by rippling outward through widespread imitation by the legislatures of the individual states.

With even greater direct and indirect impact, Congress enacted in 1986 the Omnibus Crime Reduction Act (OCRA) as a cornerstone in the Reagan Administration's War on Drugs. OCRA mandates incarceration for a variety of offenses related to the sale or possession of drugs ("controlled dangerous substances," in the Federal lexicon) or of "drug paraphernalia," the penalties for many of which had previously been left to the discretion of judges. Once again, as the "hang "em high" bandwagon coursed through the nation, OCRA elicited wide imitation by state legislatures.

The direct impact of CSRA and OCRA (and surrounding and supporting legislation) on the Federal prison system can be gauged fairly precisely by considering the data reported by the Bureau of Justice Statistics (Maguire & Pastore, 1999, p. 505) concerning drug offenders in Federal prison as a proportion of all Federal prisoners. In 1980, before either CSRA or OCRA, there were slightly more than 19,000 Federal prisoners, of whom 25% (4,749) were drug offenders. In 1990, nine years after CSRA and four years after OCRA, the total Federal prison population had more than doubled to 47,000, with 52% (25,000) drug offenders. Within the space of a single decade, during which the general population had increased by only 10% (from 226 million to 248 million), the number of Federal prisoners had increased by nearly 150%, or at a rate approximately 15 times as great as the increase in the general population. Indeed, by 1990 there were 52% more drug offenders incarcerated than the total number of inmates in Federal prisons for any and all offenses 10 years earlier. By 1998, the comparisons yielded even greater more drama, with a total of 95,000 inmates including 56,000 (57%) drug offenders. In whole numbers, the number of drug offenders confined in Federal prisons in 1998 was very nearly treble the total number of offenders serving sentences in Federal prisons for any and all offenses in 1970. Figure 33-2 depicts the relevant data at selected intervals from 1970 through 1998 (Maguire & Pastore, 1999, p. 505).

Precisely comparable data of national scope are not available for the prisons of the states. However, some approximations can be gauged by considering that, in 1980, there were 130 state prisoners per 100,000 of the general population (Maguire & Pastore, 1999, p. 491). By 1990, that rate had increased to 272 per 100,000 (approximately 110%) and, by 1998, to 415 per 100,000 (approximately 220%). In studies of limited scope, some investigators put the proportion of prisoners in state institutions with *diagnosable substance abuse or dependence disorders* as high as 74% (Peters, Greenbaum, Edens, Carter, & Ortiz, 1998), a figure that represents a substantial increase over the 54% reported by Pallone (1991) in his epidemiological inventory of mental disorders among prisoners.

Although it primarily targets adult offenders, a "get tough, hang "em high" posture extends to juvenile offenders as well, primarily by rendering certain offenses committed by juveniles at some ages (e.g., between 14 and 18) or at any age liable to prosecution and

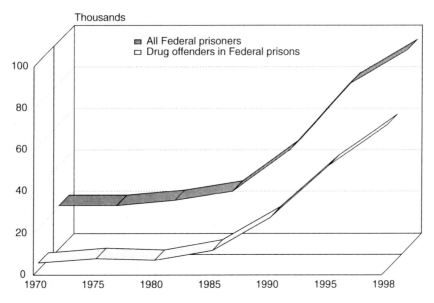

FIGURE 33-2. Drug offenders as a proportion of all Federal prisoners, 1970–98.

sanctioning under the adult, rather than under the more lenient juvenile, criminal code (Clement, 1997a; Feld, 1998; Kempf-Leonard & Peterson, 2000; Zimring, 1998).

The Pendulum Swings: Taxpayers Rebel, Judges Revolt, the Drug Czar Converts

It is generally estimated that the annual cost of maintenance for a prisoner ranges between $42,000 and $55,000. For a fully informative estimate, however, to that maintenance cost should be added the amortized costs incurred in constructing and equipping prison facilities, which may add another $15,000–$45,000 per prisoner. However much it satisfies a primordial urge toward vengeance at the visceral level, "get tough, hang "em high" as a public policy clearly imposes huge financial burdens upon the taxpayer. And therein lie the seeds of the California Taxpayers' Rebellion of 2000, the first in a string of remarkable events in late 2000 and early 2001 that appear to signal yet another major oscillation in the public attitude toward rehabilitation services for criminal offenders.

In November 2000, the voters of California, the most populous state in the union, adopted Proposition 36. California's prison system, operating at 172% capacity, had become hopelessly overcrowded, with a large proportion of inmates serving mandatory sentences for possession of controlled dangerous substances in quantities large enough to suggest nothing more sinister than personal (sometimes called "recreational") use. Serious doubts had already been expressed as to whether punishment represents an optimal societal response to such offenses (Lipton, 1994; Wexler, Blackmore, & Lipton, 1991). The key provisions in Proposition 36 repeal the mandatory sentencing provisions of relevant statutes, with the expectation that those guilty of drug possession will instead be placed on probation but required to undergo treatment in the community, whether at the offender's expense or at public expense. Proponents of Proposition 36 emphasized that, even were they to be borne by the public treasury, the annual per-person cost for outpatient treatment for drug use would consume fewer dollars per offender per year than California's current cost per prisoner per year for punitive confinement. Moreover, at least some proportion of drug offenders sanctioned in this way could be expected to maintain employment and continue to pay taxes, thus adding to rather than depleting the public treasury; and, finally, in some proportion of the cases, the costs of outpatient treatment might be borne by third-party medical insurers or health maintenance organizations or even paid by the offender rather than by the public treasury.

Almost simultaneously, a cadre of criminal court judges in New York declared themselves essentially to be on a "wildcat" strike, asserting that they would hear no further cases involving drug offenses for which incarceration is legislatively mandated until the state made provision for alternate, community-based drug treatment, whether through the by-then burgeoning Federally financed "drug courts" that provide pre-trial diversion (Peters & Murrin, 2000) or elsewhere. Some observers saw in the declaration by the judges a prospective rebirth of the pre-trial intervention strategies (Matthews, 1980) pioneered in the early 1960s by the New York State Narcotics Addiction Control Commission (and imitated elsewhere), through which criminal charges lodged against an accused offender who is demonstrably drug-involved are held in abeyance until he/she has completed a course of treatment for addiction, in much the same fashion in which first-time driving while intoxicated (DWI) offenders are dealt with in traffic courts (Lucker & Osti, 1997). If treatment is successful, criminal charges are dropped. In the 1960s version, treatment was typically provided under the auspices of a correctional agency in a "secure" facility through long-term inpatient (nine-month) care and outpatient (24-month) aftercare, but the 1990s version appears to favor shorter-term outpatient treatment in the community (Jenkins, 1995; Peters & Hills, 1999; Rose, 1997).

The judges of New York and the voters of California served as the early heralds of the swing of the pendulum, nowhere better illustrated than in what was widely perceived as a wholesale change in strategy toward substance use and abuse proposed in the waning days of the Clinton Administration by General Barry McCaffrey, the nation's "drug czar." McCaffrey had presided over a "war on drugs" with its genesis in the early days of the Reagan presidency. The governing policies of the "war on drugs" placed its greatest emphases, (1) on the "supply" side, on the interdiction of controlled dangerous substances at points of origin (replete with American paratroopers conducting raids on coca growing fields in Colombia and U.S. aircraft and patrol boats assiduously guarding the nation's permeable borders) and, (2) on the "demand" side, on the punitive incarceration of substance users in American prisons. But, as he prepared to leave office, McCaffrey recommended that emphasis shift emphatically to prevention and treatment. The war on drugs, he proposed, should be supplanted by a "crusade against drugs." In a published account of his unexpected conversion, *New York Times* writer Christopher Wren (2001) described McCaffrey as "the drug warrior who would rather treat than fight."

McCaffrey's conversion appeared to become contagious across party lines when the Republican Governor of New York proposed in mid-January 2001 a tripartite change in the way in which that state deals with illicit drug use. The key elements in the Governor's plan provided for (1) "shorter prison terms for . . . nonviolent drug offenses"; (2) "replacing mandatory imprisonment with treatment"; and (3) "giving judges greater discretion in handling drug-related criminal charges" (Perez-Pena, 2001). Given the enormous aggregate population of California and New York, accounting for nearly 25% of the nation's total, there seemed little question that what had started life as a taxpayers' rebellion had rather rapidly given rise to a major change in policy with substantial implications for rehabilitation services for offenders both in the community and within correctional institutions. Nor has it escaped notice that the pendulum began to swing not as the result of an emergent flood tide of sentiment favoring humanitarian values over punitive postures; instead, the pendulum swing has been motivated largely by financial considerations. Implicitly, however, the new focus on rehabilitation for drug offenders recognizes that punitive incarceration has simply failed to reduce recidivism, a position that echoes the long-standing conviction in the literature on penology that prisons are themselves schools for the perfection of the skills associated with crime and hardly harbors for their extirpation (Pallone, 1991).

A CATALOG OF SERVICES FOR OFFENDERS

Without question, that pendulum swing spotlights drug offenders primarily. It is thus to be expected that, as correctional rehabilitation re-energizes, principal emphasis will be placed on regimens that directly address drug use and abuse. But inevitably attendant, supportive, and ancillary services will experience a "coat tail" effect. For one offender, effective drug treatment will require support via educational programming and job placement; for another, effective treatment will require support via self-enhancement experiences, social skills training, and parenting skills training; and so on, as the ripples widen.

Physicians working in correctional settings or with members of the correctional population in the community need *either* to be able to deliver an array of services, techniques, and strategies relevant to emergent medical problems "in-house" *or* to have ready access to resources within the community capable of rendering specialized services upon referral. The prison physician may treat flu and strep throat in the prison infirmary, but he/she is likely either to refer the offender who requires cardiac surgery to specialized resources outside the correctional setting, or, less often and only in the largest prison facilities with reasonably well equipped surgical suites within in-house infirmaries, to "import" specialists from the community. Specific medical services provided within correctional facilities, then, are contingent not only on the health status needs of the clientele but also on such issues as the size of the institution and the availability of responsive resources in the community.

There are strong parallels to be drawn for correctional rehabilitation services. This section thus presents an inventory of mental health, social, and educational services relevant to, and appropriate for, a correctional clientele. In an array of permutations and combinations, varying sets of services are to be found in large and comprehensively organized institutions with varied levels of security; other sets are to be found in specialized correctional settings for juvenile offenders, sex offenders, or women; yet other sets are to be found in agencies in the community with links to probation and parole or which serve pre-trial diversion or intervention regimens. It is unlikely that the entire panoply of services here litanized is to be found in any single setting. Quite apart from the strictures of professional licensure and certification, it is also improbable that any single practitioner can have mastered the knowledge base and clinical skills required to deliver each of so broad a range of services efficaciously—and absolutely certain that no university-based program of professional preparation can have prepared practitioners to range so widely across professional roles and functions. (The reader should further be aware that, owing to space limitations, citations are provided only to (1) sources that are regarded as historically pivotal or (2) recent publications which offer comprehensive treatments of the particular service in focus.)

Alcohol and substance abuse intervention, sometimes modeled after the principles of "rational recovery" (Cox, 1979) but more often following the "Twelve Step" model of the

Alcoholics Anonymous (AA) movement, is provided either within correctional settings or in the community by rehabilitation specialists and/or by members of such groups as AA and/or Narcotics Anonymous (NA) (Glatt, 1974; Peters, May & Kearns, 1992; Ronel, 1998) and adapted, with somewhat lesser relevance, by Gamblers Anonymous (GA) (Anderson, 1999). Although he examined only a sample of states and the Federal prison system, Lipton's (1998) review of effectiveness data shows generally positive results for such intervention provided within correctional institutions; Peters and Hills (1999) reached similar conclusions in a review of data bearing upon programs in community settings. In addition to the Twelve Step model anchored in "talk therapy," alternate and supplemental interventions include psychodidactic components (Newbern, Danserau, & Dees, 1997) to educate offenders about the biochemical effects of habituation to substances of various sorts and covert measures for sensitization and desensitization (Daniel & Dodd, 1990). In "last chance" cases refractory to milder treatment and in which life is imminently threatened, pharmacotherapy with substance-specific chemical antagonists (e.g., Antabuse in the case of alcohol addiction) may be medically prescribed (Bailey & Praderio, 1994). In such cases the role of the mental health or social service specialist may change to supportive counseling aimed at compliance with medical directives, following the "mental health care" model enunciated in *Pugh*. However, Twelve Step programs are prized for their strong emphasis upon self-help and upon extension of help to others who have more recently engaged the process of recovery (Scott, Hawkins, & Farnsworth, 1994). Whatever the modality, focus is sharply on relapse prevention (Knight, Simpson, & Danserau, 1994) rather than on the antecedents to addiction or its past criminal consequences. Special attention is often given to the differential pathways to addiction pursued by women (Clement, 1997b). In view of the massive needs for such intervention among correctional clientele, pilot programs have been undertaken to train probation and parole officers to provide substance abuse treatment (Cunningham, Herie, Martin, & Turner, 1998).

Anger management and aggression control intervention, for adult or juvenile offenders (McCarthy-Tucker, Gold, & Garcia, 1999), with a primary focus on control of hostile and injurious behavior, whether directed toward other inmates (Finn, 1995; Hemmens & Marquart, 1999; Richards, Kaplan, & Kafami, 2000; Vaughn, 1997; Wright, 1991) or security officers (uniformly called "corrections officers," or COs) within correctional institutions (Morrissey, 1997); towards specific or generalized victims in the community, or even inwardly through self-mutilation or worse (Beasley & Dolin, 1998; Plutchik & van Praag, 1994; Smyth & Ivanoff, 1994). Such interventions utilize an array of stratagems, including age regression (Eisel, 1988), behavior therapy (Hillbrand & Waite, 1992) and cognitive (Escamilla, 1998) and cognitive–behavior therapy (Valliant, Ennis, & Raven-Brooks, 1995) techniques, bibliotherapy (Daniel, 1992), group counseling (Napolitano & Brown, 1991), and psychodidactic methods (Larson, 1992).

Assessment, testing, and evaluation services are required at various junctures and sites (Pelc, 1977): To determine whether a suspected but untried offender is likely to complete pretrial intervention (Van Whitlock & Lubin, 1998) or abscond; prior to the sentencing decision (McGrath, 1993) to determine whether to sanction the offender to incarceration or to place him/her on probation, with or without such requirements as community service, electronic monitoring of movements, outpatient treatment, or participation in self-help groups such as AA and NA; whether he/she is likely to satisfy attendant conditions and complete probation satisfactorily (Morgan, 1995); at a "diagnostic and reception center" within a correctional system, universally the "first stop" after sentence to incarceration, where an offender is evaluated for placement with regard to custody level (high, medium, low; lock-up, prison farm, prison camp, etc.), probability of escape, and adjustment to institutional routines (Walters, 1998), with special focus on assaultive and/or self-injurious propensities (Hillbrand, 1996; Traver & Rule, 1996); within correctional institutions, at the point of eligibility to advance from one security level to another (Beck, Palmer, Lindau, & Carpenter, 1997); at the point of eligibility for parole (Anderson, Schumacker, & Anderson, 1991; Hanlon, O'Grady, & Bateman, 2000; Pallone & Hennessy, 1977); in the case of sex offenders, at expiration of term to ascertain whether community notification is required under the provisions of "Megan's Law" or even post-release civil commitment to a forensic psychiatric hospital because there is demonstrable risk for re-offense (Langevin & Watson, 1996; Pallone, Hennessy, & Voelbel, 1999; Prentky, Lee, Knight, & Cerce, 1997; Quinsey, Rice, & Harris, 1995). In each such evaluation, both an offender's "aptitude for" and his/her willingness are important considerations in assignment and placement determinations, whether within institutions (Jackson & Innes, 2000), in non-correctional residential placement (Knight, Hiller, Broome, & Simpson, 2000), or in the community. Evaluations utilize standard psychometric instruments, both actuarial and group administered (e.g., the Minnesota Multiphasic Personality Inventory, the Millon Clinical Multiaxial Inventory, the Hartford–Shipley Intelligence Scale); actuarial and individually administered (e.g., the Wechsler Adult Intelligence Scale); and clinical and individually administered (e.g., the Rorschach Psychodiagnostic Plates, the Thematic Apperception Test); clinical interviews, preferably following a standard format such as the Diagnostic Interview Schedule developed with the support of the National Institute of Mental Health; codification of case history material, including prior record of arrests, convictions, and incarcerations, if any, and prior mental health treatment, if any; and sometimes behavior samples (Waite, 1994).

Counseling on an individual or group basis (Day, 1993), focused principally on acclimating to the demands and requirements to the correctional institution or those concomitant with placement on probation (e.g., for participation in community service, for outpatient mental health, or substance abuse treatment) or on the development of coping skills to achieve optimal functioning in the here-and-now despite underlying psychopathology (Valentine, 2000). Some efforts have been made to involve security staff as first-line caregivers, particularly in regard to issues of acclimation (Hobbs & Dear, 2000; Joss & Sechrest, 1996), while models for PEER COUNSELING (Schema, 1999; Scott et al., 1994) within correctional institutions have also been developed.

Educational programs are offered within correctional institutions at a variety of levels (Gerber & Fritsch, 1995), ranging *from* basic literacy training (Anderson & Anderson, 1996; Roberts, Cheek, & Mumm, 1994) and the remediation of learning disorders among cognitively limited offenders, whether among juveniles or adults (Traynelis-Yurek & Giacobbe, 1988); *through* improvement in basic communication (conversational) skills (Traynelis-Yurek & Giacobbe, 1988), academic training at the primary and/or secondary level in preparation for the General Equivalency Diploma (GED) examinations, and vocational and occupational training (Craig & Rogers, 1993; Koski, 1998); *to* higher education at the undergraduate and even graduate levels (Duguid, Hawkey, & Knights, 1998; Fox, 1998). Higher education programs within institutions may be expected to be curtailed sharply as a result of the decision of Federal Congress during the heady days of the "Contract with America" to withdraw eligibility for Pell grants from inmates (Tewksbury, Erickson, & Taylor, 2000). In response, in-house educational programs at the secondary and tertiary levels offered in prisons have begun to utilize a variety of "distance learning" regimens.

Family intervention services, particularly targeted toward the families of juvenile offenders, range from customary family counseling (Stringfield, 1977) and psychodidactic modalities (Sagatun, 1991) to more comprehensive, aggressive, and intensive "family empowerment programs" (Dembo, Ramirez-Garnica, Rollie, & Schmeidler, 2000) aimed at family preservation combined with parent education and reduction of recidivism. It is not infrequent that parents themselves require access to a variety of social, educational, or mental health services; the appropriate role of the correctional worker in such situations may be effective referral to responsive community resources.

Halfway house and work release programs enable prisoners near the termination of their sentences (Wozner & Arad-Davidson, 1994), or in some states already approved for parole or on parole (Twill, Nackerud, Risler, Brent, & Taylor, 1998) to live outside institutions under supervised conditions while working at jobs in the community. Some jurisdictions have even made provision for STUDY RELEASE (Shichor & Allen, 1977). Typically, an offender in a halfway house is permitted to be away from the residence a specified number of hours daily (usually, between 8 and 10); the remainder of the day (and night) is spent in participation in programs and activities designed by the staff of the residence.

Institutional therapeutic community (ITC) programs (Knight, Simpson, Chatham & Camacho, 1997; McCorkel, Harrison & Inciardi, 1998; Mrad & Krasnoff, 1976; Siege et al., 1999) apply, with appropriate modifications, principles evolved from introduction of "milieu therapy" in psychiatric institutions in the 1920s (Rosenbaum, 1976). Application of the pivotal premise that a patient's entire institutional experience, and not merely the hour or two he/she spends with a psychiatrist each week, should yield therapeutic benefit literally revolutionized the operation of psychiatric hospitals, so that a variety of functions and services, ranging from physical activities to occupational therapy and group therapy, were introduced. Because patients and staff, including nurses and ward orderlies, began to interact intensely with each other in a variety of social configurations, a sense of community typically ensued, in which each member sought to contribute to the therapeutic progress of other members. In correctional institutions, contemporary ITC units have tended to focus on drug offenders. Despite inherent hierarchical and prospectively adversarial relationships, COs as well as rehabilitation personnel are regarded as full members of correctional ITCs. Perhaps for that reason, membership in such units typically is limited to offenders who have had few prior convictions and have incurred few disciplinary infractions during the present confinement. It is normatively (and by design) the case that group discussion, whether leaderless or peer-led, comes to occupy a major portion of time that is not otherwise consumed with institutional routines.

Job placement services (Bouffard, Layton, & Hickman, 2000; Finn, 1998) are sometimes essential for inmates at or near the point of discharge from institutions, especially if they have acquired new knowledge and skills through educational programs, or at times of transition for offenders on probation or parole.

Monitoring and encouraging compliance with medical instructions, including psychotropic medication (Bailey & Praderio, 1994; Hillbrand & Young, 1994; Karper, Bennett, Erdos, & Krystal, 1994;) and NUTRITIONAL REGIMENS (Fishbein & Pease, 1994), frequently requires the combined efforts of medical and social service staff, with the latter providing the sort of "mental health care" envisioned in *Pugh*.

Parenting skills training has become an important service in correctional institutions, especially as the number of incarcerated women has increased. In-house programs most frequently are aimed at incarcerated mothers (Clement, 1993; Carlson, 1995; Harm & Thompson, 1997; Moore & Clement, 1998; Showers, 1993), but some attention has been paid to incarcerated fathers (Lanier, 1991). At least one state provides a live-in nursery in its prison for women (Carlson, 1998). In the community, parent effectiveness training is generally a component of family intervention services provided or arranged by probation or parole agencies.

Peer support groups for inmates at times of crisis, such as separation of an incarcerated mother from her children (Harris, 1993) or the death of a family member (Kaplan, 1988), are invaluable to the acculturation of offenders to institutions. In general, the role of the professional in such circumstances focuses on facilitation.

Religious programs (O'Connor, Ryan, & Parikh, 1998; Pass, 1999; Shaw, 1995; Young, Gartner, O'Connor, Larson, & Wright, 1995) are intended to serve the expressed interests of offenders in institutions. Mental health professionals often find the institutional chaplain and chaplains from the community who regularly visit the institution for worship or merely for spiritual counseling to be vital allies in the rehabilitation effort.

Self-esteem enhancement experiences assume myriad specific forms, from learning how to care for domestic animals (Moneymaker & Strimple, 1991) or even (through a "horse adoption" program) non-domestic animals (Cushing & Williams, 1995) to horticulture (Rice & Remy, 1998; Richards & Kafami, 1999). Expert technical guidance may be needed to ensure that such experiences yield positive reinforcement.

Sex offender treatment progresses in institutions and/or in the community (Wilson, 2000) through a panoply of specific techniques designed for rapists and/or child molesters (Coleman & Dwyer, 1990; Coleman, Dwyer, & Pallone, 1992, 1996; Dwyer, Amberson, & Tensley, 1988; Jenkins-Hall, 1994; Pallone, 1990; Prendergast, 1991; Prentky & Burgess, 1992; Reddon, Payne, & Starzyk, 1999; Saap & Vaughn, 1991), involving such strategies as individual and group methods, role-playing, behavior rehearsal, and relapse prevention; for incest offenders (Zuskin, 1992); for inmates who offend sexually against other inmates (Nacci & Kane, 1984); for adolescents who offend sexually, whether against juvenile or adult victims (DiGiorgio-Miller, 1994; Hagan & Gust-Brey, 2000; Hagan, King, & Patros, 1994; Mazur & Michael, 1992; Sciarra, 1999; Stops & Mays, 1991). Group counseling often intersects with psychodidactic modules dealing with sexual and psychosexual functioning (Stump, Beamish, & Shellenberger, 1999). Specific modalities now in use include cognitive–behavior therapy (Valliant, Sloss, & Raven-Brooks, 1997); group counseling and psychotherapy (Pope, Payne, & Reddon, 1997); pharmacotherapy and bioimpedance regimens leading to "chemical castration" (Coleman, Cesnik, Moore, & Dwyer, 1992; Emory, Cole, & Meyer, 1992; Federoff & Federoff, 1992; Federoff, Wisner-Carlson, Dean & Berlin, 1992); and, in Texas since 1997, surgical castration (Meyer & Cole, 1997). Mentally retarded sex offenders present particularly difficult challenges (Langevin, Marentette, & Rosati, 1996; Nolley, Muccigrosso, & Zigman, 1996). In addition, medical advances have increased longevity especially among men (e.g., the by-now common quadruple bypass cardiac surgery that renders what half a century ago would have been a fatal episode into no more than a minor inconvenience), but without simultaneously retarding the advance of senile dementia. As a result, episodes of grandfather-to-grandchild incest have reached alarming proportions, and modifications of sex offender treatment strategies have been devised to address these offenders, both within and outside correctional institutions (Watson, 1990). Assessment of progress in treatment may involve gauging physiological responses to aberrant sexual stimuli of various sorts (Earls, 1988; Quinsey, Chaplin, & Upfold, 1984) directly, by means of plethysmograph, or indirectly, through biofeedback devices that measure Galvanic skin response or vasoconstriction (Marsh & Walsh, 1995). Perhaps in consequence of renewed emphasis on pedophilia in the wake of Megan's Law and its variants, unrealistically large numbers of mental health professionals in the community have claimed expertise in outpatient treatment of such offenders (Arp & Freeman, 1997). Nonetheless, there is at present no widespread consensus about what set of knowledge, skills, and supervised experience *beyond training in a standard mental health or social service profession* are appropriate to meet reasonable standards of care for treatment of sex offenders (Coleman, Dwyer et al., 1996).

Social skills training and values clarification exercises utilize role-playing, group counseling, and psychodidactic modalities (Novotony & Enomoto, 1976; Twentyman,

Jensen, & Kloss, 1978; Dean, 1979; MacKinnon). Such exercises frequently focus on anger management (Higgins & Thies, 1981) or drug use (Anderson, Carson, & Dyson, 1997) and seem especially apt for juvenile offenders who have been reared in "dysfunctional" asocial or antisocial circumstances (Ortmann, 2000; Roundtree & Faily, 1980).

Survival and wilderness camp experiences were initially devised for use with adolescent offenders (Castellano & Soderstrom, 1992; Claggett, 1992; Houghton, Carroll, & Shier, 1996; Lambie, Robson, & Simmonds, 1997; Toombs, Benda, & Corwyn, 1997), primarily to elicit self-reliance and social cooperation. To this category of experiences can also be added shock incarceration (Camp, 1991) and "boot camps" (Salerno, 1994; Toombs, Benda, & Corwyn, 2000; Wright & Mays, 1998), regimens with similar intent.

Token economies (Ottomanelli, 1976; Toch, 1988) "reward" inmates for positive behavior and "fine" them for negative behavior. In what is likely the most ambitious token economy ever implemented (Ault & Weston, 1975), inmates confined in the prisons of Georgia were permitted to "earn" release on parole by accumulating the requisite number of tokens.

SUMMARY

This chapter has had two purposes. In the first instance, we have reviewed the oscillating posture of the American public toward rehabilitation services in corrections. Following Beccaria in the 18th century and the Quakers of Pennsylvania a century later, by the middle of the 20th century in the United States, rehabilitation had become widely recognized as *primus inter pares* (alongside punishment, deterrence, and incapacitation) as the governing purpose of the corrections enterprise. Promulgation of the decision of a Federal court in *Pugh* v. *Locke*, later upheld by the Supreme Court, seemed to seal permanently the position of rehabilitation in state prisons at least. Yet, with the publication of the Martinson Report in 1974, a period of therapeutic nihilism dawned, in which rehabilitation became essentially sidelined. Therapeutic nihilism combined with a "just deserts" position prompted, during the early 1980s, wholesale changes in Federal and state legislation governing corrections. In particular, eligibility for parole became securely anchored to serving a "mandatory minimum" proportion of the sentence imposed, with no attention paid to successful participation in whatever rehabilitative programs may have survived the "nothing works" onslaught. In addition, sentences to confinement were mandated for drug offenses of various sorts. Such public attitudes and public policies continued to hold sway until the century ended, when clear evidence of a swing of the pendulum was signaled by a revolt of the taxpayers of California, a "wildcat strike" by the criminal court judges of New York, the "conversion" of the Federal "drug czar" in the final days of the Clinton administration to a preference for treatment rather than punishment, and the Governor of New York calling for wholesale reform in the correctional handling of drug offenders. With the two largest states in the union apparently speaking with a single voice, there can be little doubt that a new era for correctional rehabilitation looms on the horizon.

Our second purpose has been to present a comprehensive catalog of rehabilitation services of varying types that, collectively and singly, are relevant to the corrections enterprise. Which services, and what programs incorporating which services, are appropriate in each segment of the correctional system will perforce vary. The capital point is not that any single installation should endeavor to incorporate each of the myriad services litanized, but rather that these services should be accessible in one configuration or another as the case-by-case need arises, whether services are rendered to offenders in confinement or on probation or parole.

We conclude with a comment about the "needs" and "wants" of correctional offenders. To the mental health or social service professional, the rehabilitation services that offenders "need" may not be difficult to discern. But that is not to say that offenders "want" these services. Indeed, there is reason to believe that offenders more frequently than not prove resistant to rehabilitation services, for a variety of reasons ranging from the ego-syntonic character of certain disorders prevalent in correctional populations (e.g., mania, psychopathic deviation) to a fixed perception that whatever is offered under the benefice of the correctional authority will ultimately prove punitive. For such reasons, offenders are likely to perceive even the most non-intrusive, non-invasive treatment modalities as coercive and to be resisted (Shearer, 2000). In addition to the technical skills appropriate to his/her profession, therefore, the rehabilitation services specialist in correction needs both the clinical skill and the patience to address client resistance.

REFERENCES

American Friends Service Committee (1971). *Struggle for justice*. New York, NY: Hill & Wang.

Anderson, D. B. (1999). Problem gambling among incarcerated male felons. *Journal of Offender Rehabilitation, 28*(3/4), 113–128.

Anderson, D. B., & Anderson, S. L. (1996). Educational needs of juvenile offenders. *Journal of Offender Rehabilitation, 23*(1/2), 153–166.

Anderson, D. B., Schumacker, R. E., & Anderson, S. L. (1991). Releasee characteristics and parole success. *Journal of Offender Rehabilitation, 17*(1/2), 133–146.

Anderson, J. F., Carson, G., & Dyson, L. (1997). Drug use and shock incarceration outcome. *Journal of Offender Rehabilitation, 25*(1/2), 97–102.

Arp, P. O., & Freeman, B. (1997). A national survey of NAPN treaters of adolescent sex offenders. *Journal of Offender Rehabilitation, 26*(1/2), 109–124.

Ault, A., & Weston, P. (1975). *Project PERM [Permanent Earned Release Model]*. Atlanta: Department of Corrections and Offender Rehabilitation.

Bailey, D. S., & Praderio, N. H. (1994). Propranolol. In M. Hillbrand & N. J. Pallone (Eds.), *The Psychobiology of aggression: Engines, measurement, control* (pp. 223–230). New York, NY: Haworth Press.

Bayse, D. J., Allgood, S. M., & Van Wyk, P. C. (1992). Locus of control, narcissism, and family life education in correctional rehabilitation. *Journal of Offender Rehabilitation, 17*(3/4), 47–64.

Beasley, T. M., & Dolin, I. H. (1988). Factor analyses of the Chronic Self-Destructiveness Scale among delinquent adolescent males. *Journal of Offender Rehabilitation, 26*(3/4), 141–156.

Beck, H. P., Palmer, R. M., Lindau, W. D., & Carpenter, P. L. (1997). The use of a discriminant function to improve prison promotion decisions. *Journal of Offender Rehabilitation, 25*(3/4), 123–130.

Bouffard, J. A., Layton, D. L., & Hickman, L. J. (2000). Effectiveness of vocational education and employment programs for adult offenders: A methodology-based analysis of the literature. *Journal of Offender Rehabilitation, 31*(1/2), 1–42.

Bowman, G., Hakim, S., & Seidenstat, P. (Eds.) (1993). *Privatizing Correctional Institutions*. New Brunswick, NJ: Transaction.

Camp, D. C. (1991). Shock incarceration in Georgia: An analysis of task performance and training needs among corrections officers. *Journal of Offender Rehabilitation, 16*(3/4), 153–176.

Carlson, J. R. (1995). Usefulness of educational, behavior modification, and vocational programs as perceived by female inmates. *Journal of Offender Rehabilitation, 22*(3/4), 65–76.

Carlson, J. R. (1998). Evaluating the effectiveness of a live-in nursery within a women's prison. *Journal of Offender Rehabilitation, 27*(1/2), 73–86.

Castellano, T. C., & Soderstrom, I. R. (1992). Therapeutic wilderness programs and juvenile recidivism: A program evaluation. *Journal of Offender Rehabilitation, 17*(3/4), 19–46.

Claggett, A. F. (1992). Group-integrated reality therapy in a wilderness camp. *Journal of Offender Rehabilitation, 17*(3/4), 1–18.

Clements, M. (1993). Parenting in prison: A national survey of programs for incarcerated women. *Journal of Offender Rehabilitation, 20*(1/2), 89–100.

Clement, M. (1997a). *Juvenile justice system: Law and process*. Newton, MA: Butterworth-Heinemann.

Clement, M. (1997b). New treatment for drug-abusing women offenders in Virginia. *Journal of Offender Rehabilitation, 25*(1/2), 61–82.

Coleman, E., Cesnik, J., Moore, A.-M., & Dwyer, S. M. (1992). An exploratory study of the role of psychotropic medications in the treatment of sex offenders. In E. Coleman, S. M. Dwyer, & N. J. Pallone (Eds.), *Sex offender treatment: Psychological and medical approaches* (pp. 75–88). New York, NY: Haworth Press.

Coleman, E., & Dwyer, S. M. (1990). Proposed standards of care for the treatment of adult sex offenders. *Journal of Offender Rehabilitation, 16*(1/2), 93–106.

Coleman, E., Dwyer, S., & Pallone, N. (1992). *Sex Offender Treatment: Psychological and Medical Approaches*. New York: Haworth Press.

Coleman, E., Dwyer, S., & Pallone, N. (1996). *Sex Offender Treatment: Biological Dysfunction, Intrapsychic Conflict, Interpersonal Violence*. New York: Haworth Press.

Coleman, E., Dwyer, S. M., Abel, G., Berner, W., Breiling, J., Hindman, J., Knopp, F. H., Langevin, R., & Pfafflin, F. (1996). Standards of care for the treatment of adult sex offenders. In E. Coleman, S. M. Dwyer, & N. J. Pallone (Eds.), *Sex offender treatment: Biological dysfunction, intrapsychic conflict, interpersonal violence* (pp. 5–12). New York, NY: Haworth Press.

Cox, S. (1979). Rational behavior training as a rehabilitative program for alcoholic offenders. *Offender Rehabilitation, 3*(4), 245–256.

Craig, D., & Rogers, R. (1993). Vocational training in prison: A case study of maximum feasible misunderstanding. *Journal of Offender Rehabilitation, 20*(1/2), 1–20.

Cullen, F. T., & Gilbert, K. E. (1982). *Reaffirming rehabilitation*. Cincinnati, OH: Anderson.

Cunningham, J. A., Herie, M., Martin, G., & Turner, B. J. (1998). Training probation and parole officers to provide substance abuse treatment: A field test. *Journal of Offender Rehabilitation, 27*(1/2), 167–178.

Cushing, J. L., & Williams, J. D. (1995). The wild mustang program: A case study in facilitated inmate therapy. *Journal of Offender Rehabilitation, 22*(3/4), 95–112.

Daniel, C. (1992). Anger control bibliotherapy with a convicted murderer under life sentence: A clinical report. *Journal of Offender Rehabilitation, 18*(1/2), 91–100.

Daniel, C., & Dodd, C. (1990). Covert sensitization treatment in the elimination of alcohol-related crime in incarcerated young offenders. *Journal of Offender Rehabilitation, 16*(1/2), 123–137.

Day, A. (1993). Brief prescriptive psychotherapy for depression with an incarcerated young offender: An application of Barkham's 2 + 1 model. *Journal of Offender Rehabilitation, 20*(1/2), 75–84.

Dean, D. G. (1979). Some correlates of social insight in adult incarcerated males. *Journal of Offender Rehabilitation, 3*(3), 257–270.

Dembo, R., Ramirez-Garnica, G., Rollie, M. W., & Schmeidler, J. (2000). Impact of a family empowerment intervention on youth recidivism. *Journal of Offender Rehabilitation, 30*(3/4), 59–98.

Demone, H. W., & Gibelman, M. (1990). "Privatizing" the treatment of criminal offenders. *Journal of Offender Counseling, Services & Rehabilitation, 15*(1), 7–26.

DiGiorgio-Miller, J. (1994). Clinical techniques in the treatment of juvenile sex offenders. *Journal of Offender Rehabilitation, 21*(1/2), 117–126.

Duguid, S., Hawkey, C., & Knights, W. (1998). Measuring the impact of post-secondary education in prison: A report from British Columbia. *Journal of Offender Rehabilitation, 27*(1/2), 87–106.

Earls, C. M. (1988). Aberrant sexual arousal in sexual offenders. In R. A. Prentky & V. L. Quinsey (Eds.), *Human sexual aggression: Current perspectives* (pp. 41–48). New York, NY: New York Academy of Sciences.

Eisel, H. E. (1988). Age regression in the treatment of anger in a prison setting. *Journal of Offender Counseling, Services & Rehabilitation, 13*(1), 175–182.

Emory, L. E., Cole, C. M., & Meyer, W. J. (1992). The Texas experience with DepoProvera, 1980–1990. In E. Coleman, S. M. Dwyer, & N. J. Pallone (Eds.), *Sex offender treatment: Psychological and medical approaches* (pp. 125–140). New York, NY: Haworth Press.

Escamilla, A. G. (1998). A cognitive approach to anger management treatment for juvenile offenders. *Journal of Offender Rehabilitation, 27*(1/2), 199–208.

Federoff, J. P., & Federoff, I. C. (1992). Buspirone and paraphilic sexual behavior. In E. Coleman, S. M. Dwyer, & N. J. Pallone (Eds.), *Sex offender treatment: Psychological and medical approaches* (pp. 89–108). New York, NY: Haworth Press.

Federoff, J. P., Wisner-Carlson, R., Dean, S., & Berlin, F. S. (1992). Medroyx-progesterone acetate in the treatment of paraphilic sexual disorders. In E. Coleman, S. M. Dwyer, & N. J. Pallone (Eds.), *Sex offender treatment: Psychological and medical approaches* (pp. 109–124). New York, NY: Haworth Press.

Feinberg, S., & Gramsbach, P. (1979). An assessment of the accuracy of "The effectiveness of correctional treatment." In L. Sechrest, S. O. White, & E. D. Brown (Eds.), *The rehabilitation of criminal offenders: Problems and prospects* (pp. 119–147). Washington, DC: National Academy of Sciences.

Feld, B. C. (1998). Juvenile and criminal justice systems' responses to youth violence. In M. Tonry & H. Moore (Eds.), *Youth violence*. Chicago, IL: University of Chicago Press.

Finn, M. (1995). Disciplinary incidents in prison: Effects of race, economic status, residence, prior imprisonment. *Journal of Offender Rehabilitation, 22*(1–2), 143–156.

Finn, P. (1998). Job placement for offenders in relation to recidivism. *Journal of Offender Rehabilitation, 28*(1/2), 89–106.

Fishbein, D. H., & Pease, S. E. (1994). Diet, nutrition, and aggression. In M. Hillbrand & N. J. Pallone (Eds.), *The psychobiology of aggression: Engines, measurement, control* (pp. 117–144). New York, NY: Haworth Press.

Foucault, M. (1978). *Discipline and punish: The birth of the prison*. New York, NY: Pantheon.

Fowler, R. D. (1976). Sweeping reforms ordered in Alabama prisons. *APA Monitor, 7*(4), 1, 15.

Fowler, R. D. (1987). Assessment for decision in a correctional setting. In D. R. Peterson & D. B. Fishman (Eds.), *Assessment for decision*. New Brunswick, NJ: Rutgers University Press.

Fox, T. A. (1998). Adult education practices in a Canadian Federal prison. *Journal of Offender Rehabilitation, 27*(1/2), 107–122.

Gendreau, P., & Ross, B. (1979). Effective correctional treatment: Bibliotherapy for cynics. *Crime & delinquency, 25*(4), 463–489.

Gendreau, P., & Ross, B. (1981). Offender rehabilitation: The appeal of success. *Federal Probation, 43*(3), 45–47.

Gerber, J., & Fritsch, E. J. (1995). Adult academic and vocational correctional education programs: A review of recent research. *Journal of Offender Rehabilitation, 22*(1/2), 119–142.

Glaser, D. (1976). Achieving better questions: A half century's progress in correctional research. *Federal Probation, 39*(3), 3–9.

Glatt, M. M. (1974). *Drugs, society, and man: A guide to addiction and its treatment*. New York, NY: Wiley.

Golann, S., & Fremouw, W. J. (1976). *The right to treatment for mental patients*. New York, NY: Irvington.

Gormally, J. G., Brodsky, S. L., Clements, C. B., & Fowler, R. (1972). *Minimum mental health standards for the Alabama correctional system*. University of Alabama, AL: Center for Correctional Psychology. University of Alabama.

Hagan, M. P., & Gust-Brey, K. L. (2000). A ten-year longitudinal study of adolescent perpetrators of sexual assault against children. *Journal of Offender Rehabilitation, 31*(1/2), 117–126.

Hagan, M. P., King, R. P., & Patros, R. L. (1994). Recidivism among adolescent perpetrators of sexual assault against children. *Journal of Offender Rehabilitation, 21*(1/2), 127–138.

Hanlon, T. E., O'Grady, K. E., & Bateman, R. W. (2000). Using the Addiction Severity Index to predict treatment outcome among substance abusing parolees. *Journal of Offender Rehabilitation, 31*(3/4), 67–80.

Harm, N. D., & Thompson, P. J. (1997). Evaluating the effectiveness of parent education for incarcerated mothers. *Journal of Offender Rehabilitation, 24*(3/4), 135–152.

Harris, J. W. (1993). Comparison of stressors among female vs. male inmates. *Journal of Offender Rehabilitation, 19*(1/2), 43–56.

Hemmens, C., & Marquart, J. W. (1999). Straight time: Inmates' perceptions of violence and victimization in the prison environment. *Journal of Offender Rehabilitation, 28*(3/4), 1–22.

Higgins, J. P., & Thies, A. P. (1981). Social effectiveness and problem-solving thinking of reformatory inmates. *Journal of Offender Counseling, Services & Rehabilitation, 5*(3–4), 93–98.

Hillbrand, M. (1996). Validity of two measures of suicidal risk: MCMI-II self-destructive potential "noteworthy" items vs. the suicidal risk scale. *Journal of Offender Rehabilitation, 23*(1/2), 1–10.

Hillbrand, M., & Waite, B. M. (1992). The social context of anger among violent forensic patients: An analysis via experience sampling method. *Journal of Offender Rehabilitation, 18*(1/2), 81–90.

Hillbrand, M., & Young, J. L. (1994). Anticonvulsants. In M. Hillbrand & N.J. Pallone (Eds.), *The Psychobiology of aggression: Engines, measurement, control* (pp. 231–243). New York, NY: Haworth Press.

Hobbs, G. S., & Dear, G. E. (2000). Prisoners' perceptions of prison officers as sources of support. *Journal of Offender Rehabilitation, 31*(1/2), 127–142.

Hollin, C. R. (1990). *Cognitive-behavioral interventions with young offenders*. New York, NY: Pergamon.

Houghton, S., Carroll, A., & Shier, J. (1996). A wilderness program for young offenders in western Australia. *Journal of Offender Rehabilitation, 24*(1/2), 183–202.

Jackson, K. L., & Innes, C. A. (2000). Affective predictors of voluntary inmate program participation. *Journal of Offender Rehabilitation, 30*(3/4), 1–20.

Jenkins, L. A. (1995). Pre-trial diversion strategies for drug involved offenders: Focus on social work involvement. *Journal of Offender Rehabilitation, 22*(3/4), 129–140.

Jenkins-Hall, K. (1994). Outpatient treatment of child molesters: Motivational factors and outcome. *Journal of Offender Rehabilitation, 21*(1/2), 139–150.

Joss, D. A., & Sechrest, D. K. (1996). Treatment vs. security: Adversarial relationship between treatment facilitators and correctional officers. *Journal of Offender Rehabilitation, 23*(1/2), 167–184.

Kaplan, M. F. (1988). A peer support group for women in prison for the death of a child. *Journal of Offender Counseling, Services & Rehabilitation, 13*(1), 5–14.

Karper, L. P., Bennett, A. L., Erdos, J. J., & Krystal, J. H. (1994). Antipsychotics, lithium, benzodiazepines, beta-blockers. In M. Hillbrand & N. J. Pallone (Eds.), *The psychobiology of aggression: Engines, measurement, control* (pp. 203–222). New York, NY: Haworth Press.

Kempf-Leonard, K., & Peterson, E. S. L. (2000). Expanding realms of the new penology: The advent of actuarial justice for juveniles. *Punishment & Society, 2*(1), 66–97.

Knight, K., Hiller, M. L., Broome, K. M., & Simpson, D. W. (2000). Legal pressure, treatment readiness and engagement in long-term residential programs. *Journal of Offender Rehabilitation, 31*(1/2), 101–116.

Knight, K., Simpson, D. W., Chatham, L. R., & Camacho, L. M. (1997). An assessment of prison-based drug treatment: Texas' in-prison therapeutic community program. *Journal of Offender Rehabilitation, 24*(3/4), 75–100.

Knight, K., Simpson, D. W., & Danserau, D. F. (1994). Knowledge mapping: A psychoeducational tool in drug abuse relapse prevention training. *Journal of Offender Rehabilitation, 20*(3/4), 187–206.

Koski, D. D. (1998). Vocational education in prison: Lack of consensus leading to inconsistent results. *Journal of Offender Rehabilitation, 27*(3/4), 151–164.

Lambie, I., Robson, M., & Simmonds, L. (1997). Embedding psychodrama in a wilderness camp program for adolescent sex offenders. *Journal of Offender Rehabilitation, 26*(1/2), 89–108.

Langevin, R., & Watson, R. J. (1996). Major factors in the assessment of paraphilics and sex offenders. In E. Coleman, S.M. Dwyer, & N.J. Pallone (Eds.), *Sex offender treatment: Biological dysfunction, intrapsychic conflict, interpersonal violence* (p. 39–70) New York, NY: Haworth Press.

Langevin, R., Marentette, D., & Rosati, B. (1996). Why therapy fails with some sex offenders: Learning difficulties examined empirically. In E. Coleman, S.M. Dwyer, & N.J. Pallone (Eds.), *Sex offender treatment: Biological dysfunction, intrapsychic conflict, interpersonal violence* (p. 143–157) New York, NY: Haworth Press.

Lanier, C. S. (1991). Dimensions of father–child interaction in a New York state prison population. *Journal of Offender Rehabilitation, 16*(3/4), 27–42.

Larson, J. D. (1992). Anger and aggression management techniques through the *Think First* curriculum. *Journal of Offender Rehabilitation, 18*(1/2), 101–118.

Lindner, R. M. (1949). *Handbook of correctional psychology.* New York, NY: Philosophical Library.

Lipton, D. (1994). The correctional opportunity: Pathways to drug treatment for offenders. *Journal of Drug Issues, 24*(4), 331–348.

Lipton, D. (1995). CDATE: Updating *The effectiveness of correctional treatment* 25 years later. *Journal of Offender Rehabilitation, 22*(1/2), 1–20.

Lipton, D. (1998). Treatment for drug abusing offenders during correctional supervision: A nationwide overview. *Journal of Offender Rehabilitation, 26*(3/4), 1–46.

Lipton, D., Martinson, R., & Wilks, J. (1975). *The effectiveness of correctional treatment: A survey of treatment evaluation studies.* New York, NY: Praeger.

Lucker, G. W., & Osti, J. R. (1997). Reduced recidivism among first-time DWI offenders as a correlate of pre-trial intervention. *Journal of Offender Rehabilitation, 24*(3/4), 1–18.

Maguire, K., & Pastore, A. L. (Eds.) (1999). *Sourcebook of criminal justice statistics.* Washington, DC: U.S. Department of Justice, Bureau of Justice Statistics.

Marsh, R. L., & Walsh, A. (1995). Physiological and psychosocial assessment and treatment of sex offenders: A comprehensive victim-oriented program. *Journal of Offender Rehabilitation, 22*(1/2), 77–97.

Martinson, R. (1974). What works?—Questions and answers about prison reform. *Public Interest, 35*(1), 22–54.

Martinson, R. (1976). California research at the crossroads. *Crime & Delinquency, 12*(2), 189–199.

Matthews, W. G. (1980). Pretrial diversion screening: An analysis of differential labeling categories on sentencing outcomes. *Journal of Offender Counseling, Services & Rehabilitation, 4*(4), 369–380.

Mayer, C. (1990). *Survey of case law establishing constitutional minima for the provision of mental health services to psychiatrically involved inmates.* Albany, NY: Albany Law School.

Mazur, T., & Michael, P. M. (1992). Outpatient treatment for adolescents with sexually inappropriate behavior. In E. Coleman, S.M. Dwyer & N.J. Pallone (Eds.), *Sex offender treatment: Psychological and medical approaches* (p. 101–204) New York, NY: Haworth Press.

McCarthy-Tucker, S., Gold, A., & Garcia, E. (1999). Effects of anger management training on aggressive behavior in adolescent boys. *Journal of Offender Rehabilitation, 28*(3/4), 129–142.

McCorkel, J., Harrison L. D., & Inciardi, J. (1998). How treatment is constructed among graduates and dropouts in a prison therapeutic community for women. *Journal of Offender Rehabilitation, 27*(3/4), 37–60.

McGrath, R. (1993). Preparing psychosexual evaluations of sex offenders: Strategies for practitioners. *Journal of Offender Rehabilitation, 20*(1/2), 139–158.

Meyer, W. J., & Cole, C. M. (1997). Physical and chemical castration of sex offenders: A review. *Journal of Offender Rehabilitation, 25*(3/4), 1–18.

Moneymaker, J. M., & Strimple, E. O. (1991). Animals and inmates: A sharing companionship behind bars. *Journal of Offender Rehabilitation, 16*(3/4), 133–152.

Moore, A. R., & Clement, M. J. (1998). Effects of parenting training for incarcerated mothers. *Journal of Offender Rehabilitation, 27*(1/2), 57–72.

Morgan, K. D. (1995). Variables associated with successful probation completion. *Journal of Offender Rehabilitation, 22*(3/4), 141–155.

Morris, N. (1974). *The future of imprisonment*. Chicago, IL: University of Chicago Press.

Morrissey, C. (1997). A multimodal approach to controlling inpatient assaultiveness among incarcerated juveniles. *Journal of Offender Rehabilitation, 25*(1/2), 31–42.

Mrad, D. F., & Krasnoff, A. G. (1976). Use of the MMPI and demographic variables in predicting dropouts from a correctional therapeutic community. *Offender Rehabilitation, 1*(2), 193–202.

Nacci, P. L., & Kane, T. R. (1984). Inmate sexual aggression: Some evolving propositions, empirical findings, and mitigating counter-forces. *Journal of Offender Counseling, Services & Rehabilitation, 9*(1/2), 1–20.

Napolitano, S., & Brown, L. G. (1991). Strategic approach to group anger management with incarcerated murderers. *Journal of Offender Rehabilitation, 16*(3/4), 93–102.

Newbern, D., Danserau, D. F., & Dees, S. M. (1997). Node-link mapping in substance abuse: Probationers' ratings of group counseling. *Journal of Offender Rehabilitation, 25*(1/2), 83–96.

Nolley, D., Muccigrosso, L., & Zigman, E. (1996). Treatment successes with mentally retarded sex offenders. In E. Coleman, S. M. Dwyer, & N. J. Pallone (Eds.), *Sex offender treatment: Biological dysfunction, intra-psychic conflict, interpersonal violence* (pp. 125–142) New York, NY: Haworth Press.

Novotony, H. R., & Enomoto, J. J. (1976). Social competence training as a correctional alternative. *Offender Rehabilitation, 1*(1), 45–56.

O'Connor, T., Ryan, P., & Parikh, C. (1998). A model program for churches and ex-offender reintegration. *Journal of Offender Rehabilitation, 28*(1/2), 107–126.

Ortmann, R. (2000). The effectiveness of social therapy in prison—a randomized experiment. *Crime & Delinquency, 46*(2), 214–232.

Ottomanelli, G. (1976). Follow-up of a token economy applied to civilly-committed heroin addicts. *International Journal of Addiction, 11*(6), 793–806.

Pallone, N. J. (1990). *Rehabilitating criminal sexual psychopaths: Legislative mandates, clinical quandaries*. New Brunswick, NJ: Transaction.

Pallone, N. J. (1991). *Mental disorder among prisoners: Toward an epidemiologic inventory*. New Brunswick, NJ: Transaction.

Pallone, N. J., & Hennessy, J. J. (1977). Empirical derivation of a scale for recidivism proneness among parolees: A multivariate model. *Offender Rehabilitation, 2*(2), 95–110.

Pallone, N. J., Hennessy, J. J., & LaRosa, D. S. (1980). Professional psychology in state correctional institutions: Present status and alternate futures. *Professional Psychology, 11*(5), 755–763.

Pallone, N. J., Hennessy, J. J., & Voelbel, G. T. (1999). Identifying pedophiles "eligible" for community notification under Megan's law: A multivariate model for actuarially anchored decisions. *Journal of Offender Rehabilitation, 28*(1/2), 41–60.

Pass, M. G. (1999). Religious orientation and self-reported rule violations in a maximum security prison. *Journal of Offender Rehabilitation, 28*(3/4), 119–134.

Pelc, R. E. (1977). A primer to psychological evaluation in the criminal justice process. *Offender Rehabilitation, 1*(3), 275–282.

Perez-Pena, R. (2001, January 8). Pataki presents his plan to ease state drug laws. *New York Times*, A-1, A-10.

Peters, R. H., Greenbaum, P. E., Edens, J. F., Carter, C. R., & Ortiz, M. M. (1998). Prevalence of DSM-IV substance abuse and dependence disorders among prison inmates. *American Journal of Drug & Alcohol Abuse, 24*(4), 573–587.

Peters, R. H., & Hills, H. A. (1999). Community treatment and supervision strategies for offenders with co-occurring disorders: What works. In E. Latessa (Ed.), *Strategic solutions: The international community corrections association examines substance abuse*. Lanham, MD: American Correctional Association.

Peters, R. H., May, R. L., & Kearns, W. D. (1992). Drug treatment in jails: Results of a nationwide survey. *Journal of Criminal Justice, 20*(4), 283–295.

Peters, R. H., & Murrin, M. M. (2000). Effectiveness of treatment-based drug courts in reducing criminal recidivism. *Criminal Justice & Behavior, 27*(1), 72–96.

Plutchik, R., & van Praag, H. M. (1994). Suicide risk: Amplifiers and attenuators. In M. Hillbrand & N.J. Pallone (Eds.), *The psychobiology of aggression: Engines, measurement, control* (pp. 173–186). New York, NY: Haworth Press.

Pope, G. A., Payne, L. R., & Reddon, J. R. (1997). Change in attitude toward parents among sex offenders as a function of group psychotherapy. *Journal of Offender Rehabilitation, 25*(1/2), 175–182.

Prendergast, W. E. (1991). *Treating sex offenders in correctional institutions and outpatient clinics: A guide to clinical practice.* New York, NY: Haworth Press.

Prentky, R., & Burgess, A. W. (1992). Rehabilitation of child molesters: A cost–benefit analysis. In A. W. Burgess (Ed.), *Child trauma I: Issues and research* (pp. 417–442). New York, NY: Garland.

Prentky, R. A., Lee, A. F. S., Knight, R. A., & Cerce, D. (1997). Recidivism rates among child molesters and rapists: A methodological analysis. *Law & Human Behavior, 21*(6), 635–659.

Quinsey, V. L., Chaplin, T. C., & Upfold, D. (1984). Sexual arousal to non-sexual violence and sadomasochistic themes among rapists and non-sex offenders. *Journal of Consulting & Clinical Psychology, 52*(4), 651–657.

Quinsey, V. L., Rice, M. E., & Harris, G. T. (1995). Actuarial prediction of sexual recidivism. *Journal of Interpersonal Violence, 10*(1), 85–105.

Reddon, J. R., Payne, L. R., & Starzyk, K. B. (1999). Therapeutic factors in group treatment evaluated by sex offenders: A consumers' report. *Journal of Offender Rehabilitation, 28*(3/4), 91–102.

Rice, J., & Remy, L. L. (1998). Impact of horticultural therapy on psychosocial functioning among urban jail inmates. *Journal of Offender Rehabilitation, 26*(3/4), 169–191.

Richards, H. Q., & Kafami, D. M. (1999). Impact of horticultural therapy on vulnerability and resistance to substance abuse among incarcerated offenders. *Journal of Offender Rehabilitation, 28*(3/4), 183–194.

Richards, H., Kaplan, M., & Kafami, D. M. (2000). Progress in treatment and experienced and expressed anger among incarcerated men. *Journal of Offender Rehabilitation, 30*(3/4), 35–58.

Roberts, R. E., Cheek, E. H., & Mumm, R. S. (1994). Group intervention and reading performance in a medium-security prison facility. *Journal of Offender Rehabilitation, 20*(3/4), 97–116.

Rogers, R. (1986). APA's position on the insanity defense: Empiricism versus emotionalism. *American Psychologist, 42*(9), 840–848.

Ronel, N. (1998). Narcotics Anonymous: Understanding "the bridge of recovery." *Journal of Offender Rehabilitation, 27*(1/2), 179–198.

Rose, S. R. (1997). Analysis of a juvenile court diversion program. *Journal of Offender Rehabilitation, 24*(3/4), 153–162.

Rosenbaum, M. (1976). Group psychotherapies. In B. B. Wolman (Ed.), *Therapist's handbook: Treatment methods for mental disorders* (pp. 163–183). New York, NY: Van Nostrand Reinhold.

Roundtree, G. A., & Faily, A. (1980). An intervention model for the resocialization of a group of adjudicated delinquents. *Journal of Offender Counseling, Services & Rehabilitation, 4*(4), 331–336.

Saap, A. D., & Vaughn, M. S. (1991). Sex offender rehabilitation programs in state prisons: A nationwide survey. *Journal of Offender Rehabilitation, 17*(1/2), 55–76.

Sagatun, I. J. (1991). Attributions of delinquency by delinquent minors, their families, and probation officers. *Journal of Offender Rehabilitation, 16*(3/4), 43–59.

Salerno, A. W. (1994). Boot camps: A critique and a proposed alternative. *Journal of Offender Rehabilitation, 20*(3/4), 147–158.

Schema, P. J. (1999). Social distance between inmates, peer counselors, and program staff in a women's prison. *Journal of Offender Rehabilitation, 28*(1/2), 89–100.

Schichor, D., & Allen, H. E. (1977). Study-release: A correctional alternative. *Offender Rehabilitation, 2*(1), 7–18.

Sciarra, D. T. (1999). Assessment and treatment of adolescent sex offenders: A review from a cross-cultural perspective. *Journal of Offender Rehabilitation, 28*(3/4), 103–118.

Scott, R. F., Hawkins, R. D., & Farnsworth, M. (1994). Operation kick-it: Texas prisoners rehabilitate themselves by dissuading others. *Journal of Offender Rehabilitation, 20*(3/4), 207–215.

Sechrest, L., White, S. O., & Brown, E. D. (Eds.) (1979). *The rehabilitation of criminal offenders: Problems and prospects.* Washington, DC: National Academy of Sciences.

Shamsie, J. (1982). Anti-social adolescents: Our treatments are not working—Where do we go from here? *Annual Progress in Child Psychiatry & Child Development, 24*(2), 631–647.

Shaw, R. D. 1995. *Chaplains to the imprisoned: Sharing life with the incarcerated.* New York, NY: Haworth Press.

Shearer, R. A. (2000). Coerced substance abuse counseling revisited. *Journal of Offender Rehabilitation, 30*(3/4), 153–171.

Showers, J. (1993). Assessing and remedying parenting knowledge among women inmates. *Journal of Offender Rehabilitation, 20*(1/2), 35–46.

Siege, H. A., Wang, J., Carlson, R. G., Falck, R. S., Rahman, A. M., & Fine, R. L. (1999). Ohio's prison-based therapeutic community treatment programs for substance abusers. *Journal of Offender Rehabilitation, 28*(3/4), 33–48.

Smyth, N. J., & Ivanoff, A. (1994). Maladaptation and prison environmental preferences among inmate parasuicides. *Journal of Offender Rehabilitation, 20*(3/4), 131–146.

Stops, M., & Mays, G. L. (1991). Treating adolescent sex offenders in a multi-cultural community setting. *Journal of Offender Rehabilitation, 17*(1/2), 87–104.

Stringfield, N. (1977). The impact of family counseling in resocializing adolescent offenders within a positive peer treatment milieu. *Offender Rehabilitation, 1*(4), 349–360.

Stump, E. S., Beamish, P. M., & Shellenberger, R. O. (1999). Self-concept changes in sex offenders follow prison psychoeducational treatment. *Journal of Offender Rehabilitation, 28*(1/2), 101–112.

Taylor, W. B., & Brasswell, M. C. (1979). Reflections on penology: Retribution revisited. *Journal of Offender Counseling, Services & Rehabilitation, 4*(2), 109–120.

Tewksbury, R., Erickson, D. J., & Taylor, J. M. (2000). Opportunities lost: The consequences of eliminating Pell grant eligibility for correctional education students. *Journal of Offender Rehabilitation, 31*(1/2), 43–56.

Toch, H. (1988). Rewarding convicted offenders. *Federal Probation, 52*(2), 42–48.

Toombs, N. J., Benda, B. B., & Corwyn, R. F. (1997). Recidivism among Arkansas boot camp graduates after 12 months. *Journal of Offender Rehabilitation, 26*(1/2), 141–160.

Toombs, N. J., Benda, B. B., & Corwyn, R. F. (2000). Violent youth in boot camps for non-violent offenders. *Journal of Offender Rehabilitation, 31*(3/4), 113–135.

Traver, M. D., & Rule, W. R. (1996). Self-mutilating adolescents in secure confinement: A nationwide survey of institutional response systems. *Journal of Offender Rehabilitation, 23*(1/2), 11–22.

Traynelis-Yurek, E. & Giacobbe, G. A. (1988). Age regression in the treatment of anger in a prison setting. *Journal of Offender Counseling, Services & Rehabilitation, 13*(1), 163–174.

Twentyman, C., Jensen, M., & Kloss, J. D. (1978). Social skills training for the complex offender. *Journal of Clinical Psychology, 34*(4), 320–326.

Twill, S. E., Nackerud, L., Risler, E. A., Burnt, J. A., & Taylor, D. (1998). Changes in measured loneliness, control, and social support among parolees in a halfway house. *Journal of Offender Rehabilitation, 27*(3/4), 77–93.

Valentine, P. V. (2000). Traumatic incident reduction, I: Traumatized women inmates—Particulars of practice and research. *Journal of Offender Rehabilitation, 31*(3/4), 1–16.

Valliant, P. M., Ennis, L. P., & Raven-Brooks, L. (1995). A cognitive–behavior therapy model for anger management with adult offenders. *Journal of Offender Rehabilitation, 22*(3/4), 77–94.

Valliant, P. M., Sloss, B. K., & Raven-Brooks, L. (1997). Effects of brief cognitive–behavioral therapy on recidivism among sex and non-sex offenders. *Journal of Offender Rehabilitation, 25*(1/2), 163–174.

Van Whitlock, R., & Lubin, B. (1998). Predicting outcome of court-ordered treatment for DWI offenders via the MAACL-R. *Journal of Offender Rehabilitation, 28*(1/2), 29–40.

Vaughn, M. S. (1997). Prison officials' liability for inmate-to-inmate assault: A review of case law. *Journal of Offender Rehabilitation, 25*(1/2), 1–30.

von Hirsch, A. (1976). *Doing justice: The choice of punishments.* New York, NY: Hill & Wang.

von Hirsch, A. (1985). *Past or future crimes: Deservedness and dangerousness in the sentencing of criminals.* New Brunswick, NJ: Rutgers University Press.

von Hirsch, A. (1988). *Federal sentencing guidelines: The United States and Canadian schemes compared.* New York, NY: New York University, School of Law, Center for Research in Crime & Justice.

Waite, B. M. (1994). Sampling the experience of chronically aggressive psychiatric patients. In M. Hillbrand & N. J. Pallone (Eds.), *The psychobiology of aggression: Engines, measurement, control* (pp. 187–202). New York, NY: Haworth Press.

Walters, G. D. (1998). The lifestyle criminality screening form: Psychometric properties and practical utility. *Journal of Offender Rehabilitation, 27*(3/4), 9–24.

Watson, J. M. (1990). Legal and social alternatives in treating older child sexual offenders. *Journal of Offender Counseling, Services & Rehabilitation, 13*(2), 141–147.

Wexler, H. K., Blackmore, J., & Lipton, D. (1991). Project REFORM: Developing a drug abuse treatment strategy for corrections. *Journal of Drug Issues, 21*(2), 469–490.

Wilson, R. J. (2000). Community-based sex offender management: Combining parole supervision and treatment to reduce recidivism. *Canadian Journal of Criminology, 42*(2), 177–188.

Wozner, Y., & Arad-Davidson, B. (1994). Community hostels: An alternative to rehabilitating young offenders. *Journal of Offender Rehabilitation, 20*(3/4), 37–60.

Wren, C. S. (2001, January 8). Public lives: A drug warrior who would rather treat than fight. *New York Times*, B-1, B-4.

Wright, D. T., & Mays, G. L. (1998). Correctional boot camps, attitudes, and recidivism: The Oklahoma experience. *Journal of Offender Rehabilitation, 28*(1/2), 71–88.

Wright, K. V. (1991). The violent and the victimized in the male prison. *Journal of Offender Rehabilitation, 16*(3/4), 1–26.

Young, M. C., Gartner, J., O'Connor, T., Larson, D., & Wright, K. (1995). Long-term recidivism among Federal inmates trained as volunteer prison ministers. *Journal of Offender Rehabilitation, 22*(1/2), 97–118.

Zimring, F. E. (1998). Toward a jurisprudence of youth violence. In M. Tonry & M. H. Moore (Eds.), *Youth Violence* (pp. 477–501). Chicago, IL: University of Chicago Press.

Zuskin, R. E. (1992). Developing insight in incestuous fathers. In E. Coleman, S. M. Dwyer, & N. J. Pallone (Eds.), *Sex offender treatment: Psychological and medical approaches* (pp. 205–216). New York, NY: Haworth Press.

Index

Absenteeism, 284
Abstinence model, 286
Acceptance, 44–46
ACCESS, 2
Accessibility, 56–57, 235, 237
Accessible design, 53, 54–55, 237–238, 240, 250
Accessible design interventions, 240–243
Accidents, 255
Accommodation, xi, 62, 64, 67–70, 74, 130, 299,
    321, 340, 370, 391, 393; *see also* Reasonable
    accommodation process
Acculturation, 405
Acupuncture, 292
Acute mental health episodes, 305
Acute stress, 310–311
Adaptation to disability, 382–383
Adaptive computing, 391
Addiction Severity Index, 287
Adjustment disorder, 305–306
Administrative controls, 55
Adolescence and work, 16–17
Adult children of alcoholics, 256, 298
Adulthood and work, 17–18
Advocacy, 5, 34, 112, 113, 221–222, 270,
    338, 367, 396
Affective disorders, 67–69
Affirmative industries, 394–395
African Americans, 23
Aftercare of substance abuse, 294
Aggression control, 468
Aid to Families with Dependent Children, 433, 435
AIDS, 7, 51, 417–418
Alcohol use, 283, 312
Alcoholics Anonymous, 286, 306,
    396, 467–468
Alcoholism, 285–286, 291
American Congress of Rehabilitative Medicine, 162
American Medical Association, 286
American Psychological Association, 451
American Sign Language, 354
American Society of Addiction Medicine, 288
American Standards Institute, 53

Americans with Disabilities Act, 23, 30, 33, 34, 36,
    56–57, 62, 63–65, 78, 118, 223, 237, 249, 319,
    391, 392, 422, 434, 443
Anger management training, 263, 468
Anorexia, 445
Antiretroviral therapy, 417
Anxiety, 107, 215, 418, 421
Anxiety disorders, 256, 309–310, 449
Architectural Barriers Act, 55
Architectural modification, 391
Assertive Community Treatment, 100, 139–140, 273,
    274, 278, 298
Assertiveness training, 262, 454
Assessment
    and brief therapy, 257, 264–265
    and business planning, 325–326
    and cognitive rehabilitation, 169
    criterion-oriented forms of, 143
    and dual diagnosis, 297
    and ecological approach, 368, 388
    and incarceration, 468–469
    and integration of rehabilitation and mental health
        services, 387–388
    of interpersonal problems, 107–109
    of occupational functioning, 312
    of offenders, 468–469
    and people coping with HIV/AIDS, 429
    of performance expectations, 211
    of person-in-environment, 278
    of readiness, 148, 149, 150, 151, 154–156
    of situations, 109–110
    of strengths, 86, 275–276, 278, 368, 453–454
    and substance abuse, 287, 293
    and supported employment, 365–366
    and transition from welfare to work, 441
    and transitional work plan, 73
    of victimization, 453
    of work setting, 211, 227, 257
Assimilation, 5
Assistive listening devices, 355
Assistive technologies, 219, 372, 389–391
Assistive technology device, 57

Assistive technology professional, 390
Assistive technology service, 57
Attention and concentration, 165
Auditory controls, 241–242
Autonomy, 17, 20

Bardon-Lafollette Act of 1943, 119
Behavioral health carve-outs, 128
Behavioral healthcare, 286, 304
Benefit advisement, 199–205
Benefit advisors, 201–203
Benefits, 106, 226, 424
Bereavement, 306–307
Best practices, 7, 121, 139–140, 376
Bipolar disorder, 256, 309, 354, 442
Body image, 383, 385, 386
Brain Injury Special Interest Group, 162, 163
Brief ego supportive therapy, 263–265
Brief therapies, 257–258, 290
Bulimia, 445
Business, 51, 58, 241, 284, 320, 323–324, 393

Career, definition of, 78–79
Career assets, 79–81, 83
Career contingency theory, 81, 83
Career development
    continuous, 4
    in early childhood, 80
    improvisational quality of, 84
    influences of family on, 80
    needs of people with disabilities, 84–85
    and personal flexibility, 84–85
    and planned happenstance, 84
    serendipity of, 83–84
    as series of decisions, 80
    as social opportunities, 82
    specific strategies of, 85–89
    as strategy, 81–83, 89
Career maturity, 85, 149, 153, 210
Career planning, 369
Career preparation, 345–347
Caretaking, 447–448
Case management
    case planning in, 276–277
    comprehensive models of, 271
    and deaf persons, 360
    definition of, 270
    and dual diagnosis, 298
    goal-setting in, 276–277
    growth of, 271
    process of, 275–277
    and research on employment, 272–273
    strengths model of, 270
    and therapeutic relationship, 273–275
    and vocational performance, 272–273
    and vocational success, 275–277
Case planning, 276–277
Center for Mental Health Administration, 133

Centers of Excellence, 139
Change theories, 176
Childcare, 448
Childhood and work, 16
Choose-Get-Keep model, 278, 364, 366
Chronic illness, 417–418, 428
Chronicity, 40, 145, 429
Civil rights movement, 225
Client Assistance Program, 119
Clinical interventions
    and crisis intervention, 259–262
    and ego-supportive therapy, 263–265
    and skill development training, 262–263
    and time-limited therapies, 257–259
Clubhouses, 3, 99–100, 132, 185–189, 193–195, 299
Cocaine addiction, 292
Cognitive accessibility, 238
Cognitive assessment, 166–167
Cognitive-behavioral counseling, 290, 295, 296, 471
Cognitive demands, 54, 238, 240, 244, 249
Cognitive impairments, 106, 164–165
Cognitive issues, 238
Cognitive remediation
    clinical considerations in, 164–166
    construct of, 162–164
    and individualizing treatment, 165
    restoration versus compensation in, 163
    and strategies of employment, 166–167, 169
Cognitive requirements and work, 58
Cognitive restoration, 163
Cognitive restructuring, 112, 261, 262–263
Collaboration
    examples of, 123–124, 135–137
    and Medicaid health care delivery systems, 128
    between physicians and mental
        health professionals, 315
    between public vocational rehabilitation and
        public mental health, 121–122
    and strategies for employment, 166–167, 169
Community colleges, 138, 347
Community Mental Health Centers Act, 222
Community support, x
Community support program, 133
Community support system, 99–100, 129–130, 132
Competitive employment, x, 208
Comprehensive assessment, 387
Confidentiality, 314–315, 424
Connectedness, 43–44
Consciousness raising, 180
Consumer control, 367
Consumer-driven services, 387
Consumer involvement, 118, 121
Consumer-run business
    and aspects of the business plan, 323–329
    definition of, 320–321
    empowerment opportunities in, 321
    issues in, 321–323
    management style in, 322

Consumer-run business (*cont.*)
  mission clarification of, 323
  planning of, 322–323
  relevance of, 130
Consumers, 128, 137, 200, 225
Continuous improvement, 5, 54–55
Continuum of vocational services, 118
Controls
  and engineering, 55
  and prohibitive error, 241
  and sensory input, 241–242
  and warning error, 241
Cooperative employment, 78
Coordination
  of mental health and rehabilitation services for deaf
     persons, 360
  of role transitions, 110–111
  of transition services, 348–349
Coping skills, 98, 255
Corrections, 459, 461
  attitudes toward, 460–467
  demographics of, 460
  penance v. punishment in, 460–461
  therapeutic nihilism in, 462–463
Council of Europe Directorate of Social and Economic
     Affairs, 413
Council on Rehabilitation Education, 395
Counseling, 105, 113
Countertransference, 355
Counting, 247–248
Criminal Sentencing Reform Act, 464
Crisis intervention, 259–262, 312–313, 425
Critical Incident Stress Debriefing, 312–314;
     see also Traumatic Incident
     Stress Management
Cross-cultural issues and deafness, 356–358
Cross-training, 236
Culture and disability, 386–387
Cultural affirmation, 357–358
Cultural brokers, 357
Cultural deaf identity, 356
Cultural liaison, 410

Deaf community
  cross cultural issues in, 356–358
  and disability, 356–357
  historical perspectives of, 356
  and identity, 356
Deaf people
  and accessibility to mental health
     services, 354
  with blindness, 355–356
  and case management, 360
  with chronic mental illness, 354
  and dual sensory disabilities, 353, 355
  insufficient service of, 354–355
  and mental health issues, 354–355
  and systemic approach to services, 360

Deaf people (*cont.*)
  and transition skills, 354
  unemployment of, 351–353
  and Usher's Syndrome, 353
Deaf World, 396
Deafness and hard of hearing, 351, 353, 354
Deafness, late in life onset of, 355
Depression, 253, 256, 297, 304, 305–310,
     382, 418, 433, 440, 446, 447,
     449, 451
Depressive and Manic Depressive Association, 299
Design for assembly, 244–245
Detoxification and substance abuse, 288
Developing countries, 28
Development social work, 32
Developmental disabilities, x
Developmental Disabilities Act, 223
Differential accommodations, 67–70
Disabilities Rights Movement, 9, 34, 82
Disability
  attitudes toward, 384–385
  biological definition of, 380
  cultural context of, 386
  and deafness, 356–357
  definition of, 28–29
  and difficulties in defining, 380
  environmental context of, 383–386
  functional nature of, 333
  model of, 380–386
  multiple forms of, 193
  and physical environment, 386
  prevalence and magnitude of, 29–31, 379
  and psychological adjustment, 380–381
  psychological context of, 380–383
  social environment and, 384–385
  and transition, 340
  and work, 27–28
Disability Community Small Business Development
     Center, 393
Disability management
  definition of, 71
  principles of, 72–74
  programs of, 61
Disabled Business Persons Association, 319
Disabled Women's Network, 35
Disconnectedness, 47
Discrimination, 7, 19, 23, 27, 28, 34, 35,
     38, 39, 56, 61, 63, 137, 419,
     421–422, 446
Dispersed work cluster, 364
Divorce, 306
Domestic violence, 453–454
Donaldson v. O'Connor, 461
Dorthea Dix, 221–222
Drug testing, 289
Dual diagnosis, 296–299
Dual sensory disability, 353, 355
Dysthymic disorder, 307–308

Early and middle old age, and employment, 18
Economic Opportunity Act, 435
Education, 34, 469
Ego functions, 264
Eldercare, 22
Electronic and information technology, 57, 58
Emotional arousal, 88–89
Employee Assistance Program Inventory, 259
Employee Assistance Programs, 259, 284, 299,
        303–304, 305–306, 312
Employee rotation, 56
Employment
    and clubhouse, 192–193
    of deaf and hard of hearing people, 351–354
    and human life span, 15–18
    of newcomers, 411–413
    obstacles to, 96–98
    of people with HIV/AIDS, 421–422
    predictors of success of, 106
    and role transitions, 110–111
    and serious mental illness, 140
    and support, 225–226
Employment feasibility standard, 118
Employment specialists, 293, 411, 413, 414–415
Empowerment, 46, 226, 276, 321, 337,
        349, 386, 428
Enabling technology, 239
Enabling Technologies Laboratory, 241, 244
Enclave employment model, 364
Engineering controls, 55
English as a Second Language, 410, 411
Entrepreneurial models, 319–323, 365
Environmental awareness, 153–154, 155
Epidemiological Catchment Area Study, 296–297
Equal Employment Opportunity Commission, 23, 63,
        64, 419
Ergonomic demands, 244
Ergonomic risk factors, 55
Ergonomics, 55, 236, 238, 391–392
Error-proofing techniques, 239, 241
Error reduction, 239
Ethnic enclaves, 406–407
Experiential learning, 179–180
Extended medical benefit eligibility, 226
Extended support services, 365–366, 367, 372–373

Fair Housing Act, 423
Fairweather Lodges, 3
Family development and work, 20–21
Family education, 110
Family intervention, 469–470
Family support, 22, 299
Fitness for duty evaluation, 312
Ford Motor Company, 52
Fountain House, 185, 186–187, 188, 189–190,
        191, 194
Freedom House, 2
Functional impairments, 221

Gay men, 417, 452
Gender, 19, 20–21, 28
Gender roles, 445–446
Goals, 149–150, 152, 153, 162, 167,
        173, 257, 258, 270, 276–277,
        321, 325, 337, 429
Grameen Bank, 32
Group development, 175
Group psychotherapy, 175, 182
Groups
    and consciousness raising, 180
    and education, 177
    and experiential learning, 179–180
    and problem-solving, 181–182
    and relationship enhancement, 177–179
    and skill development, 175, 176–177
    in substance abuse treatment, 294
    and use of operant procedures, 180–181
Group work
    and corrections, 469, 470
    and critical incident stress
        debriefing, 313
    and employment, 175–182, 183
    principles of, 172–175
    and psychotherapy, 182
    in rehabilitation, 171–172
    and self-help in substance abuse treatment, 290,
        294, 468
    and social action, 182–183
    types of, 172
Group work process
    beginnings of, 173
    ending stages of, 174–175
    middle stages of, 173–174

Habilitation, 296
Halfway houses, 470
Harassment and work, 21, 446, 450,
        453, 454
Hard of hearing, 351, 353, 357
Health care access, 203–204
Hispanics, 23
HIV
    and antiretroviral therapy, 417
    and barriers to support, 426–428
    and behavioral health issues, 418–422
    and emotional and psychological aspects
        of illness, 418
    and physical aspects of illness, 419–420
    and social aspects of illness, 418–419
    and work issues, 421–422
Hope, 48–49
Hopelessness, 40, 42
Household responsibilities, 447–448
Human capital, 408
Human factors, 238
Human life span and work, 15–21
Human rights, 32, 33

Identity
  and infancy, 15
  and recovery, 9
  as worker, 8, 19–20, 149, 153, 213
Immigration
  and acculturation and language use, 403, 405–406
  and alien resident card, 402
  concepts of, 402–403
  and Diversity Visa, 403, 404, 409
  and Employer Sanctions Program, 403
  and ethnic enclaves, 406–407
  factors affecting acclimatization to
    new culture in, 403–408
  and human service challenges, 411–413
  and legal permanent residence, 402
  motivating factors for, 404–405
  and related mental health concerns, 407
  and temporary status, 402
  and undocumented immigrants, 403
  and work authorization, 402
Immigration and Naturalization Service, 402
Impairment related work expenses, 371
Inclusion, x, 208, 226
INCube, 320–321
Independence and autonomy and work, 20
Independent living, 335, 340, 342–345, 368
Independent living centers, 3
Individual assessment, 441
Individual development account, 33
Individual employment plan, 118
Individual placement and support model, 133,
    278, 364
Individual psychology, 18–21
Individual Responsibility Plans, 440–441
Individualism, 12–13
Individualized education plan, 336
Individualized plan of service, 118, 298
Individualized service planning, 388–389
Individuals with Disabilities Act, 336
Industrial revolution, 16
Infancy and early childhood, and work, 15–16
Information processing, 165
Institute for Community Inclusion, 394
Institute of Medicine, 30
Integrated Psychological Therapy, 164
Integration of services
  for people coping with HIV/AIDS, 428
  for people who are deaf, 358–360
  for people with physical disabilities, 387–395
  and rehabilitation and mental health, 387–392
Interdisciplinarity, 387, 388, 396, 428
International Association of Psychosocial
    Rehabilitation Services, 188
International Center for Clubhouse Development, 185,
    194, 196
International Classification of Impairment, Disability,
    and Handicap, 129
International Organization for Standardization, 53, 236

Interpersonal problems
  intervention into, 108–109
  on the job, 108
Intimacy, 47
ISO, 9000, 53–54

Jewish Vocational Service, 2
Job accommodation, 228
Job analysis, 65, 73
Job assets, 209
Job carving, 58, 192, 370
Job clubs, 3, 228, 374
Job coach, 73, 120, 227, 278, 346, 347, 359–360
Job design, 58, 211
Job development, 208, 367, 369–371, 392–393
Job functioning, 111
Job interview, 371
Job placement, 367, 470
Job preferences, 146
Job redesign, 236
Job restructuring, 370
Job retention, 235–237, 278
Job rotation, 236, 237
Job search, 370, 374
Job shadowing, 86, 346
Job stress
  job and role characteristics in, 254
  organizational context factors in, 255
  personal characteristics in, 254–255
  societal contributions to, 255–256
Job task analysis, 56
Job termination, 235
Job training, 367, 371–372
Job Training Partnership Act, 392
Jobs, 5
Joblessness, 21
Judgment and perception, 165
Just deserts policy in corrections, 463–464

Kaizen, 5, 54–55, 58, 238, 242, 243, 244,
    246, 248, 249, 250
Kitting, 242

Labeling, 107
Lean production, 52–53, 56, 236
Learning
  generalized strategies of, 166
  and memory, 165
Learning disability, 340
Lesbians, 450, 451–452, 455
Life style planning, 369
Life transitions, 110, 166; *see also* transition

Making Action Plans, 369
Managed care, 257, 269, 279, 286, 290, 298
Manic-Depression, 309, 442
Martinson report, 462–463
Mass production model, 236

Meaning, 18–19
Medicaid, 128, 130, 134, 137, 138, 424
Medicaid Buy-In, 203
Medicaid Rehabilitation Option, 134
Medicare, 423, 424
Medication, 49, 98, 101, 106, 110, 111, 112,
    203, 277, 279, 298–299, 417, 442; *see also*
    psychotropic drugs
Medigap, 423
Memory, 165
Mental disorders, 30, 221
Mental health authorities
    and roles in employment, 130–132
    state and local levels of, 128
Mental health disorders, 62, 442
Mental health professionals, 93, 109–110, 111, 114
Mental health services
    for deaf people, 354–356
    and employment related problems, 254–256, 304–305
    and HIV/AIDS, 418–422
    and immigration, 407–408
    for offenders, 467–472
    and welfare to work, 439–443
    for women, 450–452
Mental Health Systems Act, 128
Mentors, 48, 83, 87, 196, 209, 237, 347, 414
Microenterprises, 3
Migrant Health Promotion, 2
Migrants, 2–3
Mixed production models, 237
Multicultural practice, 357–358
Mobile work crews, 364
Mobility devices, 391
Model programs, 3, 4
Models
    in action, 2–3, 5–6
    of psychiatric rehabilitation, 99–100
    of supported employment, 223–225, 364–365
    of train and place, 119, 278
Moral development, 16
Morale, 249, 284, 285
Multiple disabilities, 193
Musculoskeletal disorders, 55, 62
Mutual aid groups, 46–47
Mutual support, 82, 171

Narcotics Anonymous, 468
National Academy of Sciences, 463
National Alliance for the Mentally Ill, 122, 135, 136,
    253, 299
National Association of County Behavioral Healthcare
    Directors, 136
National Association of State Mental Health Program
    Directors, 137
National Association of Temporary and Staffing
    Services, 393
National Black Deaf Advocates, 357
National Co-Morbidity Survey, 253, 296–297

National Cooperative Business Association, 322
National Council of Disability, 200
National Hispanic Council of the Deaf and Hard of
    Hearing, 357
National Longitudinal Survey of Youth, 22
National Survey of America's Families, 439
Natural supports, 225, 227–229, 237, 365
Natural workplace support, 237
National Task Force on Employment of Adults with
    Disabilities, 319
Negotiated jobs, 370
Non-value added activity
    catetories of, 240
    definition of, 239
    examples of, 247–248
Normalization, x, 96, 208, 222
Nutritional supplements in substance
    abuse treatment, 292

Obsessive compulsive personality disorder, 256
Occupation, 12, 311
Occupational health, 304
Occupational Safety and Health Administration, 21,
    55–56, 58, 236, 238
Occupational stress, 254
Occupation Information Network, 66
Offenders
    and alcohol and substance abuse intervention, 467–468
    and anger management, 468
    assessment, testing, and evaluation of, 468–469
    counseling of, 469
    education of, 469
    and family intervention services, 469–470
    halfway houses for, 470
    and institutional therapeutic communities, 470
    and job placement services, 470
    peer support groups for, 470–471
    self-esteem enhancement of, 471
    services for, 467–472
    and social skills training, 471–472
    substance abuse intervention with, 467–468
    token economies for, 472
    and treatment for sex offenses, 471
Omnibus Crime Reduction Act, 464
On the job training, 56
Opiate addiction, 291–292
Organizational climate, 255
Organizational culture, 208, 209, 213–214, 215, 227
Organizational membership, 208, 213–214
Organizational socialization
    overview of, 208–210
    strategies of, 210–216
Orthotics, 391
Outcomes
    and readiness, 143
    and self-efficacy, 217
    of vocational rehabilitation, 146–147, 157, 163
    of vocational rehabilitation programs, 120–121

Parenting skills training, 470
Peer counselors, 313, 469
Peer groups, 99, 367, 452, 470–471
Performance accomplishments and self-efficacy, 86–87
Performance anxiety, 211, 256
Personal development, 20–21, 105, 113–114, 175
Personal flexibility, 209
Personal futures planning, 369
Personal identity, x
Personal learning, 215
Personal Responsibility and Work Opportunity
    Reconciliation Act, 434–436
Personality disorders, 69–70, 354
Person-centered planning, 349, 369
Person-centered services, 7, 389
Person-in-environment
  assessment of, 278
  definition of, 254
  Kluckhohn's variables in, 12–13
  and matching person and environment, 208
  paradigm of, 12
Persons with disabilities, 352–353
Pharmacotherapy, 291–292, 468
Physical disability
  cultural context of, 386
  environmental context of, 383–385
  psychological context of, 380–383
Place and train model, 119, 364, 366
Plan of treatment, 258
Plans to Achieve Self-Support, 371
Poka-yoke, 240–241, 243, 247, 248, 249, 250
Positive mental health, 19
Post-employment follow-up services, 120, 122, 124, 359
Post-secondary education, 347–348
Post-traumatic stress, 255, 297, 310–311,
    312, 407, 440, 449
Poverty, 2, 13, 28, 30, 447
Power, 41, 44–48
Preparation for career and vocation, 345–347
Preparation for independent living, 342–345
Preparation for post-secondary education, 347–348
Presumption of benefit and vocational rehabilitation, 118
Problem-solving skills training, 262
Process analysis, 240
Process redesign, 245–246
Process supports, 237
Project VECTOR, 236
Prompt time, 247
Prosthetics, 163, 390
Psychiatric disability, 23, 38–39, 146, 222
Psychiatric rehabilitation
  concept of, 98–99
  models of, 99–100
  programs of, 122
Psychoeducational groups, 110
Psychosocial job analysis, 65–67
Psychotherapy, 182, 425
Psychotropic drugs, 222, 451, 452

Public vocational rehabilitation program, 95, 117–118,
    120–121, 135
Pugh v. Locke, 461–462

QS 9000, 53–54
Quality, 191, 211, 239
Quality control, 54
Quality of life, 113, 139, 276
Quality management, 211

Randolph-Sheppard Act, 393
Rational recovery, 290, 467
Readiness, x, 7, 129, 143–144, 146–152, 208, 210,
    211, 337, 375
Reasonable accommodation process;
    see also accommodation
  examples of, 70–71
  and HIV/AIDS, 426
  overview of, 65–67
Recovery
  and case management, 272
  and importance of work, 272
  and issues, 39–42
  and loss
    of connectedness, 40–41
    of hope, 42
    of power, 41
    of sense of self, 39–40
    of valued roles, 41–42
  philosophy of, 131, 367
  and reclaiming
    connectedness, 43–44
    hope, 48–49
    power, 44–48
    sense of self, 42–43
    valued roles, 48
  and substance abuse, 293–294
  as vision, 38–39, 146
Recovery, Inc.
Re-engineering, ix
Rehabilitation
  and childcare, 448
  and confinement, 459
  definition of, 98
  and economic consequences of work, 112–113
  and gender, 451–455
  and group work, 171–172
  and issues
    in HIV/AIDS, 422–428
    in services to offenders, 459–460
    in transitioning from welfare to work, 439–443
  process of, 4, 6
  and range of services in corrections, 467–472
  and readiness, 148–149, 150
  and role of counselor, 100–101
  and sexual orientation, 452, 455
Rehabilitation Act, 57, 62–63, 101, 118–119, 359,
    365–366, 423

Rehabilitation counselor
  and deaf persons, 357, 358
  role of, 100–101
  and role strain, 101
Relapse prevention, 286, 294–296, 468
Relationship, 106–107, 150, 152–154, 155, 166,
        177–179, 273–275, 279
Relationship accommodations, 212
Relationship style, 153
Residential arrangements, 226, 287, 289
Return-to-work philosophy, 72
Right to treatment, 461
Rights protection, 204–205
Role ambiguity, 216, 255
Role changes, 110–111, 148
Role clarity, 210, 216
Role demands, 99
Role disruption, 110
Role models, 48, 86, 111, 209, 277, 357

Schizophrenia, 271, 297
Schizophrenics Anonymous, 299
School-to-Work Act, 392
Secular Organizations for Sobriety, 290
Self-actualization, 20
Self-awareness, 153, 155
Self concept, 380
Self-determination, 101, 119, 225, 367
Self-efficacy
  and career, 20, 42, 85, 106, 211, 405, 414
  and case management, 277
  and disability, 383
  and emotional arousal, 88–89
  four sources of, 85–86, 89
  general form of, 85, 151, 152, 155
  and mastery, 152
  and performance accomplishments, 86–87
  and rehabilitation professionals, 207
  specific forms of, 85, 211, 217
  and substance abuse, 295
  and verbal persuasion, 87–88
  and vicarious experiences, 86
Self-employment, x, 293, 319, 393
Self-empowerment, 357
Self-help, 46, 82, 131, 286, 290, 294, 468
Self-Help Factory, 35
Self-managing workplace, 242–243
Self monitoring, 46
Sense of self, 39–40, 42–43
Sensory controls, 241–242
Service Corps of Retired Executives, 323, 325
Service systems, 7, 82, 101
Services to Enhance Potentials, 246
Serious mental illness, x, 95–96, 97, 106, 117, 127,
        129, 130–132, 134, 137, 186, 363–364,
        374–375; see also severe and persistent
        mental illness
Settlement houses, 2

Severe disability, 118
Severe and persistent mental illness, 97–98, 101,
        127, 129–130, 222, 363–364; see also
        serious mental illness
Severe psychiatric disability, 146
Sex discrimination, 446, 454
Sex offender treatment, 471
Sex roles, 16
Sexual harassment, 450, 453
Sheltered work, 224, 225, 271, 393–395, 411
Sick role, 199, 384
Skill development training, 99, 262–263
Small Business Development Center Programs, 323
Social action, 182–183, 454
Social capital, 209
Social clubs, 3
Social development, 31–32, 33
Social disengagement, 106–107
Social enterprises, 78
Social identity, 13
Social integration, x, 228
Social learning, 212, 209
Social networks and serious mental illness, 108
Social roles, 41
Social Security Act, 134, 435
Social Security Disability Insurance, 130, 204, 226, 424
Social Security Work Incentives Amendments, 319
Social skills, 66, 99, 100, 212
Social skills training, 262, 471–472
Social stratification, 15
Socialization
  coaching of, 228
  and learning about the personal consequences of
        work, 214–216
  and mastery of tasks and expectations, 210–213
  and role clarity, 216
  and understanding and accepting organizational
        culture, 213–214
  into workplace, 210–216
Souder v. Brennan, 129
Spirituality, 47
Standardized work, 243
State mental health authorities, 136, 137
State psychiatric facilities, 128
Status degradation, 384, 386
Status elevation ceremonies, 111
Stigma, x, 7, 13, 18, 35, 37, 40, 45, 61, 78,
        97, 137, 188, 454
Student Earned Income Exclusion, 371
Strengths-based practice, 273–274, 314–316, 453–455
Stress
  addressing acute and post-traumatic forms of,
        310–311
  management of, 111–112
  in occupations, 311
  on the job, 12, 17–18, 21, 22, 47, 62, 111–112,
        150, 175, 254–256
  and women, 447

Stress hardiness, 256
Stress inoculation training, 263
Substance abuse
  abstinence model of, 286
  adjunct services for, 291–294
  aftercare treatment of, 294
  ambulatory detoxification of, 288
  and corrections, 464, 465, 467–468
  detoxification in, 288
  and extended care, 289
  history of field, 285–286
  and intensive inpatient care, 289
  and intervention at the workplace, 284–285
  and level of care determination, 288–290
  and levels of care, 286–287
  and Methadone maintenance, 289
  and Minnesota model of treatment, 286
  by offenders, 464
  organizational factors in, 285
  and outpatient treatment, 286
  prevalence of, 283
  and reintegration into workplace, 299–300
  relapse prevention in, 286, 294–296
  risk factors in, 284
  and self-help groups, 290, 294
  and traditional outpatient care, 289
  and treatment planning, 287–288
  treatment process in, 286–290
  triggers of relapse in, 295
  in workplace, 283–284
Substance Abuse and Mental Health Services
    Administration, 133
Substance Abuse Disorder Schedule, 287
Supervisory style, 255
Supplemental Security Income, 130, 204, 222,
    226, 424, 441
Support
  for change, 151, 152
  components of, 428–429
  for employment, 225–226
  environmental form of, 99, 389–392
  and gender differences, 427
  information as form of, 425
  instrumental form of, 426
  and lesbians, 451–452
  limitations of, 453
  natural form of, 225, 227–229, 237
  on-going necessity of, 374
  peer groups and, 99, 367, 470–471
  for people coping with HIV/AIDS, 424,
    428–429
  psychological importance of, 412–413
  social, 46, 108, 111, 237
  types of, 108
Supported education, 48
Supported employment, x, 119, 133, 223–225, 360,
    364–365, 366–375, 393–395
Supported housing, 360

Supported work services, 293–294
Symptom alleviation, 122

Talking Scale, 246–247
Task mastery, 216
Teams, 212
Team-based learning, 212
Technology-Related Assistance for Individuals with
    Disabilities Act, 389
Telecommunications Act, 57, 237–238, 249
Telecommuting, 395
Temporary Assistance for Needy Families, 433, 434,
    443–444
Test of English as a Foreign Language, 410
Therapeutic community, 470
Therapeutic nihilism, 462–463
Therapeutic relationship, 106–107, 169, 273–275
Therapy
  cognitive-behavioral form of, 258
  and crisis intervention, 259–262
  and homework, 258
  psychodynamic form of, 258
  and skill development training, 262–263, 471–472
  time-limited forms of, 257–265
Ticket to Work and Work Incentives Improvement Act,
    134–135, 137, 199–200, 201, 203, 205, 423
Time limited therapies, 257–259
Total quality management, 54
Train and place models, 119, 278
Transference, 264, 355
Transition, 2, 5, 17, 166, 185, 199, 207, 208, 209,
    335–336, 354
Transition Life Plan, 336, 341–348
Transition open house, 340
Transition Planning Process
  components of, 342–348
  and parents, 338–339
  and preparing for independent living, 342–345
  and preparing for post-secondary education, 347–348
  and school, 336
  and service agencies, 339–340
  and students, 336–338
  and vocational and career preparation, 345–347
Transition services, 348–349
Transitional employment, 5, 72–74, 99–100,
    191–192, 278, 365
Transitional work plans, 73–74
Transitional work return programs, 72–73
Transportation, 344, 412
Trauma, 39, 310, 311
Traumatic Incident Stress Management, 313; see also
    Critical Incident Stress Debriefing
Trial work periods, 226
Twelve-step groups, 290

Uganda Disabled Women's Association, 35
Underemployment, 14, 224
Unemployment, 14, 41, 51, 61, 96, 146, 223

United Nations, 29–30
United Nations Commission for Social Development, 29
United Nations Statistical Data Base, 29
United States Census Bureau, 23, 379
United States Department of Labor, 52, 55, 66
United States General Accounting Office, 135
United States Surgeon General, 304
Usher's Syndrome, 353

Variation
    and common cause, 238
    and specific cause, 238
Verbal persuasion and self-efficacy, 87–88
Vicarious experiences and self-efficacy, 86
Vicarious learning, 171
Violence against women, 448–450
Violence and the workplace, 21, 255
Visions Unlimited, 247
Visual controls, 239, 241–242, 245
Vocational development, xi, 3, 7, 109–110, 217
Vocational education, 346, 347
Vocational exploration, 110, 293, 345
Vocational identity, 85, 89, 210, 215
Vocational performance, 272–273
Vocational personality, 96
Vocational preparation, 345–347
Vocational Rehabilitation Amendments, 95, 119
Vocational rehabilitation counselor, 93, 100–101,
        102, 118, 136
Vocational rehabilitation system, 101, 136
Vocational role, 147
Vocational testing, 129
Vocational training, 48
Volunteer experience, 110

Welfare reform, 14
Welfare work requirements, 434–439
Women
    and care-taking, 447–448, 454
    and disabilities, 28
    and economic issues, 446–447
    and family responsibilities, 452–453
    and gender roles, 445–446
    and incarceration, 470
    sexual harassment of, 450

Women (*cont.*)
    and substance abuse treatment, 290, 468
    and time out of workforce, 448
    violence against, 448–450
Work, ix–x, 6, 9, 11–12, 14, 21–22, 96
    and disability, 22–23, 27–28
    and human lifespan, 15–21
    and industry trends, 52–54
    motivation for, 146, 175, 192
    as organizing principle in life, 379
    performance of, 285
    and productivity, 235–237
    skill development for, 175
    socialization into, 210–216
    symbolic meanings of, 266
Work adjustment programs, 131
Work adjustment skills, 147, 148
Work design, 238–240
Work environment, 5, 10, 248
Work ethic, 9, 12–13
Work goal, 149
Work group, 212
Work Incentive Program, 435
Work release programs, 470
Work role, 149
Worker demographics, 52
Worker performance, 244
Workforce, 52
Workforce Investment Act of 1998, 57
Work-ordered day, 189–191
Workplace, 12, 16, 17, 21, 108, 228, 229,
        242–243, 264, 284–285, 345,
        357–358, 372
Workplace organization, 213–214, 242–243
Workplace socialization, 210–216
Workplace support, 414
Workplace training, 211
World of work, 85, 150, 153, 156,
        209–210, 215, 271–272, 275,
        345, 375
World Health Organization, 30
World Summit for Social Development, 30
Wyatt v. Hardin, 461
Wyatt v. Stickney, 461
Wyman Way Co-Op, 320